THE CLINICAL SPECIALIST IN PSYCHIATRIC MENTAL HEALTH NURSING

BOOKS OF RELATED INTEREST

Adams: **Handbook of Psychiatric Mental Health Nursing,** 1983, 0–471–86983–X

Fought: **Psychosocial Nursing Care of the Emergency Patient,** 1984, 0–471–87562–7

Koldjeski: **Community Mental Health Nursing: New Directions in Theory and Practice,** 1984, 0–471–04442–3

Howe: **The Handbook of Nursing,** 1984, 0–471–89524–5

Loebl: **The Nurse's Drug Handbook,** Third Edition, 1983, 0–471–09660–1

THE CLINICAL SPECIALIST IN PSYCHIATRIC MENTAL HEALTH NURSING: THEORY, RESEARCH, AND PRACTICE

Edited by

Deane L. Critchley, R.N., Ph.D., C.S., F.A.A.N.
Professor and Associate Dean
College of Nursing
University of New Mexico
Albuquerque, New Mexico

Judith T. Maurin, R.N., Ph.D.
Professor and Assistant Dean for Graduate Affairs
College of Nursing
University of Utah
Salt Lake City, Utah

A WILEY MEDICAL PUBLICATION
JOHN WILEY & SONS
New York · Chichester · Brisbane · Toronto · Singapore

Library of Congress Cataloging in Publication Data:

Main entry under title:
The Clinical specialist in psychiatric mental health
nursing.

(A Wiley medical publication)
Includes index.

1. Psychiatric nursing. I. Critchley, Deane L.
II. Maurin, Judith T. III. Series. [DNLM: 1. Psychiatric
Nursing. WY 160 C6397]
RC440.C544 1985 610.73'68 84–19509
ISBN 0–471–87506–6

Printed in the United States of America

10 9 8 7 6 5 4 3 2

CONTRIBUTORS

Margaret E. Armstrong, R.N., M.S.
Research Associate Professor
College of Nursing
University of Utah
Salt Lake City, Utah

Karen S. Babich, R.N., Ph.D.
Chairperson, Department of Psychiatric Nursing
Rush-Presbyterian-St. Luke's Medical Center
Chicago, Illinois

Linda S. Beeber, R.N., M.A.
Assistant Professor
College of Nursing
Syracuse University
Syracuse, New York

Virginia Trotter Betts, R.N., M.S.N., J.D.
Academic Chair, Behavioral Sciences as Applied to Nursing
Associate Professor, Mental Health Nursing
Vanderbilt University School of Nursing
Nashville, Tennessee

Maureen L. Boshier, R.N., M.S., C.S.
Executive Director
New Mexico Board of Nursing
Albuquerque, New Mexico

Bonnie C. Clayton, R.N., Ph.D.
Associate Professor
College of Nursing
University of Utah
Salt Lake City, Utah

Imelda W. Clements, R.N., Ph.D.
Professor
School of Nursing
Health Sciences Center
Texas Tech University
Lubbock, Texas

Deane L. Critchley, R.N., Ph.D., C.S., F.A.A.N.
Professor and Associate Dean
College of Nursing
University of New Mexico
Albuquerque, New Mexico

Anne J. Davis, R.N., Ph.D., F.A.A.N.
Professor
Department of Mental Health and Community Nursing
School of Nursing
University of California
San Francisco, California

Mary Ann Walsh Eells, R.N., C.S., Ed.D.
Associate Professor
School of Nursing
University of Maryland
Baltimore, Maryland

Leona L. Eggert, R.N., Ph.D.
Assistant Professor
Department of Psychosocial Nursing
University of Washington
Seattle, Washington

Margie Nicks Gale, R.N., M.S.N.
Assistant Professor, Mental Health Nursing
Vanderbilt University School of Nursing
Nashville, Tennessee

Joan M. Gibson, Ph.D.
Associate Professor of Philosophy
University of Albuquerque
Adjunct Associate Professor
Schools of Law and Medicine
University of New Mexico
Albuquerque, New Mexico

Susan M. Godschalx, R.N., M.S.
Psychiatric Nurse Specialist
Salt Lake County Division of Mental Health
Salt Lake City, Utah

Suzanne Lego, R.N., Ph.D., C.S.
Private Practice
New York, New York
Demarest, New Jersey

Judith T. Maurin, R.N., Ph.D.
Professor and Assistant Dean for Graduate Affairs
College of Nursing
University of Utah
Salt Lake City, Utah

Pamela G. Reed, R.N., Ph.D.
Assistant Professor
College of Nursing
University of Arizona
Tucson, Arizona

Roxy Schlesinger, R.N., M.N.
Gerontological Clinical Nurse Specialist and Nursing Instructor
West Los Angeles Veterans Administration
Medical Center—Brentwood Division
Los Angeles, California

Mari Siemon, R.N., M.A., C.S.
Child Psychosocial Clinical Specialist
Private Practice
Seattle, Washington

Mary Kay Simmons, R.N., M.S.
Assistant Clinical Professor
Department of Psychiatry
School of Medicine
University of California
Davis, California

Shirley A. Smoyak, R.N., Ph.D., F.A.A.N.
Professor and Graduate Director
Gero-Psychiatric Nursing Program
Rutgers, The State University of New Jersey
New Brunswick, New Jersey

Beth Vaughan-Cole, R.N., Ph.D.
Associate Professor
College of Nursing
University of Utah
Salt Lake City, Utah

Joann Weiss, R.N., Ph.D.
Associate Professor
College of Nursing
University of New Mexico
Albuquerque, New Mexico

FOREWORD

As student, practitioner, and educator, I have witnessed the dramatic evolution of the field of psychiatric nursing. The current state of the art is exemplified in this excellent book, which informs the reader of the multiple and varied domains of the psychiatric mental health clinical specialist. The book provides evidence that a critical mass of highly knowledgeable psychiatric nurses exists, a critical mass so necessary for the continuing growth and development of the specialty. The book is a testament to the changes that have occurred in nursing in less than 50 years. These changes are manifest in the breadth, scholarship, and clinical acumen of the contributors, whose expertise brings pride and satisfaction to this one-time participant and now peripatetic observer of the field.

It is true that entire books have been devoted to some of the chapter topics in this text. Some readers may fear that the broad approach will be at the expense of depth. Can an overview on such topics provide depth as well as breadth? My positive response to this question is based on the erudition of the authors in their areas of expertise, which results in effective probings of relevant subject matter.

Despite the number of authors and the huge amount and variety of subject matter, the book has cohesiveness and integrity. The authors are clear in their identification of issues and provide the broadest possible theoretical approaches to their discrete areas. Further, the authors are not dogmatic with regard to theory or technique and permit the reader to form independent judgments.

While serving as a major reference for the field, the book will fulfill yet another purpose. The authors' scholarly approach to data and their use and citation of original source materials will help the student, faculty, and practitioner reader follow up on particular areas of interest. Each chapter in itself and the book as a whole will be a superb resource for nursing students, educators, and practitioners of the theory and practice of the clinical specialist in psychiatric nursing.

Claire M. Fagin, Ph.D., F.A.A.N.
Professor and Dean
University of Pennsylvania School of Nursing
Philadelphia, Pennsylvania

PREFACE

The role of the clinical specialist in psychiatric mental health nursing has changed markedly since the concept was first introduced. The use of the term *clinical specialist* implies a nurse prepared by education and experience to provide a superior quality of nursing. As the science of nursing has developed, so too has the role of the psychiatric mental health clinical nurse specialist. However, there are few contributions to the nursing literature that specifically address theoretical, research, and practice issues at the advanced level appropriate for the clinical specialist.

This book is intended for psychiatric mental health clinical specialists and graduate students in the field. Consequently, since the reader is assumed to have the beginning level of knowledge required for practice, the book focuses on more advanced discussions of the theoretical knowledge and clinical competencies required in working with diverse clinical populations using a broad range of treatment modalities. The editors' intent and hope is that this book will provide some common themes and a common ground for identifying psychiatric mental health nursing clinical specialist practice.

While the focus of the book is clinical practice, the content reflects strong agreement with the American Nurses' Association's *Standards of Psychiatric and Mental Health Nursing Practice* (1982); these standards are based on appropriate theory verified and refined through research. The book does not address all the standards, but individual chapters relate to many of them, especially those describing the use of theory and research, specific psychotherapeutic interventions with different populations, and ethical issues facing the clinical specialist. Authors of each chapter were free to use whatever theoretical framework they judged to be most meaningful and useful to them in their clinical decision making and practice. Although the result is the absence of a unifying conceptual framework, there is a demonstrable link between theory and practice. Such is the current state of knowledge about the phenomena and the direction urged by the ANA standards.

A book of this length could not be exhaustive, however, so the editors have chosen to include discussions of issues and clinical populations they believe critical to specialist practice. Of necessity, then, there are several areas that have been omitted. It speaks positively to the growth of knowledge and to the contributions that psychiatric mental health nurses have to offer and are willing to share in such a diverse field that such decisions were even necessary.

Unit I explores the role of the psychiatric mental health nursing specialist and the knowledge upon which it is based. The relevance of both nursing and nonnursing theories, neurophysiological theories, and developmental theories is discussed. Nursing and neurophysiological theories are relatively underused theories in psychiatric mental health nursing practice. Also included is a discussion of research as it interfaces most directly with practice. The case study is examined as an underused method that could be valuable to the specialist committed to critical analysis of his or her clinical work. Models for research utilization are also discussed. The reader is directed to other texts for explanations of research methodology appropriate to the study of psychosocial phenomena.

Unit II focuses on clinical intervention issues encountered as the psychiatric mental health specialist uses a variety of treatment modalities in the care of various populations. In all of the chapters, the authors identify the specific theoretical perspectives that guide their practice in both prevention and intervention. The authors also imply or identify criteria for minimal performance skills demonstrative of theoretical and clinical knowledge at the clinical specialist level.

Unit III deals with the social/professional dimensions of accountability of the psychiatric mental health nursing specialist. The ethical-legal dilemmas in clinical practice, the issues facing psychiatric mental health nursing as a professional specialty, and the issues and process of providing responsible clinical supervision for specialist practice are all addressed.

In Unit IV, the editors reflect on the implications for the specialty of the material presented in the previous chapters. They discuss the impact on the field of advances in knowledge in such areas as neurophysiology and psychopharmacotherapy and expansion of the clinical specialist role as well as greater integration of nursing theory into clinical research and practice. Finally, the editors present their views on the viability of the specialty and the measures required of psychiatric mental health nurse clinical specialists to ensure that viability.

The chapters in this book attest to the valuable contributions adult and child psychiatric clinical specialists are making to the field. It is hoped that this book will provide models of advanced practice and stimulate new generations of psychiatric mental health clinical specialists to join in the challenge of delineating the clinical specialist role as a major health care provider of the future.

The editors wish to express their appreciation to Dr. Maeona Jacobs, Dr. Kathy McCance, and Margaret Armstrong, who read selected chapters and offered thoughtful suggestions. We are especially grateful to Gerald Bennett, R.N., Ph.D., whose careful reading, pertinent comments, and encouragement helped immensely. Thanks must also be expressed to Mrs. Eleanor Orth for typing our manuscripts with such speed and careful attention to detail. Finally, thanks go to Irving and Ken for their support, understanding, and unfailing faith that this project would see completion.

Deane L. Critchley
Judith T. Maurin

CONTENTS

UNIT I
KNOWLEDGE BASE

PART ONE DEVELOPING THE KNOWLEDGE BASE FOR SPECIALIST PRACTICE

Part One emphasizes Standards I and XI of ANA's *Standards of Psychiatric and Mental Health Nursing Practice* (1982). Advanced psychiatric mental health nursing practice is informed by a scientific theoretical base. The authors who have contributed to this book model that standard as they share their experience with various treatment modalities and client populations. However, advancement of the field demands more. It demands continuing development and verification of that knowledge base. Part One explores various facets of this endeavor.

Chapter 1 provides a historical overview of the development of psychiatry and psychiatric nursing. It explores the following questions: what is psychiatric mental health nursing and what is clinical specialist practice in psychiatric mental health nursing? The chapter builds a case for a bridging role between the medical and nonmedical fields on the part of the clinical specialist, based on the unique preparation of the psychiatric mental health nurse specialist.

Chapter 2 examines theory development in nursing and discusses the extent of interface between this area and psychiatric mental health nursing. Psychiatric mental health nurses' contribution to theory development is reviewed and the debate about the need for a unique perspective for psychiatric mental health nursing is examined. One of the contemporary nursing models, Orem's Self-Care Deficit Model, is examined for the strengths and limitations of its use in psychiatric mental health nursing practice.

In Chapter 3, an overview of neuroanatomy and physiology, which helps to clarify the biological dynamics that underlie behavior, is presented. An overview of the brain is discussed first, followed by more specifics of the structure and function of the central nervous system. Examples of the circular interplay between mental status and physiology are provided. While the chapter offers some implications for psychiatric mental health nursing practice, it is clear that we are still in the stage of discovery. There is much work yet to be done to integrate neurophysiological knowledge with psychiatric mental health nursing practice. An exciting next step would be interspecialty nursing research.

Chapter 4 discusses research application with the argument that the case study is a neglected but potentially valuable tool for psychiatric mental health nurses committed to thoughtful inquiry about their practice. It examines the process by which a research problem is formulated for study with this method and describes the various types of case studies and the issues central to each. Ethical issues in the case study approach are also addressed.

Chapter 5 concludes the discussion of research application with an examination of research utilization models. It presents an overview of research dissemination models used in nursing and explores the clinical specialist's role as a knowledge broker.

Participation in the processes of knowledge development and verification on the part of clinical specialists active in practice is a goal that psychiatric mental health nursing has set for itself. The demands of this goal present numerous challenges, but the promise is relevant practice theory.

CHAPTER 1 EVOLUTION OF THE ROLE

Deane L. Critchley

This chapter provides a brief historical overview of the care of the mentally ill, the development of psychiatry and child psychiatry, and psychiatric and child psychiatric nursing. The chapter focuses on the questions: what is psychiatric mental health nursing and what is clinical specialist practice in psychiatric mental health nursing? The chapter concludes with a brief discussion of how the unique preparation of the psychiatric mental health nurse clinical specialist based on knowledge from the biological, medical, and social sciences enables the nurse to serve a bridging role between the medical and nonmedical fields. Such a role can both provide strengths and present problems for psychiatric mental health clinical nurse specialist practice.

HISTORICAL OVERVIEW

Since humans have kept records, there have been descriptions of individuals who were considered "mad," "possessed," or "lunatics" or were given some other adjective describing their condition. It is important to remember that from antiquity through today the prevalent social, moral, and religious attitudes of society have influenced the identification, understanding, and "treatment" of the mentally ill. Before the inclusion of psychiatry within the field of medicine during the seventeenth century, mental illness had been considered within the realm of philosophy. Depending on society's prevalent attitudes, the mentally ill were ignored, avoided, sheltered, punished, or exorcised by clergy, medicine men, and the public.

Early Concepts of Mental Illness

Certain universal concepts appear to have been prevalent in early cultures. A widespread belief was that all illnesses, including mental illness, were sent by supernatural forces such as gods or demons. This belief created the need for many different rituals to propitiate the cause and to absolve the patient of wrongdoing or illness. Many illnesses or misfortunes were attributed to devils or demons and thus white (permissible) magic and black (forbidden) magic rituals were used to exorcise or control the devils or appease the gods (Middleton, 1967).

Stemming from these beliefs about the nature of illness and principles of intervention, "treatment" of the mentally ill was based on a combination of magical and religious actions. Thus, exorcism or ritual ceremonies were often combined with the use of drugs made of combinations of secret ingredients and prepared according to rituals.

Greek and Roman Concepts

It was only with the rise of the Greek and Roman cultures that concepts of mental illness began to change. Belief about madness in the Greek culture was derived from several sources:

popular opinion, medicine, and literary and philosophical writings. Each viewpoint prevailed at different periods and each influenced the others (Mora, 1975).

The popular view was characterized by the belief that supernatural forces caused mental illness as a punishment for angering the gods. There was no treatment, as it was believed that those the gods made mad the gods could also cure. The mentally ill were thus objects of abuse, ridicule, and fear, and were either kept at home, if violent, or cast away. They held no legal status so that if convicted of a crime by reason of insanity the criminal was relieved of any legal responsibility for his actions although he could be banished from his community.

The medical concept of madness arose from beliefs about the interactions of four bodily humors: blood, black bile, yellow bile, and phlegm, which resulted from combinations of the four basic qualities of nature: heat, cold, moisture, and dryness. These concepts were elaborated by Hippocrates into a theory of illness and mental illness. Significantly, this was the first time illness was ascribed to natural rather than supernatural causes and could thus be treated by physicians rather than priests (Singer, 1928).

Many of the Roman concepts of mental illness were derived from the Greeks and therefore were similar. It is with regard to the legal aspects of mental illness that the Romans made their major contributions. Previously, terms used to describe the mentally ill had been used interchangeably. Roman law detailed the various types of conditions that, if present when the individual committed a crime, might lessen his responsibility for the crime. The determination of the individual's competency was determined by judges, not by physicians. The Romans, in some cases, also admitted the mentally ill to institutions for the poor in addition to placing them in the custody of relatives as had previously been the practice (Mora & Brand, 1970).

Many approaches were used to treat the mentally ill in these ancient cultures. The three methods that appeared to be most widely used were the interpretation of dreams, ritual purification coupled with sleep induction, and use of the spoken work in prayers, magic charms, and exhortations (Lain, 1970).

The Middle Ages

During the Middle Ages, in Western European cultures there was little advancement of the clinical understanding of mental illness as derived from the Greeks and the Romans. The treatment of the mentally ill lost its humanism and became punitive or neglectful (Jackson, 1972).

Arabic cultures are supposed to have derived most of their understanding of mental illness from the Greeks. However, because of their belief that the mentally ill are loved by God and are chosen by him to reveal truths, the insane were often worshipped. Arabic treatment of the mentally ill was remarkably humanitarian. They were housed in spacious asylums built in pleasant surroundings. Each asylum had an outpatient facility and attached medical school. While much of their clinical knowledge was derived from the Greeks and the Romans, its application in the treatment of the mentally ill was combined with their own mystical and religious beliefs in unique and original ways (Wilson, 1967).

Conflicting Attitudes Toward the Mentally Ill

Increasing secularization led to increasing conflict between those who held the world view that existence had meaning in itself and those who held that life on earth was to prepare for one's return to God. The Renaissance is noted for the rise in the incidence and persecution of those identified as witches. Historians of the period speculate that as many as 100,000 men, women, and children were executed for witchcraft in Germany alone and a similar number in France. Several treatises on witchcraft appeared during this period which only enhanced belief in the phenomenon (Kors & Peters, 1972).

Social psychologists point out that Western civilization's belief in witchcraft, based on religion and magic common to all cultures, underwent a transformation from a probable fertility cult to a ritual prohibited by religious leaders. This transition occurred during a period of great social upheaval. People subjected to severe frustrations use scapegoats as targets of their aggression. So too, the appearance of witchcraft permitted the emergence of a system of counter witchcraft as a means of maintaining the status quo (Hemphill, 1966).

During this same period, a more humanistic outlook developed toward humankind including those considered less fortunate—the mentally ill. It was during this time period that Johann Weyer (1515–1588) made his contributions to psychiatry. His clinical acuity enabled him to explain convincingly a variety of the supposedly supernatural signs by which witches were identified as the result of natural causes. His extensive clinical experience led to descriptions of diagnostic problems with their associated symptoms. Weyer's greatest contribution was to psychotherapy. His approach to the mentally ill combined scientific knowledge with a benevolent, humanistic approach. He stressed the importance of the therapeutic relationship and recognized the necessity for both kindness and understanding on the part of the therapist. As a result of his contributions, Weyer has come to be considered the first psychiatrist (Binz, 1969). However, Weyer's approach was so radical that it was initially greeted with hostility and then ignored. Following Weyer, there was a growing trend in the development of scientific ideas, as opposed to those of religion or tradition, as a basis for knowledge and understanding of mental illness.

By the fourteenth century, several institutions had been established for the custody of mental patients. The prevailing attitude toward the mentally ill was to contain them and even to profit from them by putting them on view to the public for pennies or auction them off to work. During the Renaissance, the image of the mentally ill as fools gave way to a more human picture of them as troubled human beings who were different in degree but not in kind from their fellows (Foucault, 1965).

Contradictions in attitudes toward the mentally ill remained. As reason and logic became increasingly admired and sought after, evidences of the irrational were less tolerated philosophically, culminating in the rejection of the mentally ill. On one level, learned societies including medicine rejected the mentally ill. On another level, impressive social and scientific accomplishments led to the establishment of modern science.

Treatment Reforms

Social and moral reforms, begun during the sixteenth and seventeenth centuries, impacted on the care of the mentally ill. In France, Philippe Pinel, in England, William Tuke, and in Italy, Vincenzo Chiarugi all worked unswervingly for more humane treatment of the mentally ill. Of all the pioneers during this period, Pinel gained and continues to enjoy the greatest recognition. Pinel's greatest accomplishments were thought to be freeing the mentally ill from their chains in the institutions he directed, his straightforward analysis and categorization of psychiatric symptoms, and his application of "moral treatment" based on Aristotle's concept that mental illness was caused by an imbalance of the passions (emotions) (Pinel, 1962). Recently, Jean Pussin has been identified as initiating most of the reforms for which Pinel received credit (Weiner, 1979).

Many of the ideas of Pinel and Tuke were accepted in the United States. During the Colonial period under the influence of Puritanism, insanity was linked to superstition of all kinds, including witchcraft. Care of the mentally ill was cruel and punitive. Many were cast out by their families and placed in the poorhouse or jail. Treatment was at best rudimentary and at worst brutal, using handcuffs and leg irons to restrain patients and, following the European custom, exhibiting the patients to the public for a fee.

During the late eighteenth and early nineteenth centuries, the Quakers played an important role in humanizing the care of the mentally ill in the United States. The first general hospital in the United States, the Pennsylvania Hospital, was founded by Benjamin Franklin in 1756 and the mentally ill were accepted as patients. The first public mental hospital was established in 1773 in Williamsburg, Virginia (Deutsch, 1937; Szasz, 1973).

Through the influence of the Quakers, the care for the mentally ill reflected respect for the individual and a humanistic approach. Moral treatment was the concept espoused and it meant the use of kindness in a friendly atmosphere in a small hospital with pleasant surroundings. Amusements, games, opportunities for learning, and religious observance were accepted practice.

Despite the humanitarian movement and improved treatment of patients, the belief that mental illness was incurable was widespread. As the century drew to a close, approaches to mental illness changed again. Functional insanity was associated with faulty life habits. New forms of treatment were introduced: diet, massage, hydrotherapy, electrotherapy, family care, and the cottage system. For the first time, training courses for psychiatric nurses and attendants were initiated by institutions.

The Twentieth Century

Early in the twentieth century, a small number of psychiatrists interested in research founded the Pathological Institute of New York Hospital, which later became the New York State Psychiatric Institute. In 1902, Adolf Meyer (1866–1950), a Swiss psychiatrist, joined its staff, where he remained until 1913 when he left to head the first psychiatric clinic at Johns Hopkins University (Hall, 1944).

In 1908, Clifford Beers published *A Mind That Found Itself,* a description of his own mental breakdown and subsequent treatment in mental institutions (Beers, 1948). He capitalized on the response to the book and founded the mental hygiene movement, whose purpose was to increase public awareness of the needs of the mentally ill. Increasing public awareness led to the development of child guidance clinics.

At the beginning of the twentieth century, Emil Kraepelin (1855–1926) identified definite clinical syndromes by recording their signs, course, and outcome (Kraepelin, 1921). Kraepelin differentiated between manic-depressive psychosis and dementia praecox, his term for schizophrenia. He also characterized dementia praecox patients as incurable and this pessimistic outlook continues to be associated with schizophrenia. Despite being a contemporary of Freud, Kraepelin has come to be regarded as the last of the predynamic psychiatrists. The emphasis on clinical classification reached its peak in his work. In later years a Swiss psychiatrist, Eugen Bleuler (1857–1939), renamed dementia praecox to be schizophrenia and differentiated the illness into several forms. Bleuler was also far more optimistic about treatment outcomes for schizophrenic patients than was Kraepelin.

Sigmund Freud (1856–1939) is considered to be the founder of psychoanalysis. While Freud practiced as a neurologist for several years, his interests ranged well beyond neurology and he studied with many outside that field. In 1896, Freud described free association and first used the term psychoanalysis to describe his method of treatment. Summarized briefly, Freud's major contributions to psychiatry are as follows. He clinically documented an explanation of human behavior based on the psychological concept of the dynamic unconscious. His exploration of the unconscious led to such concepts as primary process, dream interpretation, the defense mechanisms, the libido theory, and a psychosexual theory of development. While many of Freud's ideas were uniquely original, others can be traced to earlier cultures. However, his ideas were so different from the prevailing beliefs and attitudes of his society that he and psychoanalysis were subjects of much criticism and hostility.

MODERN TRENDS IN PSYCHIATRIC THOUGHT

World War II with its tremendous number of psychiatric casualities highlighted the problem of mental illness. To meet the treatment and rehabilitation needs of the many soldiers and veterans, the Veteran's Administration established large psychiatric facilities. In 1946, the National Mental Health Act was passed authorizing the National Institute of Mental Health (NIMH), which since 1949 has delegated funds for research, training, and assistance to the states in providing preventive, therapeutic, and rehabilitative services (Rossi, 1962).

From the mid-1940s to the mid-1950s in this country, psychiatry developed in two different directions, the biological and the dynamic (Ellenberger, 1970). Proponents of the biological approach focused research on the hereditary and neurological bases of mental illnesses. From this research grew an interest in psychosomatic illness and the biological factors in functional psychiatric disorders. In the dynamic direction, attention was focused on the mother-child relationship. David Levy, Leo Kanner, and Rene Spitz studied the effects of a lack of maternal involvement and maternal deprivation on the child. Concurrently in England, John Bowlby identified three phases of emotional reactions of children to separation from their mothers. He related these responses to grief, mourning, and to later psychopathology.

During the 1940s and 1950s, a significant shift in psychoanalytic thought occurred. Heinz Hartmann identified two groups of ego functions, one group that normally develops without conflict and one that is specifically involved in conflict. His contributions heralded a beginning focus on the ego rather than on the unconscious and led to a school of modified psychoanalytic thought known as ego psychology.

During this same period, psychiatry became more aware and responsive to the social influences on personality development and dysfunctional modes of behavior. A significant person in this regard is Harry Stack Sullivan (1892–1949), an American-born psychiatrist who founded the interpersonal school of psychiatry (Sullivan, 1953).

Sullivan is remembered chiefly for his concept of anxiety as related to interpersonal disapproval by others. For example, he believed that personality development is an outgrowth of interpersonal experiences and that psychopathology is the result of disturbed communication resulting from disintegrating forces of anxiety. Sullivan was a pioneer in his method of psychotherapy with the psychoses, notably schizophrenia, in which the therapist as a participant observer helps the client correct his or her parataxic distortions of others.

Sullivan focused on understanding and correcting the patient's distorted communication process within the context of the therapeutic relationship. His work broke new ground and excited interest in others to work with the psychotic individual.

In 1956, Erik Erickson introduced his concepts of ego identity, ego diffusion, and identity crisis in explaining the transition from childhood to adulthood. Erikson's theory of psychosexual development heralded a greater integration of cultural and social factors in the approaches to personality and psychopathology (Coles, 1970).

In the 1960s, a theoretical approach emerged that has continued to exert a great influence on the health sciences. Ludwig von Bertalanffy introduced general system theory (GST) related to living systems. GST postulates a reciprocally influencing system of homeostasis, transaction, and communication among all living beings leading to either optimal functioning or, within particular circumstances, dysfunction. A second influential occurrence was the introduction of behavior therapy, a combination of Pavlovian theory and the instrumentalism of Thorndike, Hull, and Skinner. In retrospect, the period from the end of World War II to the mid-1970s was a golden age for psychiatry. People were aware, interested, and optimistic about treating mental illness. Monies for research, training, and service delivery were relatively plentiful.

A number of events occurred that impacted on the mental health movement. The Vietnam conflict, civil rights movement, racial unrest, urban violence, the disillusionment of college age youth, the women's movement, and the epidemic in drug use all presented multiple and complex problems for society to recognize and meet. For a substantial period, mental health professionals attempted to remain aloof from these problems, seeing them as separate from their own professional goals and responsibilities (Goldston, 1965).

Increasingly, however, more and more mental health professionals have come to see these issues as directly relevant to themselves as professionals and as individuals. As a result, an increasing number of professionals have become more actively involved in local, state, and national concerns, more concerned with what works than with the reason why it works, and working more closely with other professions and the public in attempting to resolve problems. At present, mental health theories and psychiatry are in a state of uncertainty and restlessness, neither ready to abandon traditional theoretical approaches nor totally prepared to face the complex social issues at stake.

CHILD PSYCHIATRY

The first documented major contribution to the study of children was, at the close of the eighteenth century, by a Frenchman, J. M. G. Itard, who sought to "civilize" and train a young child who had been found living with wolves (Itard, 1932). A student of Itard, Seguin, came to the United States in 1848 and encouraged development of facilities for the retarded. He became the superintendent of the first training school for mentally retarded children.

The first psychological clinic for emotionally disturbed children was begun at the University of Pennsylvania in 1896 by a psychologist, Lightner Witmer. This clinic in its organizational structure and functions had some of the features inherent in the yet to be developed child guidance clinics. Witmer, noting the difficulties involved, still sought to distinguish whether a child's retardation was caused by organic problems in the central nervous system or from severe emotional disturbance. He published the first paper on work with a schizophrenic boy, which originally appeared in the *Ladies' Home Journal* (Witmer, 1920).

In 1905, De Sanctis identified the childhood form of dementia praecox, which he termed dementia praecocissima. Concurrently, Heller applied the term "dementia infantilis" to six children with mental deterioration without neurological abnormalities (Heller, 1954).

In 1909, William Healy established a clinic in Chicago, The Institute for Juvenile Research, whose major purpose was to evaluate and diagnose the delinquent, abandoned, and abused children who passed through the Cook County legal system (Healy & Bronner, 1936). This agency established a model for mental health treatment involving an interdisciplinary mix of physicians, psychologists, and social workers. The agency also served as a training center; those interested in child care from other parts of the country would study at the

Institute and then return to establish similar centers in their own communities. Both Witmer's and Healy's work provided the model of treatment later used by the child guidance movement in the 1920s and 1930s and a model for social and health interagency consultation around the treatment of an individual child. About this time, Freud was publishing his work with a phobic 5-year-old boy whom he treated by making recommendations to the father based on the father's records and reports of the child's behavior (Freud, 1946). Somewhat later, Freud described his concept of infantile sexuality and the parents' influences on the child's personality development.

With the growing awareness of the problems of children, the pioneers in the work with children felt a need for closer communication with their colleagues. The American Orthopsychiatric Association was established as a multidisciplinary organization in 1924 to promote and exchange ideas, concepts, and methods relevant to child mental health.

It was not until 1953 that the American Academy of Child Psychiatry was established and only since 1957 has child psychiatry been recognized as a subspecialty of psychiatry and a subspecialty Board of Child Psychiatry established by the American Board of Psychiatry and Neurology.

PSYCHIATRIC NURSING

While care of some sort for the mentally ill had occurred for centuries, prior to the mid-eighteenth century those who were ill and well-to-do were cared for by family members or members of religious orders. Such care, while not ideal, maintained some level of comfort for the patient. For the poor, the situation was quite different. Their care was minimal or nonexistent and they were kept in filthy surroundings.

In the United States in the 1800s with industrialization and increased immigration, the population increased markedly, especially in the urban areas. The small mental hospitals and humanitarian treatment of the mentally ill began to change. At this time, institutions admitted only the middle and upper classes. The poor and the black were sent to the poorhouse, workhouse, jail, or large custodial institutions, depending on the nature of their illness and the violence of their behavior. Insanity became connected with poverty and the thought was that the patient was insane because he was poor and that he was poor because he came from inferior stock.

There were some who tried to change these conditions. A leader in these efforts was Dorothea Dix (1802–1887), who, although not a nurse herself, devoted her life to improving the care of the mentally ill (Marshall, 1937). She was appointed the Superintendent of Women Nurses during the Civil War and was given the authority to select and assign women nurses to general or military hospitals.

However, nursing as a discipline only emerged in the late nineteenth century. Earlier, in Germany, a school of nursing was established in 1836. While in England, Florence Nightingale established a training program for nurses, after demonstrating the principles of sound nursing care during the Crimean War. Nightingale emphasized cleanliness, good hygiene, and systematic observations of patients. She identified nursing as an honorable profession and recommended that the direction of hospital nursing departments should be through nurses rather than physicians (Nightingale, 1860).

Psychiatric Nursing in the United States

In the United States, several American schools of nursing were established in the late 1800s patterned after the Nightingale model. Linda Richards, a graduate from one of these schools, spent most of her nursing career promoting better nursing care in psychiatric hospitals (Richards, 1915). In 1880, McLean Hospital in Massachusetts opened the first American school to train nurses to care for the mentally ill. At the beginning of the twentieth century, trained nurses were found in many psychiatric hospitals dispensing medications and overseeing others who provided physical care to the patients. Since the nurse-patient ratio was often 1 nurse to 100 or more patients, nursing care was custodial, physically oriented, and totally directed by physicians (Goodnow, 1938). Nurses made no attempt to deal with interpersonal or psychodynamic issues with patients. Nursing, as a discipline, became organized during this period with the creation of the American Society of Superintendents of Training Schools for Nurses in 1893. Its successor was the National League of Nursing Education in 1912, which in 1952 became the National League for Nursing.

In 1896, the Nurses' Associated Alumnae of the United States and Canada was organized for all nurses. It then became the Nurses' Associated Alumnae of the United States in 1899 and in 1911 became the American Nurses' Association. This was and continues to be the principal professional organization for nurses and from its founding has been concerned with setting high standards of patient care and better welfare for nurses.

Between 1900 and 1930, psychiatry became more dynamic as a result of Freud's contributions and those of the English and American schools of psychiatry. In 1920, the first text on psychiatric nursing, *Nursing Mental and Nervous Diseases* by Harriet Bailey, was published (Bailey, 1920). This book became the standard text in psychiatric nursing, went through four revisions, and only went out of print in 1954. In 1937, Katharine McLean Steele published *Psychiatric Nursing,* which outlined the role and functions of the psychiatric nurse (Steele, 1937). These first nursing books were published before Freud's or Sullivan's work had any impact on psychiatry in this country, which, particularly Sullivan's, began to be felt only in the 1930s. Sullivan's concept of the interpersonal influence on individual behavior and his analysis of the therapeutic and nontherapeutic effects of staff-patient relationships exerted tremendous influence on identifying a place for psychiatric nursing in milieu treatment and one-to-one relationships with patients. Psychiatric nurses were no longer primarily responsible for the physical care of patients but became instrumental in creating a therapeutic environment for them.

Besides philosophical changes in treatment, the introduction of somatic treatments such as Metrazol, insulin, electroshock, and chemotherapy all combined to make patients more accessible and responsive to interpersonal work. Public awareness of mental health problems was heightened by the psychiatric problems resulting from World Wars I and II.

In 1943, there were three university-linked graduate programs in psychiatric nursing. World War II profoundly affected psychiatric nursing. Nurses returning from service were eligible under the GI Bill for advanced education. The existing programs were unable to meet the demand. In 1946, with the passage of the National Mental Health Act research and training funds were provided for the core mental health disciplines. Psychiatric nursing was designated a core discipline and thus received federal funds for both undergraduate and graduate nurse education. The National Mental Health Act provided funding and influenced the scope and direction of nursing and psychiatric nursing education.

Educational Trends

Prior to 1946, less than 1% of psychiatric nurses had advanced preparation in psychiatric nursing and baccalaureate programs accounted for less than 5% of all undergraduate nursing programs. Eight universities were given NIMH funds to expand and improve graduate nursing programs in 1947. In the same year, Render published *Nurse-Patient Relationships in Psychiatry,* a textbook for psychiatric nurses (Render, 1947). In 1950, psychoanalytic concepts were first reflected in a nursing textbook by Kalkman, *Introduction to Psychiatric Nursing* (Kalkman, 1950). This book, along with Muller's work (1950), gave impetus and direction to the field. A short time later, Peplau's book (1952), *Interpersonal Relations in Nursing,* provided for the first time a conceptual framework for nursing and psychiatric nursing. Concurrently, Tudor (1952), using an interpersonal framework derived from psychoanalytic concepts, described the use of the nurse-patient relationship to develop an intensely positive bond that broke the mutual pattern of withdrawal between the staff and a patient on an inpatient unit. These works together with Peplau's subsequent writings and teachings have had a tremendous influence on graduate psychiatric nursing education and practice.

The result of the National Mental Health Act and initial publications by psychiatric nurse educators and clinicians had an impact on psychiatric nursing in many ways. The pool of well-educated clinicians, teachers and administrators was increased, and psychiatric nurses became leaders as clinicians, teachers, and administrators. With their impetus, in 1955, undergraduate nursing programs for the first time required psychiatric nursing as part of the basic preparation in nursing. Beginning in 1956, NIMH made funds available to integrate psychological and behavioral concepts into undergraduate nursing programs. Integration has been a mixed blessing. While it has sensitized nurses to the emotional components present in all illness and has strengthened nurses' knowledge and skill in interpersonal communication, it has also created problems. In many nursing programs, the integration of social and psychological theories throughout the program was at the expense of minimizing the presentation of discrete psychopathology content and student clinical experiences with identified psychiatric patients in a psychiatric setting.

By 1960, a body of psychiatric nursing knowledge was accumulating and being used by nurses in all areas. While delineating specific concepts, principles, and practices, psychiatric nurses were beginning to explore new areas of practice within the field.

The practice of psychiatric nursing was changing. There was a major shift from custodial care to assuming leadership roles in the care of psychiatric patients in inpatient and outpatient settings. Psychiatric nurses were preparing themselves to assume new and challenging roles in the decades ahead.

Psychiatric Mental Health Nursing

The Community Mental Health Centers Act of 1963 further emphasized a shift in graduate psychiatric nursing education from a focus on inpatient care to a focus on knowledge and clinical competencies, such as the one-to-one relationship, family and group therapy required for treatment within the community, and the prevention and early intervention of psychiatric problems. With this act, large amounts of federal monies became available for states to use in planning, building, and staffing community mental health centers (Freedman, 1967). Psychiatric nurses were seen as integral service providers in these settings.

During this era, psychiatric nursing joined forces with public health nursing to develop psychiatric mental health nursing (PMHN). The molding of the two developed both psychotherapy and mental health consultation as areas of interest and expertise for the psychiatric mental health nurse. As more and more psychiatric nurses moved into community mental health centers, certain issues related to their preparation and role were voiced (Sills, 1973).

These issues focused on where and how psychiatric nurses could best be prepared for practice in community mental health centers. There were those who believed that nurses were best prepared by first learning and working with the severely psychiatrically ill so that they could clearly identify and understand the pathology involved and its treatment. Others believed that since nurses would be working in the community, their education and experience should be in community-based programs as this would better prepare them to recognize and intervene with the more common everyday stresses and crises that people encounter. Both types of preparation have advantages but, ideally, a blend of the two is required if psychiatric nurses are to function appropriately in the treatment of the mentally ill, as well as in mental health maintenance and promotion. The issue of how best to prepare the psychiatric nurse educationally and experientially remains an unresolved issue.

Another issue of concern then and now is whether in fact there needs to be some type of generic mental health program that would prepare all those who work in community mental health since many of the functions interweave and overlap. A second point of view believes in maintaining the multidisciplinary experiences in order to break down the stereotypes that currently exist among disciplines.

It is important to remember that it was only in 1965 that the American Nurses' Association (ANA) took the position that nursing education was within the control of the nursing profession. However, it was 1968 before this stand was accepted by the American Psychiatric Association. Only then were nurse training programs in mental hospitals no longer controlled by the American Psychiatric Association as they had been since the early 1900s. As a direct result, psychiatric nursing hospital programs closed and nursing education's move to educational institutions was accelerated (Dolan, 1978).

Child and Adolescent Psychiatric Nursing

As we have noted, child psychiatry itself is a very recent addition to the mental health professions. Child guidance clinics that focused on identifying and assisting children with emotional problems only began in the 1920s and 1930s. The disciplines involved in this movement were psychology, psychiatry, and social work. There was little evidence of nursing interest or activity in the field. As state psychiatric hospitals established units for children, nurses became involved only minimally in their physical care. Although NIMH has encouraged and supported graduate education in nursing since 1946, the earliest nurses seeking advanced work in child psychiatric nursing had only "adult" psychiatric nursing programs from which to choose. Nurse educators and clinicians recognized the inadequacies of these programs to prepare nurses for a career in working with mentally ill children and adolescents. Recognition of the need spurred the establishment of graduate programs designed specifically to give nurses the knowledge and experience they required to work with children and adolescents. The first graduate program in child psychiatric nursing was established at Boston University in 1954. Other graduate programs in this field followed until there were eight by 1967.

Nurses prepared in child psychiatric nursing have not increased in large numbers for several reasons. Child psychiatric nursing graduate programs have had limited funds since the majority of funding has gone to adult programs. Beyond this, however, there are other issues. There has never been the interest or priority for work with mentally ill children and adolescents in this country as there has been for working with the disturbed adult. Because of the limited number of treatment programs for mentally ill children and adolescents, there have been fewer opportunities for nurses to have exposure to such programs either as students or as part of their work experience. Consequently, few nurses have been aware and/or interested in the possibilities in the field.

With few graduate programs and small numbers of graduates from such programs, child and adolescent psychiatric nurses have worked in a variety of roles in widely different settings. In most cases, these nurses have had to "sell" prospective employers the fact that they were educated and equipped to fulfill the work responsibilities better than nurses and others prepared in more traditional ways. However, scarcity in numbers and diversity of roles have meant that there have never been sufficient numbers in a particular role or setting to enable those prepared in child and adolescent psychiatric nursing to have a major impact on mental health services or nursing education. This is doubly unfortunate in that their clinical interests and educational preparation make them uniquely qualified and outstanding contributors in the treatment of mentally ill children and adolescents.

The ANA has not yet established standards of practice for child and adolescent psychiatric nursing. Currently, an ANA task force is working on such standards. One hopes that they will be identified soon. Such standards would make the current certification in child and adolescent psychiatric nursing more meaningful and certainly more worthwhile.

It can be seen from the foregoing discussion that there are a multitude of roles and settings where adult and child psychiatric nursing specialists can practice. They can function in primary, secondary, or tertiary settings with clients and families experiencing both psychiatric and physical illnesses. They can serve as consultants to nurses in other areas and to other disciplines. They are a valuable although as yet a largely untapped resource in mental health promotion and treatment.

THE KNOWLEDGE BASE FOR CLINICAL SPECIALIST NURSING PRACTICE

There is general agreement about the areas of knowledge and skill required in psychiatric mental health nursing although the line dividing the generalist and the specialist in psychiatric nursing remains in dispute.

The knowledge base for psychiatric mental health nursing contains the following: marital and family dynamics and pathology, psychopharmacology, crisis intervention theory and therapy, psychopathology, intake assessment/diagnosis, theories of individual therapy, self-awareness, personality theory, developmental theory, prevention and early intervention, treatment planning and goals, community resources and referral, psychobiological theory, research methodology and statistics, and management and organizational issues.

The skill areas required in psychiatric mental health nursing include establishing short- and long-term treatment goals; designing, conducting and analyzing research; effective use of community resources; evaluation of intervention strategies; integrating social, psychological, and medical treatment models; individual, group, family, and milieu treatment; stress and crisis management; assessing suicide potential; group processes; making differential diagnoses; assessing physiological and neurological aspects of symptomatology; knowledge of psychotropic medications; therapeutic effects and nontherapeutic side effects; and interpersonal skills to facilitate relationships with other professionals and nonprofessionals. The focus of psychiatric mental health nursing is broad in that it addresses the prevention, treatment, rehabilitation, and maintenance activities for people at different developmental stages of life. Its orientation covers all diagnostic categories and it is practiced in diverse settings from the inner city to the small rural community, the university medical center to the long-term residential facility.

Definition of the Clinical Specialist

The ANA Division on Psychiatric Mental Health Nursing Practice and the Council of Specialists in Psychiatric Mental Health Nursing define psychiatric nursing as a specialized nursing practice area focusing on prevention, treatment, and rehabilitation of the mentally ill. Clinical specialists use the nursing process to assess need, to diagnose, and to evaluate treatment. Treatment modalities used by the psychiatric mental health specialist include individual and group psychotherapy, family therapy, screening and evaluation, house calls, conducting health teaching activities, providing support and medication monitoring, and responding to client needs through community action as necessary. A psychiatric mental health clinical specialist is a nurse with a master's degree in psychiatric and mental health nursing; additional supervised clinical experience; and depth of knowledge, competence, and skill in the practice of psychiatric and mental health nursing. She or he has ANA specialist certification or eligibility for such certification. Educational standards at the graduate level, the ANA Standards of Psychiatric Mental Health Nursing Practice, and ANA specialist certification all provide means for evaluating the preparation of the individual against the accepted standards of knowledge and skill required of the clinical specialist.

ANA Standards of Psychiatric Mental Health Nursing Practice

In 1982, a committee of the ANA completed a revision of the psychiatric mental health nursing practice standards that apply to all settings where psychiatric mental health nurses practice (American Nurses' Association, 1982). The 1982 revision is significantly more encompassing and detailed than the 1973 standards. In addition, they are written to include both generalist and specialist practice. The 1982 standards are divided into two broad areas: professional practice and professional performance. Within the professional practice section, nursing theory and nursing diagnoses are included. Additionally, Standard V, dealing with intervention, has been expanded into substandards delineating in detail appropriate psychiatric mental health nursing interventions. The standards focusing on psychotherapy and community health systems relate specifically to specialist practice.

The section on professional performance includes standards on peer review, continuing education, interdisciplinary collaboration, community health systems, and research. All standards include a rationale as well as structure, process, and outcome criteria that are critical to determining whether a given criterion has or has not been met. The standards represent a major and needed revision that more precisely delineates the psychiatric nurse clinical specialist's responsibilities to his or her clients and profession, as well as accountability to self, client, peers, profession, and to the public. These are the most complete and descriptive Standards of Psychiatric Mental Health Nursing Practice to date and are well suited to measure and provide guidance to achieve excellence in care.

Clinical Nurse Specialist Roles

With the knowledge and skills that psychiatric mental health clinical nurse specialists have as a group, they have moved into leadership positions in service and education. They have provided highly visible role models, ranging from liaison-psychiatric nurses in general hospitals, integrating social and psychological content into undergraduate nursing education, to individual psychotherapists. By the close of the 1960s, a number of graduate-prepared psychiatric nurse specialists whose roles as individual, group, family, and milieu therapists had been clearly established were able to obtain direct third-party reimbursement for these services.

Psychiatric mental health nurses were the first clinical group to identify minimal educational and clinical criteria for functioning as clinical specialists. They were also the first specialty group to establish certification at the specialist level, initially through the New Jersey and New York state nursing organizations and then through the ANA certification process.

It is clear that psychiatric mental health nursing, though young as a specialty, has had many accomplishments. It has been in the vanguard of nursing for most of the last 30 years. It has been a major influence in nursing and has established itself as equal with the other mental health disciplines.

Yet one hears on every side that psychiatric nursing is a vanishing specialty. How can this be so? With the past accomplishments and present leaders, why the pessimism? The following is a discussion of the current and future issues for the specialty.

Current Issues

An ongoing issue is the multiple names given this area of nursing. The uncertainty about what these health professionals are called may reflect a deeper uncertainty about who these people are.

What should this specialty be called? There are many names in current usage for what once used to be called *psychiatric nursing.* Many were dissatisfied with that name, believing it too narrow in focus, illness oriented, and medicine dominated. Philosophical and conceptual changes in nursing led increasingly to the use of the term *psychiatric mental health nursing.* Advocates for this title contend that the name implies a broader focus including concepts related to both mental illness and health. Advocates also believe the title reflects the current shift in nursing to include a focus on prevention of illness. There are others who believe the term *psychosocial nursing* is more apt in that nurses in the field are well grounded in social and behavioral sciences. Proponents of this term contend that psychosocial nursing is much broader in focus even than psychiatric mental health nursing in that it focuses far less on disease and more on life stresses and environmental and cultural factors (Leininger, 1973).

A major criticism of the psychosocial label is that it gives insufficient priority to the biological or psychopathological areas. Psychosocial advocates retort that nursing cannot possibly keep abreast with the biological field and, in any case, they would prefer to drop the biological aspects from psychosocial nursing. There have been other terms that have been proposed, such as mental health nursing and behavioral nursing.

More recently, Koldjeski (1984) differentiated the field of psychiatric nursing into three areas of nursing practice: community mental health nursing, mental health nursing, and psychiatric nursing. Koldjeski reserves to the first two areas work with groups and families who are less disturbed and healthy and limits the area of psychiatric nursing to seriously mentally and emotionally ill individuals.

Additionally, in the past, there has been much discussion and some confusion regarding the use of the terms clinical specialist, nurse clinician, and even nurse practitioner. Since the late 1970s, however, *clinical specialist* has been accepted as the term describing those nurses holding Master's degrees in nursing and who are primarily clinicians with a high degree of knowledge, skill, and competence in one area of nursing. It was in 1979 that the ANA Council of Advanced Practitioners in Psychiatric and Mental Nursing changed the group's name to the Council of Specialists in Psychiatric Mental Health Nursing.

The editors have chosen the name *psychiatric mental health nursing* as being most representative of their own thinking about where the specialty is today. The term bridges the historical heritage and indicates the future direction. It stresses a dedication to treatment of the ill and to health maintenance and promotion. The term *clinical specialist* is the most appropriate one to describe the level of psychiatric mental health nurses for whom this book is written. Throughout the book this term will be used to refer to nurses with the appropriate preparation to work with children, adolescents, and/or adults.

A second issue of note is that enrollment in psychiatric mental health nursing graduate programs has decreased in the last 10 years and continues to decrease in comparison to enrollment in all nursing graduate programs. More information is needed regarding the number of graduate-prepared psychiatric adult and child psychiatric nurse specialists who are currently working in these fields. In what roles and in what numbers do specialists work in these roles? How have employment opportunities for these specialists changed? Despite years of continuous federal support for specialty training, a data base for psychiatric mental health nursing is lacking. It is not possible to identify numbers, distribution, or even all points of entry into the health care system for these nurses with any degree of accuracy.

Another issue relates to the current state of psychiatry. As medicine moves toward increasing specialization and more complex technology, it increasingly requires specialized clinical knowledge and skills. Together with specialization comes more impersonal and even dehumanizing health care.

Both the psychiatric mental health and child and adolescent psychiatric clinical nurse specialist can play a vital role in dealing with the problematic interpersonal aspects of physical and mental illness with children, adolescents, and adults, including the elderly, and their families; in intensive care units for infants, children, or adults; in liaison nursing; and in ambulatory treatment and prevention areas—all in addition to the more familiar psychiatric settings. In all settings, the treatment modalities of individual, group, family, and milieu can be used effectively. There is a growing need for psychiatric mental health clinical nurse specialists prepared to work with the elderly and the chronically mentally ill in a multitude of settings.

With increasing family stress and disruption affecting large numbers of children, there is an urgent need for school nurses to have greater knowledge of psychopathology, crisis intervention theory and intervention, as well as individual, group, and family therapy. School nurses need additional skills in the areas of individual, group, and family supportive therapy, assessing stress and abuse potential, and in involving significant others in treatment.

In addition, there are a multitude of areas where the needs of the mentally ill and emotionally stressed are unmet. The provision of humane, supportive care in the least restrictive environment remains a goal yet to be attained. Alternatives to inpatient care remain few and fragmented, reflecting haphazard planning, limited funding, and erratic monitoring. State and county hospitals and other continued care facilities require changes in treatment goals and staffing patterns that are readily apparent. Nursing has the largest number of health care providers in hospitals. Hospitals are a major source of employment for nurses. There should be room for interdisciplinary sharing with nursing colleagues to identify alternatives that might improve hospital care and residential care in a cost-effective manner.

Other unmet needs of the mentally ill include deinstitutionalization and aftercare. Utilization reviews and decreasing insurance coverage have contributed to earlier discharge with fewer provisions for aftercare. Limited adaptive capacities and chronic dysfunction are increasingly a problem with discharged mental patients. There is a need to explore monitoring, maintenance, and support services that are accessible, adequate, cost effective, and available. There is a growing concern that in a society with greater health needs than resources, the focus on meeting mental health needs will mean an abandonment of the mentally ill. Still others believe that mental health care reflects health care in our society. The focus is on treating the acutely mentally ill rather than on the maintenance and promotion of mental health and the treatment of the less acutely ill.

Psychiatric mental health nursing has been shaped by social and cultural forces throughout its evolution. For the most part, this process has been beneficial; however, this has not or may not always be the case.

Currently, psychiatric mental health nursing is struggling with issues and problems that will shape the specialty in perhaps even more different configurations. But clarity in decisions and direction will only be achieved if psychiatric nurses continue to actively identify and work together toward shared goals that are congruent with the larger goals of nursing.

THE BRIDGING ROLE IN PSYCHIATRIC MENTAL HEALTH NURSING

For many years, nursing practice relied heavily on the biological-medical model for identification and direction of the nursing role. This same reliance has been true for psychiatric nursing as well. Psychiatric nursing and nursing in general has come to realize that much of the knowledge basic to nursing practice is common knowledge shared with many other disciplines. However, that knowledge needs to be modified to serve the purpose and practice of psychiatric mental health nursing.

Thus, the biological-medical model requires examination in order to select those aspects that can be reformulated into concepts more relevant to nursing and to discard those concepts that are logically inconsistent with theories of nursing practice.

Biological-Medical Model

For example, the biological-medical model is based on certain assumptions: that mental disorders will be found to have an organic basis; that behavioral manifestations of a mental disorder are evidence of an underlying pathology; that because the disorder is organic or biochemical in nature, the individual is not responsible for behaviors resulting from the disorder; and that ordering or classifying the symptoms into syndromes is the best way to understand them.

There are values inherent in these assumptions that need to be made explicit in order to evaluate their implications for nursing. These values include the beliefs that

1. Mental illness ultimately will be found to be organic in nature. Thus, there is no role for maladaptive learning or environmental stress as precipitating factors.
2. The behaviors symptomatic of the disorder are merely reflecting underlying cellular pathology so that treating the symptom alone will not cure the disorder.
3. The individual cannot and should not be held responsible for thoughts and acts that are the result of the disorder. These thoughts and acts are outside the individual's free will. This value is directly counter to the idea of free will and accountability.
4. Categorizing and labeling bring order out of chaos, identifies disorder more accurately, and pinpoints treatment more precisely. However, categorizing and labeling also create arbitrary and artificial distinctions that may force individuals into inappropriate classifications.

Most psychiatric mental health clinical nurse specialists would take issue with some or all of the values implied in the biological-medical conceptual framework. There are advantages, however, for psychiatric mental health nursing in using the model judiciously. The nurses' familiarity with and understanding of the model permits them to assist clients to understand the model and its implications for treatment. The nurses can also understand and intelligently carry out medical treatments such as administering medications or somatic treatments. Last, but by no means least, this particular model is widely used for labeling and treatment. Understanding the model and the process permits the nurse to engage with colleagues using a commonly understood language. Thus, the nurse can use an understanding and application of the model to literally "bridge the gap" that frequently exists between physicians and patients and physicians and their nonmedical colleagues. At the same time, knowing the limitations of the model, nurses can use their own holistic perspective of nursing to assess the emotional and physical needs of clients and to assist both clients and families to achieve the necessary adjustments in their life-style rather than focusing only on adjustment to the disorder.

The biological-medical model has become less functional for nursing education as theory development in nursing has progressed. The model is still useful and appropriate in organizing disease-related course content of which psychiatric nurses must be well informed. In addition, the medical model is still the principal organizing framework used in most clinical practice settings, especially those involving acute care.

The greatest danger for psychiatric mental health nursing in using the biological-medical model is in curtailing the autonomy and accountability of the behavior of those individuals who interact with the physician as patients or colleagues. However, this danger can be avoided and psychiatric mental health nursing practice can be strengthened if nurses clearly understand that theories borrowed from other disciplines must be assessed, evaluated, and reformulated so that they are logically consistent with nursing theory and practice.

Psychiatric Nursing Theory Development

One hopes that the clinical specialists in both adult and child psychiatric nursing will be among those in the profession who will struggle to bring synthesis to the many dichotomous explanations of human behavior, such as biological, psychodynamic, systems, and social labeling theories, to name only a few. While this may seem to be an overwhelming task, it is a critical component of nursing's struggle to define its unique perspective on the diagnosis and treatment of human responses to actual or potential health problems.

The unique modification of these theories from other disciplines to meet nursing's purposes will serve as a stimulus for psychiatric nursing theory development. It is important that psychiatric mental health clinical nurse specialists continue to publish information about the clinical concepts and the theories used in their practice. Only with published data available can nursing theorists select and modify appropriate concepts and their relationships for psychiatric nursing theories. It will be critical to continue testing these theories empirically. PMHN specialists are eminently prepared to conceptualize practice theory and to test it. Both of these tasks are vital to the continued existence of the speciality.

SUMMARY

The goal of this chapter was to enhance the reader's appreciation of psychiatric mental health nursing's heritage through highlighting the care of the mentally ill from antiquity to the present. The emergence of psychiatric mental health nursing as a professional speciality and some major forces influencing its development were described.

The future of the speciality is interdependent with the needs and resources of society.

Psychiatric mental health and child and adolescent psychiatric clinical nurse specialists will need to actively work together to shape the speciality's future role in nursing and society or else the direction of the speciality will be determined by forces outside the profession.

REFERENCES

American Nurses' Association. *Standards of psychiatric and mental health nursing practice.* Kansas City, MO: American Nurses' Association, 1982.

Bailey, H. *Nursing mental and nervous diseases.* New York: Macmillan, 1920.

Beers, C. *A mind that found itself* (rev. ed.). Garden City, NY: Doubleday, 1948.

Binz, C. *Doctor Johann Weyer* (2nd ed.). Heidelburg: Springer, 1969.

Coles, R. *Erik H. Erikson. The growth of his work.* Boston: Little, Brown, 1970.

Deutsch, A. *The mentally ill in America.* Garden City, NY: Doubleday, Doran & Co., 1937.

Dolan, J. *Nursing in society: A historical perspective.* Philadelphia: W. B. Saunders, 1978.

Ellenberger, R. *The discovery of the unconscious. The history and evolution of dynamic psychiatry.* New York: Basic Books, 1970.

Foucault, M. *Madness and civilization: A history of insanity in the age of reason.* New York: Pantheon Books, 1965.

Freedman, A. Historical and political roots of the community mental health centers act. *American Journal of Orthopsychiatry, 1967, 37,* 487.

Freud, S. *Collected Papers:* Vol. 3. *Analysis of a phobia in a five year old boy.* London: Hogarth, 1946.

Goldston, I. Community psychiatry, its social and historic derivations. *Journal of Canadian Psychiatric Association,* 1965, *10,* 461.

Goodnow, M. *Outline of nursing history* (6th ed.). Philadelphia: W. B. Saunders, 1938.

Hall, J. (Ed.). *One hundred years of American psychiatry.* New York: Columbia University Press, 1944.

Healy, W., & Bronner, A. *New light on delinquency and its treatment.* New Haven: Yale University Press, 1936.

Heller, T. About dementia infantilis. *Journal of Nervous and Mental Disease,* 1954, *119,* 471–477.

Hemphill, R. Historical witchcraft and psychiatric illness in Western Europe. *Proceedings of the Royal Society of Medicine,* 1966, *59,* 891.

Itard, J. M. G. *The wild boy of Aveyron (G. Humphrey & M. Humphrey, Trans.).* New York: Appleton-Century, 1932.

Jackson, S. Unusual mental states in medieval Europe 1. Medical syndromes of mental disorders, 400–1100 A.D. *Journal of Historical Medicine,* 1972, *27,* 262.

Kalkman, M. *Introduction to psychiatric nursing.* New York: McGraw-Hill, 1950.

Koldjeski, D. *Community mental health nursing.* New York: John Wiley & Sons, 1984.

Kors, A., & Peters, E. *Witchcraft in Europe, 1100–1700, a documentary history.* Philadelphia: University of Pennsylvania Press, 1972.

Kraepelin, E. *Manic-depressive insanity and paranoia.* Edinburgh: E. & S. Livingstone, 1921.

Lain, E. *The therapy of the world in classical antiquity.* New Haven: Yale University Press, 1970.

Leininger, M. Winds of change. In M. Leininger (Ed.), *Contemporary issues in mental health nursing* (pp. 1–21). Boston: Little, Brown, 1973.

Marshall, H. *Dorothea Dix: Forgotten Samaritan.* Chapel Hill, NC: University of North Carolina Press, 1937.

Middleton, J. (Ed.). *Magic, witchcraft and curing.* Garden City, NY: Natural History Press, 1967.

Mora, G. Historical and theoretical trends in psychiatry. In A. Freedman, H. Kaplan, & B. Sadock (Eds.), *Comprehensive textbook of psychiatry* Vol. 1 (2nd ed.) (pp. 1–21). Baltimore, MD: Williams & Wilkins, 1975.

Mora, G., & Brand, J. (Eds.). *Psychiatry and its history.* Springfield, IL: Charles C. Thomas, 1970.

Muller, T. G. *The nature and direction of psychiatric nursing: The dynamics of human relationships in nursing.* Philadelphia: J. B. Lippincott, 1950.

Nightingale, F. *Notes on nursing.* London: Harison, 1860.

Peplau, H. *Interpersonal relations in nursing.* New York: G. P. Putnam, 1952.

Pinel, P. *Treatise on insanity.* New York: Hafner Press, 1962.

Render, H. *Nurse-patient relationships in psychiatry.* New York: McGraw-Hill, 1947.

Richards, L. *Reminiscences of America's first trained nurse.* Boston: Whitcomb & Barrows, 1915.

Rossi, A. Some pre World War II antecedents of community mental health theory and practice. *Mental Hygiene,* 1962, *46,* 78.

Sills, G. Historical developments and issues in psychiatric mental health nursing. In M. Leininger (Ed.), *Contemporary issues in mental health nursing* (pp. 125–136). Boston: Little, Brown, 1973.

Singer, C. *A short history of medicine.* Oxford: Clarendon Press, 1928.

Steele, K. *Psychiatric nursing.* Philadelphia: F. A. Davis, 1937.

Sullivan, H. *The interpersonal theory of psychiatry.* New York: W. W. Norton, 1953.

Szasz, T. *The age of madness: The history of involuntary mental hospitalization.* Presented in selected texts. Garden City, NY: Doubleday, 1973.

Tudor, G. Sociopsychiatric nursing approach to intervention in a problem of mutual withdrawal on a mental hospital ward. *Psychiatry,* 1952, *15(2),* 193–217.

Weiner, D. B. The apprenticeship of Philippe Pinel: A new document, observations of Citizen Pussin on the insane. *American Journal of Psychiatry,* 1979, *136(9),* 1128–1134.

Wilson, J. Mental diseases of ancient Mesopotamia. In D. Brothwell & A. Santison (Eds.), *Diseases of antiquity* Springfield, IL: Charles C. Thomas, 1967.

Witmer, L. Orthogenic cases, XIV—Don: A curable case of arrested development due to a fear psychosis the result of shock in a three-year-old infant. *Psychological Clinic,* 1920, *13,* 97–111.

BIBLIOGRAPHY

Ackerknecht, E. *Short history of psychiatry* (2nd ed.). New York: Hafner Press, 1968.

CHAPTER 2

NURSING CONCEPTUAL MODELS

Judith T. Maurin

There is a growing literature in nursing concerned with the development of a theoretical base for nursing practice. Nurses are writing about theory development and offering conceptual models in the hope that these will eventually guide nursing practice and research. This chapter will review psychiatric mental health nurses' contribution to theory development and discuss the debate about the need for a unique nursing perspective for psychiatric mental health nursing. Finally, Orem's Self-Care Deficit Model of Nursing will be applied to a clinical situation to explore the advantages and disadvantages such a model might hold for psychiatric mental health nursing practice.

THEORY DEVELOPMENT IN PSYCHIATRIC NURSING

Historical Contribution to Theory Development

Psychiatric nursing made an early contribution to theory development in nursing through the concept clarification engaged in during the 1950s and 1960s. Concepts representing symptoms and patient problems were identified in clinical practice, described, and analyzed (e.g., Gregg, 1955; Peplau, 1955; Tudor, 1952). Under the influence and mentorship of Hildegard Peplau this work continued (Burd & Marshall, 1963; Smoyak, 1975). Peplau taught hundreds of nurses the importance of documenting their practice and refining their conceptualization of that practice. In these efforts, the relationship between clinical practice and theory development was unquestionable. Theory development was not pursued as an end in itself. The phenomena operationalized and emerged from clinical practice and the relevance for practice was readily apparent. The increased understanding resulting from this theoretical work facilitated recognition of the phenomena in clinical practice and often suggested points for intervention. For example, the description of the process of mutual withdrawal provided by Tudor (1952) encouraged recognition of this phenomenon in the practice of others. Furthermore, identification of mutual withdrawal as an interpersonal process in which the nurse is involved provided the practitioner with a framework for intervention.

On the other hand, this immediate payoff may have reduced the incentive to push for theory development at higher levels of abstraction. One did not find psychiatric nurses suggesting relationships between and among the many concepts operationalized.

Current Theory Development Efforts in Nursing

During the past few years, nurse scholars have increased their efforts to deliberately tackle the work of theory development for nursing. Some have attempted to delineate the processes of theory development, analysis, and application. Others have offered theoretical frameworks deemed useful for the profession.

One of the early contributors to the work of defining nursing was Peplau. In *Interpersonal Relations in Nursing,* Peplau (1952) identified the nurse-patient relationship as central to an understanding of nursing and articulated several nursing roles through which patients are assisted. This work was not limited in scope to psychiatric mental health nursing, but made a statement about nursing wherever and for whatever patient group it was being performed. Despite this early contribution to the definition of nursing, psychiatric nursing as a specialty has made little effort to apply the nursing models to its phenomena of concern. A few exceptions include Underwood (1980), Schmidt (1981), Whall (1981), Buckwalter & Kerfoot (1982), and Clements & Roberts (1983).

Notable exceptions to the tendency for psychiatric mental health nurses to ignore the nursing models being developed can be found in the works of Whall (1980) and Fitzpatrick, Whall, Johnston, & Floyd, (1982). These authors believe that nursing brings a unique perspective to psychiatric mental health and that it is important to explicate the difference. They have selected concepts and propositions from borrowed theories that psychiatric nurses frequently use (e.g., System Theory, Crisis Theory, Freudian Theory) and explored the degree of congruence between these ideas and the statements about person, environment, health, and nursing found in contemporary nursing models. They argue for the need to reformulate borrowed theories to achieve congruence with nursing models.

The suggestion that borrowed theories may need reformulation by nurses may at first sound arrogant and presumptuous. However, theories are meant to be evaluated and questioned. That is how they are refined and made to reflect more adequately the world as nurses experience it. Nursing could contribute to both theory refinement and the creation of more useful theory for practice if nurses reflected on the congruence of borrowed theory and the phenomena of concern.

For example, Orem's Self-Care Deficit Model describes the individual as a holistic being who can be viewed as functioning biologically, symbolically, and socially. Suppose a nurse who was using Orem's framework came upon an article about operant conditioning derived from the experimental psychology of Watson and Skinner and thought these ideas may have application in his or her practice. However, this nurse would find that operant conditioning (which focuses on observable and measureable phenomena: behavior, responses, stimuli) is incongruent with Orem's framework, which assumes that humans function symbolically. To state that humans function symbolically means that they attribute meanings to things and these meanings are influenced by their unique points of view. Failure to take symbolic ability into account would result in one missing the tendency to select what is stimuli and/or rewards in the environment as a result of the meanings attributed to selected phenomena. The nurse is more likely to develop a successful behavior modification program for a client if this symbolic ability is considered.

A UNIQUE PSYCHIATRIC NURSING PERSPECTIVE?

The Debate

People who practice psychiatric mental health nursing as a clinical specialty are clearly undecided as to whether to participate in defining nursing theory with a unique perspective or to work within other models. Some authors urge psychiatric nurses to adopt a framework for clinical practice that would facilitate the ability to communicate and participate with the interdisciplinary mental health team. This point of view has been strengthened by the availability of the latest edition of the *Diagnostic and Statistical Manual of Mental Disorders* (American Psychiatric Association, 1980), commonly known as DSM-III.

DSM-III reflects a descriptive, phenomenological perspective of mental health problems and deliberately avoids theoretical (etiological) frameworks. While this is a controversial aspect of DSM-III, the atheoretical approach was in recognition of the lack of theoretical consensus in psychiatry today and of the inadequacy of all the etiological explanations available. Williams & Wilson (1982) have argued for the advantages of DSM-III in that it incorporates a more holistic array of variables and provides a framework for interdisciplinary communication. They acknowledge the current debate about whether psychiatric mental health nursing should strive for uniquely "nursing diagnoses," which would provide the basis for therapeutic nursing intervention. Their conclusion supports the use of DSM-III rather than that of a separate nursing framework. They urge nurses to use their expertise to define and develop Axis IV (Psychosocial Stressors) and Axis V (Adaptive Functioning) or to extend DSM-III to incorporate yet a sixth axis should the current five prove insufficient to encompass the nursing perspective.

Tarell (1982) urges psychiatric mental health nursing to develop a nursing diagnostic taxonomy that will correspond to what the rest of the mental health professions are using. Whether nurses work within or outside of DSM-III definitions, the atheoretical nature of DSM-III suggests that the search for etiological understanding of mental health problems will continue. The ways in which nurses can contribute to defining and explicating the phenomena of concern are numerous. Nurses may use DSM-III categories in their research, focus on certain axes as suggested by Williams & Wilson, or explore the relationship between DSM-III categories and nursing diagnoses as recommended by DSM-III and Nursing Diagnosis Nexus at the Portland, Oregon conference, "Stigmatized Groups: Needs and Interventions" (Snyder, 1981). For example, Axis V (Highest Level of Adaptive Functioning Past Year) is a potentially useful piece of information to have about a client. However, this axis is very underdeveloped. Clinicians are asked to consider the client's social relations, occupational functioning, and use of leisure time to derive a rating from 1 = Superior to 7 = Grossly Impaired. It might be interesting to consider if Orem's Self-Care Requisites concepts could be used to develop and refine this category of adaptive functioning and, in turn, further develop Orem's concepts (e.g., the self-care requisite of promotion of normalcy). Axis IV (Psychosocial Stressors) is also underdeveloped and like Axis V lacks diagnostic criteria.

Other authors have emphasized the need for psychiatric mental health nursing personnel to articulate their distinct approach (Fagin, 1967; Mellow, 1968; Ujhely, 1973). The point counterpoint debate by Kohnke and Lego (1980) regarding whether or not there is a difference between nurse psychotherapists and psychotherapists educated as psychologists or psychiatrists is an example. Kohnke argued there is no difference, while Lego argued that nurses are unique in their holistic approach, orientation to crisis situations, and knowledge of general health. Fitzpatrick et al. (1982) also argue for the uniqueness of psychiatric nursing. They argue that while the core mental health professions tend to use the same theories, there is a distinctiveness about psychiatric nursing. Therefore, these borrowed theories are applied in individual ways by individual nurses. Fitzpatrick et al. urge that nursing models be used to reformulate borrowed theories for the unique purposes of nursing.

The adoption of a theoretical perspective is not a neutral act. It is influenced by social and intellectual issues. Psychiatric mental health nurses were one of the first groups of nursing specialists to participate in the private practice mode of health care delivery and to enter the competitive arena for third-party reimbursement. Fagin (1981, p. 36) points out that psychiatric nursing success has been through substituting for other reimbursed providers. "In general, psychiatric nurses have not tried in rhetoric or behavior to have nursing services added to reimbursed services but have rather claimed reimbursement for performing generic roles in psychotherapy." The fact that DSM-III (American Psychiatric

Association, 1980) has become the dominant framework for diagnostic decisions in most mental health facilities and the basis on which third-party payors often make decisions about reimbursement means that many psychiatric mental health nurses are motivated and/or required to use that framework. At the same time, the paradigmatic crisis in psychiatry embodied in DSM-III may free nurses to entertain unique perspectives.

Is this simply a status search, or could the work to articulate the uniqueness of nursing have payoff for nursing practice? When considering the relation between theory and nursing practice, it is important to stop and consider the characteristics of practice theory and its relationship to the work of a profession.

Theory for Nursing

Dickoff, James, & Wiedenbach (1968) have proposed a scheme by which theory can be ordered on the basis of what it does. Level One, factor-isolating theory, isolates factors (phenomena/concepts) and describes and names them. Level Two, factor-relating theory, suggests connections or relationships between and among concepts, for example, the theory that abusive behavior on the part of a parent is related to having been abused as a child. Abusing is connected with having been abused. However, it does not explain the connection as Level Three would. Level Three, situation-relating theory, actually predicts causal or explanatory relationships that can then be confirmed or tested. Each succeeding level of theory makes use of the information from the preceeding level(s). According to Dickoff et al. (1968), the level of theory needed by a profession is situation-producing or prescriptive theory. The latter is Level Four theory, which uses the knowledge from all preceeding levels not merely to predict outcomes, but also to provide prescriptions for activities to bring about the goals defined within the theory. Another term used to refer to this fourth level of theory is practice theory.

Situation-producing theory has three components: (a) a goal, (b) a prescription, and (c) a survey list (Dickoff et al., 1968). The goal is the desired outcome: the aim toward which the professional acts. It is a valued state. The prescription is the activity that will achieve the goal—nursing intervention. The survey list calls attention to those other aspects of the situation that contribute to the complexity of action in the practice arena. The goal statement is an important distinguishing feature of this level of theory and makes it qualitatively different from the three previous levels.

Walker (1971) argues that use of the term *theory* to refer to practice directives that include a goal statement and procedure only causes confusion. Theory provides an understanding of phenomena by description, explanation, and/or prediction. It is a separate activity altogether to place a value on a certain outcome. Developing a strategy to achieve that outcome of course draws upon theoretical understanding of the phenomenon, but draws upon ethics and a cost-benefit analysis as well.

The professional, as compared to the academician, is action oriented. The sociologist will observe the interaction between a mother and her son, a diagnosed alcoholic, to understand the structure of the situation in which the deviance of excessive alcohol is used or threatened or to understand under what circumstances alcohol use is defined as deviant. The ability to describe and explain this event and eventually to predict under what circumstances such behavior will occur is the aim of the sociologist's observation. The result would be a theoretical understanding of this form of human behavior. The professional, however, upon observing the same interaction, makes a judgement about it. Very early in the educational career of a student of nursing, she or he is taught to use the nursing process to generate a problem list. "Problems" are not self-evident in raw data. Judgments must be made about the data using some criteria before a problem is defined. It is here that the profession's unique perspective or concerns will be revealed. Borrowed theory cannot provide this.

To say that nurses need to attend to the business of developing nursing theory does not mean that nurses must rediscover basic knowledge about people or that people within nursing's perspective are different than they have ever been described before. Fawcett (1984) identifies nursing theory as that which explains or links the metaparadigm concepts of person, environment, health, and nursing in specific terms and propositions. As such theories are developed, directives for nursing practice ought to be derivable and nursing will contribute to the public domain of knowledge about human phenomena.

Theory by its very nature is abstract. It provides guidance to the professional by providing an explanation of clinical phenomena. It is the professional, however, who must make the link between abstract theoretical formulations and the particular practice situation. Consider the following illustration.

The Labeling Theory of deviance (Scheff, 1966) holds that an essential aspect of social deviance is that select behavior is labeled as deviant by persons in the social environment. Furthermore, once an individual is labeled, there are consequences of the social role behaviors and self-concept of the person labeled as deviant that tend to fix the deviant behavior. Now this understanding of deviance can be most helpful to psychiatric nurses, but it cannot be expected to provide a problem definition or goal statement for any specific instance where deviance has been labeled. In one situation, the psychiatric mental health nurse will use his or her knowledge of Labeling Theory and child growth and development theory to decide that "the problem" is the parent's unrealistic expectations for a child of a given age. The nursing goal would be to alter the expectations and behavior of the labelers. In another situation, the nurse may use his or her knowledge of Labeling Theory and family system theory to decide that the identified patient is expressing and bearing a family problem. The nursing goal would be to have the family recognize "the problem" as the family's rather than the individual's and institute new behaviors to deal with it. Such a change in the interaction field would free the identified patient to meet basic needs in ways that meet with acceptance and approval. In this situation, both the labelers and the labeled patient need to alter their behavior. Finally, in yet another situation, where an elderly nursing home resident has been labeled as behaving strangely and suspiciously during the night, the psychiatric mental health nurse may decide that Labeling Theory is not useful at all. Instead, pharmacology and physiology may prove more useful for defining the problem. Directions for nursing action cannot come from Labeling Theory or any other theory. However, within an identified scope of practice, theories yield the understanding required to make professional decisions in practice.

Ultimately, many nurses would like a theory base sufficiently developed to suggest interventions that would reliably lead to desired outcomes. The CURN Project is an example of such work in nursing. Project personnel reviewed the nursing literature for scientifically sound and clinically useful research that could be transformed into a clinical protocol. The purpose of the clinical protocol is to transform the knowledge, methods, and technology inherent in the research studies into knowledge, methods, and technology useful to clinicians. As a result of this search, clinical protocols have been written for structured preoperative teaching, preventing decubitus ulcers, and mutual goal setting in patient care, among others (see, for example, Horsley, 1982). This is a modest but significant beginning.

O'Toole (1981) has suggested that the reason for the lack of research on practice in the psychiatric field in general may be related to the lack of technological sophistication of our interventions. In considering her observation, one must understand technology in its broad definition to mean not only things (machines, chemicals) but also processes and strategies that can be brought to bear on achieving an end. It may be that in the field of mental health, none of the core disciplines has a unique technology that works to their satisfaction because theories about the phenomena of mental health and mental illness are not sufficiently developed. For example, there is ample evidence in the literature to argue that uncertainty exists regarding the characteristics of the phenomena with which the field is concerned. One recent issue alone of *Schizophrenia Bulletin* contained two excellent examples of the huge knowledge gap in spite of which the mental health disciplines are attempting to work. Strauss, Bowers and Keith (1982) are editing a series of essays on schizophrenia in which they state, "Although no one may yet be able to provide the definitive answer, at least this collection of informed opinions may help clarify the major questions" (p. 433). Buckley (1982) discussed clinical research evidence for a subgroup of schizophrenic patients who should not be treated with neuroleptics. He also stated that to date there is no reliable way of identifying this subgroup and urged studies of patients' psychological experience during the acute and recovery phases from psychosis in an attempt to better describe and hopefully differentiate subtypes. Both of these articles represent calls for better Level One theory about a concept, schizophrenia, which has been around a long time.

This discussion has not answered the debate as to whether psychiatric mental health nursing ought to articulate its unique perspective on mental health problems or participate with the other core mental health disciplines in the search for theory. Probably the answer is that our specialty would benefit from both.

The Responsible Use of Theory

As eager as nurses are to generate a theory-based practice and to be granted the social mandate to exercise it, there is one word of caution. Medicine has been criticized for the degree of autonomy it has exercised in defining problems for patients. Medicine's single-minded focus has resulted in social control that has had negative consequences for some (Freidson, 1970; Zola, 1972). One has also been made aware of the fallacy of assuming a value-free technology (Habermas, 1970). No profession whose technology is sufficiently developed and who has won a social mandate to use it could rest assured that it would not have the same potential for abuse. It is essential that nursing maintain its commitment to validate problems of living with clients, to engage in mutual goal setting, and to insist that nurses clarify and examine the values on which their decisions and theories are based. Otherwise, nursing could have the same potential for abuse that has been evident in other professions using other technologies.

Psychiatric mental health nurses must systematically observe the phenomena encountered in their practice and the consequences of their interventions. Here the methodology of the case study as discussed by Weiss in Chapter 4 would be valuable.

The Significance of One's Theoretical Framework

A closer look at the debate between Kohnke and Lego (1980) as to differences among psychotherapists is interesting because of their points of agreement. Lego argued that nurse psychotherapists are different because of their holistic approach to people (see also Lego, 1973). Kohnke believed that most graduate programs in psychiatric nursing patterned themselves on the medical-psychological model and so the graduates were like psychotherapists from other disciplines. "It is only when nursing patterns and defines itself according to holistic principles that differences become evident, and the nurse-psychotherapist is qualitatively distinct from other types of psychotherapists" (Kohnke and Lego, 1980, p. 38). Both Kohnke and Lego agree that the theoretical framework learned as a graduate student is a key ingredient. Both also agree that a holistic approach to people is desirable and unique among psychotherapists. They disagree on the extent to which they believe nurse psychotherapists bring such a perspective to their practice.

Clement and Boylan (1982) provide a dramatic example of the difference made by the theoretical framework within which a situation is considered. They present two clinical situations: one is discussed from an Interpersonal Theory viewpoint and the other from the viewpoint of Minuchin's Family System. Many readers will be surprised to learn that the identified patient in both situations is the same, but the lens worn by each therapist in the form of her theoretical framework led each to focus on certain variables and to ignore others. This same impact of conceptual frameworks is evident in the book on family theories edited by Clements and Roberts (1983). In this book, authors of nursing models discuss clinical case studies from the perspective of their particular models. The emphasis on certain data and selective inattention to other data, which is encouraged by the use of a given model, is quite clearly demonstrated.

> [All of these examples vividly remind us that] . . . theory serves as the clinician's frame of reference to (1) provide structure and direction for assessement; (2) determine what of the behavior observed constitutes data; (3) guide the analysis of the data selected to formulate a working diagnosis; (4) direct hypothesis formation; (5) establish the rationale for intervention; and (6) dictate the criteria by which outcome of the selected interventions can be judged. (Clement & Boylan, 1982, pp. 126–127)

APPLICATION OF A NURSING MODEL

In view of the significant consequences of one's frame of reference, it is worth exploring the view made visable through the lens of a nursing model. A new look at an old scene often yields unanticipated discoveries. Toward this end, the remainder of this chapter will explore the advantages and disadvantages of using one of the contemporary nursing models as the framework for psychiatric mental health nursing practice. Orem's Self-Care Deficit Model was selected for this task because the focus on self-care activities and self-care deficits seemed compatible with the clinical goals of psychiatric mental health nursing. Also, while Orem's concept of self-care seemed intuitively meaningful for psychiatric nursing, extending its application beyond the care of the physically ill seemed an interesting challenge.

To assure a baseline of familiarity with Orem's nursing model, a summary of the major concepts and principles will be presented (Orem, 1980). Subsequent to this presentation, Orem's concepts will be used to consider a clinical situation in psychiatric mental health nursing practice. Should this discussion stimulate others to explore the applicability of Orem's model to their own practice, they are urged first to consult the source. Orem's model is far more complex and rich than a summary can portray.

Orem's Model of Nursing

The Self-Care Deficit Model of nursing is a complex theoretical system made up of three articulated theories: (1) the theory of self-care, (2) the theory of self-care deficit, and (3) the theory of nursing systems. The theory of self-care describes a necessary human endeavor which entails actions aimed at maintaining conditions essential for human functioning and development. This theory also includes dependent care which is the self-care actions provided by responsible adults for dependents. The theory of self-care deficit describes the conditions under which individuals are in need of nursing. The theory of nursing systems describes the nursing roles and relationships that emerge in response to the self-care agency (capacities) and self-care demands brought by the patient.

The concepts and ideas inherent in these three theories will be organized around the four core concepts central to nursing models: person, environment, health, and nursing (Fawcett, 1978).

Person

A person in Orem's theoretical system is a psychophysiological organism with rational powers who makes decisions affected by his or her learned values and goals. One aspect of a person's repetoire of behavior is self-care activities learned relative to the beliefs, habits, and practices of the culture of the group to which the person belongs. Adults normally deliberately initiate and perform these activities on their own behalf in maintaining life, health, and well-being. Adults also normally initiate and perform self-care activities for dependents under their care. A person's ability to engage in self-care or dependent-care activities is conditioned by age, developmental state, life experience, sociocultural orientation, health, and available resources.

Self-care activities are performed to maintain three kinds of self-care requisites: universal, developmental, and health-deviation. Universal self-care requisites arise from basic human needs. These include the maintenance of, or provision for (1) sufficient air; (2) sufficient water; (3) sufficient food; (4) elimination processes; (5) a balance of activity and rest; (6) a balance between solitude and social interaction; (7) prevention of hazards to human life, functioning, and well-being; and (8) normalcy. Developmental self-care requisites are associated with processes and conditions specific to human developmental stages aimed at (1) supporting and promoting development toward maturation and (2) preventing or mitigating the effects of conditions that may be deleterious to human development. Health-deviation self-care requisites arise from disease, injury, disfigurement, disability, and from medical interventions prescribed or performed to treat the former conditions.

Environment

Of the four central concepts, environment is the least developed in Orem's theoretical system. It has physical and symbolic dimensions, and person and environment form an integrated, interrelated system. It provides the context within which self-care is learned and performed. It affects and is affected by persons and nursing. It also affects health. Society and the family are subconcepts of environment.

Health

Health is, in part, a value judgement made by individuals about their well-being. It is a state of integrated human functioning. It is living as a whole human being and achieving some measure of the potential of human life. Illness is a state where integrated human functioning is disrupted.

Nursing

Nursing is a helping or assisting service to people unable to meet their own self-care needs. Legitimate patients of nursing are those with deficit relationships between their current or projected capability for providing self-care or dependent care and the qualitative and/or quantitative demand for care. There are at least five general methods for giving assistance: (1) acting for or doing for, (2) guiding, (3) supporting physically or psychologically, (4) providing an environment conducive to individual development, and (5) teaching.

Three nursing systems are identified that reflect the role relationships of nurse and patient necessitated by the patient's health state and self-care deficits. The characteristics of the nursing systems stem from the method of assistance emphasized. The three nursing systems include wholly compensatory, partly compensatory, and supportive-educative systems.

A wholly compensatory system is one where the patient has no active role and the nurse assists primarily by acting for and doing for the patient. In the partly compensatory system, the nurse and patient share in the performance of self-care activities. All five methods of assisting may be used. In the supportive-educative system, the patient's need for assistance is relative to decision making, behavior control, and/or acquiring knowledge and skills. The nurse provides assistance in the form of support, guidance, provision of a developmental environment, and/or teaching until the patient can provide self-care of a therapeutic quality on his or her own behalf.

Orem identifies nursing's unique concern and goal as follows: "Nursing has as its special concern the individual's need for self-care action and the provision and management of it on a continuous basis in order to sustain life and health, recover from disease or injury, and cope with their effects" (Orem, 1980, p. 6). Nursing problems within this conceptual model are self-care and/or dependent-care deficits. The source of the deficit may be limitations of action, knowledge, skills, or willingness.

A Clinical Case Study

The following is a vignette presenting a clinical situation to which Orem's theoretical system will later be applied.

Mrs. Roberts came alone to the outpatient clinic of a mental health center because she needed help to manage the behavior of her youngest son, Bill. Bill, 11 years old, had shot his BB gun in the living room last evening, putting holes in the walls and through pictures and damaging an overstuffed chair. During the interview with a psychiatric nurse specialist, Mrs. Roberts sat rigidly on the edge of her chair and frequently made the sign of the cross. When the nurse inquired about what prompted her to cross herself, she would look straight ahead and ignore the nurse, never responding to the inquiry. The following information was obtained regarding the current family situation and relevant history.

Mrs. Roberts is 34 years old, divorced two years and working full time on a factory assembly line, a job she has held for a little over one year. She has two sons, Tim, age 13, and Bill, age 11. Both sons live with her. She described Tim as a loner who does not have many friends but who is her "helper." Bill is a "problem child." He is active, independent, prefers to be with his friends rather than at home, and is hard for her to manage. The episode with the BB gun last evening was preceeded by an argument between Mrs. Roberts and Bill over his going out with friends. It was 4:00 P.M. and Mrs. Roberts wanted Bill to help around the house. While Bill has always been hard to manage in Mrs. Robert's opinion, he had never done anything as violent before.

When asked if Mrs. Roberts was normally home at 4:00 P.M., it was learned that she had not gone to work for three days because she had been "nervous." When the nurse inquired about support systems, it was learned that she had no contact with, or source of support from, her former husband. Her parents lived in the same town, but she did not view them as supportive. In fact, she stated that they spied on her.

Mrs. Roberts stated that she had been hospitalized twice with the diagnosis of paranoid schizophrenia. The first time was during her freshman year in college and the second time was following Bill's birth. She was currently taking no medication.

When asked if there was anything different in her life recently over which she might be concerned, she revealed that she was four months pregnant by a man who had ended their relationship and left town. She has not yet sought prenatal care.

Areas in which the nurse's interview yielded data indicating that self-care demands were not being adequately met are summarized in Table 2.1. The nurse noticed that there was much in the current situation that represented recent changes in behavior coinciding with Mrs. Roberts' loss of the significant relationship within which her pregnancy occurred. The nurse, therefore, used Family and Crisis Theory to provide explanations for some of the self-care deficits observed and to suggest intervention strategies. Based on her knowledge of Family System Theory, she hypothesized that there was a relationship between Mrs. Roberts' personal crisis and Bill's violent behavior. Also, based on Crisis Theory, the nurse hypothesized that Mrs. Roberts could be supported toward health if helped to cope successfully with this crisis. The nurse decided to go home with Mrs. Roberts to facilitate further data gathering and initiate interventions.

The home visit revealed the living room to be in a state of disarray as had been described by Mrs. Roberts. However, it also revealed that there were several day's dirty dishes in the sink, very little food in the cupboards, and the bathroom and bedrooms also in disarray. Mrs. Roberts had clearly been unable to do her normal activities of daily living while staying home from work. The nurse began doing the dishes and involving Mrs. Roberts in this chore. Using this shared activity to facilitate conversation, the nurse gained a greater understanding of Mrs. Roberts' concerns and view of the situation. She also helped Mrs. Roberts problem solve where she would obtain prenatal care and supported her while she called for an appointment. When Tim and Bill came home from school, the nurse conducted a family interview and then organized all family members in attending to the activities of daily living that had been neglected. An appointment was made with the family for the next family interview and a separate appointment was made to see Mrs. Roberts following her prenatal visit to reinforce the health teaching needed and to encourage her keeping the appointment.

This family eventually coped successfully with this crisis and dealt with family problems in therapy sessions, which eventually included Mrs. Roberts' parents, who were more involved in the family interaction than was first apparent.

Strengths and Limitations of Orem's Model

The major strengths of Orem's Self-Care Deficit Model for psychiatric mental health nursing that were found in the above attempt to apply it to a clinical situation were (1) the ability to also collect the data needed to make a DSM-III diagnosis, (2) the holistic model of person, and (3) an identified scope of practice that focuses on functioning.

Examination of Table 2.1 reveals that while the data are reorganized, all the data needed to make a diagnosis on the five Axes of DSM-III can be collected using Orem's framework. Responding to Williams and Wilson (1982), it would appear that nurses certainly could contribute to the development of Axes IV and V. While Table 2.1 referred to Axis V in conjunction with deficits found in the universal self-care requisites of normalcy, in fact a decision about Axis V is based on data regarding all the universal self-care requisites. Also, one must remember that Axis V refers to Adaptive Functioning During the Past Year. A sixth Axis may be important for nursing that would reflect the *current* level of

Table 2.1 Nursing Care Plan Following Home Visit

	Self-Care Deficits	*Self-Care Agency*	*Planning and Implementation*	*Theoretical Rationale*
Mrs. Roberts	I. Universal Requisites			
	A. More data needed regarding knowledge about and adequacy of *food intake* for pregnancy	Feeds self; shops for self and family	Will address in subsequent follow-up visits	Theory of Anxiety: Severe anxiety disrupts cognitive functioning
	B. Change in *activity/rest:* unable to work because of "worry"; unable to do household activities	Ordinarily cares for house; held job over 1 year	Use supportive role while doing dishes with Mrs. Roberts; facilitate family's doing household tasks by organizing their efforts	Crisis Theory: Provide support to help the family mobilize to deal with concrete problems; Orem: Self-care is a human capacity
	C. Recent termination of a significant relationship which lasted one year. No adult social support, *solitude, and social interaction*	Formed significant relationship which lasted one year. Sought help.	Explore meaning of event; nurse initial source of social support; develop self-care in this area in subsequent individual work	Crisis Theory: Termination of the significant relationship appears to be precipitating event; DSM-III, Axis IV: 5 (severe)
	D. Behavior in interview would not be defined *normal* in her social group		Support and interventions aimed at reducing anxiety and organizing behavior	Theory of Anxiety: Behavior manifestation of severe anxiety; DSM-III, Axis V: 3 (good)
	II. Developmental Requisites			
	A. Has not sought prenatal care	Has had 2 children	Support to make appointment for prenatal care and see individual patient immediately after	Physiology of Pregnancy, DSM-III, Axis III: pregnancy; social support to encourage compliance
	B. Self-care unsuccessful in mitigating effect of recent loss and pregnancy upon maturation	Sought help	Addressed through interventions above	Crisis Theory: Success in coping with events will be growth promoting
	III. Health-Deviation Requisites			
	A. Change in behavior and stereotyped behavior suggest psychiatric deterioration	Long period between episodes; sought help at Mental Health Center	Interventions above deal with the manifestations of health deviation	DSM-III, Axis I: Paranoid Schizophrenic; chronic with acute exacerbation
	IV. *Dependent-care deficits*			

Table 2.1 ***(continued)***

	Self-Care Deficts	*Self-Care Agency*	*Planning and Implementation*	*Theoretical Rationale*
Tim, 13	I. Universal Requisites			
	A. Few friends; mother's helper, *solitude and social interaction*	Attends school regularly	Family therapy to change relationship	Family Theory: Attempting to play age and generationally inappropriate role to try to meet mother's needs
	II. Developmental Requisites			
	A. Above suggests inadequate psychosocial development toward maturation for age		Collect data from school about peer relations and course work; consider adolescent group and/or big brother	Growth and Development Theory
	B. Mitigate effect of divorce, mother's new relationship, and pregnancy on psychosocial development		Explore meanings of events in family therapy	Family Theory: Behavior and roles of one individual in family will affect all members
Bill, 11	I. Universal Requisites			
	A. Conflict relationship with mother; *solitude and social interaction*	Attends school regularly; has peer relations	Family therapy to change relationship	Family Theory
	B. Episode with BB gun; *prevent Hazards*	Damaged only inanimate objects	Immediate: Help mother set limits; family therapy	Family Theory: Child will often express in behavior that there is a family problem
	II. Developmental Requisites			
	A. Above suggests inadequate psychosocial development toward maturation for age		Collect data from school about peer relations and course work; consider group or individual work and/or big brother	Growth and Development Theory
	B. Mitigate effect of divorce, etc.		Explore meanings of events in family therapy	Family Theory

adaptive functioning. It is with current behavior that the nurse works, and behavior is seldom specifically inferrable by the medical diagnosis. A taxonomy of nursing diagnoses could articulate with Axes IV and V (and VI?) and also contribute to the refinement of Orem's framework. For example, Table 2.1 reveals that a variety of situations can evidence a self-care deficit in Solitude and Social Interaction. Mrs. Roberts was experiencing an absence of adult social supporters. For his age, Tim was inappropriately related to his mother. Bill evidenced a conflictual relationship with his mother. Nursing diagnoses could be developed to express the types and degrees of deficits specific to each self-care requisite.

Physical and psychosocial aspects of the individual are brought into focus by the three categories of self-care requirements identified (universal, developmental, and health-deviation). The inclusion of symbolic functioning in the definition of person allows for individuality in the perception of events and the attribution of meaning, which is very important for psychiatric mental health nursing. Thus, while self-care activity is conceived to include decision making and deliberate action, it is not a simplistic rational model. There is room for decision making based on private meanings for events resulting from lessons learned in social interaction. Because of the concept of holism and the importance of the social context, Fitzpatrick et al. (1982) find Orem's model congruent with many points of Peplau, Sullivan, and Erikson.

Psychiatric nursing has long been primarily concerned with the consequences of mental illness for the personal and social functioning of the individual rather than with the mental illness itself. Orem's focus on self-care activities and self-care deficits is compatible with the focus of psychiatric mental health nursing. As stated above, the use of Orem's model by psychiatric mental health nurses could potentially lead to greater refinement, especially of the universal self-care requisites of maintenance of a balance between solitude and social interaction; prevention of hazards to life, functioning, and well-being; promotion of normalcy; and the developmental self-care requisites.

The limitations of Orem's model for psychiatric mental health nursing that are illustrated in this attempt to apply it were (1) its failure to suggest specific explanations for the deficits found that would, in turn, suggest interventions and (2) the individual focus of the model.

The former limitation is likely to be particularly frustrating to many psychiatric mental health nurses. However, it is a limitation inherent in conceptual models. Fawcett (1984) draws a distinction between a conceptual model and a theory based on the level of abstraction of each. Because a conceptual model is more abstract than a theory, there are differences in the way each can be used.

> Thus, a conceptual model guides all aspects of clinical practice. The model tells the clinician what to look at when interacting with clients and how to interpret observations. It also tells the clinician how to plan interventions in a general manner and provides beginning criteria for evaluation of intervention outcomes.
>
> The specifics of nursing assessment, diagnosis, intervention, and evaluation, however, must come from theories. Although the conceptual model may, for example, direct the clinician to look for certain categories of problems in adaptation, theories of adaptation are needed to describe, to explain, and to predict client manifestations of actual or potential problems in particular situations. Similarly, theories are needed to direct the particular nursing interventions needed in such situations. (Fawcett, 1984, p. 27)

Orem provides an identified scope of practice and a framework that accommodates a rich array of variables. The nurse must bring other theories to bear to account for a relationship among specific variables and specific theories must be developed to provide a better understanding of the concepts and relationships in the model. Examples of how borrowed theory articulates with the nursing model are as follows. In the above vignette, the nurse used her knowledge of Family System Theory to establish a relationship between Bill's self-care deficit in the area of preventing hazards and Mrs. Roberts' self-care deficit in the face of events in a significant interpersonal relationship that threatened her psychosocial integrity and development. Also, the nurse used her knowledge of crisis theory to account for Mrs. Roberts' self-care deficits in the face of these events. It also suggested the strategy of lending support to deal with concrete, here and now problems. The Crisis perspective, plus Mrs. Roberts' response to crisis intervention, prevented an automatic intervention of hospitalization for "a recurring psychotic episode in paranoid schizophrenia." Finally, the nurse used her knowledge of psychosocial growth and development to alert her to concern for the "good" eldest son. The holistic framework of Orem, however, helps prevent the nurse from losing sight of the broader picture while zeroing in on specific intervention points.

A second limitation of Orem's theoretical system, which is evident in Table 2.1, is that the unit of analysis is clearly the individual. One can assess all individuals in the family, but one cannot use Orem's framework to assess the family as a unit. As in this vignette, the nurse can identify self-care deficits in individual family members that the nurse may hypothesize are interrelated. However, then the nurse would need to use another framework to assess the family as a functioning unit.

In the preface of the second edition of Orem's book, she states, "The mastery of the concepts should enable nursing students and nurses to place in perspective other descriptions of nursing, including those in areas of nursing specialization" (Orem, 1980, p. viii). A reciprocal effect of such use would be the verification, refinement, or modification of the nursing model as diverse nursing realities are taken into account. Only in this way can the nursing models move beyond ideological statements to nursing theory.

NURSING'S COMMITMENT TO HOLISM

The decision to limit the exploration of the applicability of just one nursing model admittedly leaves much work still to be done. Psychiatric mental health nurse specialists need to explore the utility of all the available models. Fitzpatrick et al. (1982) have begun this work.

One observation repeatedly made by those analyzing nursing models is that models tend to contain a holistic view of man which is usually cited as a strength. Psychiatric mental health nursing has tried to maintain a multidimensional, holistic view of people. This has been difficult, however, when the theories used to guide practice emphasized either the psychological or social dimensions of humans and usually failed to explain the biological, psychological, and social interrelationships. Recognizing and caring for the psychological and physical conditions of individuals as facilitated by DSM-III or Orem's model is certainly a start toward holism. However, the concept of holism could have a more revolutionary implication for psychiatric mental health nursing than that. If this specialty is to remain true to the conceptualization of holism, it must abandon the almost exclusive reliance upon psychosocial theories. As a discipline, psychiatric mental health nursing has largely failed to maintain currency with the research exploring endocrinological, biochemical, and/or neurophysiological corralates of behavior. A commitment to holism demands that this level of human functioning not be ignored or the holistic synthesis toward which nursing is striving will be impossible to achieve. Roy's Adaptation Model of Nursing may hold the promise of such a synthesis.

Roy (1983) views the person "as an adaptive system with regulator and cognator control processes acting to cope with internal and external changing stimuli to produce adaptive and ineffective responses that are manifested in behavior related to physiological function, self-concept, role-function, and interdependence" (p. 266). The regulator and cognator referred to above are subsystems of the person that serve adaptive mechanisms. The regulator receives input from the internal and external environments of the person and processes it through neural-chemical channels.

> Chemical stimuli travel through the circulatory system and may be transduced into neural inputs. The spinal cord, brainstem, and autonomic reflexes act through effectors to produce an automatic, unconcious effect on the body responses. Chemical stimuli at the same time influence the endocrine glands to produce appropriate hormones. Target organs or tissues respond to the hormones also to effect body responses. Physiologists believe that by some unknown process, the neural inputs become conscious perceptions in the brain. (Roy, 1983, p. 264)

The cognator is also a subsystem of the person and receives the same inputs as the regulator. However, the inputs received by the cognator are processed through cognitive-emotive pathways. Four basic cognitive-emotive pathways have been conceptualized: perceptual/information processing, learning, judgement, and emotion (Roy & Roberts, 1981).

As all subsystems of a system, the regulator and cognator are interrelated. They appear to be linked together in the process of perception. "Inputs to the regulator are transformed into perceptions, yet perception is a process of the cognator. Responses of both the regulator and cognator following perception are fed back into both subsystems" (Roy, 1983, p. 265).

Use and refinement of such a model could realize nursing's focus on the person as a whole and reunite the mind and body in psychiatric mental health nursing practice. Researching such social, psychological, and physiological interrelationships for the knowledge base of psychiatric mental health nursing practice is one of the many exciting frontiers waiting for the attention of the clinical specialist.

SUMMARY

Psychiatric mental health nursing's debate over the need for a unique nursing perspective was discussed in this chapter. The characteristics and contributions of models and theories and their relation to clinical practice have also been explored. Finally, the potential strengths and weaknesses for psychiatric mental health nursing practice of operating within the framework of Orem's model were assessed. This self-conscious search for the most appropriate framework for practice is not a frivolous endeavor. Theory does more than provide explanations to guide practice. Theory (as language) also facilitates communication and serves a boundary maintenance function. By means of theoretical perspectives, one defines one's world and identifies the insiders and outsiders.

REFERENCES

American Psychiatric Association. *Diagnostic and statistical manual of mental disorders* (3rd ed.). Washington, DC: American Psychiatric Association, 1980.

Buckley, P. Identifying schizophrenic patients who should not receive medication. *Schizophrenia Bulletin,* 1982, *8,* 429–432.

Buckwalter, K. C., & Kerfoot, K. M. Teaching patients self care: A critical aspect of psychiatric discharge planning. *Journal of Psychosocial Nursing and Mental Health Services,* 1982, *20,* 15–20.

Burd, S. F., & Marshall, M. A. (Eds.). *Some clinical approaches to psychiatric nursing.* New York: MacMillan Co., 1963.

Clement, J. A., & Boylan, S. R. Actualizing theory in practice. *Perspectives in Psychiatric Care,* 1982, *20,* 126–133.

Clements, I., & Roberts, F. *Family health: A theoretical approach to nursing care.* New York: John Wiley & Sons, 1983.

Dickoff, J., James, P., & Wiedenbach, E. Theory in a practice discipline: Part I, practice oriented theory. *Nursing Research,* 1968, *17,* 415–435.

Fagin, C. M. Psychotherapeutic nursing. *American Journal of Nursing,* 1967, *67,* 298–304.

Fagin, C. M. Concepts for the future: Competition and substitution. *Journal of Psychosocial Nursing and Mental Health Services,* 1981, *21,* 36–40.

Fawcett, J. The "what" of theory development. In *Theory development: What, why, how.* New York: National League for Nursing. 1978.

Fawcett, J. *Analysis and evaluation of conceptual models of nursing.* Philadelphia: F. A. Davis Co., 1984.

Fitzpatrick, J., Whall, A., Johnston, R., & Floyd, J. *Nursing models and their psychiatric mental health applications.* Bowie, MD: Robert J. Brady Co., 1982.

Freidson, E. *Profession of medicine.* New York: Dodd, Mead & Co., 1970.

Gregg, D. Reassurance. *American Journal of Nursing,* 1955, *55,* 171–174.

Habermas, J. *Toward a rational society.* Boston: Beacon Press, 1970.

Horsley, J. A. *Mutual goal setting in patient care: CURN project.* New York: Grune & Stratton, 1982.

Kohnke, M., & Lego, S. Point/counterpoint: A psychotherapist is a psychotherapist. *Perspectives in Psychiatric Care,* 1980, *28,* 26–27, 38–39.

Lego, S. Nurse psychotherapists: How are we different? *Perspectives in Psychiatric Care,* 1973, *11,* 144–147.

Mellow, J. Nursing therapy. *American Journal of Nursing,* 1968, *68,* 2365–2369.

Orem, D. E. *Nursing: Concepts of practice* (2nd ed.). New York: McGraw-Hill Book Co., 1980.

O'Toole, A. W. When the practical becomes theoretical. *Journal of Psychosocial Nursing and Mental Health Services,* 1981, *19,* 11–19.

Peplau, H. E. *Interpersonal relations in nursing.* New York: G. P. Putnam, 1952.

Peplau, H. E. Loneliness. *American Journal of Nursing,* 1955, *55,* 1476–1481.

Roy, S. C. Roy adaptation theory of nursing. In I. Clements & F. Roberts (Eds.), *Family health: A theoretical approach to nursing care.* New York: John Wiley & Sons, 1983.

Roy, S. C., & Roberts, S. *Theory construction in nursing: An adaptation model.* Englewood Cliffs, NJ: Prentice-Hall, 1981.

Scheff, T. J. *Being mentally ill: A sociological theory.* Chicago: Aldine Publishing Co., 1966.

Schmidt, C. S. Withdrawal behavior of schizophrenics: Application of Roy's model. *Journal of Psychosocial Nursing and Mental Health Services,* 1981, *19,* 26–33.

Smoyak, S. (Ed.). *The psychiatric nurse as a family therapist.* New York: John Wiley & Sons, 1975.

Snyder, M. DSM-III and nursing diagnosis nexus. *Pacesetter,* 1981, *6,* 4.

Strauss, J. S., Bowers, M. B., Jr., & Keith, S. (Eds.). What is schizphrenia? *Schizophrenia Bulletin,* 1982, *8,* 433–437.

Tarell, J. D. *Use of the DSM-III in the formulation of a nursing diagnostic system based on self-care deficits.* Paper presented at the Psychiatric/Mental Health Nursing Conference, Los Angeles, Ca. November, 1982.

Tudor, G. E. Sociophychiatric nursing approach to intervention in a problem of mutual withdrawal on a mental hospital ward. *Psychiatry,* 1952, *15,* 193–217.

Ujhely, G. B. The nurse as psychotherapist: What are the issues. *Perspectives in Psychiatric Care,* 1973, *11,* 155–160.

Underwood, P. Facilitating self-care. In P. Pothier (Ed.), *Psychiatric nursing: A basic text.* Boston: Little, Brown & Co., 1980.

Walker, L. O. Toward a clearer understanding of the concept of nursing theory. *Nursing Research,* 1971, *20,* 428–435.

Whall, A. L. Congruence between existing theories of family functioning and nursing theories. *Advances in Nursing Science,* 1980, *3,* 59–67.

Whall, A. L. Nursing theory and the assessment of families. *Journal of Psychosocial Nursing and Mental Health Services,* 1981, *19,* 30–36.

Williams, J. B. W., & Wilson, H. S. A psychiatric nursing perspective on DSM-III. *Journal of Psychosocial Nursing and Mental Health Services,* 1982, *20,* 14–20.

Zola, I. K. Medicine as an institution of social control. *Sociological Review,* 1972, 487–504.

CHAPTER 3 NEUROPHYSIOLOGICAL THEORIES

Margaret E. Armstrong

This chapter will provide a summary of developments in the knowledge of neuroanatomy and physiology that will help to clarify the biological dynamics that underly behavior. As this body of knowledge continues to develop, health professionals attempting to help people afflicted with mental illness will increasingly be able to refine their therapeutic approaches to obtain more specific goals. This process will become more feasible as one gains a clearer grasp of the details of the normal functioning brain, the specific pathophysiology involved in a given mental or behavioral dysfunction, and, as a result, the correction that must be made to regain maximum function.

Not long ago, such a chapter could not have been written. Those attempting to understand the dynamics of mental illness were forced to treat the brain as a "black box." It was an entity viewed as such a mystery that efforts to include consideration of its function in conceptual frameworks used for therapeutic approaches were precluded. Therefore, it was common practice to consider the inputs into the brain and to assess the resultant outputs or behavior, bypassing what went on in the brain itself, and then to decide what therapeutic approach would be appropriate. It is quite remarkable that this method resulted in as much positive results as it did. The success of this approach probably resulted in part because the brain uses those observable inputs in large part to make decisions as to what behaviors to enact.

There is no rational excuse to continue using this black box approach to mental health clinical practice. During the past two decades, there has been a phenomenal increase in research of the brain. The result of this research has been knowledge that helps health professionals understand what in the past was often both too complex and diffuse to use in clinical approaches with patients. Although there is much yet to learn, this developing knowledge can be used to better understand the specifics of normal human functioning, individual differences, pathological details of common mental illnesses, and the bases for our approaches to therapy.

Currently, there are over 100,000 articles published in the neuroscience literature yearly. It is impossible in a single chapter to provide a complete discussion of all research findings that have relevance for psychiatric mental health nursing practice. Therefore, an attempt has been made to summarize a few examples of relatively new information that have particular application possibilities for nursing practice.

An overview of the brain's functioning will be given as a basis for understanding general types of normal behavior. The following section will cover more specific topics related to the structure and functioning of the central nervous system. Finally, examples of the circular interplay between physiology and behavior will be given. The chapter concludes with speculations about what the future may hold for the use of neurobiology in psychiatric mental health nursing.

OVERVIEW OF BRAIN ORGANIZATION AND FUNCTION AND THE TRIUNE BRAIN

The brain provides the vital functions of receiving, processing, evaluating, and storing information. Based on the information derived from these processes, the brain then determines the behavioral response. This process includes consideration of relevant past experiences, meanings, symbolisms, current related emotions and thoughts, as well as a myriad of other factors. Only a fraction of the variables that the brain evaluates before intiating a behavior response are visible to an external observer. It is therefore possible to understand why a person's behavior may not be totally explainable (rational) to the most careful observer.

The full details of the process involved are certainly not yet understood. However, we do have a clearer picture than we once had. Information inputs from a variety of internal and external sources constantly bombard the brain. These messages are basically coded according to an electrical frequency. The more important the message, the higher the frequency of action potentials or firing rate of the neuronal pathway carrying the message. The electrical code is interrupted by a temporary chemical coding whenever one neuron has to relay the message to another neuron in the sensory pathway. The message is carried across the space or synapse between the connecting neurons, coded as to importance by the amount of neurotransmitter released from the presynaptic membrane of the first neuron.

Since the brain is receiving incoming messages from many different locations simultaneously, it is basically a frequency analyzer. That is, the brain receives a large number of stimuli at varying frequency rates. It then makes a complex and, hopefully, accurate analysis to decide what behavioral response is appropriate. The response usually serves to facilitate survival and to increase learning, enjoyment, and other behavior luxuries. The analogy of the hologram, a method of using several frequencies of light to produce a three-dimensional image of an object, can be used to explain some functions of the brain (Greguss, 1975). Viewing the brain in this way can be of help when trying to understand its overall purpose, as well as specific functions such as memory and automatic movements.

The holographic analogy has been added to other concepts such as those related to the telegraph, telephone, and computer, which were previously used to attempt to explain brain functions. Recalling a past experience from stored memories is one example. According to the analogy, the stored information or memory is likened to the holographic image. Once the holographic image is produced from the combination of two or more light frequencies, the image may be stored on photographic film. The image may be visualized by focusing one of the light frequencies used in its production (called the reference light). Shining the reference light onto the film results in the appearance of the holographic image in three-dimensional form. According to the analogy in the case of memory, an aspect of a current experience that has some similarity to a past situation may act as a stimulus to the brain (like the reference light in the hologram). Thus, a powerful, lifelike image of the total past experience is produced (Goleman, 1979). In this way, past experiences have the potential of significantly influencing present behavior. It is often this influence that results in different behavior by individuals having the same experience.

Automatic, learned behaviors may function in much the same way. For example, one learns the numerous, sequential steps necessary to starting a car. At first, the driver has to think consciously about each step. After some practice, the sequence of movements is accomplished rather automatically without conscious processing of each step. According to the holographic analogy, the first step of inserting the key into the ignition may serve as the reference light for the memory of the total sequence. Thus, the next steps are recalled automatically as a part of the memory (image) of the total task, making it unnecessary to recall each step. With further developments in technology, other analogies are likely to be used to enhance the understanding of brain function (Wilber, 1982).

The overall perspective of the structure and functions of the brain, developed over many years of research by Dr. Paul MacLean, helps to explain the dynamics of commonly observed behaviors (MacLean, 1975). This research provides a very useful perspective for mental health practitioners. The human brain is actually divided into three distinct compartments or brains each with its own functional responsibilities, hence the name triune brain (see Fig. 3.1).

The most basic brain functions are located in the reptilian brain, so named because reptiles have only this brain. It is also referred to as the "survival" brain since it contains all the structures necessary for survival of the organism including the brain stem structures and the basal ganglia. With this brain, the individual is able to regulate essential physiological functions such as respirations, blood pressure, and heart rate. Movement regulated by the basal ganglia is needed for seeking food, shelter, and sexual mates. Establishment and defense of territory, grooming, courtship, and mating are all survival functions that may be enacted by this brain. The formation of social groups and creation of a social hierarchy are also included within these functions. This brain may also be called the sensory brain since it provides the entrance pathways for sensory information coming into the brain. Although some preliminary processing of the incoming information may have taken place in the spinal cord and brain stem structures, the individual is not yet consciously aware of the information. The reptile brain serves to influence physiological functions and relay incoming physiological information. Both processes are normally accomplished without the conscious awareness of the individual.

The paleomammalian or emotional brain contains the midbrain limbic structures in addition to the frontal cerebral cortex. The so-called old mammals (e.g., the lemur) have this brain in addition to the first and therefore are capable of processing emotions or feelings about their experiences.

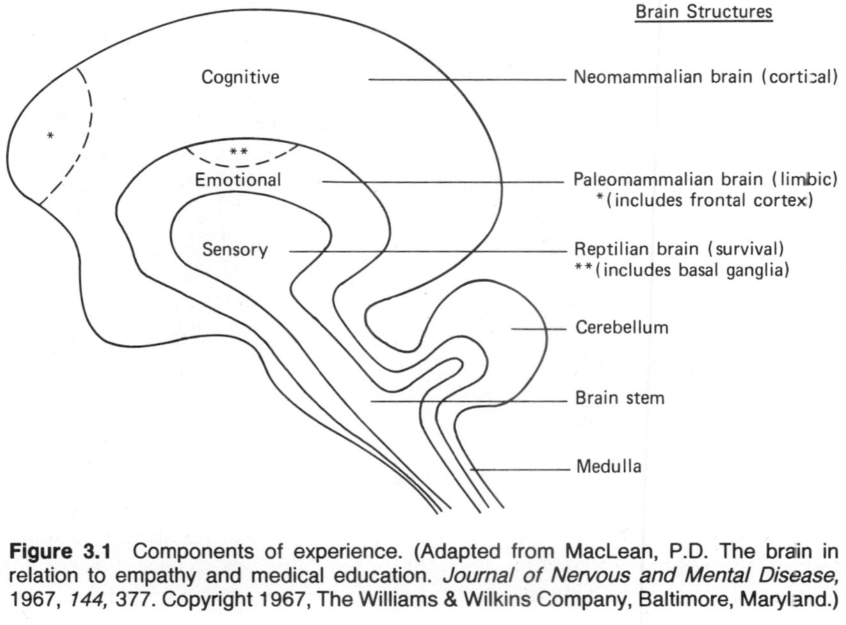

Figure 3.1 Components of experience. (Adapted from MacLean, P.D. The brain in relation to empathy and medical education. *Journal of Nervous and Mental Disease,* 1967, *144,* 377. Copyright 1967, The Williams & Wilkins Company, Baltimore, Maryland.)

The neomammalian or cognitive brain includes the cerebral and cerebellar cortex. The new mammals, including humans, have this brain as well and thus are able to have thoughts about their experiences. It is believed that the higher cortical centers may serve as a "data bank" for unconscious information while the limbic brain deals with conscious thought and reflection (Ferguson, 1983). Further research should help to clarify the anatomy and physiology of thought processes.

The three brains work in concert according to a set of functional principles that provide the three basic components of any life experience: the sensory, emotional, and cognitive aspects. These principles help to explain behavior that may otherwise be puzzling to the observer. For instance, why does the same experience invoke a variety of behaviors among a group of individuals or within the same person from one time to another? Why do we often "fall apart" emotionally after an emergency? Why is the unknown more anxiety-provoking than knowing the worst? When one's survival is threatened, why can one seemingly be overconcerned about simple physical sensation? The answers to these and other behaviors can be explained, at least partially, with the triune brain perspective.

First, all three brains receive information from the internal and external environment. Pathways exist between the three brains for comparison of their reactions to this information. It is as if a message is brought to a room of people who all hear the message and then compare notes as to their sensations, feelings, and thoughts concerning the message. Then, all three brains have the opportunity to contribute to the response to the incoming information. This response takes the form of internal and external behavior on the part of the individual.

There is a hierarchy of control among the three brains. If left on its own, the reptilian brain will function to maintain survival functions. However, the emotional brain can override the functioning of the reptile brain. This can be easily observed when someone is angry or excited; emotional expressions and limbic brain influence takes precedence over functions normally controlled by the reptilian brain. Pathways from the frontal cerebral cortex and/or other structures of the limbic brain have connecting pathways with the autonomic nervous system that affect the functioning of most internal organs such as heart rate, respiratory rate, and blood pressure. In addition, the cognitive brain can attempt to dominate behavior over the emotional and sensory brains. This hierachy can be altered in some instances, most commonly when structures in one of the brains is already active for some reason. When this occurs, the brain already active has the opportunity to dominate behavior.

Although we do not usually see behavior that is wholly enacted by one brain, it is not rare to observe dominance by intellectual, emotional, or survival behaviors any of which may or may not be appropriate at the time. MacLean's favorite example of reptilian behavior is that which is often seen in committee meetings (Holden, 1979). When facts are not provided to give the cognitive brain something to deal with and the committee members do not have emotional feelings about the task at hand, the "reptiles" within us are allowed to dominate, with behavioral displays exhibited for the purpose of establishing social hierarchy. (Behaviors for the establishment of a social hierarchy are a function of the reptilian brain.) This example demonstrates that another way to upset the hierarchy of control is to give the two higher brains nothing to deal with, thus leaving the reptilian brain to dominate.

The functional princinles of the triune brain plus the impact of past learning and cultural background, readily explain the variance observed in reponse to the same input among different people. Depending on the unique aspects of the current situation, the individual may respond to the same experience differently from one time to another. For example, if one is already upset, a seemingly insignificant event, such as breaking a glass, may result in emotionally dominated behavior when, ordinarily, one would not have responded in that way.

Another example is that of an emergency. One may function quite well until the emergency situation is over. One then attempts to relax and the cognitive brain no longer dominates behavior since its work has been completed. Now, the emotional brain has the opportunity to respond, and it will automatically do so according to the hierachy of the three brains. One may experience behaviors such as anxious giggling, trembling, or crying. Such reactions are common to everyone, and it is best to allow this expression to occur rather than inhibit the behavior. With the buildup of emotions waiting to be expressed, the emotional brain is forced to express itself internally or in an inappropriate or excessive manner later. People tend to strive for a sophisticated, intellectual, or "correct" approach to behavior, thereby overriding expression by the other two brains. However, the three brains will influence one's behavior one way or the other at some point in time, with physiological or behavioral pathology as a possible result.

When someone is dealing with the unknown as in not knowing the cause of an illness, the cognitive brain is left with no facts with which to operate, thereby allowing the emotional brain to dominate behavior. Naturally, a person would be quite anxious in this situation. Even realizing the worst possible cause gives the cognitive brain some information to process. The cognitive brain can then contribute to the person's behavior and can decrease the amount of influence by the emotional brain and, therefore, the extent of anxiety able to be expressed. Thus, cognitive functions may serve to assist in moderating emotions.

When a person's survival is threatened, for example with the awareness that he or she has a terminal disease, health professionals are sometimes surprised that the patient appears overly concerned with physical comfort factors, such as the temperature of the room, rather than expressing emotions about their prognosis. This temporary preoccupation occurs because the threat to survival alerts the reptilian brain structures that also function to relay incoming physical sensations. The increased alertness increases the individual's sensitivity to physical sensations, resulting in behavior that is difficult to understand given the circumstances.

Awareness of the general organization and functional principles of the triune brain gives the mental health professional a framework to better understand the physiological nature of behavior. Using this information, one can then choose therapeutic approaches to elicit desired behavioral changes. The triune perspective of the brain has similarities to other explanations of how behavior is organized, as in Freud's framework of the id, superego, and ego. Components of both perspectives bear a rough resemblance to each other, with the triune brain adding anatomical and physiological details. Maslow's principle of the hierachy of needs identifies physiological needs as the most basic and resembles the role of the sensory or reptilian brain. While Freud, Maslow, and MacLean are explaining different processes and functions, they share an assumption of a hierarchy of function with primitive, physiological survival needs being primary. As more is learned about the internal organization of the brain, explanations of behavior will continually be refined. Freud himself predicted that behavioral explanations would eventually be modified by the developing knowledge of neurobiology (Trotter, 1981).

ORGANIZATION OF BRAIN STRUCTURES RELEVANT TO BEHAVIOR

Emotions

The limbic brain appears to contain structures designed to process and respond to information from an emotional or feeling perspective. There is a difference in opinion about the structures responsible for these functions, but they generally include the midbrain structures: hypothalamus, thalamus, amygdala, hippocampus, septum, cingulate gyrus, and the frontal portion of the cerebral cortex. Figure 3.2 outlines the major inputs and outputs of the limbic brain. The hypothalamus provides the interface between the limbic structures and the autonomic nervous, endocrine, and immunological systems (Cox, 1978). As a result, a person's emotional state often affects physiological functioning via pathways to these systems. For example, when one is angry or anxious, physiological functions such as heart and respiratory rates are commonly affected. The specific functions of the frontal lobe are still being defined. Activities such as self-awareness, initiative, and planning are thought possibly to take place in this area (Pines, 1983).

As more details are clarified as to the pathways and mechanisms involved, there will be a much clearer picture of the complexity of the functioning of the limbic structures. Recently, a pathway was identified that indicates the route through which extreme emotions processed in the frontal cortex affect heart rate (Skinner, 1978). Continued stimulation of this pathway initially increases the heart rate. If stimulation continues, arrythmias occur, then fibrillation and cardiac arrest if stimulation is sufficiently severe or prolonged. Microscopic damage to heart tissue may result. Sudden cardiac arrest and other cardiovascular pathologies may in some instances have their origin in persistent or extremely stressful emotional experiences.

Cognition

Until the past decade, the processes underlying thinking or cognition were shrouded in ambiguity. There is evidence that the ancient Eygptians had a suprisingly accurate under-

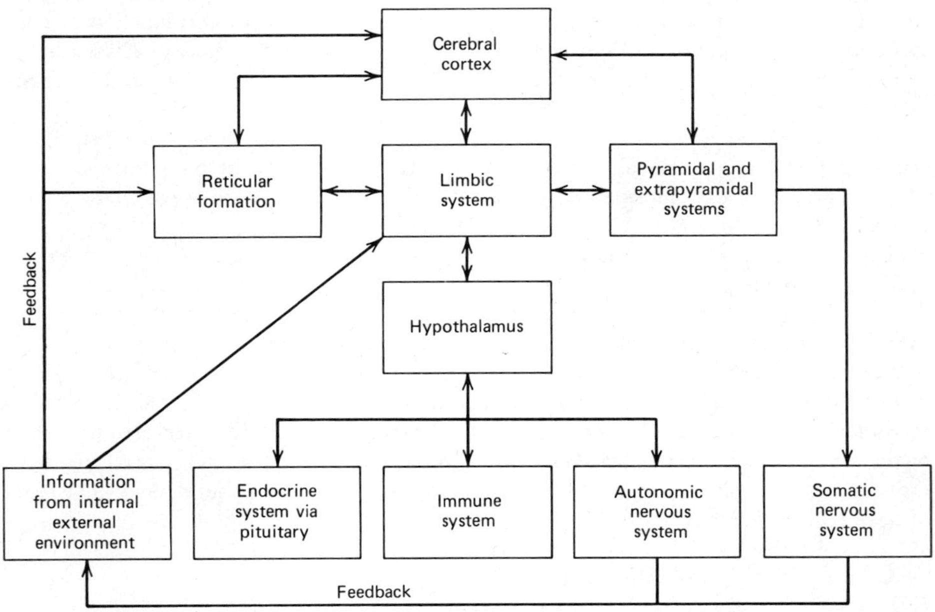

Figure 3.2 The major input and output pathways of the limbic system indicate that the hypothalamus uses information related to emotions for controlling influence of the endocrine, immune, and autonomic nervous system. (Adapted from Cox, T. *Stress.* London, Basingstoke: Macmillan Accounts and Administration, Ltd., 1978, p. 51.)

standing of some of the more important cognitive functions, such as speech. However, only recently has the way in which the two cerebral hemispheres process information been even generally understood. For a long time, the left hemisphere was designated as the dominant hemisphere, since in most individuals that side of the brain was responsible for verbal behavior. In the early 1970s, Robert Ornstein demonstrated that one hemisphere was not necessarily dominant over the other. Instead, Ornstein identified that the right and left hemispheres generally process and use incoming information differently. Each provides a unique but helpful perspective to a person's total awareness (Ornstein, 1972).

Knowledge concerning the differentiated hemispheric functioning (also called hemispheric lateralization) continues to increase. The left cerebral hemisphere generally organizes inputs in parts or units. This is helpful in activities such as mathematics, logical reasoning, and analytical thinking. In contrast, the right side of the brain generally organizes inputs in patterns or wholes that, in turn, are necessary for creative or intuitive thinking (Springer & Deutsch, 1981). Table 3.1 lists the types of thinking currently accorded to each hemisphere. The right side of the brain is thought to process new or unfamiliar experiences. Once some familiarity is gained, the left side of the brain may then take over that function if appropriate. Handling a particular type of information may change from one hemisphere to the other if the way in which the inputs are processed changes. For example, one may initially process the patterns and rhythms of music with the right hemisphere, but once one begins to learn music theory and to analyze music according to its parts, the music will then be processed by the left hemisphere. One can then no longer recall the music selections as easily as a whole (Bever & Chiarello, 1974).

The right side of the brain is usually listed as the emotional side, meaning that thoughts about emotions are processed in the right hemisphere. It is now believed that this aspect of lateralization is influenced by gender. While most males process both negative and positive emotions in the right hemisphere, most females process negative (anxious) emotions on the right side and positive emotions on the left side of the brain.

Although the reasons are unclear, knowledge is steadily building that there are several other gender differences in hemispheric lateralization. In development, the left side appears to develop more rapidly in females and the right side in males. The causative factor may be testosterone, which is known to slow left hemisphere development (Durden-Smith & DeSimone, 1984). In the adult brain, females seem to be able to use both sides of the cerebrum at the same time more easily than males. This difference may be either an advantage or disadvantage depending on the case. Females may be more easily distracted from a

Table 3.1 Hemisphere Lateralization[a]

Left		Right	
Familiar	Analytical	Unfamiliar	Integrative
Rational	Evaluative	Intuitive	Imagination
Logical	Mathematics	Nonlinear	Experiential
Linear	Science	Patterns	Synthesizing
Sequential	Reason	Wholes	Spiritual
Temporal	Intellectual	Images	Spatial
Verbal	Discriminative	Inductive	Relationships
Deductive	Digital	Analogies	Art
Explicit	Parts	Symbols	Emotional

[a] Lateralization of cerebral hemisphere functioning may be described by the different types of cognitive processing thought to be attributed to the right versus the left hemispheres.

given task while males may be better able to concentrate on one task at a time. By the same token, females may be better able to attend to different types of cues in the environment at the same time. Thus, when a man and woman compare analyses of someone's behavior, they may find that the woman is more aware than the man of the nonverbal and the verbal behaviors. An anatomical difference may account for this difference in ability. The corpus callosum is a collection of neural pathways that transfers information back and forth between the right and left sides of the brain. Without this transfer of information, as with the split brain, one side does not know what the other side is thinking. The splenium is the portion of the corpus callosum that conveys nonverbal information. It has recently been shown that the splenium is significantly thicker in the female brain. Therefore, the female is anatomically more equipped to process nonverbal information while simultaneously attending to verbal inputs (Fackelmann, 1982).

This brief description of the lateralization of cognition is true for approximately 85 to 90% of the population. Data indicate that the hand position used for writing may give a clear clue to the nature of lateralization in the person being observed (Sibatani, 1980). The lateralization described above seems to hold true for right-handed people who write with a straight wrist and those left-handed people who write with a hooked wrist. In contrast, left-handed writers who use a straight wrist and the small minority of right-handed people who write with a hooked wrist seem to have lateralization opposite to that described above. Some people are more plastic in their cognitive functioning, which means that both hemispheres tend to process all information. In these instances, lateralization is not present to any significant degree.

Two types of inhibitions typically occur in cognitive function. Ipsilateral (same side) inhibition occurs when one side of the cerebrum is attending to an input that causes other activities by the same side of the brain to be relatively inhibited during that time. The sayings "I can only think of one thing at a time" and "I have a one track mind" may come from this type of inhibition. Contralateral (opposite side) inhibition occurs when one side of the brain is active and the ability of the opposite side of the brain to attend to inputs is relatively inhibited.

These inhibition mechanisms can be used in a creative fashion by the clinician. For example, when extremely anxious, one may be unable to attend to a therapeutic activity or thought. In this case, it might be helpful to temporarily decrease the anxiety. To accomplish this via the inhibition described above, the clinician may ask the person to attend to rhythmical, happy music. If successful, this activity would use ipsilateral inhibition to take the right brain on a "brief vacation" away from the thoughts that are producing the anxiety. It is easy to see why wearing earphones to listen to music is so popular in these stressful times. If the person is not able to concentrate on the music, the clinician could use contralateral inhibition with the same therapeutic objective in mind. Engaging the person in a conversation that requires sequential thinking, such as relating the details of a baseball game, would automatically activate the left hemisphere that, by contralateral inhibition, would slow the thinking of the right brain. The better the clinician knows the client, the easier it is to choose an activity that will reach the desired objective. However, application of knowledge related to hemispheric lateralization and inhibition mechanisms can increase the therapeutic options of the psychiatric mental health nurse.

Abnormalities in the lateralization of cognitive function, as well as handedness, have been implicated in the presenting symptoms and even as part of the etiology of several mental diseases (Beale & Corballis, 1983; Segalowitz, 1983). For example, left hemisphere deficit or, in other words, right hemisphere dominance has been studied in relation to schizophrenia (Magaro, 1981). However, the problem may not be of dominance as much as a deficiency in the ability of the corpus callosum to carry information back and forth between the two hemispheres.

Right hemisphere dominance is more common among left-handed people. A number of studies have been done that illuminate the relationship between left-handedness and a number of diseases including schizophrenia, dyslexia, migraine headaches, and a variety of autoimmune disorders (Durden-Smith & DeSimone, 1984; Marx, 1982). Left-handed people have approximately ten times the rate of learning disabilities, three times the rate of autoimmune diseases, and a significantly higher rate of schizophrenia and phobias than the right-handed population. By some unknown mechanism, right hemisphere dominance over the left hemisphere tends to make one more vulnerable to these conditions.

Testosterone seems to be a common factor in these disorders. Testosterone slows the development of the left hemisphere during fetal development via a mechanism not yet fully understood. Too much testosterone during development of the nervous system contributes to the relative overdevelopment and later dominance of the right hemisphere. Testosterone also alters the expression of the immune system including the thymus gland, site of the production of some types of immune cells. Males tend to have a higher incidence of left-handedness. It is curious that females tend to suffer more from autoimmune diseases until one looks at the results of current research showing that these women seem to metabolize testosterone abnormally. Two new terms have been defined to indicate the clinical relationships described above: psychoneuroimmunity and neuroimmunoendocrinology (Ader, 1981). There is much yet to be learned about the effect of hemisphere lateralization on behavior and mental disease; however, the horizon appears to be rich in relevant possibilities.

Learning and Memory

The processes of learning and memory have long eluded explanation; however, current research is helping to clarify the problem. Learning has generally been defined as a change in behavior, but somehow this change has to be the result of an anatomical and/or physiological change at the cellular level in the brain. Memory, the retention of learning, has been hypothesized to be an electrical event in the case of short-term memory and a biochemical or structural event for long-term memory. Changes in action potentials, synaptic events and structures, neurotransmitters, dendritic growth, and specialized neuronal circuits have all been studied for their effects on learning and memory.

Current information indicates that synaptic connections are susceptible to strengthening or weakening in response to sensitizaton and habituation, respectively (Kandel, 1982) Learning may well have an effect on the structure and arrangement of neuronal circuits as they develop, but once the brain is fully formed, those circuits are probably relatively fixed. (This idea may change with more research.) However, the strength of the connections or synapses between neurons is not as rigid and is thus maleable to experience.

Neurotransmitters, the chemicals that carry information from one neuron to another across the synapse, are released from what are called active zones in the varicosities at the terminal end of the axon of the neuron. Studies of this process have shown the following about the physiology of learning. First, simple learning takes place at synaptic connections. Second, long-term memory occurs via changes in the strength of already existing connections. Third, these synaptic connections can be modified by learning with a resultant change in the amount of neurotransmitter released, thereby changing the strength of the connections between neurons.

When an animal habituates, that is, ceases to pay attention to an input, the number of active zones and thereby the amount of neurotransmitter released decreases. Therefore, the message is slowed or stopped in its transmission along the neuronal pathway. Conversely, when an animal is being sensitized to an input, that is, paying more attention to it, the number of active zones and the amount of neurotransmitter released increases. Thus, both structural and chemical changes take place during learning.

Various forms of therapeutic counseling are based on the premise that learning takes place on the part of the individual in relation to his or her abnormal behavior. Frequently, medications are given as an adjunct to psychotherapy in an attempt to correct excesses or deficits in neurotransmitters and, thereby, increase the efficacy of the counseling. The assumption is made that the counseling and medications will work together to actualize the same structural and biochemical premises. Ideally, when patterns of behavior occur that indicate that stabilized changes have occurred at the synaptic level, medication and then therapy may be discontinued. Although this is the ideal, a few of the pitfalls in using this approach are discussed in Chapter 15.

There has also been an interesting development in our understanding of the mechanism by which memories are retained and then recalled at a later time. Memories of events are apparently retained in their full context, that is, both the factual content and the emotional aspects of the experience (Bower, 1981). The details of the process are not yet well understood, but it appears that when a given memory is recalled, the process is facilitated by remembering both the factual and emotional aspects. Therefore, if one is anxious while in a particular learning situation, the anxiety will be reexperienced when attempting to recall the factual information. This concept has broad implications for the kind of approaches used in educational programs whether they be for students or patients.

An inability to remember and an exaggeration of memories may both play an important role in mental disorders. As one patient with schizophrenia stated, "Recovery comes to the patient if the brain begins to function by trying to remember" (Dawson, Blum, & Bartolucci, 1983).

Anxiety as a Neurophysiological State

The tendency to pay too much attention to incoming information rather than sorting out the important from the unimportant may trigger some forms of severe anxiety. A specific structure within the brain stem has been shown to help make that distinction. The locus coeruleus, located in the pons, functions with the raphe system to regulate sleep. This structure changes the level of consciousness from quiet drowsiness to the first stages of slow wave (REM) sleep. It also appears to help arouse the brain back to the drowsiness and from the sleep cycle back to an awake state. Once awake, the locus coeruleus is responsive to novel stimuli, alerting the brain to anything new that requires particular attention (Bloom, 1982). In this sense, the locus coeruleus may be said to act as a sympathetic ganglia in alerting its target organ, the brain. Having both the sleep-regulating and novel stimuli-alerting mechanism occurring in the same structure is helpful as one often experiences arousal from drowsiness or sleep because of an external event warrenting attention.

When routine events are taking place, the locus coeruleus is quiet. Again, this is helpful; one can imagine that being continuously alerted to all possible external stimuli without sorting out what is important would leave the brain needlessly bombarded with an overload of information. This, in fact, may be what occurs in some forms of anxiety. The locus coeruleus may not be performing its task of discrimination, thereby leaving the individual to react to all internal and external environmental stimuli, in effect overreacting and understandably anxious.

As the hypothalamus interfaces between the limbic brain structures and physiological activities of the nervous, endocrine, and immune systems, the locus coeruleus provides an important "filtering" function of incoming information before it reaches higher brain centers. Some would say that it provides the language for the interface between the brain and the behaving mind on the sensory side of behavior. Clinical implications of the triune brain and lateralization for intervention with an anxious person have already been discussed. Hopefully, this additional knowledge concerning the role which the locus coeruleus may play in anxiety will also result in suggesting and clarifying therapeutic approaches.

Other crucial brain structures may be identified that provide important links between neurophysiology and behavior. Thus, the old dichotomy between the mind and body is rapidly disappearing as more information becomes available. For example, the anatomical locations of specific aspects of memory and types of amnesia are being identified (Herbert, 1983).

NEUROCHEMISTRY AS A BASIS FOR MENTAL DISORDERS

Synapses and Neurotransmitters

We now need to examine in more detail the events that normally take place at the synapse. Abnormalities in the functioning of synaptic events are receiving increasing attention in relationship to the etiology of pyschopathology. Rather than reviewing all of the types of synapses in the nervous system, a brief overview of those aspects common to the functioning of all synapses will suffice. Figure 3.3 outlines typical events at the synapse. In all cases, the following steps are generally required for adequate synaptic function. Precursors need to be provided in sufficient amounts for neurotransmitter production. Once synthesized, the neurotransmitter is packaged and temporarily stored in vesicles (granular pools) in active zones near the presynaptic membrane of the neuron.

When stimulated to do so by the occurrence of an action potential, vesicles move to the presynaptic membrane releasing packets of neurotransmitter into the synaptic space. The amount of neurotransmitter released is dependent on the frequency of action potentials, availability of calcium, and amount of neurotransmitter available from storage. The function (e.g., excitation or inhibition) of different neurotransmitters varies according to a variety of factors, including which end of the molecule is active. For instance, one end of the neurotransmitter molecule, substance P, provides analgesia, while the other end is thought to transmit pain (Ferguson, 1983).

The neurotransmitter then diffuses across the synaptic space or cleft and attaches to the postsynaptic membrane of the second neuron at the location of receptor sites for that particular neurotransmitter. At that time, the neurotransmitter may be inactivated in several ways or reused later by the presynaptic neuron. Inactivation may be accomplished by an enzyme specific to the neurotransmitter on the postsynaptic membrane or in the synaptic space. The neurotransmitter may be lost by diffusion into the extracellular space. Lastly, the neurotransmitter may be inactivated after it has been taken up through the presynaptic membrane (as norepinephrine is inactivated by monamine oxidase, [MAO]). If not affected by any of the inactivation possibilities, the neurotransmitter may be reused after reuptake into the presynaptic neuron. Although this is a superficial summary, it outlines the steps crucial to the normal passage of messages from one neuron to another (Kandel & Schwartz, 1981).

The picture becomes much more complex when one realizes that the average adult brain contains approximately ten billion pages of information, with roughly 100 billion neurons

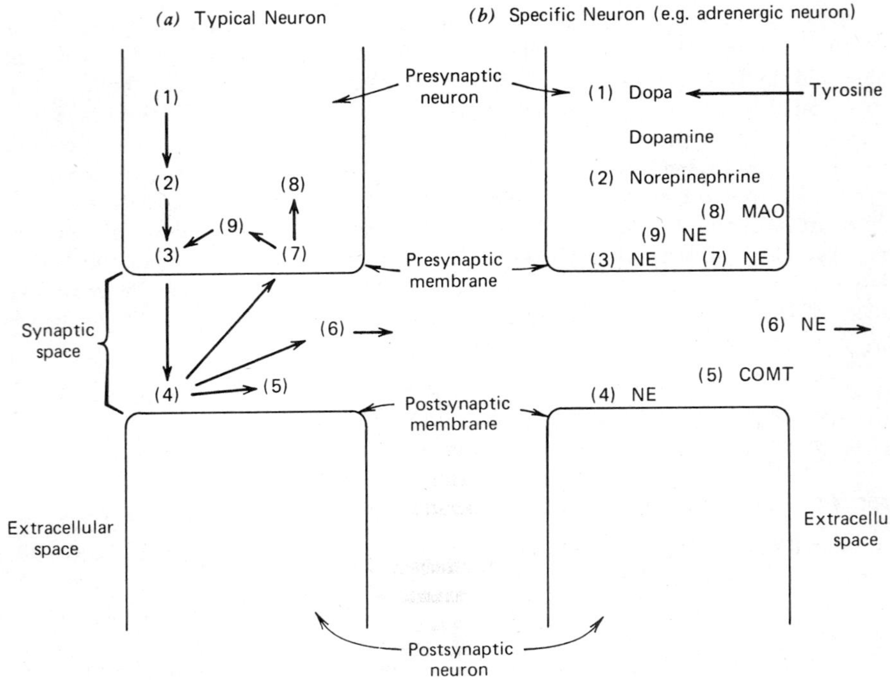

Figure 3.3 Synaptic events. (*a*) Events normally taking place at the typical synapse include: (1) precursors for the formulation of the neurotransmitter (NT), (2) NT stored in vesicles, (3) release of NT from vesicles on presynaptic membrane, (4) NT combines with receptors on postsynaptic membrane, (5) inactivation of NT by another substance, (6) diffusion of NT into extracellular space, (7) reuptake of NT into presynaptic neuron, (8) inactivation of NT in presynaptic neuron, and (9) reuse of NT by presynaptic neuron. (*b*) Synaptic events at a particular type of synapse, the adrenergic neuron utilizing norepinephrine (NE) as the neurotransmitter: (1) sequential formation of NE from the precursors tyrosine, dopa, and dopamine, (2) NE stored in vesicles, (3) release of NE, (4) NE combines with receptors, (5) inactivation of NE by catechol-O-methyltransferase (COMT), (6) diffusion of NE, (7) reuptake of NE, (8) inactivation of NE by monoamine oxidase (MAO), and (9) reuse of NE by presynaptic neuron.

communicating with one another over 100 trillion synapses (Hubel, 1979)! A given neuron may communicate with hundreds and even thousands of other neurons with simultaneous inputs that may be inhibitory or excitatory in nature. An algebraic summation of these inputs must be accomplished by the receiving neuron to determine the appropriate frequency of action potentials that should be propagated down the axon.

The action potential will not be fully described here; however, it resembles a burning fuse, moving up to 100 yards per second, and is initiatied by the influx of sodium ions into the neuron creating an electrical current. When the message thus coded according to an electrical frequency reaches the terminals, it is then changed to a chemical code according to the amount of neurotransmitter released from the presynaptic membrane and diffused across the synaptic space to the next neuron (Shepherd, 1983).

It is becoming increasingly clear that part of the etiology of many of the common mental disorders may at least partially lie within the synaptic events just described. For example, increased activity of the neurotransmitter dopamine has been implicated in the etiology of schizophrenia. In contrast, a deficit of serotonin and norepinephrine may play a role in the syndrome of chronic depression. Medications continue to be developed with the purpose of correcting these abnormalities (Cooper, Bloom, & Roth, 1982; Iverson & Iverson, 1981; Kruk & Pycock, 1983; Maugh, 1981). Table 3.2 provides examples of medications and their desired effects (see Chapter 15 for a more detailed discussion of psychopharmacotherapy).

Endogenous Chemicals

In 1973, when the receptor sites for endogenous opiates were first identified and, two years later, when the first of the endogenous chemicals was described, much surprise was expressed. However, it is reasonable to conclude that any chemical that affects brain function does so because there are receptor sites in brain tissue that are sensitive to that chemical. If receptor sites are present for a particular chemical, it also stands to reason that they are there for a functional purpose, that is, to receive that chemical. Therefore, that chemical or one very similar to it must be present via production by the nervous system or elsewhere in the body and not because the brain is waiting for society to produce and inject the chemical.

This line of reasoning is receiving further support as more endogenous chemicals, substances that the body produces, are being identified. The search is underway to locate the receptor sites and identify the chemicals that are similar to substances that we know have an effect on nervous system functioning. It is hypothesized that excessive or deficient amounts of some of these chemicals will also be found to contribute to the etiology of some mental disorders.

The first example to come to light was the excessive amount of the endogenous opiate, beta endorphin, generally found to be present in individuals with schizophrenia (Marx, 1981). At first, it was thought that the excess was a part of the disease syndrome when initial studies showed improvement with the injection of narcan (naloxone), which is a morphine antagonist. However, other studies had opposite results and showed improvement in disease symptomatology with injection of additional beta endorphin. Research findings are inconclusive and it is still a controversial point, but the excessive amount of the endogenous opiate may be a part of the body's defense against the emotional pain associated

Table 3.2 Medications and Desired Effects[a]

Medication	*Desired Action*
L-Dopa	Increases synthesis of dopamine and norepinephrine
Methyldopa	Provides synthesis of false neurotransmitter
Reserpine	Decreases supply of vesicles with neurotransmitter
Librium	Blocks release of neurotransmitter from vesicles on presynaptic membrane
Bromocriptine and isoprenaline	Increase activity of receptors on postsynaptic membrane
Chlorpromazine and propranolol	Decrease activity of receptors on postsynaptic membrane
Tricyclics	Block reuptake of neurotransmitter into presynaptic neuron
MAO inhibitors	Destroy monoamine oxidase (which normally inactivates neurotransmitter norepinephrine thereby increasing amount of neurotransmitter available for reuse by presynaptic neuron)

[a] A variety of medications are used to affect synaptic events for a therapeutic benefit for individuals afflicted with mental disorders.

with the disease (Koob & Bloom, 1983). It is a common observation that schizophrenic individuals desire excessive amounts of milk and other dairy products. Milk is one of the two richest sources (turkey being the other) of tryptophan, a dietary precursor for serotonin, a neurotransmitter associated with activation of endogenous opiates and/or a nonopiate pathway. These individuals may instinctively be seeking a substance that makes them feel more comfortable as endogenous opiates function to reduce emotional pain in the limbic brain structures, as well as physical pain elsewhere.

The search for other endogenous chemicals related to behavior has just begun, and the list is growing rapidly. Receptors, and in some cases the endogenous chemicals themselves, have already been identified for valium, PCP, and others (Starr, 1983). It is predicted that several hundred such sites and chemicals will eventually be identified. It is hypothesized that schizophrenic individuals may produce an excessive amount of endogenous hallucinogens such as LSD. The benzodiazepine receptor with its neurotransmitter gamma-aminobutyricacid (GABA) seems to be the site at which valium acts. As the endogenous valiums are identified, medications that more closely mimic the natural chemical or the endogenous chemical itself produced via genetic engineering techniques may be used without the side effects inherent in the use of the current medications.

Perhaps more importantly, therapeutic techniques may be developed to assist people to produce their own natural chemicals when appropriate. Various behavioral techniques such as imagery and biofeedback hold promise in this regard. Through techniques such as these, the potential of the brain to use conscious thought to override and control functions that are usually regulated automatically can be brought into play. For example, some people are better able than others to keep themselves calm in anxious situations probably in part by stimulating the release of their own natural valiums. Whenever possible, it would seem preferable to use this natural approach compared with the ingestion of medications. Counseling or therapy can augment the medication in facilitating the desired cellular effects. Mechanisms used to produce and release a desired endogenous chemical may be overwhelmed by experiences. If these experiences can be modified by therapy, this may enable the person's natural mechanisms to again assume control, returning the person's behavior to a more normal state.

PSYCHOLOGICAL BASIS OF PHYSICAL ILLNESS

Hypothalamus

Just as neurophysiology underlies and affects behavior, the same can be said of emotions and thoughts on physiology since the intimate interaction between the mind and body (behavior and physiology) functions in both directions. To summarize the flow of influence of the cognitive and emotional states on physical functioning and disease, we must go back to the hypothalamus interface. This small piece of brain tissue located in the floor of the third ventricle just above the pituitary is responsible for a variety of important functions. It coordinates communication among the limbic structures of the brain and in turn provides much of the control of the autonomic nervous system. This is accomplished via pathways down through the brain stem, the endocrine system via neural and hormonal messages to the pituitary, and the immune system via indirect control of thymus functioning and levels of immune cell and antibodies. The hypothalamus also provides much of the control for a variety of functions including temperature regulation, hunger, thirst, extreme emotions such as murderous behavior and extreme pleasure, sexually motivated behavior, and others.

The organization of neuronal groups responsible for various functions in the hypothalamus helps to explain relationships among certain frequently observed behaviors. For example, the neurons involved with cooling mechanisms and sleep are located in the same general area (anterior nucleus). Their proximity may help account for the observation that a drop in body temperature is associated with the initiation of sleep and a rise in body temperature is associated with waking.

Neurons involved with hunger, pleasure, aggression, and motor activity are also located in the same area (ventral medial nucleus). One can see that hunger can elicit aggressive behavior and activity to obtain food, which, if successful, is followed by pleasure behavior. The groups of neurons for the feelings of pleasure and aggression are in close approximation to each other, giving an anatomical reality to the old saying that "there is a thin line between love and hate."

Stress Response

Chemical and neuronal pathways between the hypothalamus and other structures and systems listed above provide the framework for the stress response which is often responsible for physical disorders that may have emotional and/or cognitive origins (Snyder, 1980). In any situation where internal or external stimuli have resulted in perception on the part of the individual that results in anxiety, the stress response is automatically called into play to enable the person to deal with the perceived emergency. The key to eliciting the stress response is the perception of the stimuli, incoming information, or event and not the stimuli itself. Therefore, what is stressful for one person may not be for another. Just as the anxiety-provoking stimulus may be physical in nature, such as a warm room, it may also be emotional in nature, such as an argument, or cognitive in nature, such as thoughts about an upcoming examination. No matter the stimuli, the same stress response will be called into play, initiated in large part by the hypothalamus.

In the short run, the stress response is helpful to the individual in dealing with the situation. However, when this response is initiated too often or for too prolonged a time, the same physiological results can be responsible for a variety of physical disorders. While it is not appropriate to address the details of the stress response in this chapter, recall that the hypothalamus generally initiates the following actions.

When activated, the sympathetic nervous system pathways initiate the flight or fight response. The posterior pituitary is asked to increase its secretion of antidiuretic hormone to increase blood volume, and the adrenal medulla is asked to increase secretion of the hormones epinephrine and norepinephrine. Increased epinephrine results in such useful mechanisms as pupil dilation, increased cardiac output, blood pressure, and metabolic rate. Other functions not having a priority in an emergency are decreased, such as peristalsis. Blood supply to the heart, brain, and skeletal muscles is increased. Norepinephrine increases results in peripheral vasoconstriction to the skin (which is not a priority in an emergency) and to the kidneys, resulting in renin secretion and eventual increase in blood pressure and blood volume.

Norepinephrine appears to increase more in familiar stressful situations while epinephrine increases more in unfamiliar situations. Recall that depression is usually accompanied by a deficit in norepinephrine, thereby rendering the individual less able to cope, even in situations which are familiar. The low periods for the seasonal rhythm of norepinephrine in March and October may therefore partially account for the sometimes observed increased suicide rate during those months.

The hypothalamus also sends a hormonal message (corticotropin releasing factor) to the anterior pituitary, which in turn stimulates the adrenal cortex via adrenocorticotrophic hormone (ACTH) to release increased amounts of mineralocorticoids and glucocorticoids (the most prominent being cortisol). Increased blood glucose, mobilization of fatty acids, and increased protein catabolism all result to provide energy to deal with the emergency. When ACTH is released from the anterior pituitary, beta endorphin, an endogenous opiate, is automatically released with it (perhaps to reduce the discomfort associated with the stress). It is now hypothesized that the release of these two chemicals may act to decrease function of the higher brain centers allowing the midbrain and brain stem structures to act instinctively for the promotion of survival in acute stress (Ferguson, 1983).

Increased cortisol and epinephrine also decrease functioning of the immune system, seemingly to conserve energy normally used by the immune response (Hales, 1981; Riley, 1981). Immune cells, particularly T cells, have receptor sites for these hormones and are inactivated by them. Thymus gland functioning also decreases. The hypothalamus in turn has receptor sites for hormones produced by the thymus (thymosin hormones) and is thus able to monitor the level of activity of the immune system. Overall, changes in the immune system include a decreased number of functioning T cells, macrophages, antibodies, and thymus function. Vitamin C, vitamin B-complex, and zinc also appear to be destroyed during the stress response. Prolonged stress can lessen the immune defenses against viral and bacterial pathogens, rendering the individual more vulnerable to these problems. If a person chooses to use smoking or alcohol as coping measures, the problem is compounded as these substances also chemically destroy vitamin C.

In addition to the effects on the immune system, prolonged or frequent stress will promote physical disorders owing to the nature of the stress response itself. The possibilities are numerous such as hypertension from the increased blood pressure, hyperthyroidism from the increase in metabolism, and diabetes from the increase in glucogenesis (Goldberger & Breznitz, 1982). Emotions and thoughts, acting as stressors, can therefore have a powerful impact on physical health mediated through the stress response.

Associated Disorders

There are other relationships between mental and physical disorders which are not well understood. For example, the following endocrine disorders are associated with chronic depression: hyperthyroidism, hypothyroidism, Addison's disease, Cushing's disease, diabetes, hyperparathyroidism, and hypoglycemia (Blumenthal, 1980). These and other observed associations need to be studied further. For instance, personality traits, such as those described as hardiness, that seem to increase resistance to illness are being studied (Kobasa, 1981).

Differentiation of Causes of Behavioral Symptoms

At times, it can be very difficult to differentiate between the mental and physical causes of behavioral symptoms. This problem requires astute observational skills and detailed knowledge of the underlying neuroanatomy and physiology. For example, the symptoms of visual hallucinations, paranoid ideation, slurred speech, shortened concentration span, time disorientation, and immediate memory loss may prompt the clinician to determine that the cause of these symptoms may be a type of psychosis or dementia. However, these are also classic symptoms of severe sleep deprivation in an otherwise normally functioning brain. There is much to learn regarding the interrelationships between mental and physical disorders to avoid errors in differential diagnosis and to improve the efficacy of therapeutic approaches.

THE FUTURE OF NEUROBIOLOGY AND PSYCHIATRIC MENTAL HEALTH CLINICAL PRACTICE

It might be tempting to say that the future will bring the replacement of behavioral and counseling approaches to mental illness by neuropharmaceutical techniques. However, it can be predicted that two trends will become evident with further neurobiological discoveries. First, the emerging knowledge about the functioning brain should refine and enhance rather than eliminate many of the counseling techniques used today. Health professionals should be able to delineate therapies that are more specific to the disease and the individual with increased knowledge of the normal and disease mechanisms inherent in neurophysiology and neurochemistry. In turn, the neuropharmaceuticals becoming available should promote the desired direction of behavioral therapies. Ideally, the behavioral and chemical approaches should work in concert with one another for increased efficacy.

Second, increased success in treating psychotic behavior should provide more opportunity for preventive approaches, as well as increased time and attention to the more common behavioral problems besetting the population. Both results hold significant promise for increasing the mental health of society.

Several promising developments in neurobiology have not been addressed in this chapter since their application potential has not yet been clearly defined though their potential is exciting to contemplate. One example is the recent data, although indirect, of the importance of genetic inheritance in the incidence of mental disorders. Depression, mania, and schizophrenia have received the most attention thus far, though other disorders are bound to follow (Bunney, 1982). Studies with separated twins and other genetic research techniques will continue to contribute to our knowledge in this area. As techniques are refined to analyze the histocompatibility complex, that is, the genetic abnormalities of the individual, it will be possible to determine ways to genetically treat vulnerable people with an increased potential to prevent the disorders from occuring.

New techniques in three-dimensional computerized images of the brain also offer great potential in early diagnosis of mental disorders. While computerized axial tomography (CAT scan) is used to provide an image of the anatomy of the brain and positron emission transaxial tomography (PETT) is able to visualize the metabolism of the brain, newer techniques are being refined that yield even more information without the necessity of injecting radioactive isotopes or applying Xrays to produce the image (Marano, 1982). For example, nuclear magnetic resonance (NMR) uses the application of radio waves, and the detection of the signals given off by brain tissues in response, yields images that afford clearer pictures of pathological processes than earlier methods (Durden-Smith, 1982). Another technique called brain electrical activity mapping (BEAM) uses the computer to analyze an elaborate electroencephalogram to depict the electrical activity of the brain in three dimensions (Herbert, 1982; McKean, 1981). The metabolic and electrical changes inherent in disorders such as depression, mania, schizophrenia, and dementia are now able to be studied in far more detail than ever before. By combining these techniques, earlier and more accurate diagnoses will be possible in the near future.

Last, the discovery that the brain is an immunologically privileged site has led to the realization that brain tissue may be transplanted without the problems of tissue rejection experienced with other organs (Huyghe, 1983; Marx, 1982). In some way, the brain (probably through the blood brain barrier) has the ability to accept tissue from other people and even other species without rejection of the graft. Research is now ongoing with the transplantation of tissue to replace deficient cells such as the substantia nigra for the treatment of

Parkinson's disease in which there is an insufficient production of the neurotransmitter dopamine. It should not be long before other uses of this technique are developed, and one can be most creative in thinking of the possibilities ahead.

SUMMARY

A holistic approach to the mind, brain, and body is now not only possible but imperative to make use of emerging knowledge for the prevention and treatment of mental disorders. This chapter presented an overview of neurobiological information which may help the mental health professional to refine existing therapeutic approaches. It is certain that relevant discoveries will now emerge at a rapid pace, rendering this chapter merely an introduction to the exciting merger of neurobiology and mental health practice that the future holds.

REFERENCES

Ader, R. (Ed.). *Psychoneuroimmunity.* New York: Academic Press, 1981.

Beale, I.L., & Corballis, M.C. *The ambivalent mind: The neuropsychology of left and right.* Chicago: Nelson Hall, 1983.

Bever, T.G., & Chiarello, R.J. Cerebral dominance in musicians and nonmusicians. *Science,* August 9, 1974, 537–539.

Bloom, F.E. Brain regulation of responsiveness to environment. *The science of the brain* [Audiocassette]. APA Convention, Smith, Kline, & French, 1982.

Blumenthal, M.D. Depressive illness in old age: Getting behind the mask. *Geriatrics,* 1980, *35,* 34–43.

Bower, B. Emotional rescue. *Science News,* April 18, 1981, 253–255.

Bunney, W.E. Mental illness and neuroscience. *The science of the brain* [Audiocassette]. American Psychiatric Association Convention, Smith, Kline, & French, 1982.

Cooper, J.R., Bloom, F.E., & Roth, R.H. *The biochemical basis of neuropharmacology.* New York: Oxford University Press, 1982.

Cox, T. *Stress.* Baltimore: University Park Press, 1978.

Dawson, D., Blum, H.M., & Bartolucci, G. *Schizophrenia in focus.* New York: Human Science Press, 1983.

Durden-Smith, D. Nuclear magnetic resonance. *Technology,* January-February, 1982, 32–39.

Durden-Smith, J., & DeSimone, D. Hidden threads of illness. *Science Digest,* January, 1984, 51–105.

Fackelmann, K.A. Male-female brain anatomy may differ. *Science News,* June 6, 1982, 121, 422.

Ferguson, M. New neurobiology era parallels leap in physics. *Brain Mind Bulletin,* October 24, 1983, *8,* 1–3.

Goldberger, L., & Breznitz, S. *Handbook of stress: Theoretical and clinical aspects.* New York: The Free Press, 1982.

Goleman, D. Holographic memory. *Psychology Today,* February, 1979, 71–84.

Greguss, P. (Ed.). *Holography in medicine.* New York: IPL Science & Technology Press, 1975.

Hales, D. Psycho-immunity. *Science Digest,* November, 1981, 12–14.

Herbert, W. Rememberance of things partly. *Science News,* December 10, 1983, *124,* 378–381.

Herbert, W. Schizophrenia: From adolescent insanity to dopamine disease. *Science News,* March 13, 1982, *121,* 173–175.

Holden, D. Paul MacLean and the triune brain. *Science,* June 8, 1979, *204,* 1066–1068.

Hubel, D. The brain. *Scientific American,* March, 1979, *241,* 44–53.

Huyghe, P. Exploring the unexplained. *Science Digest,* December, 1983, 68–119.

Iverson, S., & Iverson, L. *Behavioral pharmacology.* New York: Oxford Press, 1981.

Kandel, E.R. Changes in the brain produced by learning. *The science of the brain* [Audiocassette]. APA Convention, Smith, Kline, & French, 1982.

Kandel, E.R., & Schwartz, J. *Principles of neural science.* New York: Elsevier North-Holland, 1981.

Kobasa, S. The hardy personality: Toward a social psychology of stress and health. In J. Suls & G. Pardons (Eds.), *Social psychology of health and illness.* Hillsdale, NJ: Erlbaum, 1981.

Koob, G.F., & Bloom, F.E. Behavioral perspectives of opioid peptides. *British Medical Bulletin,* 1983, *39,* 89–94.

Kruk, Z.L., & Pycock, C.J. *Neurotransmitters and drugs.* Baltimore: University Park Press, 1983.

MacLean, P. *A triune concept of brain and behavior.* Toronto: Toronto Press, 1975.

Magaro, P.A. The paranoid and the schizophrenic: The case for distinct cognitive styles. *Schizophrenia Bulletin,* 1981, *7,* 632–661.

Marano, H.E. Mental turmoil in technicolor. *American Health,* May-June, 1982, 38–39.

Marx, J. Brain opiates in mental illness. *Science,* November 27, 1981, *214,* 1013–1015.

Marx, J.L. Autoimmunity in left-handers. *Science News,* July 9, 1982, *217,* 141–144.

Maugh, T.H. Biochemical markers identify mental states. *Science,* October 2, 1981, *214,* 39–41.

McKean, K. Beaming new light on the brain. *Discover,* December, 1981, 30–33.

Ornstein, R.E. *The psychology of consciousness.* San Francisco: W.W. Freeman, 1972.

Pines, M. The human differences. *Psychology Today,* September, 1983, 62–68.

Riley, V. Psychoneuroendocrine influences on immunocompetence and neoplasia. *Science,* June 5, 1981, *212,* 1100–1110.

Segalowitz, S.J. *Two sides of the brain.* Englewood Cliffs, NJ: Prentice-Hall, 1983.

Shepherd, G.M. *Neurobiology.* New York: Oxford University Press, 1983.

Sibatani, A. The Japanese brain. *Science 80,* December, 1980, 22–27.

Skinner, J.E. Heart attacks from stress, via brain. *Science News,* November 18, 1978, 94.

Snyder, S.H. *Biological aspects of mental disorder.* New York: Oxford University Press, 1980.

Springer, S.P., & Deutsch, G. *Left brain right brain.* San Francisco: W.W. Freeman, 1981.

Starr, D. Brain drugs. *Omni,* 1983, 26, 127.

Trotter, R.J. Psychiatry for the 80's. *Science News,* May 30, 1981, 119.

Wilber, K. (Ed.). *The holographic paradigm.* Boulder: Shambhala, 1982.

BIBLIOGRAPHY

Herbert, W. Melancholy genes. *Science News,* February 13, 1982, *121,* 108–109.

Herbert, W. Sources of temperment: Bashful at birth? *Science News,* January 16, 1982, 36.

Hughes, J. (Ed.). *Opioid peptides.* New York: Churchill Livingstone, 1983.

Kolata, G. Transplants as guides to brain development. *Science,* July 23, 1982, *217,* 340–344.

Snyder, S.H. Drugs, neurotransmitters and the brain. *The science of the brain* [Audiocassette]. APA Convention, Smith, Kline, & French, 1982.

Toutexia, A. A brainy marvel called PET. *Time,* September 14, 1981, 74.

CHAPTER 4

RELEVANCE OF RESEARCH: THE CASE STUDY

Joann Weiss

In the American Nurses' Association *Standards of Psychiatric and Mental Health Nursing Practice,* the importance of research as one means of improving the quality of patient care is expressed. The first standard of practice states: "The nurse applies appropriate theory that is scientifically sound as a basis for decisions regarding nursing practice" (American Nurses' Association [ANA], 1982, p. 3). Many more of the standards carry the implication that psychiatric mental health nurses should be thoughtful and inquiring observers of the nature of their clients' problems, of the interventions nurses use, and of outcomes of therapy. The final standard expresses the research mandate most directly: "The nurse contributes to nursing and the mental health field through innovations in theory and practice and participation in research" (ANA, 1982, p. 19). The issue thus appears not to be whether or not the practicing psychiatric mental health nurse should be research oriented but, rather, how to go about carrying out research that will yield useful information.

In psychiatric mental health nursing, as in other nursing areas, there is need for study of issues that nurses find most problematic in dealing with clients. Concepts need to be developed and researched that reflect the nature of nursing values and involvement with the client and the care system. Case studies are a way that nurses can focus on the problems of greatest concern to them while they refine concept development. Yet, the case study as a methodology, when discussed at all in research texts, is frequently described as if it is to be preferrably avoided. This is ironic since major theoretical paradigms have been developed from case studies in the mental health field.

A basic assumption of this chapter is that the case study has a legitimate function. As a method, it could contribute to the thoughtful inquiry of psychiatric mental health nurse specialists in relation to their clinical work. However, as any methodology, it has strengths, limitations, and design elements that must be attended to in order to have confidence in the results. This chapter will discuss the contribution to be gained from case studies and present the process by which one formulates a research problem for study with this method. Select types of case studies will be described and the central issues of each will be discussed. Finally, ethical issues in case study methods will be addressed.

WHAT IS A CASE STUDY?

In this discussion, a case study is an instance where the researcher utilizes extensive description of one unit to either gain insight into a problem or situation or to test a hypothesis. The task is to characterize this knowledge in a way that makes it useful for in-depth understanding of the case. When more than one case is used, the investigation is sometimes called a comparative case study. The kind of knowledge developed varies with the theoretical purpose of the study. Units of analysis for the case study may be individuals, dyads, encounters, social groups, organizations, or other types of networks.

The distinguishing characteristic of the case study, as the term is used here, is the intensity of the data collection and its presentation in such a way as to optimize the understanding of complexity. Beyond this similarity, case study methodology is quite broad, as will be explained.

Another feature of case studies is that the notion of probability is generally not employed in the statistical sense. The researcher is unlikely to know whether or not an individual, organization, or situation is empirically representative of the universe of units of general interest unless a great deal is already known about that population. Particularly when the researcher's interest is in process phenomena, what is most important is the explanation of unfolding events, not their typicality as an *initial* concern. If one wishes to use the explanation of those events to specifically predict other events, however, the problem of how unusual the case may have been becomes a matter for concern. Although a single case study may not be regarded as a prototype of all cases, case studies may become cumulative and generate information about a set of similar situations. The researcher's philosophical assumptions about the nature of the reality that is being studied sets the framework for whether or not what is being described is believed to be universal phenomena or limited to the specific time and space under study. These assumptions are usually a part of the theoretical framework chosen for the study, which will be discussed later.

WHAT DO CASE STUDIES CONTRIBUTE?

In the development of any scientific knowledge base, there is a need for information that provides sensitization to elements of the real world, accurate description and classification, and tests of predictions drawn from theories. One must, however, have a good understanding of what is, of some principles underlying the events that concern us, before we can predict unforeseen happenings or propose alterations that correspond with one's value system. Some of the problems of clinicians arise from the fact that they have limited understanding of the varieties of human responses to problems and therapeutic interventions. A descriptive approach to these issues should logically precede either experimentation or clinical applications. Careful descriptions need to be shared with colleagues through the professional literature for these descriptions to become useful as cumulative information. Meta-analysis, or studies that attempt to combine the findings from several studies into a conceptual whole, is possible when well-done case studies on the same phenomenon are done by a variety of researchers.

The kind of knowledge gained from case studies is not unlike clinical experience that can be recognized as expertise in the effective clinician. Experience in this sense encompasses the totality of situations and this is what the case study researcher should attempt to convey. The skill of the researcher in translating some of the ingredients of this totality as form, structure, process, or other type of regularity determines the usefulness of the case study research as a contribution to knowledge. When these regularities are expressed in ways that others can identify in similar situations, or can dispute with other instances, the knowledge base built by case study research is cumulative.

An example of form, or structure of a situation, is Bateson's "Double Bind" (Bateson, Jackson, Haley, & Weakland, 1956). It is not necessary for us to know the complete details of a case to understand these ingredients at an abstract level:

1. Two persons, one of whom is the victim.
2. A repeated experience, so that the double bind becomes a habitual expectation.
3. A primary negative injunction carrying a threat of punishment.

4. A secondary injunction conflicting with the first, but at a more abstract level. Like the primary injunction, the second threatens punishment.
5. A tertiary negative injunction prohibiting the victim from escaping from the field.

Bateson and his associates studied dyads intensively as single cases before they isolated the form of the interaction that was problematic for a victim. Repeated observations and studies of the outcomes of this process pattern led them to the viewpoint that humans developed pathological information processing patterns under such conditions. Bateson's description can be refuted by others studying dyads. It may be possible to find situations when the form exists but other outcomes occur. This could then add to the understanding of such issues as context variations for the double bind or of individual differences which may lead to alternative outcomes. In any event, while no probability statements are attached to Bateson's ideas, others may recognize the form he described and attempt verification of his conclusions.

Case studies add to knowledge using induction or deduction. Inductive case studies provide analytic descriptions. Others may challenge the conclusions, or the proposed form, by describing cases that do not fit what the first author has proposed. Deductive case studies become examples of theory verification by providing positive or negative cases. Since the case study researcher is free to describe the complexity of situations, he or she may be able to clarify *why* a theoretical formulation does or does not apply. Comparison cases presented in the literature provoke negative instances that force the refinement and specification of theory.

PRELIMINARY CONCERNS IN DEVELOPING A CASE STUDY

There are several important issues the nurse must resolve in planning a sound case study. These are primarily the substantive issues of concern, the units for analysis, the conceptual framework, and the theoretical purpose of the study. Practical considerations of time and resources and ethical considerations are additional factors to be dealt with at the design phase of the case study. Decisions about these issues are made either consciously or by default at the point of selection of a method of data collection and in data analysis. The more consciously these decisions can be made, the more scholarly the endeavor is likely to be. Lofland (1971) makes this point by noting that even when one intends to be purely descriptive, analysis is always involved in presentation, even by sifting through volumes of material deciding what to condense and what to expand on. He stated:

> To select some things from a larger body of materials is to make analytic judgments. If that is the case, then it is certainly more useful to go on to a conscious process of decision making about what one is doing than to obscure it under the mantle of inarticulate intuition. When the process of selection becomes conscious and deliberate, it is also possible explicitly to share one's resultant decisions with one's audience. And if one is going to share those decisions with his audience, then he can do them the elementary courtesy of being CLEAR about what he has selected and how those selections have been ordered. (Lofland, 1971, p. 7)

The Substantive Problem

The researcher needs a problem focus, which becomes the substantive issue for investigation. Substantive refers to the types of people, groups, or situations of interest and whatever is problematic to the researcher about them. For example, one might be interested in people on a particular drug regime and the problem might be how their family relationships are affected by treatment issues. Sometimes, the clinician may have an interest in a particular type of client, but no single problem focus provides a logical starting point for the case study. In such situations, a research question may be formulated that serves the purpose of focusing attention for initial data collection. Successive studies could then be based on the findings of the first case study. Lofland suggests research questions for such situations:

> What is problematic to the participants here?
> What are the things over which they fret, show irritation, desperation and the like?
> When they look out into the world, what appears to them as important, stressful, or difficult? (Lofland, 1971, p. 54).

Another way to phrase a research question which identifies the substantive concern but does not have specific variables in focus is to clarify the problem as a situation that needs classification. For example, there is a theme running through the literature on psychiatric intervention that raises the question of whether or not institutionalization of any kind is beneficial for clients. Surrounding this issue are questions of the results of labeling and what effect socialization to the patient role has on people. One might ask, out of such a general concern: "Are there regularized forms of client reactions to psychiatric institutionalization?" The resulting study would document the behavior and perceptions of such clients in the early stages of hospitalization. Obviously, a comparison of case studies would be necessary for such classification purposes.

Units of Analysis

The substantive problem and the choice of units for analysis are separate but related issues. When nurses contemplate studying clinical situations, they are faced with few discipline restrictions on what the appropriate units should be. They may choose to describe problems from a strictly intrapsychic perspective (the individual as the unit), as relationships (the dyad as the unit), as group phenomena (the family or other group as the unit), or as a large system problem (organizations, networks, or communities as the unit). The substantive problem should imply the units in the way the question is worded.

The choice of units for analysis is usually a reflection of traditions within disciplines into which the researcher has been socialized. Psychologically oriented researchers focus intensively on the intrapersonal characteristics of subjects and on their reactions to life situations, interactions, and the like. Explanations are likely to be sought that emphasize the particular traits or states of individuals such as their attitudes, perceptions, values, personality characteristics, cognitive style, level of development, intelligence, and so on. These issues are likely to be viewed as the independent variables of concern, or those things that precede the problems of interest in time. Psychologically oriented case studies may also be oriented to how these characteristics develop over time. For example, studies of "burnout" would be likely to look within the individual for explanations of why these reactions to work situations arise. Individuals would be studied for their tendencies to be "burnout prone" by the way they invest themselves in work. Studies like these occasionally suggest that individual characteristics influence adaptations to the stress of work situations.

The sociological framework focuses on the nature of dyads, groups, organizations, or the structure of situations in the social world as the "reasons" behind problems of interest. For example, a study of "burnout" from a sociological perspective would likely focus on how organizations and the structure of work influence the decreasing motivation of individuals and resultant intrapersonal symptoms of stress. An example of how social structures influence what one sometimes thinks of as personal factors, such as motivation, is portrayed in Kantor's study of work, *Men and Women of the Corporation* (1977). Even for sociologists who adopt a purely inductive approach to research, the basic nature of the concepts in the field, such as roles, networks, mobility, hierarchy, functions, power, and resources, are likely to influence what the sociologist "sees" in his or her unstructured observations.

An anthropological perspective would likely focus attention on the value systems, mores, traditions, and symbols of situations. Individuals are seen as being shaped by their attachment to groups and cultures which influence their behavior and cognition. A study of burnout from an anthropological perspective might emphasize work expectations based on group identities and cultural socialization. Burnout might be attributed to the conflict between one's value system as developed in a previous milieu and the values of the significant others in the immediate job situation. Kramer (1974) utilized the concept of "culture shock" to describe such situations for baccalaureate nurses in hospitals dominated by values other than those in which they were socialized.

In the absence of specific expertise in a contributing discipline, or a philosophical preference for the units of analysis, other considerations may be used to select this general framework. If the problem itself is practice oriented, it is probably wise to choose a level of analysis that reflects one's intervention capacity. For example, if a clinician is in a position of counseling individuals who are experiencing career crises and work burnout, it may be most salient to focus on individual issues that (1) make persons more or less suited for the work that has become problematic for them and (2) describe personal adaptations to stressful situations and means to alter one's style in this regard. If the investigator is in a position to change the work world, such as an administrator or a managerial consultant, the emphasis is likely to be on solving persistent problems of burnout by focusing on the problematic aspects of the work itself. This approach might point to such things as the structure of opportunities in the organization and identifying some of the physically or emotionally stressful aspects of the work.

The case study offers some advantages to other methods in regard to the units of analysis for investigation. In describing a case situation in its context, the researcher may choose to look beyond the immediate phenomenon to other elements of the system that appear to reflect on the problem. An example of such a case study is described in the later section, Comparing Levels of Interpretation in Systems.

The Conceptual Framework

In a survey of 25 years of *Nursing Research* literature, Batey (1977) found that the most substantial problems were not in the empirical or methodological phases of the studies but in the conceptualization of the problems. Even for the case study, which is sometimes thought of as a "loose" approach to research, the logic and consistency of the way ideas are put together substantially influence the credibility and utility of the work. In addition to identifying the substantive problem and the units of analysis, the clinician researcher needs to put intellectual energy into literature reviewing and *thinking* in order to frame the problem conceptually. Different research purposes, which will be reviewed later, put this conceptualizing at different stages of the investigation, but it is this work that distinguishes case study research from journalism.

The degree to which the theoretical framework dictates details of the problem for investigation and methodology depends on how specifically the theory can be applied to a research perspective. Most social science and nursing frameworks are not developed as a set of interrelated propositions (Jacox, 1974) even when they do seem to fit the clinical problem well. In these cases, the investigator may use the concepts identified in the theory as issues for exploration or as sensitizing concepts. Whether research proceeds from, or generates, a theoretical framework, the advance of knowledge about clinical problems is dependent on drawing theory and research together. It is important to remember, however, that theories are never proved. One can, through research, provide evidence that the theory is not incorrect. One may also demonstrate that it is inadequate to explain critical parts of a phenomenon or that it is incomplete. It is also possible to demonstrate that a theory is inaccurate.

The conceptual framework, meaning concepts and the relationships between them, becomes the lens through which the researcher chooses to view the world. The choice of a conceptual framework represents a type of "placing one's bets" in a given direction. The choice of a conceptual framework should be made after careful contemplation of what impact the choice will have on the problem formulation and data collection. Enough reading into the area should be done so that the researcher understands what the framework's assumptions are about the nature of man and personal or social pathology. In an expanded discussion of this problem, Diers cautions against "picking a theory and adopting it wholeheartedly, without tracing it back to its beginning and without carefully evaluating its fit to the problem at hand" (1979, p. 65).

Theoretical Purpose

What is meant by the term theoretical purpose is not the same as what question the study is trying to answer. The term refers to the *type* of knowledge that will be generated by the investigation. The ultimate purpose of any type of research is to generate some type of knowledge. The term theory is a way to communicate the idea of knowledge, but there are many types of theory that serve the general purpose of explaining. The question of what a proper theory consists of is a confusing matter in the social and behavioral sciences. Terms such as models, paradigms, taxonomies, typologies, and conceptual frameworks are confusingly used in the same context as the term theory in the literature. The process of scientific knowledge building uses all these forms, but in different ways and in different stages.

Axiomatic theory involves the manipulation of a set of interrelated propositions. These propositions are ordered by rules of logic as a method of explaining some class of empirical phenomena (Jacox, 1974). Research that is derived from axiomatic theory is considered deductive, sometimes referred to as theory testing or verification.

The ordering of phenomena is another purpose of science and some theories focus entirely on such classification. Others clarify developmental sequences or causal models. When "testing" theory is referred to, what is generally meant is that the theory is used to predict as yet unseen phenomena.

In another sense, theories may be applied in research when the investigator checks for similarity between the classifications of phenomena contained within a taxonomy and his or her own data. The sequence of events spelled out by a developmental sequence or a causal model may be compared with instances of the phenomena as documented by the researcher. What is being done in this latter instance is challenging the fit of the theory to the real world. Obviously, the more clarification of empirical observation that a theory can provide, the more "believable" it becomes.

Theory as knowledge is classified by Dickoff and James (1968) into levels, ranging from concept naming to prescriptive theory utilizing value systems. Diers (1979) describes corresponding types of research inquiry for each level of theory. Diers' framework is useful to the extent that it resolves some of the confusion around what constitutes "good" or "ideal" methodology by clarifying that the central issue of research design lies in the research purpose implied in the problem formulation.

While case studies are typically descriptive research aimed at developing insight and for generating theoretical perspectives by induction, they also may serve other theoretical purposes. The following discussion will provide examples of how case studies are used for a variety of theoretical purposes, such as sensitization, concept formation, testing the utility of conflicting theories, comparing levels of interpretation in systems, and testing hypotheses.

Description for Sensitization

Description, from the point of view of subjects, as an end in itself is the purpose of research guided by the philosophical orientation of humanistic phenomenology. There has been considerable advocacy for this perspective in nursing research literature recently (Oiler, 1982; Omery, 1983). The advocates of this research purpose are more concerned with an accurate representation of the world view and value orientations of their subjects than they are with whether or not the studies are labeled as scientific (Omery, 1983).

An example of a clinically relevant case study from such a perspective might involve the description of a family of refugees from another culture who are experiencing the stress of cultural displacement and physical survival. The clinician may set out to describe in some detail what the family's interaction patterns are, what their activities of daily living are, and how they interact with those from whom they acquire resources. Of particular concern would be how the family members interpret these situations. In such a study, the purpose would be to sensitize readers to the dilemmas and problems of the subjects from their vantage point. The clinician might do a parallel study of how those within the health care system who interact with the family perceive the family. Problematic encounters might be highlighted from either set of actors' point of view. The value of the study would be related to the accuracy of the portrait and the degree to which it presents new viewpoints to readers.

Denzin (1978) referred to the image of the mosaic to describe the scientific value of single descriptions of the world of individuals from the phenomenological perspective. He noted, "When any pieces have been placed, we can see, more or less clearly, the objects and the people in the picture and their relation to one another" (Denzin, 1978, p. 290). This viewpoint maintains that an understanding of the effects of such things as opportunity structures, deviant (or other) subcultures, and social norms can only be achieved through knowledge about how the situation looks to the actor, what he is contending with, and what alternatives he sees.

There are several variations of the phenomenological perspective among philosophers and social scientists. Three of them are described by Omery (1983) as having differing implications for research methodology. Despite some differences, the general implications of phenomenological studies are unique from other perspectives. These studies begin without prior theorizing or structuring of concepts. There is no expectation of duplication of behavior or perspective from repeated studies. Duplications may be found when subjects experience similar meanings or experiences but exactness of replication would be highly unexpected. Since data from any one study stand as a type of story or sensitization, seldom are generalizations attempted.

This is not to suggest that there are no hallmarks of good research from a phenomenological perspective. Lofland (1971) outlines several features of reporting on the lives of others that make such reports reasonable substitutes for personal knowledge acceptable to social scientists. First, the reporting is to be factual. This means one may not take literary license with reported material and should strive to verify what is believed to have occurred. Second, the researcher should have physical proximity with his subjects over extended time and variety of circumstances. He should have a social sense of intimacy with his subjects. Third, he should describe the reality of the setting and the people using restraint on initial interpretation. Detailed and mundane aspects of life should be included. Last, the researcher should allow the subjects to speak for themselves in the reporting. This means liberally using direct quotations, in context, in the descriptions.

Even using these guidelines, and despite the philosophical orientation in phenomenology regarding the suspension of prior theorizing, the description is never free from researcher interpretation. Therefore, the investigator should be explicit about whatever he or she can acknowledge about his or her perspective.

One way a researcher can be honest about unavoidable personal perspectives is to clarify for readers his or her particular interest in or value toward the topic. Having others provide critical questions about the data and any interpretation should also be useful in preventing systematic biasing of the data. Coobservation during interviews may help the researcher identify when he or she is leading the subjects into desired responses, which is not an atypical problem in interviewing (Truax, 1966).

Denzin (1978) reviewed the factors the researcher should incorporate into the life history study. The life history is a case study of an individual and his or her life situations through a narrative provided by the subject, as a type of phenomenological research. In doing such a study, no important facts or events should be slighted. However, the facts from the subject's viewpoint should be compared with other available evidence on situations. The subject's interpretations are to be reported honestly and in the context in which they were rendered. The researcher frames the subject's experiences by the questions that are of research concern, keeps the subject oriented, and tries to make the story relate to matters documented by other sources. Denzin's approach thus tempers a purely phenomenological approach with checkpoints from other versions of the same "reality." In these ways, the life history researcher differs from the novelist or autobiographer. The researcher who has specific questions surrounding the substantive concern has the difficult task of keeping subjects oriented to the questions while not leading their responses.

Case studies with the phenomenological perspective may use such data collection methods as observations, interviewing, and examination of artifacts or documents produced by subjects. Observation only would not suffice, however, because of the importance of having the *actor's* viewpoint on what is going on. Beyond that, the specific research problem focus and practical concerns of time, resources, and availability of written materials or subject-produced expressions are factors that dictate specifics of data collection.

The importance of keeping accurate records cannot be overemphasized in any case study reporting of this type. It is imperative to avoid the dangers of using recollection to restructure the researcher's perceptions. Several research texts provide examples of recording systems that have been useful to others (McCall & Simmons, 1969; Schatzman & Strauss, 1973).

Description for Concept Formation

The grounded theory method differs from the perspective of humanistic phenomenology even though both approaches are classified as qualitative research. The grounded theory approach begins with more assumptions about the social world, namely, that underlying processes or patterns exist in social interactions if one can but identify them. A library search before data collection and the use of sensitizing concepts are advocated. The emphasis in data collection tends to be on social (interactional) phenomena, or patterned relationships called structures, rather than on purely intrapsychic factors.

The most complete statement of research design to facilitate formulating concepts for predictions, explanations, interpretations, and applications to practice within the area of qualitative methodology is the work of Glaser and Strauss (1967). While the single case study as such is not the central thrust of the grounded theory perspective, individual cases are examined and compared in what is called a general method of comparative analysis.

Glaser and Strauss (1965) provided an example of this method in their study of dying in hospitals. The researchers first identified a problematic situation for the dying and their caregivers in hospitals: the sensitivity surrounding awareness and communication of an impending death. They then set out to identify settings where this awareness factor might be variable to see what effect this had on other aspects of interaction in the setting. They compared the general medical ward with the emergency room and the newborn intensive care with a geriatric nursing home. They also compared situations where the dying patients were young and attractive and where they were older with few social ties. Each comparison was explored to identify new meanings in the idea of social loss.

In the grounded theory approach, the comparison process stops when no new ideas or meanings are drawn from succeeding comparisons of cases or settings. This type of methodology appears to hold considerable promise for clinical researchers because of the potential for deriving constructs for applied problems. Studies from this perspective tend to require substantial time for completeness of data "saturation" to occur, and this should be planned for. It is also recommended that this approach utilize a team of researchers in order to profit from discussion and multiple observers' interpretations. Participant observation is heavily relied on as a data gathering approach, but many other methods may also be employed.

The issue of how to begin categorizing observations under a concept development, or grounded theory, approach can be problematic unless a value orientation or some noticeable regularity appears early in the study. Lofland (1971) proposes that some organizing schema may be helpful. He suggests beginning a study of the social situations by classifying observations as acts, activities, meanings, participation, relationships, and settings and moving from the more microscopic units (individual perspectives) to the more macroscopic (group or system) perspectives within each category. Within each of these six categories, the researcher may distinguish between whether his or her analysis is a static depiction or a report of phases or sequences through which a phenomenon passes over time. Some such system may then serve to order observations and to suggest other analytic approaches to data analysis. The resultant labels, taxonomies, or constructs may form the basis of propositions that may then be investigated as a form of theory.

Testing the Utility of Conflicting Theories

Another theoretical purpose of case studies is a cross between induction and deduction. Two or more theoretical models, or types of propositions about phenomena, may be applied to descriptive information in a case study and an attempt made to demonstrate which perspective provides the greatest explanation or reflection of the issues in the light of the facts accumulated. The result may be to eliminate one perspective as irrelevant to the type of problem described or to suggest ways in which the approaches may be complementary. Maurin's study (1980) of Western Birth Center is such a case study. She described the organizational development of an innovative, consumer-oriented health care setting run by nurse-midwives and a lay board. Data were collected by interviewing nurse midwives, board members, lay volunteers, and physicians in the community and by observation of group meetings and interactions at the center over an extended period of time. An initial purpose of the study was to explore the relevance of two perspectives on professional-organization relationships. Freidson's concept (1970) of "professional dominance" and the "Negotiated Order" framework drawn from symbolic interactionism as described by Strauss, Schatzman, Ehrlich, Bucher, & Sabshin (1963) were applied to the data. The midwives were observed to have strategies and ways of negotiating with their environment to get some of what they wanted in the way of resources and autonomy to direct their own health care delivery. They did this, however, not by negotiating over the norms in the professional community, but by finding ways to avoid them. The dominance of more powerful professional groups in the environment (physicians) was very important in restricting what the midwives could do. Negotiations within the organization between professionals and lay volunteers suggested that the professionals were advantaged whenever they held the material resources related to the organization under their control. Maurin found ways that each of the perspectives applied to the case study but also noted the limitations of the Negotiated Order Theory in specifying what some of the empirical factors were which limited negotiating. She also noted that a major question to ask in situations of negotiation is whether a less dominant individual or group could negotiate around the rules or *about* the rules themselves. The application of this type of approach to clinical issues utilizing case studies holds the potential of clarifying theoretical frameworks by contrasting their utility.

Comparing Levels of Interpretation in Systems

Case studies are sometimes the only way of describing interrelationships between levels in a system that on the surface do not seem to be connected. The analogy of ecological description comes to mind as a way to explain the theoretical purpose of studies that provide a demonstration of the way in which different "systems" interact. When something goes wrong in an organization or a group, unless a rather expansive description of the context of the problem is drawn, it is easy to miss the appropriate locus of the difficulty. This kind of study may be particularly useful for nurses, whose scope of concern includes the client, the client's family, and the management of the treatment milieu itself.

Maguire and Miller (1982) present this type of case study. Using an open system model of organizations, they presented the perspective that tasks, technologies, and organizational structures have the capacity to frustrate needs and arouse anxiety in participants. They describe a situation where patients of a different category (chronic schizophrenics) were introduced into a mental health center program, because of the financial needs of the organization. Before this, the client population had been mostly those with mild forms of social dysfunction amenable to psychotherapy. The therapists (mostly trainees) experienced considerable anxiety about safety and found themselves confronted with unsettling behavior from the new clientele. Supervisor-trainee sessions tended to assume an atmosphere of "emergency" requests for help by trainees regarding problems with the new clients. Supervisors, in turn, dealt with these emotions as manifestations of transference responses on the part of the trainees and tended to focus on the anger of the trainees as the "problem" to be resolved. What was ignored was the realistic anxiety of all the staff (supervisors included) owing to the generalized lack of experience of the entire system with new clients as system inputs. Due to their tendency to see problems as intrapsychic and personalistic, the staff missed the opportunity to develop a working culture based on realistic system problems.

Case studies of this nature are usually indicated when it is obvious to all that something is wrong in the system. When organizations are functioning well, it is much more difficult to see the interconnectedness of the levels. It is very important in clinical work to make appropriate assessments of system problems. To attribute problems to personal character, communication, or group processes which are substantially the result of alterations in other parts of the system results in wasted resources and personal frustrations.

Testing Hypotheses

Hypotheses used in case studies are most appropriately stated as theoretical and not statistical hypotheses. Generalization is made at the level of the logic of the evidence. Case studies may involve experimentation using hypotheses to predict relationships before data collection. Good experimental design is separable from the use of statistical tests of significance, in the opinion of Campbell and Stanley (1963). They note:

> It [experimental design] is the art of achieving interpretable comparisons and as such would be required even if the end product were to be graphed percentages, parallel prose case studies, photographs of groups in action, etc. In all such cases, the interpretability of the "results" depends upon control over the factors we are describing. (Campbell and Stanley, 1963, p. 22)

The important issue in a test of hypotheses is that the study must provide an opportunity for the facts to be contrary to what is proposed. This means that the case is selected prior to the expected events so that subjects are not simply selected as examples of positive findings after the fact or so that the findings cannot be attributable to incidental factors. Optimally, a longitudinal approach to the study is chosen where the researcher has the opportunity to watch the unfolding of events and to compare the results with what was predicted. Comparisons may also be made across time in the same individuals or between cases if several cases are used to test the same hypothesis.

An example of such a study might be the testing of particular therapeutic interventions on patient outcomes. An adolescent therapy staff may wish to try a milieu change and document the reactions of clients on a case by case basis. Comparisons might also be made of group phenomena, such as ward tension, or disruptive interaction. Since all the behavior would be unlikely to be completely predictable, a fairly complete set of descriptions under two or more milieu situations would constitute case comparisons. The comparison of outcomes under differing treatment approaches allows the hypothesis about any given approach to be challenged.

An example of using a case study to test hypotheses is Durand's study (1975) of a child with Down's syndrome and Failure to Thrive. The nurse proposed that under certain nursing interventions, the child would change in specific areas of development, in sleep measures, and in weight. Measurements were taken at the point of beginning the study and at the termination of hospitalization. The report highlights the importance of accuracy of observations and reporting. Durand notes the importance, also, of having enough control of concurrent events during an experimental hypothesis-testing case study to avoid confusing the client's responses to the intervention with other issues.

If multiple cases are to be examined, randomization procedures to select them should be considered. This would reduce the likelihood of individuals occurring as subjects who only reflect a verification of the hypothesis.

In the case of testing correlational (nonexperimental) hypotheses, the researcher needs to use multiple cases to allow for the possibility that the factors or processes identified are absent or other than what was projected. There is a decision to be made at this point between a case study approach and correlational research. The reason for utilizing case studies is that intensity of data collection is possible and complex interactions may be documented in detail. If the researcher has identified very discrete variables and is attempting to correlate them with some factor or process that is also operationalized, he or she may be better off abandoning the case study approach and selecting instead a larger sample with less intensity of data collection. This is particularly likely to be wise if the hypothesis *itself* is central to the investigator's concern. Sometimes hypotheses are set out at the beginning of a study to direct inquiry but researchers are perfectly willing to abandon them in the field if they see that they were shortsighted in some way or that they somehow missed the point of what was critical to the phenomenon. When hypotheses are used in this way, the case study method provides the benefit of offering other insights about the problem by providing much alternative information that can be explored.

SPECIAL PROBLEMS OF EX POST FACTO CASE STUDIES

Case studies are sometimes undertaken after the fact (ex post facto) when it has become clear that the unfolding of events was significant in some theoretical or practical way. This is likely to be the case in instances of suicide or problematic behavior of psychiatric clients or staff. Organizational crises are not always predictable to those inside the system. Obviously, we cannot simply ignore the analysis of these kinds of events and they are frequently the very things we are most anxious to have information about to increase our likelihood of being able to see them coming. This poses a problem for research in terms of data collection and interpretation.

As much as possible the original participants in the situation should be contacted to avoid second and thirdhand interpretations about events and perceptions. Organizational records, personal documents, films, and other types of expressions (such as drawings or poems) may provide data about past events and feelings. In the ex post facto data collection process, it is especially important that interviewing of principals or observers be broadly based. Since the researcher has to rely *entirely* on how others describe the facts, he or she has no way to judge the facts other than to compare reports of a wide variety of people who are likely to have differing perspectives.

A way to guard against selective interpretation of past events would be to view these investigations as having two stages. The first stage would involve the careful description of all that can be gleaned as information about the situation(s). Organizational and historical contexts should be included if possible. When a hunch is developed about one case, or several cases, the second stage of the investigation could be designed. Selection of cases for this next stage could then proceed as described for hypothesis testing. The factors or situations believed critical in generating some problem, or substantially contributing to it, could be the basis on which new cases for exploration were selected. One would try to find instances where those factors both were and were not present and compare the subsequent course of events in the comparative cases.

An example may serve to clarify these steps. Mestrovic and Cook (1982) described several case studies of suicides drawn from a mental health center's files. The researchers noted that many of the clients had experienced what was termed "loss of access" to treatment prior to their suicides. To logically argue that "loss of access" is a substantial factor in suicides, it must next be demonstrated that those without "loss of access" are not equally successful in suicide. This assumption would allow for checking the possibility that the subjects studied had something else in common that was equally likely to have been impacting on their suicides. One might try to identify cases of "loss of access" situations where no suicides occurred in order to clarify the issue. One might also compare the suicides from the center's files with those from another institution, or from the coroner's office, selected on some random basis, to investigate what role the treatment institution appeared to play, either in terms of recency of contact or degree of involvement.

LINKS BETWEEN LARGE SAMPLE RESEARCH AND CASE STUDIES

Thus far, the discussion has focused largely on qualitative case studies. Case studies also may serve as an adjunct methodology to quantitative studies using large samples. Frequently in quantitative analysis, there are subjects or cases of events that fall on the far ends of the measurement continuum. Sometimes, cases do not fit the model of the majority of cases in terms of the explanation provided by the independent variables. In such instances, the researcher is at a loss unless he or she can find a way to investigate the atypical cases. These subjects or situations may be reinvestigated with a case study approach to facilitate developing a more thorough explanation. This type of analysis is called "deviant case" analysis (Kendall and Wolf, 1949). Substantial theoretical insight has been developed from the study of instances where existing theoretical formulations simply did not fit a select group of cases.

Another type of relationship exists between large-sample quantitative studies and case studies. Sometimes a relationship between types of events is verified through statistical analysis but the researcher does not really understand what the dynamics of the situation are. An example of such an identified issue was reported in a study of imitative suicide (Bollen and Phillips, 1982). The authors were able to establish that there is an increased incidence of suicide up to 10 days following a major news report of suicide. They concluded that it would be valuable to study case histories of individuals who commit suicide after a publicized suicide to determine in what respects they differ from those dying in a time period without publicized suicides. Such studies would provide a vehicle for understanding the imitative process. This type of information would be very valuable for clinicians working with suicidal clients in order to recognize potential problem situations.

ETHICAL ISSUES IN CASE STUDY METHODS

The more critical ethical issues surrounding case studies are those of confidentiality of data and the anonymity of the subjects. Since the data collection is likely to be very extensive, it is possible that areas of sensitivity and conflict could prove injurious to the subjects if their identities were known. This issue has substantial bearing on how subjects are selected and the nature of the contract made with them about the study. The researcher must assess whether any reporting of information about the subjects, even in professional journals, would seriously jeopardize them. This injunction applies to groups as well as to individuals. Frequently, the type of groups that are accessible to intensive study are those that are relatively powerless vis-a-vis the researcher or other care-givers. The researcher should exercise judgment about exposing secret and extensive information about such groups that make them even more vulnerable to manipulation, control, or deprivation. The last "hold out" for powerless people (the elderly, the institutionalized, the economically deprived) is to keep people in control at bay by withholding information from them. Even in the interest of professional knowledge, the researcher should deal with his or her conscience and peers, and anticipate how to protect the vulnerable when the information may be used by others.

Whenever possible, individuals and groups should be camouflaged when reporting to protect their identity. Pseudonyms are generally used, even for organizations, unless the situation is so innocuous or so obvious as to make it unnecessary. Field notes should be protected from scrutiny by others except for those associated with the analysis.

Another consideration in intensive research on individuals or groups is the nature of the contract made with subjects before data collection begins. Informed consent as a concept applies to the case study situation whenever individuals, groups, or situations are discernible, even on an ex post facto basis. The researcher should decide in advance of the study how much of the information and analysis will be shared with the subjects. This is delicate information in some instances, particularly with psychiatric clients. It would be wise to discuss this issue with others involved in therapeutic relationships with the client to arrive at a consensus about what would serve the client's best interests. In the solicitation of consent, the researcher should make clear what his or her plans are for publication or dissemination of the information.

A last consideration has to do with whether or not the subject of an intensive case study deserves any financial remuneration if the author is successful in selling the work about that individual. The issue may apply to groups as well. This issue is not often addressed by professionals, who seem to hold the assumption that intensive information about a client belongs to them as a type of personal property. Undoubtedly, either a pro or con position could stir considerable debate in professional circles.

IMPLICATIONS FOR THE PSYCHIATRIC MENTAL HEALTH NURSE

Case study research provides the thoughtful clinician with a vehicle to document important clinical insights and share them with others. The importance of such an enterprise cannot be overemphasized, both for the future of nursing and for the advancement of therapeutic goals for clients. Nurses need the opportunity this approach provides to explore problems of the care system that form the context for their client involvement and that define client problems. By examining the context of problems, nurses are less likely to become prematurely settled into inaccurate or incomplete assessment of where problems originate.

Mental health service settings are ideal for case study research in that the client relationships are usually over an extended period of time and in sufficient depth to facilitate data collection. Longitudinal development or process issues can be documented in narrative form, which makes findings easily understood by others.

At times, case study research is the only practical way for clinicians to study a problem. There may be only one or a very small number of organizations, situations, or individuals in a category. The process under investigation may be so involved that attention can only be given to one such situation with reasonable thoroughness. Sometimes, unfortunately, limited permission for nurses' access to clients for research purposes dictates an intensive rather than extensive approach.

This approach is not for the fainthearted, however. Faulty conceptualization can be easily noted when presented in reports that are not clouded with statistical complexity. One needs to be prepared for the rebuttal case to appear in the literature that challenges one's initial conceptualization. Case studies also tend to require a major investment of time and energy. The beginning researcher would be wise to solicit supervision in the process of carrying out initial studies. Even experienced researchers need to expose their procedures and analysis to colleagues for critique during the process of the research.

The terms researcher and clinician have been used interchangeably throughout this chapter. The standards that psychiatric mental health nurses have set for themselves make it clear that that is what they intend their work to involve. The excitement of discovery and colleague interaction over ideas provides rewards for the clinician incorporating the researcher's stance into his or her work. The astutue clinician has a wealth of material at hand to facilitate the effort.

SUMMARY

The appropriate research method is determined by the question being asked. Many questions asked about psychiatric mental health nursing phenomena will require research methods suited to testing of hypotheses and the ability to generalize. However, in this clinical specialty concerned with the experience as perceived by individuals, there are also questions very appropriately explored with the case study method.

This chapter has discussed the case study method, its purposes, and the important issues in its implementation. Psychiatric mental health nurses committed to thoughtful inquiry into their clinical practice have much to gain by its utilization.

REFERENCES

American Nurses' Association. *Standards of psychiatric and mental health nursing practice.* Kansas City, MO: American Nurses Association, 1982.

Bateson, G., Jackson, D., Haley, J., & Weakland, J. Toward a theory of schizophrenia. *Behavioral Science,* 1956, *1,* 251–264.

Batey, M. Conceptualization: Knowledge and logic guiding empirical research. *Nursing Research,* 1977, *26,* 324–329.

Bollen, K., & Phillips, D. Imitative suicides: A national study of the effects of television news stories. *American Sociological Review,* 1982, *47,* 802–809.

Campbell, D., & Stanley, J. *Experimental and quasi-experimental designs for research.* Chicago: Rand McNally and Co., 1963.

Denzin, N. (Ed.). *Sociological methods: A sourcebook* (2nd ed.). New York: McGraw Hill, 1978.

Dickoff, J., & James, P. A theory of theories: A position paper. *Nursing Research,* 1968, *17,* 197–203.

Diers, D. *Research in nursing practice.* New York: Lippincott, 1979.

Durand, B. Failure to thrive in a child with Down's syndrome: A clinical nursing study. *Nursing Research,* 1975, *24,* 272–286.

Freidson, E. *Professional dominance.* Chicago: Aldine, 1970.

Glaser, B., & Strauss, A. *Awareness of dying.* Chicago: Aldine, 1965.

Glaser, B., & Strauss, A. *The discovery of grounded theory.* Chicago: Aldine, 1967.

Jacox, A. Theory construction in nursing. *Nursing Research,* 1974, *23,* 4–12.

Kantor, R. *Men and women of the corporation.* New York: Basic Books, 1977.

Kendall, P., & Wolf, K. The two purposes of deviant case analysis. In P. Lazarsfeld & F. Stanton (Eds.), *Communications research (1948–1949).* New York: Harper, 1949.

Kramer, M. *Reality shock: Why nurses leave nursing.* St. Louis: C.V. Mosby, 1974.

Lofland, J. *Analyzing social settings.* Belmont, CA: Wadsworth, 1971.

Maguire, T., & Miller, J. The professional culture of the mental health center as a defense against confronting organizational dysfunction: A case study. *Psychotherapy: Theory, Research and Practice,* 1982, *19,* 18–25.

Maurin, J. Negotiating an innovative health care service. In J. Roth (Ed.), *Research in the sociology of health care* (Vol. 1). Greenwich, CT: J.A.I. Press, Inc., 1980.

McCall, G., & Simmons, J.L. *Issues in participant observation.* Reading, MA: Addison-Wesley, 1969.

Mestrovic, S., & Cook, J. *Patient suicide and loss of access to treatment.* Paper presented at the meeting of the American Sociological Association, San Francisco, Ca., September, 1982.

Oiler, C. The phenomenological approach in nursing research. *Nursing Research,* 1982, *31,* 178–181.

Omery, A. Phenomenology: A method for nursing research. *Advances in Nursing Science,* 1983, *5,* 49–63.

Schatzman, L., & Strauss, A. *Field research.* Englewood Cliffs, NJ: Prentice-Hall, 1973.

Strauss, A., Schatzman, L., Ehrlich, D., Bucher, R., & Sabshin, M. The hospital and its negotiated order. In E. Freidson (Ed.), *The hospital in modern society.* London: Free Press, 1963.

Truax, C.B. Reinforcement and nonreinforcement in Rogerian psychotherapy. *Journal of Abnormal Psychology,* 1966, *71,* 1–9.

BIBLIOGRAPHY

Manis, J., & Meltzer, B. *Symbolic interaction: A reader in social psychology.* Boston: Allyn and Bacon, 1978.

CHAPTER 5

APPLICATION OF RESEARCH

Karen S. Babich

It is generally agreed that one of the major reasons for doing nursing research is to improve the quality of care provided to patients. Yet, as Ludemann (1979) points out, there seems to be a lack of language skills and mechanisms for facilitating the communication of findings to practitioners. This paradox between the purpose of research and the outcome is one that seems to plague all professions. Bridging the gap between those who produce the research and those who use the research is a problem that certainly is not unique to nursing but serves as a major concern to scientists, educators, and policy-making administrators. The most commonly held explanation for this gap is related to a belief that since the researcher and the clinician exist in their own worlds with their own values, language for expressing themselves, and reward systems, the communication gap between the two is inevitable and unsolvable. The researcher is guided by a search for causality and a cautiousness about generalizing beyond the data, whereas the consumer/clinician/policy maker needs immediate, specific information that pertains to his or her unique situation.

In an interesting article on information biases, Meltsner (1982) notes that this definition of the problem is deceptively simple and is based on a set of assumptions that are questionable. It is assumed by the clinician/consumer that the answers to complex problems do exist and that the researcher is just not able to communicate the information in appropriate language or through accessible channels. On the other hand, the researcher assumes that there are not political or organizational barriers to the clinician using the information. It is also generally assumed that the researcher and consumer do not have other interests and priorities, that the knowledge producers are interested in having their products "consumed," and that clinicians are interested in consuming knowledge that would benefit them.

An additional assumption that seems to be held by those measuring use of new information is that a linear relationship exists between producer knowledge and user utilization. That is, instruments developed to measure the transfer of information often assume that the information is in the exact same form as it was presented. Hence, a pre- and post-test design is used that does not give credit for information received that has been filtered through the consumer's experience and used in an altered form from that originally presented.

The questions of how, what, where, when, and why research is used are certainly of vital concern to graduate prepared nurses who are charged with the task of practicing nursing from a research base and developing and testing new knowledge and interventions. It is the purpose of this chapter to discuss the topic of application of research in the clinical area by focusing on four areas: (1) an overview of models of knowledge utilization and research on this topic, (2) research dissemination models used in nursing, (3) the clinical specialist's role as knowledge broker, and (4) techniques for improving dissemination of research findings.

MODELS OF KNOWLEDGE UTILIZATION

Defining the Concept

As a field of study, knowledge utilization is relatively new and suffers the growing pains of delineating exactly what is to be encompassed. It is clear that it involves both the creation and diffusion of knowledge as preliminary steps, but what constitutes utilization remains at issue. In addressing this concern, Weiss (1977) questions: "Is 'use' the adoption of research recommendation intact, the nudging of a decision in the direction suggested by research findings, the reinforcement of a likely decision by research, the consideration of research findings (even if these are overwhelmed by other considerations in the situation), rethinking the nature of the policy issue, redefining informational needs? What kind of use is 'real' use? And how much is enough?" (p. 213). Traditionally, researchers held the basic assumption that knowledge was used when it was implemented as a component of a program or led to a decision or course of action, the critical issue being that some specific measurable action had occurred (Larsen, 1980).

By the mid 1970s the term was broadened to include both the manifest (intended and recognized) and the latent forms (neither intended nor recognized), and then was further broadened to include types of utilization expanding beyond awareness of intended and unintended outcomes. Caplan, Morrison, & Stambaugh (1975) labeled these alternative forms of utilization as "instrumental" and "conceptual." *Instrumental utilization* applies to situations in which the subjects can cite and document the specific way in which knowledge is being used for decision-making or problem-solving purposes. An example of this form would be data obtained from course or workshop evaluations. *Conceptual utilization* refers to influencing a decision maker's thinking about an issue *without* putting information to any specific, documentable use. Thus, adding this category (acknowledging human thought processes as a component of knowledge utilization) meant that direct observation of the use of specific knowledge was no longer the sole or accepted method for measuring whether utilization had occurred. When knowledge utilization did not have to fit into a circumscribed set of predetermined variables and could include the consideration of research-based concepts and generalizations in formulating questions, setting goals, and planning activities, it greatly expanded understanding of the impact of research.

Of equal importance to understanding knowledge utilization is the examination of nonutilization. As with its counterpart, nonutilization can be conceived as intentional and unintentional. The potential user may consider the knowledge and deliberately decide not to use it, or, as in the case of conceptual nonutilization, not use the information in any obvious fashion. Larsen (1980) notes that the belief that all knowledge must result in an observable change and that nonutilization may be preferable to inappropriate utilization are recent refinements that challenge the inherent beliefs that utilization and change are good.

Based on the extensive work done by Havelock (1969), Rogers and Shoemaker (1971) and Zaltman (1973) on understanding how new ideas (innovations) are shared (diffused), knowledge utilization is believed to occur in the following stages:

1. Knowledge enters awareness and is judged on its own merits and against other information and factors (e.g., political, organizational, socioeconomic, and personal beliefs and attitudes).
2. It is implemented by the potential user (probably on a tentative basis).
3. It enters into general practice or policy.
4. It is integrated into an ongoing program so that its original identifying characteristics are no longer discernible (institutionalization).

Exactly how this process occurs and what relationship exists between the knowledge producer and the user over time has been represented by different models. The three general models described below encompass the views of most theorists in this field.

The Rational Linear Model

The *rational linear model* is perhaps the most common and well established model of knowledge utilization. It is based on the notion that one set of activities will naturally lead to another. This model, as described in Havelock's (1969) linkage model, Rogers' (1962) communication process model, and Bennis and colleagues' (1969) empirical-rational strategies model, assumes a linear transfer from knowledge producer to knowledge user in the following sequence: (1) a need is identified, (2) relevant information is presented, and (3) the information is used. The rationale underlying this model assumes that people are guided by reason and that they will utilize some rational method of self-interest in determining needed changes in behavior. It further assumes that users are relatively passive (Bennis, Benne, & Chin, 1969), and, if the researcher produces the "right" information, the linkage is made and the process can proceed to the next phase. As Larsen (1980) notes, an assumption is made that both researchers and users behave rationally and in predictable ways; thus, if relevant, understandable information is given, even from a remote resource person, chances are it will result in a decision to use it or not use it and eventual confirmation.

Although the belief that new knowledge occurs in an orderly process from research, to development, to use is now considered a naive approach and an incomplete picture of the process, it did (and still does) represent how a rather large portion of the research community viewed utilization. An example from nursing literature will help examine some of the difficulties and pitfalls of this model.

Application of the Rational Linear Model

In 1975, Ketefian designed a study to determine whether nursing research was helping to improve nursing practice. In particular, she wanted to know what happened with research findings that had been reported in journal articles. From nursing literature, she chose studies that met five criteria: (1) that the study would have been widely published, (2) that it had been in circulation for at least a five-year period to insure dissemination, (3) that the research would involve a likely nurse activity, (4) that it be reported in a manner readily applicable to practice, and (5) that the study had been replicated to assure validity.

She chose a series of studies by Nichols and colleagues on optimum measurement of temperature (Nichols, Ruskin, Glor, & Kelly, 1966; Nichols, 1967; Nichols & Verhonick, 1968). The research studies had been reported in *Nursing Research* and *The American Journal of Nursing.* Their studies suggested that the optimum placement time for rectal temperatures was two minutes when patients were in a 65°F (cool) room and three minutes in a 78°F (warm) room. Oral temperatures, however, should be in place eight minutes for men and nine minutes for women in a cool room and seven minutes for both in a warm room. Optimum placement was defined as the time needed for 90% of the subjects' temperatures to reach maximum readings (±.2°F).

Based on these studies, Ketefian devised an instrument to elicit information on nursing practice in determining oral temperatures. Of the 87 nurse respondents, only one knew the correct placement time for the oral thermometer, and this nurse used only rectal readings! The majority of nurses used oral temperatures but believed that rectal readings were more accurate.

Ketefian concluded her article by questioning why nurses practice in a routine manner if they do not believe they are taking the patient's temperature accurately. Her logic, however, suggests that the nurses were aware that the oral reading was inaccurate and hence were purposefully functioning against good practice. It is what Zaltman (1979) calls a *rationalistic bias,* meaning, what is rational and clear to you must also be rational and clear to the potential user. The first model, the rational linear model, assumes that people are guided by reason to accept the findings in toto, given that they are presented in a logical fashion. From the nurses' standpoint, even if they had known that their oral temperature readings were inaccurate, whether or not they would have changed is another question. It should be noted that nonutilization occurs for logical reasons also. It may be that the new innovation (e.g., taking oral temperatures for seven to nine minutes) would not be seen as cost-effective. That is, since the baseline from which they were determining increases or decreases in patients' temperatures was based on a three-minute reading, the additional cost in time to get the most accurate reading may not be worth it. A more exact reading may make more sense in a situation where temperature control was of prime importance, for example, in hypothermia. In normal situations, the exactness may not be necessary.

In efforts to establish a research-based practice, it would seem particularly important to be cognizant of some of the problems with trying to measure research utilization. The use of research findings in the clinical setting may not follow the linear course described or not seem to be logical, but it may still be the underlying base of practice. The assumption of a passive recipient of new information may have led researchers to incorrectly judge the effect of research on practice.

The User-Oriented Model

In this model, the user is primary and initiates use of information to interact with some decision or problem. The Zaltman, Duncan, and Holbek (1973) model, the Havelock and Havelock (1973) planned innovation model, and Carol Weiss' (1977) problem-solving model all emphasize the user system and its involvement in working out strategies of information utilization. As Weiss (1977) notes, all the models assume a decision-driven model of research use. That is, it is assumed that the policy maker and the researchers agree on the desired end and that the contribution of research will be the identification and selection of appropriate means to reach that goal. In a sequence of five steps, the researcher moves from defining the problem, to identifying the missing knowledge, to acquiring research data, to interpreting for problem solution, to making a policy choice. It is assumed that the end result will be a policy based on the research findings.

The basic notion underlying this model is a belief that change is a planned process with identifiable strategies that result in a predetermined goal. Thus, for Havelock and Havelock (1973) and Zaltman, Duncan, and Holbek (1973), heavy emphasis is placed on the role of the change agent in working with the user in defining and addressing the problem. From their work and that of others, (notably, Glaser, McKee, Watson, & Wrenn, 1972) sets of conditions in the environment (workplace) necessary for the acceptance of new ideas have been delineated. These factors, which will be examined in more detail later in the chapter, include looking at pragmatic aspects such as the credibility and practicality of the suggested changes in the work environment. This model assumes interaction between the researcher (or the change agent) and the potential user. However, it is linear to the extent that the model posits a sequence of stages that are followed when research is utilized.

The problem with this model is that it assumes that the users have a clear idea of the goals, acceptable alternatives, and the type of information that is relevant to their needs.

In truth, however, rarely are decisions the results of clear-cut choices and cooperative actions. More often they are formed from conflicts among individuals based on differences in interests, objectives, and perceptions (Weiss, 1977).

Application of the User-Oriented Model

In nursing, this particular model has received the most attention and the role of change agent is considered an integral part of graduate nursing practice. In both the Western Interstate Commission for Higher Education (Krueger, Nelson, & Wolanin, 1978) model for research utilization in nursing and the Michigan Conduct and Utilization of Research in Nursing (Horsley, Crane, Crabtree, & Wood, 1983) project, nurses were asked to define a nursing problem, seek out research and critically evaluate its quality and usability, and then apply the principles of planned change to introduce the research findings into practice. The models were built on the assumption that the research study selected was appropriate in addressing the need they had identified and that the "staff and/or administration" would be resistant to implementing the research findings. As will be noted in the next model of knowledge utilization, the heavy emphasis on one solution to the problem and resistance to change may have constricted the view of nurses' use of research.

The Interactive Model

The third model, and the one that is receiving the most attention currently, is the *interactive model.* It assumes that the user, the research information, and the situational context all have an influence on knowledge utilization. In describing this model, Larsen (1980) notes that research findings and generalizations are used to produce an effect when presented in the context of related research, beliefs, and political realities, all of which are relevant to the user. It is not the findings of a single study nor even a body of related studies that directly affect policy; rather, it is the concept and theoretical perspectives that social science research has engendered that permeate the policy-making process. Rarely can people cite a finding of a single research study that changed their behavior. Instead, the process works in the following manner: As a body of knowledge emerges, it accumulates and combines with data derived from other sources to define or redefine the issues. Nurses, like other social scientists, often fall prey to the belief that if they are not directly recognized as the idea source, or if their research findings are not accepted in the form they were presented, then they have failed to be heard.

Application of the Interactive Model

To test the belief that social scientists and decision makers exist in separate, isolated communities and view the importance of social research from totally different perspectives, Weiss and Weiss (1981) designed a study to address the issue of what factors are perceived as making social research useful for public policy. One hundred social scientists (principle investigators of grants and peer review team members) and 153 decision makers (administrators in mental health federal agencies and directors of clinical agencies) were asked to rate the importance of 26 different characteristics that make research useful.

There was general agreement between both groups that research studies were most useful for decision making in mental health when (1) they dealt with a topic of particular relevance to decision makers, (2) they examine variables that decision makers can do something about, and (3) the report is written clearly and is not overly technical.

The strongest disagreements between the groups concerned social scientists overestimating the role of political considerations and underestimating the importance to decision makers of the scientific merit of the research. The most important difference, however, was how they perceived *use* of research. Social scientists, not seeing direct application of their research, believed the problem to be that decision makers required (1) explicit recommendations with direct implications for a course of action, (2) a pragmatic focus on policies and programs, and (3) that it be compatible with the political view of the user.

Users, on the other hand, stated that they rarely used research in its pure form, but used it to bring new ideas to public attention, for framing or conceptualizing a problem, for keeping up with professional developments, for gaining information about other states or agencies, for legitimizing budget allocations, attacking established policies, or lobbying for new programs. What has been neglected by those studying research utilization is that there are multiple channels by which social science evidence and ideas may affect the behavior of decision makers. It is a multicausal, progressive relationship rather than a linear cause-effect.

Another important aspect of research utilization is the time dimension. From research conducted by Rich (1977), it appears that there are two waves or cycles of utilization. The first wave seems to occur when information is initially received and for approximately three months thereafter. Utilization in this wave is characterized by the flow of information upward through the decision-making hierarchy and the utilization of information is primarily instrumental. (*Instrumental* refers to cases in which respondents can cite or document the specific way in which they are using particular information.) The second wave of utilization generally occurs from three to six months after the information is introduced. The flow of information is primarily lateral or downward in the hierarchy with utilization primarily conceptual in nature. (*Conceptual utilization* refers to influencing someone's thinking about an issue without that person putting information to any specific, documentable use.)

Stated more simply, during the first three months after being introduced to a new way of doing something, most of the energy is directed toward convincing someone higher up on the decision-making hierarchy to use the new approach. This process requires that one convince others by quoting the research on why it should be done. After a three-month period, the idea/approach has gone through some transformations and is now considered to be the company's idea and the directive to use it moves from the boss downward.

The interactive model, then, can be used to examine the complexity of the process whereby research is translated into public policy. The process is not one of linear order from research to decision but a disorderly set of interconnections that defy neat diagrams. It should also be noted that research is only one part of the decision-making process, which also uses experience, political insight, pressure, social technologies, and judgement (Weiss, 1977).

RESEARCH DISSEMINATION MODELS IN NURSING

The WICHE Model

One of the first projects to systematically look at models for dissemination of research findings in the clinical area was the Western Interstate Commission for Higher Education (WICHE) Regional Program for Nursing Research Development (Krueger et al., 1978). This six-year project, funded by DHEW Division of Nursing, was designed to achieve two goals: (1) to create needed researcher role models in educational and service settings and (2) to provide a setting in which nurse researchers could develop a network for discussing and solving problems. To accomplish these goals, three series of workshops in different geographic areas in the West were developed. Each workshop followed a five-phase resource linkage model.

In phase 1, pairs or dyads of nurses from the same geographic area were selected to participate in the workshop. Dyads were chosen because it was believed that together nurses would serve as a unit of change and provide mutual support for the objective of incorporating research into the clinical setting. Once selection of the 133 participants was made, materials were sent to the teams for preparation for Workshop I. In the first series of workshops, the nurses were asked to define a nursing care problem that existed in their agencies and locate research helpful in solving the problem before attending the workshop. At the workshop (phase 2), they were helped by WICHE staff to locate other pertinent research and to evaluate the quality and usability of the research. Principles for management of change and strategies for coping with problems of risk-taking were taught. In addition, participants were asked to write plans for evaluating change and the effect of change on the health care system when the research findings were applied to the nursing care problem identified. During an interim period of five months, the nurse dyads were to implement their proposal for change (phase 3), and then report their progress back to the total group (phase 4). Throughout the project period, WICHE staff served as resource people to the staff providing encouragement and expertise.

One of the major frustrations noted by the WICHE staff in conducting this project was the lack of nursing clinical research and the difficulty that nurses in clinical settings had in gaining access to the information when it was available. In an effort to overcome this problem, they used three different approaches. In series 1, described above, a problem-solving (user-oriented) approach was used with the underlying assumption that, if a problem was identified, all possible resources could be used for its solution.

Because of the difficulties in locating research pertinent to the problems identified by the nurses, a second approach was used for series 2. Using the work of Rogers and Shoemaker (1971) on characteristics of innovations that are highly predictive for adoption, participants were instructed to identify research findings (rather than identify problems) that were new to them and that they believed would make a difference if used in providing client care in their setting. This second approach emphasized the importance of the social system in the adoption of an innovation. The essential components of this model include: (1) the users belong to a network of social relations that influence their behavior, (2) one's position in the network is a predictor of the rate of acceptance of new ideas, (3) informal personal contact influences the adoption process, (4) identification with a reference group will influence one's ability to adopt the new idea, and (5) the rate of adoption will follow a predictable s-curve pattern (Rogers & Shoemaker, 1971). Stated more simply, the ability to influence others to adopt a new way of doing something rests on the status and leadership of the innovator.

In the final series of workshops, the emphasis was again placed on the change agent (innovator), but, rather than asking the participants to find studies, three different bibliography packages with high potential for use (based on the other workshops) were presented to the participants. Thus, the last group served as "middlemen" in information exchange, or what Zaltman (1979) terms *knowledge brokers.*

Unfortunately, the difficulty in finding applicable research and other situational factors overshadowed the ability to determine which of the three models used was most successful in producing research utilization. Based on their experience with this project, the WICHE staff strongly believe that responsibility for reviewing, analyzing, and collating nursing research applicable to practice is the responsibility of the nursing profession, not of the individual nurse. This includes publishing research findings as well as indices of studies that have not been published (e.g., master's theses). In addition, they emphasize the need for rigorous, systematic analysis of research studies so that generalizations can be drawn and variables needing further investigation can be identified.

The CURN Model

Using a more literal translation of research utilization than is commonly held, the Conduct and Utilization of Research in Nursing (CURN) Project, funded by the Division of Nursing under the auspices of the Michigan Nurses' Association, developed and tested 10 nursing practice innovation protocols during their five-year funding period (1975–1980). In this project, research utilization was seen as a process of transferring specific research-based knowledge into actual clinical practice through a series of six distinct phases (Horsley & Crane, 1978). In the first phase, the use of research methods and planned change processes are directed toward creating an atmosphere for change and identifying specific patient care problems that have research-based solutions. The second phase focuses on evaluating the relevance of the research-based knowledge in relationship to the identified clinical practice problem, the organizational values and policies, and potential costs and benefits that would accrue from its use. The third phase is the design of the nursing practice innovation to fit between the parameters of meeting the needs of the clinical problem and not exceeding the scientific limitation of the research base. Though not seen as a replication of the studies comprising the database from which it is drawn, the innovation protocol does contain some of the rigor of the original investigation, including the use of most of the same dependent measures. However, it serves more the function of construct replication by allowing for validation of previous work, extending the findings (to the clinical setting), and offering an opportunity to test whether the methodology employed is relevant and feasible for clinical nursing (Haller, Reynolds, & Horsley, 1979).

The fourth phase is comprised of a clinical trial and evaluation of the innovation on an individual nursing unit, and the fifth phase is directed toward making a decision to adopt, alter, or reject the innovation under consideration. If the decision is to adopt the innovation, methods are developed for extending the innovation to other nursing units—phase six. In a later work (Horsley et al., 1983) a seventh step is added—developing mechanisms to maintain the innovation over time. In this step, institutionalizing mechanisms such as written procedures, incorporation of quality-assurance measures, and other methods are cited as techniques for increasing the likelihood of maintaining a new practice.

The written reports of both the WICHE Project (Krueger et al., 1978) and the CURN Project (Horsley et al., 1983) contain detailed descriptions of the procedures used in conducting their projects, copies of the instruments developed to evaluate research studies, guides for deciding the probability that the innovation will be used, and research utilization abstracts.

The NCAST Model

Since 1971, Barnard (1978), of the University of Washington School of Nursing, has been researching child-assessment techniques designed to promote early case findings and subsequent intervention/interaction by the nurse. Her findings suggest that measurements of the parent-child interaction and environmental stimulation are reliable predictors of the child's subsequent development. She developed four assessment scales that examine infant sleep patterns, behaviors, interactions with care-givers, and the environment and made these available for use by nurses throughout the country via the Nursing Child Assessment Sattelite Training (NCAST) Project.

The dissemination model used in the project was based on the diffusion-of-an-innovation framework of Rogers and Shoemaker (1971) and consisted of four components. (In this project, the researcher assumed some of the responsibility for the dissemination and utilization of the research findings.) The four interdependent and interacting components that comprise this model are (1) recruitment, (2) translation, (3) dissemination, and (4) evaluation (King, Barnard, & Hoehn, 1981).

Recruitment refers to identifying the target population one wishes to *recruit* as potential users of the innovation (e.g., the assessment scales). Initial efforts then are focused on finding nursing leaders in the community who will endorse the researcher's work or be part of the training group. King et al. (1981) point out that leaders are often the risk-takers eager to try new ideas *(innovators)* or *early adopters* who serve as role models for the *early majority* who are not considered leaders but who are willing to try new ideas.

Once the target population has been identified, the research findings must be translated into language and methods that are practical in the clinical setting. This information is then disseminated via written or oral presentations, and the effectiveness of the teaching methods is monitored through feedback to the presenters. In this particular model, participants are required to work with a preceptor to develop reliability in using the assessment tools. Thus, as participants become more knowledgable about the practical and theoretical aspects of assessment and integrate these tools into their nursing practice, they improve their ability to detect potential problems and to intervene. Likewise, the research improves because the data collected from the assessment tools is fed back to the researcher who can continue to refine and expand the variables related to health in children.

As noted earlier in describing the Rogers and Shoemaker (1971) model used in the series 2 workshop in the WICHE model, the importance of understanding the social system is a paramount factor in the success of the dissemination. The relationship between the change agent and the client's activities is interactive and interdependent.

WICHE Model II

A model used in a later WICHE project also warrants mention because it differed significantly from the other projects presented. In this project, Continuing Nursing Education to Improve Mental Health, funded by the Psychiatric Nursing Education Branch of the National Institute of Mental Health, topics pertinent to psychiatric nursing practice were elicited from clinicians. Workshops were designed to incorporate research applicable to the clinical setting, and experts in that particular area of pyschiatric nursing were selected to be knowledge brokers who would attend the workshop and then conduct similar workshops in their home states. In addition to the ripple effect produced by having the knowledge brokers presenting the new material to large numbers of nurses in both urban and rural areas of their state, efforts were made to disseminate the content of the workshops through monographs dealing with assessing violence in the health care setting (Babich, 1981), assessing the mental health of children (Babich, 1982a), and mental health issues in rural nursing (Babich, 1982b). A final publication of the project was *A Sourcebook: Research in Psychiatric Mental Health Nursing,* which was a compilation of unpublished research from master's theses, doctoral dissertations, and faculty studies (Babich, 1983).

THE CLINICAL SPECIALIST AS KNOWLEDGE BROKER

Thus far the focus has been on theoretical models and large, funded research utilization projects, but what about the role of the clinical specialist in serving as a knowledge broker of new information/ideas? The term *knowledge broker* refers to "persons actively concerned with having an item of knowledge (judged by some criteria as valid and reliable) accepted and used in some specified way by others. They are thus a type of change agent" (Zaltman, 1979, p. 85).

There can be little doubt that the clinical specialist is a key individual in improving patient care by defining clinical issues requiring systematic study and by testing new practices. Some will conduct research studies themselves, but all will be involved in some aspect of the evaluation and translation of findings to practice. The ability to evaluate the significance of the research in terms of its pragmatic implications for clinical practice and organizational soundness and/or the ability to translate the findings into a set of activities that can be taught to others are key aspects of the clinical specialist role.

Evaluating Research

The importance of evaluating research has been stressed but more from the standpoint of noting whether the research design and methodology meet specified criteria of "good research." While the emphasis of educators on familiarizing all levels of nursing students with research techniques is perhaps laudatory, it is also not without side effects that clinical specialists should be aware of either in themselves or in those with whom they work. One of the untoward side effects is that, rather than making one more skeptical of research, quoting research elevates one to the status of an expert. Nothing wins an argument like the line "I saw a research study done on that and it proved that. . . ." The other untoward side effect is that, rather than demystifying research, a few research courses can make one understand how little he or she really knows about research. At the same time, the socializing process in graduate education requires a perception of self as a researcher. Hence, there is a donning of the emperor's clothes and at the mention of research terminology there is a knowing shake of the head and an assumption that what is not clear must be above one's head yet something that one should know. It would be much healthier to question whether the research findings were naked or not.

In identifying which research is likely to be utilized by an organization, Glaser et al. (1972) identified nine factors that should be used in evaluating research. The nine factors summarized under the acronym CORRECT include credibility, observability, relevance, relative advantage, ease of understanding, compatibility, trialability, divisibility, and reversibility. *Credibility* refers to a belief on the part of the potential users that the technique suggested has been tried (and debugged) on a population similar to their own. If an institution with high status has used the innovation, there is a greater likelihood that it will be accepted. Also, if the new activity (innovation) can be seen through demonstration, is *observable,* there is a greater probability of adoption. It follows that technological innovations are adopted more readily than interpersonal innovation, but showing others the steps to use and reporting its success increases the potential of adoption.

The *relevance* of the particular innovation being suggested in addressing the problem as defined by the user is of extreme importance to its acceptance. Criteria for measuring relevance must be related to improving the operation in some manner. In addition, to make the change the new way must be seen as having a *relative advantage* over the old way. The advantage may be related to patient care outcomes, public relations, cutting costs, personnel satisfaction, and so on.

If the new innovation is presented in a clear and brief manner, there is a greater probability that the potential users will feel that they can master the new material or skill and thus will adopt it. *Ease of understanding* should be a major consideration in designing the teaching methods to be employed in sharing the innovation with staff.

The established norms, values, and practices of an organization should never be underestimated in their importance for the adoption of an innovation. The new idea or procedure must be *compatible* with the prevailing values of those expected to use it. Organizations, such as hospitals, are not necessarily homogeneous from department to department in their values and cherished ways of doing things. However, though the new innovation being introduced can deviate from established procedures, it cannot clash with the mission of the institution (Levine, 1980).

Innovations are more likely to be adopted if they can be first tried on a pilot basis or if they can be implemented in stages. The *trialability* and *divisibility* allow the individual or organization more freedom to experiment before committing themselves to a new procedure or plan of activity. Knowing that the decision to use a particular innovation is *reversible* also allows for experimentation with new ways of approaching problems.

In addition to analyzing these factors, the clinical specialists should ask a very basic question of research—so what? So what problem of significance to the clinical setting is being addressed in this study? So what difference does it make to the patients whether or not we try this? The issue of cost-benefit to the patient is of major concern in deciding whether findings should be implemented. The risk of implementing something that holds potential harm for the patient or institution is of course a serious concern. In thinking through the social consequences of an action, it may be helpful to recall the statistical outcome model presented in Table 5.1 (Monahan, 1980).

As noted in Table 5.1 there are four possible consequences that can occur. For example, if we were trying to decide the social consequences of using the NCAST screening tool in predicting healthy development in children, one outcome could be that we predict the assessment scale is correct in detecting early problems and in practice it turns out to be true (a true positive). Or we think some aspect will not be useful and in practice it is not (a true negative). Either of course is a desired outcome. However, it is important to weigh what would be the consequences if we thought the tool was useful but in practice it did not really identify those children who have problems (false positive). Is that risk major or minor? And, if it occurs, is there an easy remedy? On the other hand, what if it is a false negative—it is an excellent predictor of those who could be helped with early detection and we are not using it? Would that be a more serious error than assuming it had more value than it did? Questions such as these help the nurse and the staff with whom the nurse works make educated guesses about the consequences of new action.

Translating Research Findings

Research studies rarely come with a clearly spelled-out set of implications for practice. As King and his colleagues (1981) note, "When researchers are pressed to specify what these implications might be, they tend to become restrictive in their thinking and to cherish

Table 5.1 Four Possible Outcomes of Predictive Decisions

	Results in Clinical Practice	
Research Results	*Yes*	*No*
Yes	True Positive	False Positive
No	False Negative	True Negative

their specific findings as they stand. Whether these findings might be generalized to other populations is, to the mind of the researcher, simply another research question" (p. 164). Of the two, evaluating and translating research findings, the translation of findings into a usable form of practice seems to be more an art than a learned skill.

It is this art of being able to translate technical reports into plain English and being able to move beyond a general academic description of an issue to pull together specific policy recommendations that are prime characteristics of effective knowledge brokers (Nelson, 1982). The ability of the broker (whether researcher or someone else) to make the research come alive by using a storytelling format (presenting a theme with appropriate development of characters and their relationship to one another) increases the probability of the findings being used by those involved in policy making.

In writing research for publication, Tornequist (1983) gives a number of excellent pragmatic suggestions. Among them are: describe the data first. If you observed a difference between groups or a change, state what it was rather than bury it in statistical reporting. Tell whether the difference was statistically significant and indicate (in parentheses, preferably) how you tested for significance. The point that she makes, as do others concerned with research dissemination, is to make research readable and usable and save academic presentations for academic audiences.

As a final note in discussing techniques of disseminating research findings to audiences who are potential users, the importance of networks should be mentioned. According to Nelson's (1982) survey, informal networks were the single most important source of useful information to policy makers, ranking above all formal organizational sources. If one wants to know the state of the art, one calls someone who knows a professional expert in that area. For nurses wanting to influence the quality of care provided to patients, this means being part of networks that are concerned with these and related issues. It is important to be a part of nursing networks, but it is even more vital to develop networks outside of nursing if nursing research will have an impact on improving patient care.

SUMMARY

In this chapter, the focus has been on theoretical models of how new ideas or methods of doing something are transferred from the creator to the users. It should be clear to the reader that the original notion of a simple linear relationship between knowledge and use is instead a very complex relationship with multiple factors interfacing to affect the adoption or nonutilization of the innovation.

Four different projects on research utilization in nursing have been described. Each approaches its objectives and target populations from a different perspective. The success of any of the projects depends upon the standards by which it is measured. Should research utilization be measured by the numbers of people using a particular innovation (e.g., the child assessment scales) or the ability to use concepts derived from exposure to research workshops (e.g., an increase in numbers of researchers) or by the activities designed to create a climate for change (e.g., construct validity studies)?

The importance of evaluating factors in the environment to check for a CORRECT match between the findings and the innovation has been underscored throughout this chapter. Translating the findings into a usable form that allows one to measure the social consequences of the change has also been discussed. Lastly, it has been stressed that the ability to influence the quality of patient care rests not only on being able to do research, but on being a part of a number of networks that serve as knowledge brokers to those in policy-making positions.

REFERENCES

Babich, K. *Assessing violence in the health care setting.* Boulder, CO: Western Interstate Commission of Higher Education, 1981.

Babich, K. *Mental health issues in rural nursing.* Boulder, CO: Western Interstate Commission of Higher Education, 1982 (a).

Babich, K. *Assessing the mental health of children.* Boulder, CO: Western Interstate Commission of Higher Education, 1982 (b).

Babich, K. *A sourcebook: Research in psychiatric/mental health nursing.* Boulder, CO: Western Interstate Commission for Higher Education, 1983.

Barnard, K., & Hoehn, R. E. Nursing child assessment satellite training. In *Biomedical communications experiment using the communications technical satellite, symposium proceedings.* Washington, DC: National Technical Information Service, U.S. Department of Commerce, December, 1978.

Bennis, W., Benne, K., & Chin, R. *The planning of change.* New York: Holt, Rinehart & Winston, 1969.

Caplan, N., Morrison, A., & Stambaugh, R. *The use of social science knowledge in policy decisions at the national level.* Ann Arbor: Institute for Social Research, University of Michigan, 1975.

Glaser, E., McKee, M., Watson, G., & Wrenn, G. *Planning for creative change in mental health services: A manual on research utilization.* Rockville, MD: National Institute of Mental Health, 1972.

Haller, K., Reynolds, M., & Horsley, J. Developing research-based innovation protocols: Process, criteria, and issues. *Research in Nursing and Health,* 1979, *2,* 45–51.

Havelock, R. *Planning for innovation through dissemination and utilization of knowledge.* Ann Arbor: University of Michigan, 1969.

Havelock, R., & Havelock M. *Training for change agents.* Ann Arbor: Institute for Social Research, University of Michigan, 1973.

Horsley, J., & Crane, J. Research utilization as an organizational process. *Journal of Nursing Administration,* 1978, *8,* 4–6.

Horsley, J., Crane, J., Crabtree, M., & Wood, D. *Using research to improve nursing practice: A guide.* New York: Grune and Stratton, 1983.

Ketefian, S. *Translation of theory into nursing practice and education.* Paper presented at the Seventh Annual Clinical Sessions, New York University, School of Education, Health, Nursing, and Art Professions, New York, NY, 1975.

King, D., Barnard,K., & Hoehn, R. Disseminating the results of nursing research. *Nursing Outlook,* 1981, *20,* 164–169.

Krueger, J., Nelson, A., & Wolanin, M. *Nursing research: Development, collaboration and utilization.* Germantown, MD: Aspen Systems Corporation, 1978.

Larsen, J. Knowledge utilization. *Knowledge: Creation, Diffusion, Utilization,* 1980, *3,* 421–442.

Levine, A. *Why innovation fails.* Albany, NY: State University of New York Press, 1980.

Ludemann, R. The paradoxical nature of nursing research. *Image,* 1979, *11,* 2–8.

Meltsner, A. Information biases: Attitudes and expectations. *Policy Notes,* Institute for Research on Educational Finance and Governance, Stanford University, 1982, *3* (2), 7–8.

Monahan, J. The role of research in changing the legal system. In R. Price & P. Politser (Eds.), *Evaluation and action in the social environment.* New York: Academic Press, 1980.

Nelson, L. Bridging the gap between research and policy. *Policy Perspectives,* Institute for Research on Educational Finance and Governance, Stanford University, Spring, 1982, 1–4.

Nichols, G. Time and temperature. *American Journal of Nursing,* 1967, *67,* 2304–2306.

Nichols, G., Ruskin, M., Glor, B., & Kelly, W. Oral, axillary and rectal temperature determinations and relationships. *Nursing Research,* 1966, *15,* 307–310.

Nichols, G., & Verhonick, P. Placement times for oral thermometers: A nursing study replication. *Nursing Research,* 1968, *17,* 159–161.

Rich, R. Uses of social science information by federal bureaucrats: Knowledge for action versus knowledge for understanding. In C. Weiss (Ed.), *Using social research in public policy making.* Lexington, MA: Lexington Books, 1977.

Rogers, E. *Diffusion of innovations.* New York: The Free Press, 1962.

Rogers, E. & Shoemaker, F. *Communication of innovations.* New York: Free Press, 1971.

Tornequist, E. Strategies for publishing research. *Nursing Outlook,* 1983, *31,* 180–183.

Weiss, C. *Using social research in public policy making.* Lexington, MA: Lexington Books, 1977.

Weiss, J., & Weiss, C. Social scientists and decision makers look at the usefulness of mental health research. *American Psychologist,* 1981, *36,* 837–847.

Zaltman, G. *Processes and phenomena of social change.* New York: Wiley & Sons, 1973.

Zaltman, G. Knowledge utilization as planned social change. *Knowledge: Creation, Diffusion, Utilization,* 1979, *1,* 82–105.

Zaltman, G., Duncan, R., & Holbek, J. *Innovations and organizations.* New York: Wiley Interscience, 1973.

PART TWO CRITICAL DEVELOPMENTAL FACTORS

In Part Two, Standards I, II, and III of the American Nurses' Association *Standards of Psychiatric and Mental Health Nursing Practice* (ANA, 1982) are emphasized. This part focuses on the use of developmental theory as an appropriate component of the knowledge base required in data collection, assessment, and treatment planning for individuals of all ages.

Psychiatric mental health clinical specialists are constantly required to use their knowledge of the variety and vicissitudes of human development to understand and appreciate both the humanness and the uniqueness of each individual client. In Part Two are highlighted those aspects of development throughout the developmental stages and their relevance for advanced psychiatric mental health nursing practice. It is worth noting that despite the multiple authors and approaches, a common focus emerges in this part that examines human development from an interactionist perspective. All of the authors describe the mutual interaction between individual and environment and the importance of using this perspective for any type of intervention.

The historical, philosophical, and psychological origins of current child developmental models are examined in Chapter 6. Then developmental sequences that, although different, are highly adaptive are discussed. The author presents special developmental problems of childhood in terms of their identification, meaning, and purpose. The chapter is concluded with the implications of childhood developmental issues both for prevention and treatment and possible interventions are offered.

The complex, often confusing periods of preadolescence and adolescence are discussed in Chapter 7, in which are highlighted the impressive developmental strides made during this period, as well as the disturbances of development that are problematic for adolescents and their worlds. Some of the major adolescent problems including psychophysiological disorders, psychotic disorders and depression are presented. The discussion underscores the concept that knowing the dynamics of adolescence and its potential problems clarifies one's understanding of the issues of adulthood.

In Chapter 8, early and middle adulthood in terms of the relational or interactional developmental model are discussed. This model is particularly relevant to psychiatric mental health nursing's focus on the interactional nature of mental health and illness. Using the relational model, the major characteristics and challenges of these developmental stages, which provide opportunities for both achievement and potential problems for the individual, are identified.

A few of the myths that are prevalent about old age and their effects on the attitudes of health professionals and the general public are discussed in Chapter 9. The author provides insight into the nature and incidence of psychiatric disorders among the elderly despite the problems of measurement. Aging is viewed within the historical and societal contexts in which it is experienced.

Each of the authors in Part Two emphasizes a biopsychosocial model of human development in which the influence of the biological, the psychological, and the social are explored. The mutually interdependent influences at all developmental stages are highlighted. Taken together, the chapters emphasize the resiliency and flexibility in human development and a person's potential for change. The view that emerges is that there are many different ways to be a human being. This fact lends hope and help to clinicians and scholars who are seeking ways to assist individuals and families make adaptive changes in their lives.

CHAPTER 6 INFANCY THROUGH SCHOOL AGE

Mari Siemon

Child development can be characterized as an endless process of discovery and growth, stimulated by the question, "What is man?" From this question came others so old they are scrawled in caves and painted in cathedrals.

From the time humans first drew pictures on the walls of caves, poets, artists, and writers have marveled at the richness and intricacies of human beings. Scientists have reached similar conclusions from their studies of children using diverse perspectives. Because human beings are so complex, they cannot easily be defined, categorized, or predicted.

Recently, questions have been raised about whether current models of child development are too limiting for our complex society. Perhaps it is time to determine new directions for the future. The historical, philosophical, and psychological origins for current models of child development are examined in this chapter. Each framework has influenced in some way how society currently conceptualizes the developing child. In the chapter will also be explored current models of child development and their implications for pathology. Finally, directions to which the future may lead in promoting optimal development will be contemplated.

PERSPECTIVES ON DEVELOPMENT

Traditionally, scientific disciplines develop through a quest for knowledge. While child development shares many characteristics with other sciences, it has one significant difference that sets it apart. Rather than developing out of a desire for knowledge, child development grew as a result of pressure from social forces (Sears, 1975).

Historical Perspective

"Childhood" as a distinct phase of development is a relatively recent idea. For centuries, there was no awareness that the nature of children was essentially different from that of adults. Awareness of the historical antecedents of the modern concept of childhood is important to aid understanding of the directions taken in developing the idea that children are special people with unique needs. Emancipation for children was based on a series of historical conditions, assumptions, and trends which will be reviewed to assist our understanding of contemporary models of development.

Prevailing social and economic conditions kept early societies from recognizing the special needs of children. One barrier to the enhancement of children's development can be attributed to the prevailing belief that children were miniature adults or the property of adults. Children were dressed in imitation of adults and fully participated in adult life and work but without adult privileges, rights, or protection. During apprenticeship to learn a trade, they suffered extreme hardships and were subjected to the harsh discipline and cruelty characteristic of early authoritarian societies.

The Industrial Revolution, beginning about 1760, brought other forms of exploitation of children. Lacking public laws that defined and protected the rights of children, children were used and abused as sources of cheap and expendable labor. The social concept of specialized care for children required an ideological change, acknowledging children as separate and different from adults. Such ideas developed slowly.

The first movement in this direction came with the establishment of schools for children, creating a means of escape from the drudgery of daily life. In the 1700s, an emerging sense of need for an educated populace enabled children to move into a specialized role within society. Commitment to public education grew from the seeds of democratic thought, which would be an important force in liberating children.

The humanitarian movement of the eighteenth and nineteenth centuries further raised the status of children. A shift in societal values from authoritarianism to empathy and kindness occurred toward the end of the eighteenth century. There was reawakening of empathy toward the weak and helpless who had been mistreated and misunderstood (Sears, 1975). Orphanages were founded, and delinquent children were given care and help rather than punishment for their "wickedness." Recognition of the plight of children was further enhanced by the Factory Act of 1802. This act attempted to protect children from unsafe working conditions and to limit the kind and amount of work that could be expected of them. Compulsory education followed child labor reform laws and further safeguarded children's welfare by challenging the absolute rights of parents. Children could no longer be exploited for economic gain, but were compelled to attend school. Important changes in ideas about the rearing and education of children occurred in the nineteenth century. Enlightenment and the accompanying societal changes fostered both the desire and the social pressure to better the health of children and to improve their legal status and work conditions. For the first time, childhood was understood as a distinct developmental period and children as having special needs to be nurtured. The time was ripe for philosophers to think seriously about the nature of the child.

Philosophical Perspectives

Philosophers have studied the nature of humans and their freedom to become what they will. Through the centuries philosophers have questioned: Is man basically good or evil? Are children born with predestined personalities, or are they molded by parents and society? It is a truism that how children are understood and raised is profoundly affected by the dominant philosophy of a given period?

The enlightened attitudes of the humanitarian era paved the way for the redefinition of childhood by Jan Amos Comenius (1592–1670), an educational philosopher and realist. Comenius proposed ideas that were a radical departure from the currently held beliefs that children were miniature adults. He believed that children went through stages of development and advocated education based on development (Lugo & Hershey, 1974).

Redefining the nature of children was further enhanced by the philosopher and empiricist John Locke (1632–1704). He challenged the Puritan belief in the inherent wickedness and depravity of children, releasing them from ideas of demonic origins and control. Locke proposed a new perspective, suggesting that a child's mind was a "tabula rasa" waiting to be inscribed with a life pattern by experience.

The idea that change was possible was reinforced by the American Revolution. Independence as a nation brought the promise of self-fulfillment. This concept, coupled with the spirit of humanitarianism that was spreading across Europe, resulted in a hope for a better future and a belief that people could improve their lives. Such a spirit was reflected by Jean Jacques Rousseau (1712–1778). Rousseau regarded childhood as a time important in itself. A romantic and a naturalist, Rousseau supported the idea that children were born essentially "good," free of original sin, and products of nature with unsuspected possibilities. He saw the child not as a passive recipient of instruction, but rather as an active explorer of the world with an innate, unique nature that must be understood so that education could respond to individual needs.

Humanitarianism, combined with technical and scientific advances which occurred between 1830 and 1880, gave rise to the vision of Charles Darwin (1809–1882) that humans were infinitely perfectable. Using observations of his own child, Darwin saw children as representations of the species' capacity to perfect itself by selection.

In the latter stages of the era of humanitarianism and technology that spawned Darwin's ideas, the pragmatist John Dewey (1859–1952) proposed other ideas that profoundly influenced both education and parenting practices. Dewey deplored the idea of stereotyping and believed in the uniqueness of the individual. Above all, he valued the ability to think and to cope with a changing environment in a flexible way, advocating positive and internal discipline rather than blind conformity out of fear (Lugo & Hershey, 1974). Thus, the prevailing attitudes on the nature and treatment of children were modified dramatically by avant-garde individuals who championed the idea that children had unique natures and special needs. Philosophical recognition of children's rights and emphasis on childhood as a time important in itself paved the way for psychologists to identify forces that affected growth and development.

Psychological Perspectives

Modern child psychology was spurred by the ideas of early leaders such as Comenius, Locke, and Dewey. The first attempts to understand mental development of children by Preyer in 1882 and G. Stanley Hall in 1883 were landmarks in the development of child psychology. The Humanistic Psychology movement made other significant contributions to the study and understanding of children. Based on existential philosophy, humanists believe in understanding the uniqueness of individual responses rather than determining predictive patterns to which all persons conform. Humanistic psychologists opened the door for the direct study of human behavior through their belief that animal analogies were inadequate to explain human behavior.

Since its inception, child psychology has broadened and expanded, overlapping with other disciplines. Its focus continues to be on the biological, social, cognitive, and affective forces that interact to shape behavior. A multitude of psychological theories have resulted that have helped to identify variables that promote or hinder growth and maturation, shape theories of child rearing and guide prevention and treatment programs. The ultimate goal of child psychology has been to help children achieve their full potential.

APPROACHES TO CHILD DEVELOPMENT

For years, theoreticians in child development have searched for a framework within which to direct research and describe the nature of the developing child. Modern theories of child development emerged from the ideological conflict between nativistic beliefs that each child has capacities that unfold in a unique way and empiricist beliefs that a child's behavior can be modified through learning and environmental manipulation.

Nativism and Empiricism

A constant action-reaction cycle occurs over time that stimulates research. In the mid-nineteenth century, John Locke's empiricist views were challenged by Darwin's nativism.

More recently, a resurgence of empirically based research on early childhood education and the use of social systems to enhance a child's capacities has reactivated nativistic research on stages of cognitive development and genetic contributions to intelligence (Sears, 1975). The fact that neither empiricism nor nativism alone is enough to explain the determinants of child behavior maintains the debate. Since World War II, the conflict between these ideological positions has given rise to three major trends in child development.

Nature Versus Nurture

One of the ways in which the nativism-empiricism debate has been expressed is in the controversy over the influence of nature versus nurture on development. The earlier moral philosophical idea that people were born evil was later partially subsumed in the nature-nurture conflict through debates regarding whether genetic endowment or upbringing determines the limits of a child's achievement.

A principal issue in child psychology was, and continues to revolve around, the question of intelligence. Binet's development of the intelligence test gave strong support to the nature hypothesis. Assumptions were made by many that the poor and members of minority cultures were innately of lower intelligence. Such stereotypes contributed to a self-fulfilling prophecy for thousands of children who became tracked into curricula with goals for those with lesser abilities (Chess & Hassibi, 1978). Similar assumptions about other human attributes have been used to justify sexual and racial discrimination.

Since no conclusive evidence can be offered supporting either side, most professionals today hold that neither position has exclusive control. Growing recognition of the plasticity of development has modified the rigid positions that characterized debate in the past. Currently, an understanding that a child's personality and intellectual capacities are affected at each stage of development by the interplay of heredity and environment is the more generally accepted view.

The conflict regarding the relative contributions of nature and nurture has broadened to related issues: What influences have the greatest impact on a child's development? Which years have the most profound influence on determining a child's future abilities? Research on bonding in the last decade challenged the accepted ideas that the first three years of life were crucial to development or that infancy is *the* critical period. A more recent belief holds out for a more optimistic "second chance." Growing knowledge of the concept of vulnerability has lent support to the idea that children can adapt and learn, offering the promise of positive and corrective change (Anthony, 1974; Thomas, 1981).

Active Participant Versus Passive Recipient

The nativism-empiricism conflict also debates whether the child is an active agent or a passive object. For many years the presumption guiding childrearing practices and education represented infants as psychologically incompetent and incapable of organizing or influencing the world. They were thought to exist in a state of confusion and disorganization until the regularity of experiences provided by parents brought order to the chaos (Schafer, 1977). More recent evidence points to the contrary, and the trend is toward nativism. There is a greater understanding and respect for the innate and uniquely individual aspects of neonates' social functioning and their ability to influence their care. New knowledge has stilled the older question of when infants change from a biological to a psychological organism. They are both at birth. They need nothing more to become human because they *are* already that at birth (Thomas, 1981). Growth is a continual interaction and mutual exchange between infant and caretakers, with infants actively participating in screening stimuli and signaling needs.

Stage Theory Versus Continuity Theory

The nativism-empiricism conflict is also expressed in whether developmental models should be based on fixed stages or continuous process. The nativistic approach of stage theories constitutes the bulk of child development research (Erikson, 1963; Freud, 1949; Gesell, 1940; Kohlberg, 1964; Piaget, 1963). Implied in stage theory is the idea of a "critical period" for acquiring a skill. Research on intelligence illustrates the devastating consequences that can come as the result of rigid adherence to stage theory. Despite early research that intellectual ability can be influenced by environmental stimulation at various ages, there was no immediate reversal of the inequities in educational settings. Rather, the pessimistic idea prevailed that environmental stimulation needed to occur before a specified age or it was ineffective. The result was the belief that children from environmentally deprived backgrounds were doomed to inferiority. Eventually, a more enlightened attitude prompted the development of the Head Start Program to enhance opportunities for children to achieve their potential. Historically, stage theories have contributed to anxiety in parents who religiously track their child's development and become alarmed when he or she does not achieve the expected landmarks at the specified times.

In recent years, the trend in developmental and educational psychology has been away from stage theory. Rather than using a linear model, which is limiting and nonindividualized, the trend is toward looking at the *process* of development through an interactional model. How the developing child interacts with and is impacted by the environment is the current focus of developmental theory and research. Interest in stages of development has been replaced by a more empirical interest in the interplay between biological, psychological, and social processes as they uniquely combine in each individual. The debate between proponents of nativism and empiricism stimulated a shift from the social learning theories of the 1940s and 1950s to an emphasis on cognitive stages and genetic determinism of sex and race difference in the 1960s and 1970s. A reversal has again occurred in the 1980s with social learning theories enjoying increased popularity.

The empiricist direction in which child development is moving is both exciting and familiar to nurses. We have traditionally emphasized the person-environment interaction, working with each individual as a unique entity and as a part of a larger system.

THE TWENTIETH-CENTURY CHILD

Historically, the twentieth-century child can be understood as the product of centuries of economic, religious, educational, and technological upheavals. Moralistic and authoritarian models of child development were replaced by democratic and humanitarian theories. Advances in knowledge have enhanced models of care and parenting. Eliminating barriers to health and enabling children to reach their full potential fostered gains in prevention. Trends in the fields of sociology, anthropology, and psychology may provide a perspective for the future. Briefly, let us consider those ideas that have emerged in recent years that illustrate trends in child development and that may serve as an impetus for future directions.

Contemporary Trends in Sociology

A sociological perspective integrates information from history, philosophy, and anthropology to describe the social influences that affect beliefs, values, and prejudices. Although causal relationships are elusive, it is important to understand the complex interaction of many variables that impact and shape a child's life.

There are many forces that provide the backdrop against which the child grows: genetic, physiological, and environmental. Interacting with these variables, the child develops answers to such questions as: Who am I? What is of value to me? Am I of value? What opportunities does life hold? Answers to these and other questions influence the emerging personality of the child and help shape individuality.

An influential addition to our understanding and treatment of children came from Havighurst (1953), who identified socializing tasks of children within a developmental framework. In addition to the traditional focus on the family as the socializing agent, Havighurst suggested that education plays an important role in socialization, providing a means of social mobility by which people could positively change their economic and social status. Havighurst's ideas have contributed to the modern concept of plasticity in development.

Increased understanding of the complexities involved in each child's development has also lent a new perspective to the process of socialization. Currently, socialization is viewed as a means of *promoting* innate tendencies rather than of *transforming* a child from an asocial to a social being. This view of fostering innate potential has brought about increased recognition of the role the milieu plays in supporting or inhibiting a child's readiness for skill attainment.

The milieu's impact on socialization has also led to the identification of deviant patterns of socialization. According to deviance theory, children raised by a group who ascribe to mores that differ from the major population, such as professional thieves and racketeers, follow patterns of socialization that are deviant rather than pathological. Such children are considered to be dissocial rather than antisocial because they have identified with a group's norms and have essentially intact personality structures. Although these children are psychiatrically normal, they display behavior that is outside society's norms. Such behavior is thought to be a product of their culture rather than inherent to the child (American Psychiatric Association, 1981).

One of the more controversial aspects of sociology is the area of sociobiology. Applying the results of animal studies to human development, sociobiological research has returned full circle to genetic determinism. Sociobiologists hold that many aspects of social behavior are the result of genetic rather than environmental influences (Barash, 1977; Wilson, 1975). As might be expected, their assertions that altruism, incest taboos, and certain phobias are genetically determined have evoked criticism from a variety of disciplines. Such ideas do have some compelling attributes. As Thomas (1981) points out, genetic transmission theories are useful in explaining the recently acknowledged capacity of newborns for social behavior. Sociobiologists state that since social behavior in newborns precedes experience, it is the result of biological programming. Newborn social behavior is seen as an adaptive response retained through natural selection that is necessary for bonding to a caretaker. Criticism of sociobiological theories focuses on the emphasis placed on genetic inheritance rather than on learning and experience to describe complex social functioning.

Contemporary Trends in Anthropology

Ethology, a new branch of anthropology, has impacted on child development. Like sociobiology, ethology has also extrapolated from animal studies to human behavior, emphasizing instinctual drives and fixed patterns of action. Ethologists have also emphasized the permanent effects of early life experience, asserting there are "critical periods" for learning after which a child cannot make up deficits. This assertion is closely related to the sociobiological belief of biological programming. Recent research which recognizes the adaptability of children has cast these ideas in doubt (Thomas, 1981).

Contemporary Trends in Child Psychology

The post-World War I years of the 1920s were energetically directed toward healing. Well-baby clinics, child guidance clinics, and school health programs were established. Child development as a separate focus of study was born in this enthusiasm, with research in personality development stimulated by the emergence of psychoanalytic theory. Major advances in child psychology profoundly increased our understanding of how to nurture and enhance a child's development. These advances included (1) acquiring normative data on development; (2) understanding the role of play in development; (3) a changing view of the neonate from a disorganized, psychologically incompetent being to an organism capable of structured learning and perceiving; and (4) developing concepts of risk and vulnerability.

Normative Data

Little was known at the beginning of the twentieth century about children's behavior, interests, abilities, motives, or capacities. Binet and Simon made a significant contribution in 1907 by identifying children not capable of regular schoolwork. Their research sensitized psychologists to the relationship between thought processes and mental age and provided a substitute for moral blame. For the first time there was a measurable aspect of a child that accounted for differences in ability (Anderson, 1956).

Research in the years following World War I focused on collecting data to answer the question: "How do children normally behave at different stages of development?" The initial normative question of "How?" was then expanded to "What is the sequence of a child's development?" Piaget (1963), Erikson (1963), Freud (1949), and Gesell (1940) contributed their research to answering this question. Today, research addresses the more complex problem of: "Under what conditions do children behave in given ways?" For the past two decades, the influence of environment on the acquisition of skills has dominated normative studies.

The Role of Play in Development

Only in relatively recent history have games and songs specifically for children been developed. Since 1900 there has been increased recognition of the importance of play in growth and development. Classical theories of play viewed the specific *content* of play behavior as incidental to the *cause* of play. As a result, they provided an inadequate reference for understanding the significance of particular types of play (Herron & Sutton-Smith, 1971). Developmental theories of play provided a way to understand the content of children's play (Erikson, 1976; Freud, 1949; Piaget, 1962). Only during the past 50 years has play been understood as a biological imperative. When play is arrested, intellectual, social, and emotional growth remains immature and underdeveloped. Current thinkers believe that how well the child plays significantly influences how productively the adult works

Changing View of the Neonate

Past assumptions regarding the confused, disorganized state of neonates have been modified with increased knowledge. Recent detailed observational studies have provided surprising evidence that neonates are competent to perceive and learn (Bower, 1977; Connolly, 1972; Kagan, Kearsley, & Zelano, 1978; Thomas, 1981). Thomas has concisely summarized new information available on neonate competence. Among the points he cites are the ability to preferentially respond to visual patterns and sound, the ability to learn through both conditioned reflexes and imitation, and the capacity to actively participate in social communication. Bonding and maternal attachment have been enhanced by the knowledge that infants respond to environmental input and that there is reciprocity in communication. An understanding that the character and quality of parental responses are influenced by the responses an infant returns has led to the concept of "cueing." Far from being psychologically incompetent, infants immediately begin to influence and be influenced by their environments.

Risk and Vulnerability

Another aspect of child-environment interaction is a paradox recognized early in the twentieth century, that is, that some children find a means for healthy development in spite of detrimental environments, and others succumb to physical or emotional illness in apparently ideal environments. Resilience to illness began to be associated with the relationship between personal characteristics and environmental factors rather than with events themselves. Research identifying personal and environmental factors associated with increased frequency of health problems freed parents from blame and guilt for their child's problems.

Initially, the term "at risk" was used to describe children prone to illness, which reinforced the "tabula rasa" empiricism of Locke that assumed children were passive recipients. Growing evidence that children actively shape their environments necessitated a change in the conceptualizations of risk and vulnerability. A distinction has been made between "risk," referring to environmental hazards to health, and "vulnerability," used to characterize the individual factors that interact with the environment (Anthony, 1974; Kessler, 1979).

Disagreement continues over definitions of "at risk" and "vulnerable." However, there is consensus that a child's degree of vulnerability changes over time, determined by the complex interplay of constitutional endowment and environmentally acquired factors such as disease, trauma, or family experiences (Kessler, 1979; Murphy & Moriarity, 1976; Zubin & Spring, 1977). There is also a growing awareness of the plasticity of both child and environment, which enables the continuous learning and adjustment necessary for congruence and decreased vulnerability (Lerner, 1978; Sameroff, 1975).

THE DEVELOPING CHILD

Definitions of child development have been discussed by many but agreed on by few. Rather than selecting a particular orientation to development, a variety of perspectives, congruent with the growing recognition that there is no one process that singly underlies growth and development, is presented in this chapter. Next, selected areas of child development will be discussed to illustrate elements and assumptions about development that many theories have in common.

Basic Assumptions in Developmental Theories

Three theoretical frameworks about child development developed during the twentieth century expanded our understanding of the process by which a child develops. These three theories are psychoanalytic theory, behavioristic theory, and developmental theory (Caldwell & Richmond, 1970). Psychoanalytic theory (Erikson, 1963; Freud, 1949) claims that a child is in continual conflict between actively pursuing natural instincts and passively accepting societal constraints. Although controversial, these ideas have influenced our understanding of the interactions between child and environment. Watson (1928), Skinner (1971), and Miller and Dollard (1953) were influential in developing social learning theories. Social learning theory describes the child as a reactive organism with innate potential waiting to be shaped by learning. Behaviorists made a significant contribution to our understanding of how early learning experiences could shape later behavior. Gesell (1940), a developmentalist, increased our understanding of maturation as a hierarchical series of stages.

While in each of these frameworks a different facet of developmental learning is highlighted, all seek to describe and predict the result of the interaction between a child and the environment. All these approaches share common assumptions of development as a continuous, sequential process, with skill mastery progressing from the simple to the complex. Since skill acquisition builds on previous achievements, each level of mastery contains within it both consolidation of past achievements and beginning mastery of more complex skills (Thomas, 1981). There is no final point of achievement toward which one strives, but rather there are ever-expanding circles of competence, confidence, and relationships with others. Although traditional theories of child development fail to acknowledge individual natures and the reciprocal relationship between child and environment, they provide a valuable base from which to expand our understanding of the developing child.

Basic Tasks of Early Development

The overall purpose of development is to acquire the skills necessary for fully independent functioning using the process of socialization. The nature, processes, and effects of socialization may vary among generations and across cultures, but the goal of independent functioning remains constant. There are four areas of task mastery that are essential if a child is to achieve independence: (1) attachment, (2) separation-individuation, (3) gender identification, and (4) establishing relationships outside the family.

Attachment is an adaptive behavior of infants to ensure care and protection. Infants are active participants, using social smiling to draw parents into close proximity and to intensify the relationship (Bowlby, 1973, 1978). Differences in individual attachment relationships profoundly impact on all areas of development and have a tremendous long-term effect on future adjustment (Spitz, 1946). Two recent areas of research have further enhanced understanding of the process of attachment: father-infant attachment (Greenberg & Morris, 1974; Lamb, 1976; Lynn, 1974) and parent-child fit (Brazelton, 1969; Lewis & Rosenblum, 1974; Thomas & Chess, 1977). Knowledge in these areas increases our appreciation of the complexities of human development.

Attachment lays the groundwork for the infant to establish the self as separate and autonomous. At four to five months of age, an awareness of the self as separate from the environment replaces initial perceptions of symbiotic nondifferentiation (Mahler, Pine, & Bergman, 1975). This growing awareness in turn increases feelings of dependency on others for need gratification and arouses the stranger anxiety first noted by Spitz (1965). The term "wariness" has replaced "anxiety" as a more accurate description of infant responses (Stroufe, 1977; Thomas, 1981). Sensorimotor development enhances individuation and the increasing capacity to function independently. Weaning represents a significant psychological advance acknowledging the infant as an individual who can assume limited self-care responsibility. Locomotion and the semantic "no" gesture of the toddler period further aid separation and individuation, which is essential for independent functioning (Escalona, 1968).

The third major aspect of socialization is development of gender identity and the related process of sex-role socialization. There is no consensus about why and how gender identification occurs. Theorists do agree that it is influenced by the unique relationships each child forms with parents, siblings, peers, and social systems.

Establishing relationships outside the family is the final component of socialization essential for independence. Although the process begins in infancy, the majority of learning in this area occurs during school age when a child moves into the extrafamilial world. The child absorbs new information regarding different cultures, races, religions, and family styles. Children use this knowledge to expand their repertoire of communication and negotiation skills and to enhance their empathy with and understanding of others.

DIFFERENT DEVELOPMENTAL SEQUENCES

In keeping with the emphasis on individualism presented in this chapter, it is important to acknowledge developmental sequences that, though different, are both normal and highly adaptive. Traditionally, child development has been committed to a theoretical position that acknowledged primarily one "normal" sequence of development. Many children have been subjected to this destructive presumption and have been unfairly judged as inferior when they fail to follow the prescribed pathway.

Movement toward a more individualized model of development has freed children and health professionals from the narrow and futile belief in one acceptable developmental track. There has been increased acknowledgement of the ability of children to overcome and adapt to barriers to development.

Children with Handicapping Conditions

The flexibility and adaptability of human beings is no more evident than in children with handicapping conditions. While their developmental course deviates from what we have learned to expect, such children demonstrate a dramatic ability to compensate for deficits.

Children born with a hearing impairment do not develop as quickly in cognitive and affective functioning, as they cannot learn communication through the spoken word. However, as soon as they develop a communication system using visual cues, such as sign language, to replace hearing, their abstract thinking, problem-solving, and language development increases rapidly (Chess, 1978; Thomas, 1981).

Similar patterns of compensation and adaptation occur in congenitally blind children. Initial difficulties with neuromuscular and cognitive development owing to lack of visual stimulation can be eventually overcome. Blind children are capable of normal affective and social development, but they achieve those abilities by alternate routes, often in a sequence different from sighted children (Adelson & Fraiberg, 1974; Thomas, 1981).

Motor handicaps in children interfere with sensorimotor experience, long thought to be essential for cognitive development (Piaget, 1963). However, just as the blind child is capable of normal social and affective development and the deaf child is capable of language development, so too is the motoric-handicapped child capable of cognitive and social development. Again, while the end result is the same, the sequence and timing of skill acquisition is individually determined.

Twin Development

Twins represent another group for whom the course of development deviates from expected patterns. Traditional theories of development are based on single births. The psychological environment in which twins, whether they are identical or fraternal, develop is quite different. With twins, the novel factor is the constant interaction with another of the same age, with similar appearance and skills. The intimacy which is created facilitates bonding and identifying with each other, as well as with a parent. An essential part of development for twins involves separating from each other and from the parents. However, there is no natural process that facilitates separation between twins as there is between parent and child. The developmental features that encourage differentiation from parents, such as sensorimotor development and going to school, only reinforce the twin bond since they turn to each other for support during these and other times of stress. Although different from the developmental sequences in children from single births, identification with and separation from each other is a normal and predictable aspect of twin development (Siemon, 1980).

What Special Children Have Taught Us About Development

Traditionally, the predominant model of development has been a deficit model that labeled anything other than rigid age and stage norms as "deviant." "Critical stages" developmental theory also presumed children from impoverished or inadequate environments to be psychologically abnormal or inferior in their development. Special groups of children have shown us the resiliency and adaptability of human beings. The blind, the deaf, the physically handicapped, and the child of a multiple birth all develop at different paces. All, however, move toward the goal of functional independence. The sequence and timing of the developmental course followed is individually determined by the interaction of biological, social, and psychological capacities within limits unique to each child. Task mastery may be accomplished at a slower or more accelerated rate or may follow a more tortuous and convoluted route. The goal of independence is ultimately achieved because of the adaptive plasticity of the brain (Thomas, 1981). Early life experiences that produce barriers to full human functioning do not necessarily cause permanent and irreversible damage.

IMPLICATIONS FOR PATHOLOGY

Despite the widely diverse assumptions from which each developed, both psychoanalytic and behavioristic theories stress the importance of early life experiences in shaping psychological development in later years. Although children are born with potentially self-actualizing natures, these can be facilitated or suppressed by environmental factors and individual characteristics.

Children can frequently develop new and creative solutions to manage stress and continue on their developmental way. The aim of the psychiatric mental health clinical nurse specialist is to prevent a developmental period from being so disagreeable or painful that developmental progress is compromised.

Common Developmental Problems

Normal stresses are accentuated during times of developmental transitions, increasing a child's vulnerability to social, biological, and psychological problems. Difficulties associated with integrating and adjusting to developmental demands often lead to behaviors that are upsetting to a child or parent. Such behaviors are a means of communicating that a child's ability to cope with change or demands is being overwhelmed. Skills that are temporarily blocked are usually those that have been most recently acquired or are still incomplete. Although developmental problems may not be serious in themselves, they can become intensified or more intractable without sensitive management.

With the ambiguity that exists between what is normal and abnormal, how can one reassure parents that their child is developing as expected? The difference between normal and abnormal problems is one of degree and duration. Normal developmental problems involve age-appropriate behavior, are of limited duration and frequency, and interfere with overall development and adjustment to a minor extent. Children themselves also help to distinguish between normal and abnormal problems. Most children are able to protest in their own behalf against excessive demands or restructure an unacceptable situation to make it acceptable. In addition, if the child responds to comforting and attempts by parents to relieve the stress with positive results, it is indicative of the child's inherent strengths which have temporarily been overwhelmed.

A final issue in recognizing normal developmental problems is in distinguishing behavior that might be within the norms but is not necessarily healthy. Infants and children who make no demands on their environment, who create no "problems," may be considered "good" because they do not disrupt the lives of adults. Generally, behavioral excesses are those that demand attention. Children with behavioral deficits who do not call attention to themselves may go unnoticed until great damage has been done.

Immature Behaviors

Immature behaviors are those that are characteristic of an earlier developmental stage. They are usually indicative of a child's ineffective coping skills. An extended inability to cope may lead to lack of confidence, increased dependence, and a lowered sense of self-worth.

REGRESSION. Regression is common in two- to four-year-olds when the stress of achieving autonomy results in a temporary loss of abilities. Conflict between the desire for independence and the need for security produces periods of doubt during which a child retreats to the safety of more familiar behaviors. Clinging, tantrums, thumb sucking, wetting and soiling, and wanting a bottle may reappear intermittently. To avoid feeling overwhelmed, children need independence congruent with abilities and tempered with reasonable limits. A balance needs to be struck between gratifying earlier needs and encouraging exploration of new experiences.

NEGATIVISM. A toddler's use of the word "no" to assert individuality is a common source of frustration to parents. If parents can appreciate rebellion as a developmental move toward independence, children will not become management problems. When parents need to "show them who's boss," children eventually conform, but the cost is to their personal integrity. Acquiescence to authority becomes associated with loss of integrity. Extreme responses are either absolute submission at the cost of personal worth or rebellion against any kind of norm or rule, as is evident in delinquency. Children who never assert their individuality also experience problems. Failure to become separate will result in pathological symbiosis and can be the groundwork for crippling psychological disorders.

AGGRESSION. Aggression is a normal reaction of children to threats to their safety, happiness, or individuality. Between the ages of three and seven years, children gain increased control of impulses and aggression. Continued frequent, excessive, or unprovoked aggression in older children requires immediate parental action to curb the behavior. Poor impulse control and aggression is often associated with lax discipline owing to parental indulgence or neglect, parental hostility and harsh punishment, and imitation of parental styles of conflict resolution. Effective methods to resolve the problem include rewarding positive social behavior, ignoring aggression, and strengthening assertiveness and social skills (Schaefer & Millman, 1981). Clear limit setting and consistent follow-through by adults are essential ingredients to helping children learn self-control.

SENSORY AND LEARNING DYSFUNCTIONS. Sensory defects interfere with a child's ability to accurately perceive and understand the environment. The results of impaired judgment create problems in relating to peers and family. Children with learning dysfunctions are often described as "always doing the wrong thing at the wrong time." Problems in symbolic and abstract thinking, dyslexia, dyscalculia, limitations in auditory or visual perception, sequencing, or synthesizing may be the result of organic deficits. Other learning dysfunctions are the result of emotional factors within the child or family such as tension, discord, unrealistically high expectations, or inadequate control and discipline that interfere with learning. Treatment is specific to the etiology and requires extensive diagnostic assessment to determine the most appropriate school programs (Hawke & Lesser, 1977).

Insecure Behaviors

Insecurity occurs in children who are less adaptive and self-confident. They experience fear and anxiety that can be incapacitating.

EXTREME MISTRUST. Sometime during the first two years of life all children go through a period of wariness to strangers. When the environment is predictable with consistent, positive experiences with adults who gratify an infant's needs, feelings of trust, security, and safety generalize to others. Chronic disappointment and anxiety can lead either to an amplified need for nurturing or to an avoidance of relationships with others altogether. Failure in overcoming anxiety will lead to later restrictions of personal freedom such as insecurity and overdependence on others. An inability to develop trusting relationships at all leads to crippling personality disorders such as chronic depression and antisocial personality.

Habit Disorders

Habit disorders are automatic reactions that have persisted for so long and are so overlearned that they are resistant to change.

FEEDING DISTURBANCES. The most commonly accepted etiology of feeding disturbances is an anxiety response in the mother that elicits distress in the infant. Reassurance and guidance for parents generally results in feeding disorders that are self-limiting and disappear by the time a baby is three or four months old (Warme, 1977).

SLEEP DISTURBANCES. Disturbing dreams and restlessness in sleep are common reactions to the insecurities of growing up in children aged two to five. Fear, anxiety, overstimulation, and situational stress are some of the underlying causes. Parental support, reassurance, and comfort are vital elements in helping children through the uncertainties of maturation (Schaefer & Millman, 1981; Warme, 1977).

SPEECH DISTURBANCES. Piaget emphasized the interdependence of speech and socialization. Functional delayed speech may be the result of environmental isolation and neglect that deprive the child of the social context and positive reinforcement necessary for speech acquisition. Or, a parent or siblings may be so oversolicitous that a child never has to develop speech for need gratification. Prevention and intervention strategies involve encouraging speech as an exciting and useful tool by talking and listening with a child and rewarding efforts at speech.

Stuttering is repetition of the first sound in a word, as distinguished from word repetition characteristic of toddler speech. It usually occurs during the early school years, five times more frequently in boys than in girls. It affects only 1 or 2% of children, most frequently those who have a familial tendency toward stuttering (Warme, 1977). Children who stutter often have associated reading and writing problems, are less sure of themselves, and are sensitive to disapproval and criticism. Increased pressure, tension, or worry may provoke stuttering. Four out of five stutterers recover spontaneously in an environment of low pressure, with patient and approving people who avoid embarrassing the child.

THUMB AND FINGER SUCKING. Sucking is an innate reflex that is a common source of self-gratification and tension reduction in children up to three years of age. When thumb sucking persists beyond the age of four, it may be an indication of immaturity or insecurity caused by inadequate attachment or individuation. Older children may revert to this source of comfort in the face of new or challenging situations. Thumb sucking usually requires no intervention. Children progress to more mature behaviors in a positive atmosphere of encouragement and support rather than punishment and embarrassment (Schaefer & Millman, 1981; Warme, 1977).

FUNCTIONAL ENURESIS. Enuresis is considered a problem in children over the age of four, by which time toilet training has usually been achieved. It occurs twice as often in boys as in girls. Daytime enuresis is considered to be a more serious problem, since children usually first achieve control during waking periods. In children who have never achieved control, there is usually a physiological explanation, such as small bladder capacity. Enuresis can be a transitory regressive symptom following a stressful or traumatic event. When children have established bladder control and become enuretic, the cause is usually psychogenic, related to anger and disturbed family relationships. Effective management includes regular toileting, restricting fluids at night, emphasizing successes through a reward system, avoiding punishment and ridicule, and resolving family conflicts (Warme, 1977).

CONSTIPATION/ENCOPRESIS. Factors that contribute to constipation are exaggerated in encopresis. If organic factors are ruled out, constipation is not usually a concern, except when younger children develop functional megacolon due to fecal retention. Encopresis occurs five times more often in boys than in girls. It is usually accompanied by other problems, such as enuresis, tantrums, and learning disabilities. In a child over the age of four, encopresis generally indicates significant disturbance in a child and family and requires psychiatric intervention. Issues of control, power, and rebellion are thought to underlie the behavior. Although there is disagreement about the most effective treatment of encopresis, there is consensus that manipulative procedures should be kept to a minimum to avoid the risk of intensifying the frightening fantasies already present (Schaefer & Millman, 1981).

Special Developmental Problems

When demands on a child are overwhelming or occur over a long period of time, barriers to self-fulfillment develop. If the hurt is severe or sufficiently prolonged, personality problems may develop in later life. Three examples of abnormal conditions under which children are reared that may intensify or exaggerate developmental issues and may lead to long-term developmental problems will be discussed.

Separation-Individuation Problems in Twins

Barriers to the establishment of individual identities in twins have been discussed. Identical and fraternal twins are equally prone to separation problems since the key issue is not physical similarity, but whether they are perceived as a unit by themselves and by the environment. When the satisfaction of the twin bond outweighs environmental or individual differences, a crippling nonindividuation occurs that compromises ego development. This psychological fusion can take two directions. Either the twins will perceive themselves as intimately connected and undifferentiated parts of an inseparable social unit, or each twin develops capacities that complement the co-twin so that the two personalities blend into one harmonious whole, each incomplete without the other (Terry, 1975). When separation does not occur until adulthood, a process similar to grief occurs (Siemon, 1980). Since the twinship is the prototype for other intimate relationships, resolution of the separation-individuation phase of development has implications for marriage, competition, and other relationships outside the twinship.

Distorted Perceptions in Handicapped and Disabled Children

The course toward achievement of functional independence for handicapped or disabled children is arduous and frustrating. Although adaptive compensation may enable development to proceed, there are damaging influences on personality formation that may also occur. Parental attitudes exert the greatest influence on whether a child develops innate potential or remains in a state of crippling dependency. Parental apprehension, rejection, and disapproval contribute to the child's feelings of incompetence, insecurity, isolation, anxiety, and depression. In addition, parents may compensate for their own feelings of guilt, helplessness, and intolerance by creating unnecessary helplessness in a child through insufficient expectations for self-care. Children react to the stress of being unable to cope with normal demands, or to inappropriate handling by parents, with behaviors designed to dominate and control the environment. They may either be passive, helpless, easily frustrated, or tyrannical. The crippling aspects of these distorted perceptions about love, relationships, and personal worth are all too apparent. While some children's temperament leads them to overcompensate for inadequacies in one area, others are left with a dissatisfaction and bitterness that produces barriers to normal development (Chess & Hassibi, 1978).

Results of Parental Privation

Spitz (1946) first drew attention to the degree to which failure to meet children's emotional needs can impair their development. For many children, the quality of parenting to which they have been exposed has been so inconsistent and unsatisfactory that attachment to parental figures never developed. Chronic neglect of their emotional needs leaves these children lonely, sad, and with a deep sense of hurt. They may describe their sense of isolation as "I'm like the universe, mostly empty." Their feelings of having no substance are portrayed by this description: "It's like somebody rubbed invisible cream on me and I disappeared." If the hurt is profound, the capacity to form mutual relationships with others is grossly impaired. These children live with chronic sorrow for the lost potential they could have developed in a more nurturing environment.

IMPLICATIONS FOR PREVENTION AND TREATMENT: REDUCING BARRIERS TO SELF-ACTUALIZATION

It is neither desirable nor possible to think of prevention in terms of eliminating stress from the lives of children. The skills that children need to achieve independence include the capacity to cope with stress and solve problems. Children who have survived disasters have taught us that the strongest people are those who have been challenged by lives that are not easy. The key to healthy development is that the challenges come in doses commensurate with a child's ability to master them. Selected ways to enhance self-actualization or to minimize the barriers children have in reaching their full potential will be discussed briefly.

Anticipatory Guidance for Parents

More than ever before, there is a recognition of the importance of the quality of the parent-child relationship in predicting later development. Unfortunately, no major trend in childrearing has lasted more than two decades. Not even one generation of children has had the opportunity to grow up with and validate as adults the consequences of a particular childrearing trend before it has changed. Parents are understandably confused about how to foster optimal development for their children. The challenge for the future is to develop environments that maximize growth through congruence between a child's needs and environmental demands (French, Rodgers, & Cobb, 1974; Thomas, 1981). Environments that encourage optimal health and development are those in which parents are sensitive to a child's cues, are able to alleviate distress, and provide opportunities to foster social, emotional, and cognitive growth (Barnard, 1975). While all parents need guidance at some time or another, teenage parents, single parents, and parents who are potentially abusive may need extra support and guidance.

Early Identification and Intervention in Developmental Delays

Supporting optimal child development through enhancing the child-parent-environment interaction requires that children with special developmental needs be identified early, before their progress has been seriously affected. While primary prevention is the concern of all health professionals, it is the sole responsibility of none. Nurses, physicians, teachers, and all child care personnel need to screen vigilantly for developmental delays if they are to maximize the potential of future generations.

Parental Developmental Problems That Impact on the Child

The consequences of parental privation have already been discussed. There are many reasons why parents cannot provide for their children's basic emotional needs. Few parents maliciously set out to hurt their children. Most do the best they can, bringing into parenting their own unique assets and liabilities, self-concepts, past successes and failures, physical and mental health, and their own models for parenting. Just as children are affected by the increased demands of development, parents have similar reactions to the developmental crises of adulthood, such as marriage, parenthood, work promotion, unemployment, or aging. Any combination of these variables impact on the quality of the parent-child relationships. Some parents are too inadequate, helpless, or physically or mentally ill to nurture children. Others give priority to meeting their own needs for self-esteem to the exclusion of their children's needs. The blame and anger traditionally directed toward these parents by professionals need to be tempered and replaced by effective problem identification and intervention.

Stimulation Programs to Facilitate Development

Children whose innate capacities or environment inhibit optimal learning can be stimulated in special programs. Stimulation programs for handicapped or disabled children and Head Start programs for socially or economically deprived children are two examples. One can only hope that support for social programs that promote development through additional experiences will be increased although the current outlook is bleak.

There are many ways of influencing the development of children. Perhaps most importantly, more attention needs to be paid to how to support and maintain strengths and to sustain the healthy integration that is already within a child. One needs to recognize the child and parent as active participants in their own health by appreciating and supporting their strengths. The direction for the future is to identify the kinds of parenting, education, and social programs necessary to enhance individual growth and remove barriers to personal fulfillment.

Direction for the Future

The query, "What is man?", which stimulated early child development research, has become "What is man capable of becoming?" The traditional view held that the child's innate abilities and characteristics could not be influenced by the environment. Early efforts to identify and measure finite characteristics have been replaced by a sensitivity to the child's infinite potential for development, which is expressed in individual ways and influenced by learning and interaction with the environment. The current trend is toward expansion, offering opportunities to extend the vistas of human potential rather than to narrowly define them. The future holds unexplored capacities for adaptation and change. People may modify their own destinies.

What, then, is the key to promoting healthy development in children? Children are the product of many forces brought together in a myriad of combinations. Because no single factor can ensure a child's future, no single prescription holds the key for describing, protecting, or promoting a child's health.

Psychodynamic models of emotional disturbance focus on factors within a child, as do biophysical models. Behavioral models focus on learning patterns of behaving, and sociological models look at the environment. What seems to respond to more individualized needs is an ecological model that is dynamic and interactive in nature. It is the interface between the child and the significant environment and how well they fit together that provides the insight about how to enhance children's abilities to be fully functioning people. One model that encompasses the essence of what is needed is "goodness of fit" (Chess, Fernandez, & Korn, 1980; Thomas, 1981). The term implies a congruence between environmental demands on a child and personal resources available. Also implied is a dynamic quality of person-environment match that recognizes the constant adaptability of human beings and their ability to modify or change patterns of behaving or feeling in response to new life experiences (French et al., 1974). Children learn from experiences and add to their repertoire of coping skills so there is continual growth and readjustment of the "fit" (Lerner, 1978).

Throughout time there have always been, and will continue to be, conditions that cannot be eliminated that are detrimental to development. Change is a characteristic of our lives, as are the multitude of stresses that bombard us daily. Another condition is that children are raised by other human beings, with all the accompanying imperfections and limitations. Children are resilient and have a natural tendency to develop in a healthy way when the stresses of life are consonant with their abilities to manage stresses and when there is sufficient harmony and order to offset the traumatic changes which take place. They are capable of strength, flexibility, and creativity to actively participate in and cope with the movement toward independence. It was this belief in the personal powers of children that led Erik Erikson to say: "Children fall apart; but, unlike Humpty Dumpty, they fall back together again" (1950, p. 83). The challenge and responsibility for the future are clear: to help children use stressful situations in a growth-stimulating way so that development is not compromised and they can achieve their full potential.

SUMMARY

Throughout much of history, children were considered to be the property of their parents, to be sold, apprenticed, abused, or cherished as economic conditions and cultural values dictated. Thankfully, in each generation, people championed the rights of children by challenging and modifying the attitudes and beliefs held toward them by society. Gradually, childhood came to be acknowledged as a separate period of development and the special needs of children were recognized and addressed. The twentieth century was welcomed as a hopeful era for the child. Normative developmental data and knowledge of child environment interaction increased recognition and respect for a child's capacity to grow and change.

The process through which current ideas of child development have evolved gives us a perspective for the future. Reflection on past developments helps to refine current models and determine future possibilities for extending the vistas of child development and potential.

REFERENCES

Adelson, E., & Fraiberg, S. Gross motor development in infants blind from birth. *Child Development,* 1974, *45(1),* 114.

American Psychiatric Association. *Diagnostic and statistical manual of mental disorders* (3rd ed.). Washington, DC: American Psychiatric Association, 1980.

Anderson, E. Child development: An historical perspective. *Child Development,* 1956, *27(2),* 181.

Anthony, E. The syndrome of the psychologically invulnerable child. In E. Anthony, C. Koupernik, & C. Chiland (Eds.), *The child in his family: Children at psychiatric risk.* New York: John Wiley & Sons, 1974.

Barash, D. *Sociobiology and behavior.* New York: Elsevier, 1977.

Barnard, K. Trends in nursing care and prevention of developmental disabilities. *American Journal of Nursing,* 1975, *75(10),* 1700.

Bower, T. *A primer of infant development.* San Francisco: W. H. Freeman, 1977.

Bowlby, J. *Attachment and loss I: Attachment.* New York: Basic Books, 1973.

Bowlby, J. Attachment theory and its therapeutic implications. *Adolescent Psychiatry,* 1978, *6,* 5.

Brazelton, R. *Infants and mothers.* New York: Delacorte Press, 1969.

Caldwell, B., & Richmond, J. The impact of theories of child development. In F. Rebelsky & L. Dorman (Eds.). *Child development and behavior.* New York: Knopf, 1970.

Chess, S. The plasticity of human development. *Journal of American Academy of Child Psychiatry,* 1978, *17(1),* 80.

Chess, S., Fernandez, P., & Korn, S. The handicapped child and his family: Consonance and dissonance. *Journal of the American Academy of Child Psychiatry,* 1980, *19(1),* 56.

Chess, S., & Hassibi, M. *Principles and practice of child psychiatry.* New York: Plenum Press, 1978.

Connolly, K. Learning and the concept of critical periods in infancy. *Developmental Medicine and Child Neurology,* 1972, *14(6),* 705.

Erikson, E. Conference on the problems of infancy and childhood: Growth and crises. In M. Senn (Ed.), *Symposium on the healthy personality.* New York: Josiah Macy, Jr. Foundation, 1950.

Erikson, E. *Childhood and society* (2nd ed.). New York: Norton, 1963.

Erikson, E. Play and actuality. In J. Bruner, A. Jolly, & K. Sylva (Eds.), *Play: Its role in development and evolution.* New York: Basic Books, 1976.

Escalona, S. *The roots of individuality: Normal patterns of development in infancy.* Chicago: Aldine, 1968.

French, J., Rodgers, A., & Cobb, S. Adjustment as person-environment fit. In G. Coelho, D. Hamburg, & J. Adams (Eds.), *Coping and adaptation.* New York: Basic Books, 1974.

Freud, S. *An outline of psychoanalysis.* New York: Norton, 1949.

Gesell, A. *The first years of life.* New York: Harper & Bros., 1940.

Greenberg, M., & Morris, N. Engrossment: The newborn's impact upon the father. *American Journal of Orthopsychiatry,* 1974, *44(4),* 520.

Havighurst, R. *Human development and education.* New York: McKay, 1953.

Hawke, W., & Lesser, S. The child with a learning disorder. In P. Steinhauer & Q. Rae-Grant (Eds.), *Psychological problems of the child and his family.* Toronto: Macmillan, 1977.

Herron, R., & Sutton-Smith, B. *Child's play.* New York: John Wiley & Sons, 1971.

Kagan, J., Kearsley, R., & Zelano, P. *Infancy, its place in human development.* Cambridge, MA: Harvard University Press, 1978.

Kessler, P. A strategy for studying differential vulnerability to the psychological consequences of stress. *Journal of Health and Social Behavior,* 1979, *20,* 100.

Kohlberg, L. Development of moral character and moral ideology. In M. Hoffman & L. Hoffman (Eds.), *Review of child development* (Vol. 1). New York: Russell Sage Foundation, 1964.

Lamb, M. *The role of father in child development.* New York: John Wiley & Sons, 1976.

Lerner, R. Nature, nurture, and dynamic interactionism. *Human Development,* 1978, *21,* 1.

Lewis, M., & Rosenblum, L. (Eds.). *The effect of the infant on its caregiver.* New York: John Wiley & Sons, 1974.

Lugo, J., & Hershey, G. *Human development.* New York: Macmillan, 1974.

Lynn, D. *The father: His role in development.* Monterey, CA: Brooks/Cole, 1974.

Mahler, M., Pine, F., & Bergman, A. *The psychological birth of the human infant.* New York: Basic Books, 1975.

Miller, N., & Dollard, J. *Social learning and imitation.* New Haven: Yale University Press, 1953.

Murphy, L., & Moriarity, A. *Vulnerability, coping, and growth.* New Haven: Yale University Press, 1976.

Piaget, J. *Play, dreams, and imitation in childhood.* New York: W. W. Norton, 1962.

Piaget, J. *The origins of intelligence in the child.* New York: International University Press, 1953.

Sameroff, A. Early influences on development: Fact or fancy? *Merrill-Palmer Quarterly,* 1975, *21,* 267.

Schaefer, C., & Millman, H. *How to help children with common problems.* New York: Van Nostrand Reinhold, 1981.

Schafer, R. *Mothering.* Cambridge, MA: Harvard University Press, 1977.

Sears, R. Your ancients revisited: A history of child development. In E. Hetherington (Ed.), *Review of child development research* (Vol. 5). Chicago: University of Chicago Press, 1975.

Siemon, M. The separation-individuation process in adult twins. *American Journal of Psychotherapy,* 1980, *34(3),* 387.

Skinner, B. *Beyond freedom and dignity.* New York: Bantam, 1971.

Spitz, R. Anaclitic depression. *Psychoanalytic Study of the Child,* 1946, *2,* 313.

Spitz, R. *The first year of life.* New York: International University Press, 1965.

Stroufe, L. Wariness of strangers and the study of human development. *Child Development,* 1977, *48(3),* 731.

Terry, G. The separation-individuation process in same-sex twins: A review of the literature. *Maternal-Child Nursing Journal,* 1975, *4(2),* 121.

Thomas, A. Current trends in developmental theory. *American Journal of Orthopsychiatry,* 1981, *51(4),* 580.

Thomas, A., & Chess, S. *Temperament and development.* New York: Brunner/Mazel, 1977.

Warme, G. Childhood development problems. In P. Steinhauer & Q. Rae-Grant (Eds.), *Psychological problems of the child and his family.* Toronto: Macmillan, 1977.

Watson, J. *Psychological care of infant and child.* New York: Norton, 1928.

Wilson, E. *Sociobiology: The new synthesis.* Cambridge, MA: Harvard University Press, 1975.

Zubin, J., & Spring, B. Vulnerability: A new look at schizophrenia. *Journal of Abnormal Psychology,* 1977, *86(2),* 103.

BIBLIOGRAPHY

Ainsworth, M. The development of infant-mother attachment. In B. Caldwell & H. N. Ricciuti (Eds.), *Review of child development research* (Vol. 3). Chicago: University of Chicago Press, 1973.

Bell, R. Four new research approaches to socialization: An evaluation of their advantages and disadvantages. *Journal of Abnormal Child Psychology,* 1981, *9(3),* 299.

Berkowitz, L. (Ed.). *Advances in experimental social psychology* (Vol. 8). New York: Academic Press, 1975.

Bowlby, J. *Attachment and loss II: Separation.* New York: Basic Books, 1973.

Bruner, J., Jolly, A., & Sylvan, K. (Eds.). *Play: Its role in development and evolution.* New York: Basic Books, 1976.

Campbell, S., & Taylor, P. Bonding and attachment: Theoretical issues. *Seminars in Perinatology,* 1979, *3(1),* 3.

Chess, S. Developmental theory revisited: Findings of a longitudinal study. *Canadian Journal of Psychiatry,* 1979, *24(2),* 101.

Chess, S., & Thomas, A. (Eds.). *Annual progress in child psychiatry and child development.* New York: Brunner/Mazel, 1978.

Cline, F. The second year of life. *Nurse Practitioner,* 1981, *6,* 45.

Colombo, J. The critical period concept: Research, methodology, and theoretical issues. *Psychological Bulletin,* 1982, *91(2),* 260.

Erikson, E. Conference on the problems of infancy and childhood: Growth and crises. In M. Senn (Ed.), *Symposium on the healthy personality.* New York: Josiah Macy, Jr. Foundation, 1950.

Escalona, S. Intervention programs for children at psychiatric risk: The contribution of child psychiatry and developmental theory. In E. Anthony & C. Koupernik (Eds.), *The child in his family: Children at psychiatric risk* (Vol. 3). New York: John Wiley & Sons, 1974.

Freud, A. *The ego and the mechanisms of defense.* New York: International University Press, 1946.

Grostein, J. The significance of Kleinian contributions to psychoanalysis, II: Freudian and Kleinian conceptions of early mental development. *International Journal of Psychoanalytic Psychotherapy,* 1980, *81(8),* 393.

Guerrero, A. The superego concept, part I: Historical review; object relations approach. *Psychoanalytic Review,* 1981, *68(3),* 321.

Hetherington, E. (Ed.). *Review of child development research* (Vol. 5). Chicago: University of Chicago Press, 1975.

Kagan, J., & Klein, R. Cross-cultural perspectives on early development. *American Psychologist,* 1973, *28,* 947.

Kamhi, A. Developmental vs. difference theories of mental retardation: A new look. *American Journal of Mental Deficiency,* 1981, *86(1),* 1.

Lamb, M. A re-examination of the infant social world. *Human Development,* 1977, *20,* 65.

Lewis, M. Child psychiatry perspectives. Child development research and child analysis. *Journal of American Academy of Child Psychiatry,* 1981, *20(1),* 189.

Mahler, M. On the first three sub-phases of the separation-individuation process. *International Journal of Psychoanalysis,* 1972, *53,* 333.

Matteson, A. Long-term physical illness in children: A challenge to psychological adaptation. *Pediatrics,* 1972, *50,* 801.

Monroe, R., & Monroe, R. *Cross-cultural human development.* Monterey, CA: Brooks/Cole, 1975.

Parten, M. Social play among pre-school children. *Journal of Abnormal Social Psychology,* 1932, *27,* 243.

Rutter, M. The long-term effects of early experience. *Developmental Medicine and Child Neurology,* 1980, *22(6),* 800.

Shapiro, D. (Ed.). *Psychobiological approaches to social behavior.* Palo Alto, CA: Stanford University Press, 1964.

Siemon, M. Mental health in school-aged children. *Maternal-Child Nursing Journal,* 1978, *3(4),* 211.

Simeonsson, R. Review: Research on handicapped children: Sibling relationships. *Child: Care, Health, and Development,* 1981, *7,* 153.

Spitz, R. Anxiety in infancy: A study of its manifestations in the first year of life. *Bulletin of the American Psychoanalysis Association,* 1950, *6,* 66.

Stone, L., Smith, H., & Murphy, L. (Eds.). *The competent infant.* New York: Basic Books, 1973.

Taylor, R. Black youth and psychosocial development: A conceptual framework. *Journal of Black Studies,* 1976, *6,* 353.

Taylor, R. Psychosocial development among black children and youth: A reexamination. *American Journal of Orthopsychiatry,* 1976, *46(1),* 4.

Tooley, K. Johnny I hardly know ye: Toward a revision of the theory of male psychosexual development. *American Journal of Orthopsychiatry,* 1977, *47(2),* 184.

Tudor, M. (Ed.). *Child development.* New York: McGraw-Hill, 1981.

Williams, T. Infant development and supplemental care: A comparative review of basic and applied research. *Human Development,* 1977, *20(1),* 1.

Wolff, S. *Children under stress* (2nd ed.). Baltimore: Penguin Books, 1973.

CHAPTER 7 PREADOLESCENCE AND ADOLESCENCE

Beth Vaughan-Cole
Bonnie C. Clayton

> Our youth now love luxury. They have bad manners, contempt for authority, disrespect for older people. Children nowadays are tyrants. They no longer rise when their elders enter the room. They contradict their parents, chatter before company, gobble their food and tyrannize their teachers.
>
> Socrates, in Plato's *Republic*

No other human condition has captured the interest of society and been more widely discussed in the literature than adolescence, particularly since the turn of the century. The frequently quoted complaint of Socrates about the misconduct and lack of respect of the young for their elders 2300 years ago has found relevance for many generations of adults. Authors of fiction from Dostoevski to Salinger have expressed the bittersweet joys and agonies of youth. There is an old truism that the recall of one's own adolescence is selective and frequently distorted because of the protective function of the adult ego. In one's reminiscence, one is apt to reconstruct adolescence in shades softer than the harsh tones of reality. The recalled adolescent experiences of adults are always accompanied by recall of one's peers of the earlier era and encompass a wide range of appropriate and inappropriate behavior. Such recall has sometimes led to restrictive, often insensitive efforts to exert a level of more or less protective control over the youth of each succeeding generation.

In this chapter, the most complex and lengthy of the stages of childhood development, preadolescence and adolescence, is presented, as a unified period. The long years between puberty and young adulthood cover enormous variations in the physical, psychological, social, and cognitive characteristics of the individuals in this range. Redl (1969) states:

> The very custom of using a single term for as wide a stretch of development as we do reaching from "latency" into young adulthood leads to a most misleading and dangerous abbreviation. Usually, although we are well aware of this risk, we forget about it in the course of a discussion and then end up not talking about the same people at all (p. 80).

Another word of caution is that this chapter is divided into sections in which different aspects of adolescence are discussed. This is an approach of convenience and is inconsistent with the belief that the individual ought not to be fragmented if understanding is the goal. The marvellously complex young person who is neither child nor adult should be regarded with reverence as a whole being, interrelated with family and community. Nevertheless, this chapter presents physiological, psychosocial, and other aspects of the adolescent separately.

PHYSICAL DEVELOPMENT

In the most dramatic differentiation of the sexes since prenatal development, the onset of puberty presents an interplay of physiological forces that changes children into their adult forms. There is no single model of normal adolescence (Petersen & Offer, 1979); however, there are some very important facts that should be recognized as one conceptualizes the physiological development of adolescence and preadolescence. This section will focus on adolescents in the United States, except where noted.

First, there is enormous variation within sex-type and between sex-types. This variability of the onset and rate of growth has a strong impact on the developing psyche and self-image and on social development of the child. The onset of puberty for girls is usually between the ages of 10 and 13 with menarche shortly after the twelfth year. Within that span of four years, at any point in time, one girl may have completed the entire adolescent physical development, whereas another may not have begun. The onset of puberty for boys usually is two years later than for girls. By age 13, some changes have begun in boys (Malmquist, 1979). As in girls, the secondary sexual characteristics occur first followed by the primary characteristics.

The second fact of importance in adolescent physical development is that the orderly sequencing of growth and development assists the human organism to fulfill the species-mandated genotype. Recognition of the sequence of physiological development assists the clinician in anticipatory guidance and assessment of preadolescents and adolescents.

The third fact of significance is that there is an overlap in the beginning and ending of the many physiological changes that are occurring. This overlapping yet asynchronous variation for physiological changes accounts for the awkward, often gawky appearance of young adolescents (see Figure 7.1).

The fourth fact of importance in conceptualizing the physiological phenomena of adolescence is recognition that the biological changes are initiated by the hypothalmus (which is part of the central nervous system) rather than the pituitary as was previously thought.

Ages Ten to Thirteen

Preadolescence is probably a misnomer. It suggests that there is a distinct stage of development prior to adolescence that has specific properties applicable to all individuals of that group. Deutsch (1947) looks at this age period as "the last stage of latency" whereas Blos (1971) considers it the "earliest phase of adolescence." Because the physiological changes are more dramatic for girls at this time than for boys, the biological substrate for a category of preadolescence is inconsistent across the sexes.

Beginning about the age of 9 or 10, four major changes occur in girls. The budding of the breasts is considered the first sign of puberty in females, although the appearance of pubic hair may occur first (Tanner, 1962). Together with these two changes is a skeletal growth spurt and a fifty-fold increase in estrogen secretion (Goldings, 1979).

At the time of the endocrinological changes, there is a remolding of the bony pelvis. This broadening of the hips along with breast development removes the young girl from her childlike form to the adult figure she will carry as a young woman. The endocrine changes stimulate the increase in growth of the uterus and vagina, including the labia and clitoris. The skeletal growth spurt peaks shortly after the twelfth year of age followed shortly by axillary hair and menarche. While menarche suggests that the uterus is mature, it usually does not have full reproductive capacity for another 12 to 18 months, during which time irregular and anovulatory cycles occur (Goldings, 1979).

From ages 10 to 13, there are less obvious and dramatic changes occurring in males. The major change is in the size of the testes (4 grams at age 9 to 17 grams at age 14). The penis also increases in size with an accompanying appearance of downy pubic hair. Together with those changes comes an enlargement of the nipples and areolae (Young,

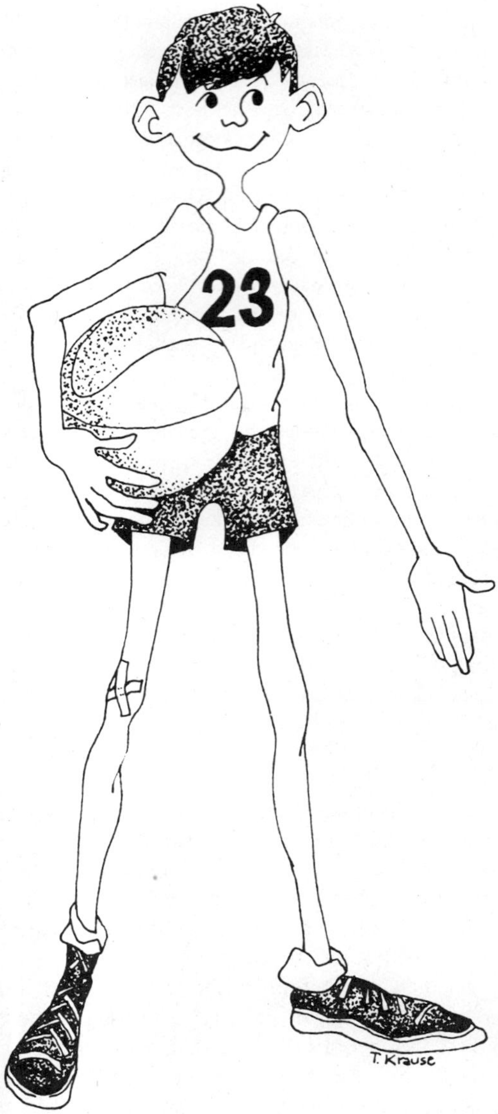

Figure 7.1 (Drawing by Teddie Krause.)

1971). Following these external changes are the internal changes, including an increase in prostatic activity and excretion of urinary gonadotropins.

Ages Thirteen to Fifteen

According to various longitudinal studies (Tanner, 1968), the onset of menarche in girls has changed markedly over the last 40 years. Menarche is now occurring for British girls shortly before age 13, compared to age 15, 40 years ago. By the age of 14½, most of the physiological changes of adolescence will have occurred for girls. The skeletal growth spurt will have been completed just as the male growth spurt begins. The proportion of muscle tone to fat is not as marked in girls as it is in boys. Regular menstrual cycles will coincide with the termination of the skeletal growth. The breasts will assume a stable size and shape as will the other primary and secondary reproductive characteristics. Aside from pregnancy, alterations in these characteristics can signal physiological dysfunctioning

It is during this time period that boys usually experience their most prolific growth. Approximately one year after the first testicular acceleration, the growth in height begins. The skeletal and muscle changes do not occur proportionately. The head, hands, and feet achieve adult size first, followed by arms and legs, with shoulder girth and trunk length last. With skeletal growth there comes an increase in the proportion of muscle to fat. The basal metabolism rate declines from the latency rate, but it declines less for boys than girls. Boys retain a higher rate due to the greater muscle mass and, therefore, a higher consumption of oxygen (Malmquist, 1979).

Prior to puberty, boys and girls have similar strength except for the hands and forearms. During adolescence, the male's strength increases markedly. According to Tanner (1962), the initial stimulus for greater height and strength is due to the increase of testosterone in the body. These changes in body strength often correspond to strong environmental pressures to participate in sports programs.

In this period, there is an increase in the size of the seminal tubes and the "sertoli cells" and spermatozosina develop. The size of the penis increases as well as the size of the prostate and bulbo-urethra glands. Research on first ejaculations suggests that they are situationally determined after biological readiness. It generally occurs one year after the acceleration of penile growth. Beginning one to two years after the onset of puberty, nocturnal emissions may occur. The associated dreams, loss of control, and fear of discovery may cause a great deal of anxiety and feelings of guilt, even in boys who are reasonably well informed about their physiology.

Two years after the growth of pubic hair, axillary and facial hair appear. Skin changes occur in both sexes with acne and "roughening" becoming a distressful experience for some. Statistically, acne occurs more often in males than females. There is rapid gland development in adolescents especially in the axilla, genital, and anal areas. These alterations lead to changes in body odors. A multimillion dollar industry has capitalized on this fact.

Ages Sixteen to Nineteen

Though most girls will have achieved adult physiological growth by 16, some may not. The uterus is the major organ in females that continues to grow through this third period of adolescent development.

The average age for males to have completed their growth in height is 16. During this period, strength continues to increase progressively. Testicular and penile growth is usually completed by 16. Axillary hair has begun to grow, but the heaviest amount of growth is not accomplished until about 30. This is true for both sexes. This is also true for facial hair for males. Frequently, the last male secondary sex characteristic to be attained is hair on the chest. Again, hair distribution may not be finalized until the late 20s, but usually by 16 males will look like men. The last change to occur is the male's voice.

In summary, each adolescent must adapt and cope with physiological changes. The mixture of bodily sensations, social responses, and altered body image requires large amounts of emotional energy, as well as large amounts of food. The newness of some of the feelings experienced together with the sometimes painful sensations associated with menses and erections can confuse the already ambivalent strivings of the adolescent.

Correct and complete information about physiological progression can relieve a great deal of the adolescent's confusion and anxiety. For this reason, anticipatory guidance is very important. Physiological maturation is only one facet of the developmental mosaic. How the adolescent develops a sense of self in the process of accommodating to significant physiological body changes comprises the psychosocial aspects, that is, development of the ego or of the self, cognitive development, and the complex nuances of peer and family relationships.

PSYCHOSOCIAL DEVELOPMENT

Anthropologists report that rites-of-passage ceremonies in primitive cultures, some of which are frightening demonstrations of adult power, are created to control the young and to formalize progress toward maturity. These expressive practices often demonstrate cultural values and describe the texture of society. In each instance, they are conservative, that is, designed to preserve the values and traditions of the culture. For example, elaborate rituals of female and male circumcision not only induct the adolescent into social, functional adulthood, but do so with cruelty and bravado, thereby establishing behavioral expectations for the new "adult."

The more sophisticated ceremonies and practices specific to adolescents in our culture include confirmation, the bar mitzvah, and commencement ceremonies at graduation from high school or college. Forced union apprenticeships and other social restrictions are designed to inhibit entry of the adolescent into adult society as a wage earner. On a less formal level, being regarded as mature enough to drive a car is a coveted developmental milestone, restricted by the minimal age requirement for taking "driver education" and becoming licensed and, of course, the adolescent must also gain permission to drive the family car. Social control of the not-quite-adult is obvious in each instance of these regulatory, transitional practices. What is it about the adolescent that requires such elaborate measures of control?

There has been a scholarly controversy, spanning at least four decades, over the nature of adolescence centered around the issue of whether adolescence is a transitional stage between childhood and adulthood, characterized by stress, turmoil, and emotional crisis, or a developmental period of rapid physical growth and change that is weathered by a majority of individuals without significant difficulty. Data have demonstrated over the last 20 years instances of high stress behaviors among segments of the adolescent population, sometimes overt rebellion and vicious forms of antisocial behavior. There are equally significant data supporting the more optimistic belief that many young people are outraged over social conditions and will ultimately provide leadership for positive change.

Central to the theory of adolescence as a tumultuous transitional period are the psychodynamically oriented authors who elaborate on the psychoanalytic theory of Sigmund Freud. The disruptive impact of increased sexual and aggressive drives associated with the physiological changes of puberty is the major theme. Unable to manage formerly repressed impulses under the hormonal onslaught of puberty, the ego of the adolescent is described as vulnerable to the point of psychopathological symptom formation. Indeed, this wrenching about of the personality is regarded by classical analysts as not only typical, but as a necessary experience for future adult adjustment.

The psychologist G. Stanley Hall (1904) was the earliest author to explore adolescence as a distinct, identifiable period. Using the phrase "storm and stress" to describe the typical emotional climate of adolescence, he is credited, together with theorists of the analytical tradition, with broadly influencing clinicians, educators, developmentalists, and even legal scholars toward regarding adolescence as a period of irresponsibility, faulty reasoning, and questionable mental health (Bakan, 1975; Proefrock, 1981). Hall saw adolescence as a period in which the personality was radically disrupted, but one which carried the potential for a new birth.

The "storm and stress" authors dominated developmental theory until midcentury when Erikson's *Childhood and Society* (1950) was published, carrying a powerful impact that continues into the 1980s. Erikson, a psychoanalyst, regarded adolescence as one of eight normal life-stage crises that collectively describe the individual's progress through life. Erikson believed that the search for identity was the major task of the adolescent period. Identity, "a subjective sense of an invigorating sameness and continuity" (Erikson, 1950, p. 19), was the focus of continuing study for Erikson. The concern of the adolescent about how he is seen by others and the waivering doubt about the validity of his or her own perceptions of self and others reflect the sometimes troubled preoccupations and curiosity of the adolescent about both the internal and external world.

Adolescence should be understood as a developmental stage distinct and describable in the same sense that infancy and maturity are considered to be stages of development. According to Proefrock (1981), the search for identity requires the adolescent to "reestablish the continuity and sameness of childhood in the post-pubescent body" (p. 854). The tentative security of the young person has been described as a sense of being uprooted, a forced letting go of the safe "sureness" of childhood and being propelled toward an unsteady grasp on adulthood. The negative alternative to identity formation in Erikson's formulation is role confusion. It should be recalled that Erikson rejected any interpretation that the outcome of the bipolar developmental crises was absolute. Role confusion persists to some degree in all individuals just as some aspects of identity formation are established in each individual no matter how tentative the process. Resolution of the developmental crisis of adolescence finds the individual more or less moving on to the next stage in which developing the capacity for intimacy or mature, interpersonal love is the major task. The adolescent who has a sense of his or her own identity is able to declare, "*This* is the real me!"

Adolescence is a psychological stage that occurs in response to the physiological event of puberty. Following that definition, preadolescence must be defined as the developmental stage of childhood that precedes the onset of puberty. Obviously, the end stage of preadolescence, and of childhood, occurs with the onset of puberty and of early adolescence in the vast majority of instances. The upper limit or endpoint of the psychological stage of adolescence is much more obscure and has no physiological signpost. Lacking the theoretical nicety of such a signpost, speculative theorists and researchers use arbitrary indicators to demarcate the chronology of adolescence.

Stating that the stage of adolescence ends at the time when the individual has attained a reasonable degree of independence from his parents, Offer & Offer (1971) note that current social phenomena extend adolescence in this country well beyond the norm either of 20 years ago in the United States or of current European standards. This change has occurred because young people in the United States increasingly attend schools of higher education and therefore remain somewhat dependent on parents well into late adolescence and early adulthood. The extension of adolescence beyond age 18 or 20 can be forced by such external factors as well as by internal or interpersonal situations.

Sullivan (1953) believed that developmental problems of adolescence were related to the extraordinarily difficult tasks of managing three urgent and frequently conflicting needs: the need for intimacy or interpersonal love, the need for sexual gratification, and the need to maintain a sense of security. Establishment of relatively enduring patterns for meeting these needs is necessary before proceeding to the tasks of late adolescence. Sullivan said, "Late adolescence extends from the patterning of preferred genital activity through unnumbered educative and eductive steps to the establishment of a fully human or mature repertory of interpersonal relations" (Sullivan, 1953, p. 297). Failure to achieve the interpersonal tasks of adolescence is common and that failure may result in the individual being caught, developmentally stalled, in a neurotic inability to achieve true interpersonal intimacy.

Development of the Ego: Development of the Self

The psychoanalytic view of adolescence as a period of near chaos describes the ego struggling to control the resurgent forces of the id, held in repression throughout latency, but now fortified by the energy of instinctive impulses directed toward genital expression. Anna Freud (1958), who described adolescence as the stepchild of psychoanalysis, wrote:

> More than any other time of life, adolescence with its typical conflicts provides the analyst with instructive pictures of the interplay and sequence of internal danger; anxiety, defense activity, transitory or permanent symptom formation, and mental breakdown (p. 258).

Nevertheless, adolescence also provides a picture of how the ego masters disruptive id impulses.

Analytic theory holds that repressed oedipal strivings resurface at adolescence and that resurgence of this infantile conflict is partially responsible for the "storm and stress" character of parent-child relationships. Ultimately, the young person leaves the conflictual arena of the home, initiates a new family unit, and proceeds into adulthood with the ego as the executive of his or her being.

The long developmental period of adolescence should be a time of ego development toward maturity and assumption of the autonomy, opportunities, and responsibilities of adulthood. It involves mastery of sexual drives, accommodation of a remarkably changed image of the self in relationship to one's own body, to family, peers, and community, and the shifting of major, but not total, energies from homosexual to heterosexual affectional relationships. Management of the individual's defenses necessitates abandonment of some patterns that were effective in childhood but may be awkward hindrances in the new relationship opportunities of adolescence and adulthood. The remarkable changes in cognition toward abstract thought make synthesis of the many inner and outer experiences possible.

Social norms and the educational system in our culture are meant to be instrumental in assisting the child to gain mastery of his or her impulses. Adolescent boys are expected to be actively involved in competitive sports or in other energy-consuming forms of social interaction. School and community athletic programs provide for healthy activity and socialization with the all-important peer group and further prized athletic characteristics.

Adolescents between ages 12 and 14 need opportunities to form new peer groups that are adjusted to the growth spurts typical of the age. This reforming of groups and of new close friendships is an important, sometimes painful experience that occurs when old relationships are no longer satisfying to the youngster who has experienced a growth spurt. Lidz (1968) points out that early maturation is usually a positive advantage for a boy. The values of male strength and prowess give the early maturer a distinct social advantage over his peers. Quite the opposite may be true for a girl who is apt to question the advantage of a fully developed figure when her friends are still little girls in appearance. The late-maturing boy may be forced into interests other than competitive sports because of his size, whereas the late-maturing girl frequently finds herself an outsider among her friends who have matured physically.

Expansion of interest toward the opposite sex is as unpredictable as physical growth. Romantic crushes are common, often involving a member of the same sex who is in the young adult age group. The likelihood for actual physical gratification is probably dependent on the degree of apprehension of the adolescent over the emerging sex role. The object of a crush can be as close as a teacher or next door neighbor or can be as distant as a rock star. The object of the crush is idealized and fulfills the position of the fantasized sex partner, often in pristine scenarios.

Since girls mature earlier than boys, the early approaches that precede dating are usually made by the girl. A boy of 15 may enjoy the flattery (although he may grumble about being pestered) of long telephone calls from girls for a full year before making the move toward anything like arranging a real date. The importance of the telephone to socialization of the early adolescent should not be overlooked even though the family may be annoyed by the long, ritualized conversations that are so woefully lacking in substance to the adult ear. The telephone provides physical distance during an important testing of new heterosexual interpersonal relationship skills.

Cognitive Development

The change in cognitive ability of the adolescent is not simply a matter of greater intellect. It is rather that the gradual increase in intellect accrued throughout childhood leads to a *qualitative* change at about the time of puberty. This is described by Piaget as a new stage of cognitive development, the period of formal operations. This change follows the stage of concrete operations that is characteristic of the prepubescent child (Inhelder & Piaget, 1958). The period of formal operations begins at 11 or 12 and the cognitive capacity is consolidated at 14 or 15.

The latency-age child develops considerable cognitive competence during six or seven years of formal schooling. "The preadolescent child has acquired a coherent cognitive system with which he can understand his world and work on it, and into which he can fit new experiences" (Lidz, 1968, p. 85). It should be kept in mind that many individuals in our culture never proceed beyond the concrete operational level of cognition, their capability being limited by genetic or accidental factors or by the extent of formal education and/or the quality of environmental stimulation.

Piaget (1969) described the cognitive development of the typical adolescent as the achievement of logical thought, the capacity to conceptualize and to reason on hypotheses or propositions—that is, the ability to grasp the "if-then" concept. This stage is in contrast to the concrete operations of the child of age 8 or 10 who discovers relationships of objects and is able to classify, serialize, observe one-to-one correspondence of objects or multiple features of objects, numbers, and spatial operations. As this novel capacity of adolescent thought becomes more refined, concrete logic can be detached from the object itself and can function on verbal or symbolic statements alone.

In considering Piaget's orientation to cognitive development, it should be kept in mind that his theory holds that cognition is a process of constant, dynamic developmental reorganization. For example, the process of "decentering" or the gaining of a proper perspective of events begins in infancy and continues throughout life. Decentering involves the gradual giving up of egocentrism until, in adolescence, the individual learns that the manipulation of ideas in his own fantasy is not the same as convincing others who have differing orientations and convictions (Lidz, 1968). Through this process, the adolescent accommodates to the universe and to the present time in history and discovers where and how his or her ideas fit into abstract systems of logic and thought.

Piaget noted that the intellectual transformations typical of adolescent thought were critical in moving the young person into social and intellectual relationships with adults. Piaget (1969) speculated that the formal operations of the adolescent-adult mind are not found in primitive cultures and might be manifested only on a "vocational level" among manual workers and technicians in an advanced society such as ours. Implicit in his speculation is the notion that such a vocational level of formal operations is different from the verbal or experimental level found in adolescents with literary or scientific training.

The ability to evaluate one's own behavior, as well as how one's ideas concur with the ideas of others, makes it possible for the adolescent to develop the necessary ego strength to keep powerful sexual and sometimes aggressive impulses within socially and personally acceptable limits. If, as Piaget suggests, progression toward formal cognitive operations is dependent on educational training, the troubled young people of urban and rural poverty in our society are doubly deprived. Due to poor education and to dysfunctional family and community environments, such young people may lack the cognitive ability to conceptualize the consequences of their actions.

It must be recognized, however, that educational and environmental advantage do not ensure optimal cognitive development of the young person. There is staggering evidence to the contrary among families of middle and upper levels of income. Poverty is not the determining factor in producing troubled youth. Whatever the cause, adolescents who fail to achieve formal operational cognitive ability are vulnerable to temptations to drop out of school and seek immediate gratification of impulses and needs. They may be prone to experience repeated disasters in living, arising from failure to put things together in any clear, logical, systematic fashion.

It was Longfellow who said, "and the thoughts of youth are long, long thoughts." The ability of the adolescent to explore the wisdom of the ages and to find the courage to challenge the values of the wise is contingent upon his or her ability to use formal operations in thinking. Erikson (1968) recognized the rich cultural resource of the young neohumanist in our society, the thoughtful, adolescent "philosopher" who rages against injustices of whatever political persuasion, and who may reassemble forgotten values and ideologies into a better society. The capacity to create poetry, art, music, and new philosophies finds genesis in the intellectural development of the adolescent.

On a less lofty and more frequently observed level, the adolescent is able to organize the disparate elements of his own existence into a logical framework. Though tentative to be sure, it is one that incorporates the values of parents and community into his or her own unique view of the world. Lidz (1968) provides a summary:

> The new abilities enable youths to embrace ideologies to challenge the status quo, to envision a better world, to gain gratification through fantasy while waiting to become able to achieve in reality and in general to soar above the prosaic world with its plodding inhabitants (p. 317).

Adults who are perceived to be the "plodding inhabitants" of the world of the adolescent are apt to be parents, too often the youngster's own. Critical scrutiny of parents ordinarily is evidence of developmental progress of sorts, all the more distressing to parents who are compared unfavorably with the young peers of their children.

Family and Peer Relationships

> In the simplest terms we can say that, with the advent of sexual maturation, cognitive leaps to higher levels, and new physical capabilities, a thrust away from infantile family dependencies into the wider social milieu becomes not only feasible but mandatory. (Blos, 1979, p. 5)

The tasks to be accomplished by the adolescent are complex. This complexity provides an explanation for the protracted time period required for achieving developmental tasks and for the many instances of frustration and real anguish encountered by the adolescent and his or her family in the process. Separation from parents can be conceptualized as the central personal and interpersonal accomplishment with which all other tasks of adolescence are interrelated. The complementary nature of these developmental tasks defines the process as one of separation-individuation. Separation from parents occurs in counterpoint to individuation and the eventual outcome is a sense of oneself as an individual capable of functioning autonomously in physical and emotional distance from the parents. It is practice in becoming one's own person.

Ability to manage the very real losses associated with separation-individuation depends greatly on earlier learning. The ideal family experience is one that reinforces the child's self-esteem through love and respect and, in addition, provides him or her with the internalized love object. As a result, the child carries the permanent mental equivalent of the parents in his or her mind and the parenting experience becomes a part of the self. Thus reinforced, the youth may be alone but is not so apt to languish in loneliness in the extended absences integral to growing up, such as the summer job away from home or going away to school. Nevertheless, the losses incurred during adolescence are very real and exact an emotional response. Mourning for the lost security of childhood and for the providers of that security is responsible for much of the melancholy experienced poignantly by young people and is often expressed in their music and literary efforts and in their clinging to each other as protection against anxiety and loneliness.

The family is a system that provides for the physical, psychological, spiritual, and social needs of its members. It is an open system since there is always an interchange of information, energy, and even members with the larger community. As is true with any system, the family is more than a sum of its parts and has its own sense of being, which is shared by its members. The shared sense of being is rich in verbal and experiential history, in family myths, autistic understandings, and in all the nuances of intimate knowing that can never be truly communicated to an outsider. The family with an adolescent member is required to tolerate a gradual loosening of the entire system, with an eventual dissolution of some dependent ties and often a reintegration of others on a more mature basis. Tight alliances formed over many years of close association will resist such change.

One of the more painful complications of adolescence is management of old intrafamilial alliances. A mutually dependent mother-son alliance that excludes the father is particularly destructive and has been widely discussed in the literature (Ackerman, 1980; Berger, 1978; Miller & Janosik, 1980). Equally destructive but less common is the intense father-daughter alliance with concomitant isolation of the mother. Cultural prohibitions against father-daughter incest are closer to conscious recognition, perhaps because the potential for acting-out of the impulse is greater. The power of the prohibition may influence distorted alliance formation in the normal family. In either event, the son or daughter who is caught in a mutually dependent web with a parent will be handicapped in achieving independence.

The nature and goals of professional intervention to assist the family with an adolescent member will be influenced greatly by the age of the young person. For example, the 14-year-old must remain an integrated member of the family for several years, whereas the 18-year-old may need assistance in loosening the ties and making plans to move to a more independent living arrangement. Accommodating the ultimate developmental goals of achieving individuation of the adolescent and separation from parents, the professional family counselor or therapist is often challenged to reintegrate the young son or daughter back into the family in order to allow the inevitable parting to occur in a positive way. To bring the adolescent back into the family may involve breaking a pattern of running away from home, one of the most frightening and increasingly prevalent examples of adolescent acting-out behavior.

An even more symbolic expression of the drive toward separation-individuation is the alienation of the adolescent from the values of the family. The family counselor in this instance is challenged to reintegrate a rebellious, defiant child back into the interpersonal family system in order to support the adolescent in becoming his own person, a paradoxical situation at best. The objective of maintaining the young person in the family is to reduce the collective pain of the inevitable separation and to encourage the weaving of more mature ties between the adolescent and the family.

The affectional attraction of peers increases dramatically as the attraction of parents decreases (Lidz, 1968; Smart & Smart, 1977). The typical adolescent will spend more and more time with friends and will often feel better understood by friends than by parents. The dynamic parallel between this developmental shift and actual alienation between the generations is apparent.

By early adolescence, the need for peer acceptance becomes very strong. Wearing the "in" clothes or having the "right" haircut become symbolic manifestations of mutually reinforced peer approval. Strong social alliances are formed outside of family relationships and the absence of peer relationships during adolescence is a significant warning that the youngster may be having real difficulty. In preadolescence, the best friend or chum is usually of the same sex; however, by middle or late adolescence best friends include members of the opposite sex. The early chum relationship allows the time to practice truly intimate, interpersonal experiences. Sullivan (1953) writes about the chum relationship:

> Because one draws so close to another, because one is newly capable of seeing oneself through the other's eyes, the preadolescent phase of personality development is especially significant in correcting autistic, fantastic ideas about oneself or others (p. 248).

The singular friendships of preadolescence progress toward heterosexual relationships that involve both interpersonal intimacy and sexual elements as a prelude to the marital relationship.

Adolescence is often described as a period that includes reworking of the major psychodynamic tasks of previous stages. Solidifying one's gender identity is one task, while at the same time the adolescent is encouraged to relate to the opposite sex. Dating becomes an important activity for many psychosocial reasons: (1) peer acceptance, (2) development of gender identity, (3) social adeptness, and (4) personal identity. When one person's gender identity is defined in terms of acceptance by an opposite sex person, sexuality, often mistaken for love, becomes the focus of the relationship. That focus may precipitate a teenage pregnancy. Teenage pregnancy and teenage marriage pose a heavy strain on the developing adolescent. Otto (1979) presents a model of antecedents and consequences of marital timing, including the interaction of premarital pregnancy and marital timing as two major interacting variables. The combination of premarital pregnancy and teenage marriage dramatically interferes with post-high school aspirations, socioeconomic attainments, and marital outcomes.

Some high schools offer adequate information to students regarding future career roles and family responsibilities. With careful attention to anticipatory guidance, adolescents can make better decisions and avoid the pitfalls of impulsive actions. Anticipatory guidance includes an information component as well as a supportive relationship component.

VARIATIONS ON THE THEME OF ADOLESCENCE

It would be reassuring to report that young people are a sound lot, proceeding toward adult status without significant turmoil; however, the bittersweet nature of adolescence persists in each generation. Changes that involve separation and loss are not easy. Health professionals must be alert to the needs of this very special segment of our society. It is with this in mind that one examines the wide variations within the normal range of behavior and takes another step beyond that wide range of normalcy to consider the true pathologies that sometimes occur in adolescence. Adolescence is a period of restlessness, conflict, and change when the young person is subject to more or less transitory periods of anxiety and depression. The action-oriented adolescent may relieve his or her anxiety through the excitement of antisocial or delinquent behavior. Other youngsters somaticize the stresses of the period and develop psychosomatic problems. In short, the responses of adolescents to stress are as diverse as the coping patterns of adults. A significant difference between the two age groups is the greater potential for successful preventive or primary intervention during the volatile, vulnerable period of adolescence.

There are obstacles that will interfere with the usual resolution of adolescence and keeping these obstacles in mind will help the care-giver in assisting adolescents and their families. Common obstacles are interruptions of family stability, physical illness or accident, learning disabilities, mental retardation, and cultural influences.

Separation, divorce, and death account for major family disruptions. In many cases, these disruptions are managed constructively by family members; however, the usual assault to self-esteem that occurs in major family disruptions takes time and energy. Energy needed for resolution of adolescent developmental tasks may be drained off to deal with the family disruption; therefore, adolescence may be prolonged or insufficiently resolved. The young person who is forced prematurely to assume adult responsibilities due to family stress or disruption is in obvious jeopardy, since normal developmental tasks must be given reduced priority.

Mastery of the major tasks of adolescence may be compromised by limitations of physical health. Loss of function in a major organ, loss of a limb, or impairments of sight or hearing can be major obstacles to a functional resolution of adolescence. Chronic pain can compromise the person's capacity to cope with the many developmental tasks. All areas of adolescent development would not necessarily be compromised; however, when large amounts of time and energy are required to meet assaults on one's physiological health, the time and energy for other tasks may not be available.

An adolescent with a learning disorder can be greatly handicapped through adolescence. An adolescent who is classified as having a learning disorder must have a significant disparity in one or more (but not all) of the basic psychological processes of listening, thinking, talking, reading, writing, spelling, or arithmetic. Educational institutions are more aware of these students and make some attempt to meet their educational needs. The same psychological processes that interfere with academic performance are major components of interpersonal relationships. Most learning-disabled students have had many negative educational and interpersonal experiences and the assault to their self-esteem is powerful and can interfere with the many tasks of adolescence.

For most moderately, severely, and profoundly retarded adolescents, the usual needs of adolescence are modified by their impairment. However, the mildly retarded, who make up nearly 90% of those classified as retarded, have the same basic strivings and adjustments as other adolescents. Because of the retarded adolescent's social and intellectual limitations, he is often easy prey to sexual exploitation. In addition, the stigma of incompetence that often surrounds this group of adolescents has a strong impact on their self-esteem and ego functioning. The physiological and psychosocial resolutions of adolescence can be mastered by mildly retarded persons in a mature, functional way, especially if they are assisted by mature, functional adults who can respect them and recognize their capabilities, as well as their limitations.

A major barrier to the successful resolution of adolescence may be the constraints imposed by cultural elements. Racial, ethnic, religious, and economic factors can foster or impede the adolescent's course toward maturity. Basic needs of survival can interfere with long-range goals of education or career. Religious rites and requirements can interfere or limit the choices of youthful members. Religious structures and constraints can foster adolescent development for some, and for others they can retard or jeopardize developmental progress.

This brief discussion of barriers to resolution of adolescent tasks is to alert the clinician to additional mediating areas that influence adolescent development. Barriers can also be examined as positive influences that challenge adolescents. Overcoming the problems or barriers they encounter can provide some adolescents with the experiential field for becoming more mature and sensitive to the nature of being human.

ADOLESCENTS WITH PSYCHOPHYSIOLOGIC DISORDERS

The discussion of disorders that have strong physiological and psychological factors reminds one again that people are multifaceted systems of interrelated elements. Thus, the assessment of a presenting problem must be analyzed from many angles to obtain a clear picture of the human condition.

Anorexia Nervosa (DSM III 307.10), (American Psychiatric Association, 1980)

In general, there are few psychological or physiological disorders that are specific to adolescence; however, anorexia nervosa is one. The average age of onset is 17 years, although it may be seen earlier or even up to age 30. The nature of the psychological conflict is fraught with the typical conflicts of adolescence.

Anorexia nervosa occurs nine times more frequently in females than males. The most obvious symptom is the emaciated appearance. The person's weight is not merely abnormally low but approaches physiological starvation. The gaunt, skeletal appearance is in dramatic contrast to their own perception of their bodies. In the mind of the anorectic, she is overweight. The distorted perception of reality makes it difficult to treat the individual with the disorder. Because of the extreme distortion in perception, anorectics usually cannot be responsible for their own food intake.

The anorectic does not generally just refuse to eat but, in her ambivalence will, at times, eat voraciously followed by episodes of vomiting to eliminate the offensive calories. Food becomes the central focus of her interpersonal interactions. Unable to enjoy eating and retaining food, the anorectic will talk incessantly about aspects of food: the preparation of food, the amount of calories a food may have, and the nutritional values of specific foods (Crisp, 1980).

Along with her slavish devotion to a diet regime, the anorectic will proceed with a vigorous exercise routine until she is so weak she is unable to continue. The diet and physical exercise are efforts to control her perceived excess weight.

Because the disorder can be life-threatening, aggressive therapy must be instituted. In addition to the emaciated appearance, these girls develop amenorrhea. This symptom is attributable to the extreme physiological disequilibrium and, at the same time, highlights one of the central issues of the psychological conflict. The anorectic's anxiety around sexual maturity and parental dependency form the core of the psychological conflict. As part of the family system, the anorectic often is sacrificing her body to maintain a tense balance within the family. Treatment is often sabotaged by uncooperative family members (Crisp, 1980).

Bulimia (DSM III, 307.51)

This eating disorder is often associated with anorexia nervosa but may exist without the starving quality of the syndrome. Bulimia refers to eating binges that are frequently followed by episodes of vomiting. In most cases, there is an accompanying depression. The frequency of binge eating averages three to four episodes per week. Over one-third have episodes of daily binges. Usually there is not an accompanying denial of one's behavior as abnormal, but there is a feeling of a lack of self control (Minkoff, Bergman, Beck & Beck, 1973).

Ulcerative Colitis

This disorder, like anorexia nervosa, has life-threatening physiological consequences. While the usual onset of the disease occurs between the ages of 20 and 40, this inflammatory bowel disease is often seen in younger people.

Differentiating ulcerative colitis from other inflammatory bowel diseases such as Crohn's disease is very important (Derezin, 1982). An interdisciplinary team approach with the medical and/or surgical physicians will be necessary to provide the therapy for these patients.

Though ulcerative colitis is not presumed to be psychogenic in origin, the precipitation and course of the disease are strongly related to psychological stress (Derezin, 1982; Engel, 1973). Most cases fall into the mild category where there are episodes of frequent diarrhea with or without gastrointestinal bleeding, abdominal cramping, pain, weight loss, anorexia, fever, and fatigue (Derezin, 1982). Ulcerative colitis proceeds with periods of exacerbations and remissions. The disease can quickly become life-threatening when the colon becomes severely inflamed and the walls become thin and paralyzed. This can result in perforation of the bowel, which can lead to peritonitis, sepsis, and death. For the severely ill person, surgical repair may be necessary to preserve life. Segmental colostomies and ileostomies may be done (Prugh & Eckhardt, 1979).

Adolescents with ulcerative colitis struggle with the same developmental issues as other adolescents. Because these adolescents have a sensitive target organ, the colon, psychological conflicts aggravate the inflammatory disease process. The psychological conflicts center around the adolescent's ambivalence toward sexual maturity and the normal strivings for independence from parental dominance. There is a strong core of depression that must be addressed as well (Engle, 1973; Prugh & Eckhardt, 1979).

Other Psychophysiologic Disorders

In adolescence, as well as in other developmental stages, the interplay of physiological and psychological processes can produce varying degrees of dysfunctional behavior. Asthma, peptic ulcers, migraines, and diabetes, together with many other apparent physiologic problems, have strong psychological concommitants that influence the manifestations and course. The interplay of intrapsychic forces and familial and social forces qualify and mitigate the person's physiological responses through adolescence. The exacerbation of physiological problems can be triggered by the physiological changes that are occurring as well as the psychosocial tensions of the stage.

The psychiatric nurse clinical specialist is in a key position to assess and treat in a holistic frame adolescents with psychophysiologic problems. As a health care provider who has knowledge of normal physiology as well as normal and dysfunctional psychosocial processes the nurse can provide an integrated approach to the health care of these adolescents.

Depression: The Affective Disorders

Music and the other arts provide for vicarious expression of emotions that might otherwise be left unanswered and restless in some unknown recess of the mind. Sadness, melancholy, loss, depression, and pain are expressed in rock music as surely as expressions of rebellion, aggression, sexual abandon, religious ecstacy, or love. Listening to the music of the adolescent is one way to discover the momentary meaning of existence for the young person and the message is often one of melancholy (see Figure 7.2).

Loss and reactive depression are linked in a cause-and-effect relationship in the literature. The losses incurred during adolescence are ordinarily compensated for by positive gains in personal, interpersonal and social realism. For example, the adolescent's social horizons expand to new dimensions of friendships, as well as toward romantic relationships with real people. Enhanced cognitive abilities encompass the worlds of science, technology, philosophy and esthetics. Nevertheless, the adolescent experience is overwhelming to too many young people. Depression and suicide are profoundly serious problems among the adolescent population (Haim, 1974; Hendin, 1976).

Kraft (1983) reported that more than 5600 young women and men under 25 committed suicide in 1981, the most recent data available from the Suicide Research Unit of the National Institute of Mental Health. There was an alarming 66 percent increase of suicide for that group during the 1970s, excluding the sharp increase in self-destructive automobile and other "accidental" deaths. In 1982, suicide was second only to accidents as the leading cause of death among adolescents (Rush, 1982). The contagious nature of suicide among adolescents was cited by Kraft (1983) as being a particularly frightening phenomenon and one susceptible to intervention by alert school personnel, mental health workers, and family members. As a reflection of current social unrest, suicide often seems like an easy way out to the young person who finds the world crowded, impersonal, devoid of career opportunities, and generally sterile.

According to psychoanalytic theory, depression occurs in response to the real or imagined loss of a love object. Depression can be defined as the emotional expression of a state of helplessness and powerlessness of the ego, irrespective of the actual cause of collapse of the esteem-maintaining mechanism. What may be experienced as the greatest loss may be the sense of self-esteem or well-being that is contingent on the interpersonal relationship, rather than the loss of the object itself. This theoretical notion accounts for the self-degradation that is such a painful aspect of depression (Rush, 1982; Sandler & Joffe, 1965).

The response to loss in preadolescence and adolescence is often anger and aggression expressed in acting-out behavior. An evil self-image is a frequent source of negative, delinquent behavior. The self-fulfilling prophesy is completed when the negative behavior earns the disapproval of parents and others, reinforcing the adolescent's already low self-image. In late adolescence, hostility is much more apt to be directed inward, thereby reducing the incidence of acting-out or delinquency and increasing the likelihood of serious depression and the danger of suicide. Hendin (1976) found that many suicidal college students used suicidal preoccupations as a means to manage rage and frustration.

Suicide is an act of despair. It is sometimes a mistake or an impulsive act meant only to be a cry for help; but all too frequently it is an act of lethal intent to escape from depression or feelings of hopelessness (Bedrosian & Beck, 1979; Minkoff, et al, 1973; Wetzel,

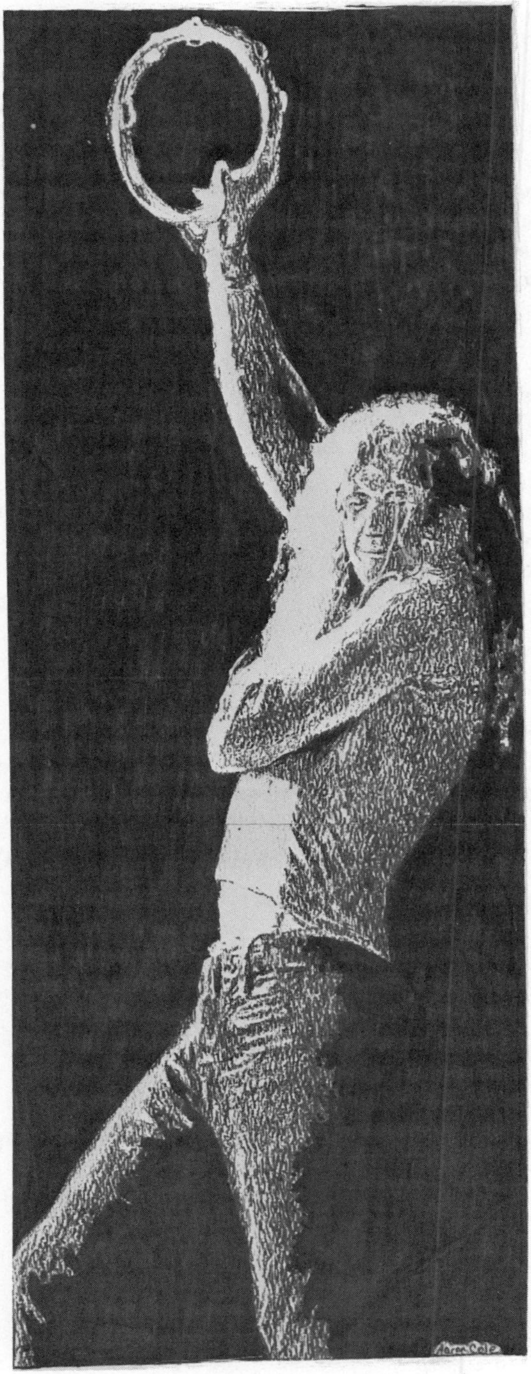

Figure 7.2 (Drawing by Aaron Cole.)

1976). Indications of depression or expressions of hopelessness or death may seem to be the only solution to the chronic problem of living for the troubled youngster (Teicher, 1979). Suicidal fantasies may preoccupy the adolescent boy or girl and are particularly painful to recognize in retrospect following a suicide attempt or an actual suicide.

Research in predictive-preventive factors in suicidal behavior over the last two decades has produced many clues for the clinician, but true predictability continues to be elusive (Capodanno & Targum, 1983). The following behaviors are cited as warning clues, which are particularly significant when an adolescent exhibits two or more: (1) dysphoric mood; (2) worrying obsessively about issues of life and death; (3) significant weight loss or weight gain; (4) giving away treasured possessions or other indications of loss of interest in usual activities; (5) ending important relationships, in effect telling a best friend he or she is free to go on alone; (6) fatigue, insomnia; (7) securing the means of suicide, even such an apparently innocuous item as an over-supply of aspirin; and (8) the most dangerous of all, actually threatening suicide or making a suicidal gesture.

The new manual of classification of mental disorders, DSM III, 296.2X and 296.3X, APA, 1980 includes depression of children and adolescents under the general description of the affective disorders for all age groups; nevertheless, clinicians are often apprehensive in trying to discriminate the mood swings of the healthy adolescent from dangerous depressive states. Seen much more frequently than the classical picture of depression are "depressive equivalents" that conceal the true mental state behind a facade. Depression in the young is often cloaked or masked and the task of the clinician is to recognize the clue for what it is.

The depressive equivalents of adolescence can be grouped according to physiological, psychological, or social masking patterns (Toolan, 1971).

Physiological Masks of Depression

Fatigue that is inordinate for the particular individual should be monitored carefully, particularly if the youngster has reasonable periods of sleep and no obvious reason for fatigue. Hypochondriasis, psychosomatic disorders, or phobias in adolescence also have been associated with development of overt depressive reactions (Lesse, 1981).

Psychological Masks of Depression

Denial is a common defense adopted by depressed adolescents in an effort to hide feelings from self as well as others. The result is a "smiling depression." From a psychodynamic perspective, helplessness and despair are associated with fear of regression to infantile dependency on the parents. False happiness based on denial may account for much of the hilarity and frenzied activity of adolescence.

Boredom alternating with restlessness is endemic in adolescence and may mask depression. Lack of interest, flat response, and short attention span in the ordinarily responsive teenager may be warning signs. The depressed adolescent often needs something to occupy every minute as a defense against loneliness.

A sudden drop in grades is frequently a key to depression in the school-competent student. Inquiry will often disclose difficulty in concentration on school work.

Hostility and anger, often directed to the person who is closest to the adolescent, are probably the most familiar psychological masks of depression. The significance of anger and rage is often confounded by the typical lability of the adolescent's mood.

Social Masks of Depression

Action is the language of adolescence. Acting-out of conflict is not limited to adolescence; however, it has become the catchword for all the hedonistic, destructive, outraged, and outrageous acts of youth. Delinquency is the ultimate of acting-out behavior, an overt demonstration of the adolescent's inability to face an impoverished self-image in the real world. The delinquent suffers from a sense of emptiness that is relieved by antisocial activity, often dangerous, illegal, or both. Drug and alcohol use can mask an underlying depression, with addiction and abuse being a predictable outcome if the depression is not interrupted.

Antisocial Behavior—Conduct Disorder

Description of the DSM III category, Conduct Disorder, requires consideration of the degree of aggression and socialization or lack of those qualities. The V codes, in contrast, accommodate and describe many difficulties experienced during the adolescent period, such as isolated antisocial acts (V 71.02), academic problems (V 62.30), or parent-child problems (V 61.20). Whatever the diagnostic system, issues of severity and chronicity are important in planning intervention and in prediction of outcome (APA, 1980).

Over a decade ago, Anthony (1970) discussed progress in theory, research, and treatment of the behavior disorders of children. He described two types: (1) a phase-specific, circumscribed, time-limited disorder, corresponding to the psychoneuroses and (2) a diffuse behavior disorder, corresponding to the primary behavior disorders and frequently persisting through every stage of development. In the first instance, the child or adolescent was evaluated as an essentially normal child usually from a nonpathogenic environment who was having transitory difficulty in coping with developmental or other stress. In the second case, the environment was apt to be both pathological and pathogenic, and the child's or adolescent's constitution resulted in vulnerability to failures in coping with developmental and other stressess.

The concept of internalization-externalization is useful in considering conduct disorders in comparison to other pathologies of adolescence. Internalization identifies the response to stress that is directed inward. In contrast, externalization flows out into the environment. "Anxiety states, phobias, depressions and obsessions involve suffering mainly for the individual, whereas delinquency, truancy, aggressive behavior and destructiveness inflict suffering on the environment" (Anthony, 1970, p. 719). Externalization of personal pain can be understood as a defensive escape from feelings of helplessness and frustration. Inflicting pain on family and community may literally save the life of a young person who might otherwise be overwhelmed by depression, the ultimate of internalization of stress.

Blos (1979) discussed a multitude of delinquencies, all of which share two characteristics, the engagement of an action system in problem solving and the use of the environment as tension regulator. Agonizing over one's problems is not an issue for the delinquent who simply acts out the problem. Action is the favored means of communication. The form of the delinquent act is influenced by the task of adolescence that is dominant at the time. The 13-year-old, Rose E., provides an example.

> Rose was the eldest of five children of a woman whose husband abandoned the family three years earlier. The mother was a dependent, sometimes euphoric woman who tip-toed precariously between reality and fantasy as a way of life. Rose slept occasionally with her mother following her father's disappearance.
>
> Rose was exhilirated by her own sexual stirrings and fantasized about having dates, looking sexy, and being "popular" with peers of both sexes; however, she had few friends. Mrs. E would not permit Rose to date and told her why in explicit sexual terms. She began to "allow" Rose to sleep regularly with her, and developed a pattern of having her daughter rub her back when she was unable to sleep.
>
> There was a powerful regressive pull for Rose toward a symbiotic, dependent, and sensual

relationship with her mother. A counterforce was the girl's budding heterosexual interest. In the absence of a father who might have afforded a more age-appropriate love object to counter the threat of maternal engulfment, Rose's love object became "the boys," two 18-year-old school dropouts. The conflict culminated one summer night when Rose saw "the boys" cruising slowly by her home with the car's headlights turned off. Barefoot, with her nightgown tucked around her hips, the girl crawled out the window of her sleeping mother's bedroom. Rose spent the next three days and nights with "the boys," declaring her heterosexual preference in explicit action.

The struggle of the early adolescent girl for sexual expression is frequently confounded by an intense regressive pull to return to the uncomplicated safety of the mother's arms. Conflict generated by developmental forces may then create feelings of opposition, aversion, or estrangement and lead to marked ambivalence in the girl's relationships with her mother. Flight to an intense relationship with the father or to "boy crazy" escapades are common defensive measures against the severe regressive pull toward the mother (Blos, 1979).

The delinquent act reflects the adolescent's efforts to manage aggressive impulses, rebellion against authorities, school or social failure, or any other developmental conflicts. A particularly virulent form of acting-out behavior in this country is substance abuse. It involves externalization of inner conflict and is destructive to individuals, families, and communities.

The report of the Joint Commission on Mental Health of Children (1973) invites reflective consideration of the decade since its publication. Of particular interest is a section on the use of drugs by the young in which a prediction was made that the "peak rates of drug use have yet to be attained across the nation" (p. 323). A particular cause for alarm was the trend of drug usage by increasingly younger students. There is no question that the grim prediction has been realized and that the trend toward drug use even among grade school children has increased (Lettieri & Ludford, 1981). Interestingly enough, consumption of alcohol was not mentioned in the 1973 report but is currently reported as the most frequently abused drug among adolescents.

A national survey found an alarming percentage of adolescents report having established drinking patterns. Over 20 percent of all tenth, eleventh, and twelfth graders contacted reported drinking once a week or more often. Over 8 percent said they drink three to four days every week, and 2 percent drink every day. One-fourth of the age group were "abstainers," but a shocking 14.8 percent described themselves as heavy drinkers. The trends are toward increased alcohol consumption among both boys and girls. Indeed, 87 percent report they have had experience in drinking alcohol. A special report to the U.S. Congress, which included the report of the survey of adolescents, noted the profound impact of increasing alcohol consumption on all segments of our society (De Luca, 1981).

A large segment of the youthful population continues to experience alienation and to look for relief, not only through drinking but in taking drugs. Since the adult segment of our culture is so thoroughly oriented toward seeking relief from even the mildest discomfort through chemical agents, reflection of that practice among our children is distressing but should not be surprising.

Warnings in the 1973 report that marijuana laws must be altered have gone unheeded and illegal production of the drug in the United States is of such magnitude that it now ranks as one of the top four cash crops in several states including California. This situation confirms the conviction of the young, and many of the not so young, that continued inclusion of marijuana under federal narcotic regulatory statutes is an example of abusurdity in the law derived from wrong information. As a result, information about illegal drugs continues to be met with skepticism or worse.

Adolescents are notorious for reacting to double standards and doubletalk. It is rarely mentioned that people take psychoactive addictive and nonaddictive drugs because the drug makes them feel good. The action of marijuana and the hallucinogens to enhance fantasy and allow expression of inhibited feelings may fill a transitory need for some youngsters (Proskauer & Rolland, 1975).

Does drug abuse indicate either conduct disorder or psychological deficit? The stereotype of the young drug user being a thoroughly antisocial "head" who is alienated from traditional social values and who has lost interest in anything beyond finding the next "fix" applies to a very small number of users (Pennington, 1973; Shopper, 1979). The majority of youths become involved with drugs believing their personal problems will be relieved by drug use, and a majority of young drug users spontaneously discontinue all involvement with drugs rather than continue beyond experimentation whether marijuana or hard drugs are involved.

The young people who only experiment with drugs are in the overwhelming majority according to Proskauer & Rolland (1975). Drawing on their clinical work with adolescents in an outpatient psychiatric court clinic at a large inner-city center, the authors described three groups of adolescent drug users:

1. *Experimental drug users.* These young people are strongly influenced by their peers to try drugs. It is unlikely that a fixed pattern of drug use will be the outcome *if* the inner need for the drug is not compelling, if the use of the drug is ego-alien to the individual or if drug use is strongly disapproved of by the important others in his or her life.
2. *Depressive drug users.* Drugs are taken by this group to relieve the intense feelings of emptiness, hopelessness, and loneliness that are experienced by most people during the long period of adolescence. Drugs are taken to reduce the feelings of depression. Since the drug abuse is a symptom, treatment should be directed toward the depression itself.
3. *Characterological drug users.* There is a relatively small number of adolescent drug users who have had severely disturbed personality development and who would be regarded by Anthony (1970) as having a primary behavior disorder. These young people are those who often have had serious difficulties throughout childhood, suffered deprivation during infancy, experienced traumatic losses, and have had pathological relationships with parents. Particular care should be exercised in discriminating between the users who are depressed and those who are characterological since their treatment programs should be different.

Psychotic Disorders

The ideal approach to the major psychoses (schizophrenias, DSM III, 295.1x–9x, and affective disorders DSM III, 296.2x–3x) is primary prevention; however, scientific progress has yet to provide a general basis for genetic counseling that would make that ideal a reality (Berlin, 1979). There has been no greater area of research activity in mental health over the past 40 years than the schizophrenias and, barring a breakthrough that would establish clear direction for primary prevention through genetic counseling, studies will continue into the psychobiological factors, family dynamics, psychopharmacology, and other aspects of this most prevalent of psychiatric disorders. Eisenberg (1979) calculated one million episodes of patient care yearly for *each* of the major psychoses, the schizophrenias and affective disorders. Adolescence is a period of particular vulnerability.

Adolescence has been defined as a psychological and social opportunity, a possibility for an experience of personal growth that may or may not occur after puberty. Among the children for whom that possibility is jeopardized or for whom the challenges of adolescence pose insuperable difficulties are those who suffer from one of the psychotic disorders.

Admissions of teenagers to state mental hospitals increased a shocking 150% during the decade of the 1960s. Even more grim were statistics showing that the young patients became sicker during hospitalization with a ricidivism rate of 30 to 50 percent and sometimes even higher (Pennington, 1973). There is no question that early diagnosis and treatment are essential to a favorable prognosis. Unfortunately, adolescence will often mask the warning signals of a psychotic episode.

Citing the fact that adolescence is the most complex maturational phase in the normal individual's development, the Joint Commission on Mental Health of Children (1973) identified the major problem in early diagnosis:

> There is no symptom of the disturbed adolescent that does not in one way or another fit into the category of normal adolescence; it is the degree, the crippling, and the unchangeableness of the symptoms that should be the criteria for evaluating whether the individual's behavior is that of a normal adolescent or indicative of something at least potentially going awry (p. 343).

In contrast to the acting out youngster, the adolescent whose ego collapses in a psychotic state internalizes his or her conflict. Self-punishing preoccupations with personal deficiencies cause morbid depression, which progresses beyond the normal periods of withdrawal common to the adolescent.

Emotional lability is a source of aggravation for the adolescent and for his or her family and friends; however, for some adolescents, marked irritability and episodes of despair may be the outward expressions of a chaotic attempt to manage the unmanageable: confusion over challenged values, conflict generated by attempts to identify career goals, or mastering sexual strivings. The youngster who is in an extraordinarily precarious psychological state may be treated tolerantly or he may be unsympathetically censored for his immaturity, his attention-getting devices, his laziness, or his irresponsibility. Psychosis may be the outcome, demonstrating failure of the system to respond before the strain reaches a level serious enough to destroy effective integration.

Regression is regarded by Blos (1979) as an essential component of normal adolescent psychic restructuring. The tendency toward action language is an example of regression as is the intense attraction to heroes and famous men and women. The latter is a reflection of the early idolization of the parent and, just as the parent is rejected at adolescence in the service of separation-individuation, the posters and other paraphernalia of the teenage crush disappear when real relationships take the place of fantasy. Regression in this instance is actually growth-promoting.

The young person who has a weak ego because of misfortunes during childhood or because of genetic predisposition may be unable to manage the strain of regression and indeed may become overwhelmed and lost in the regressive state. Without the parental support typical of childhood, the vulnerable adolescent may become psychotic. As might be expected, children who suffer from schizophrenia or other psychoses of earlier childhood are particularly vulnerable to regressive ego collapse during the adolescent phase and supportive therapy should be provided. However, a reactive psychotic episode may occur one time in adolescence or later and be followed by full recovery. The following incident occurred 25 years ago in a small community where psychiatric services were not available.

> Amy K., the youngest of four children, was socially popular and academically superior. She was indulged by her parents and three brothers and had a steady boyfriend. The pace of Amy's life accelerated during her senior year in high school and she responded with frenetic social activity, barely adequate progress at school, and frequent bursts of hilarity alternating with bouts of the blues.

Amy's best friend became pregnant. The two girls agonized for three weeks over the dilemma of an unwanted pregnancy; however, neither family was aware of the problem. Amy slipped into one of her blue moods and withdrew to her room. She missed school for four days, refused phone calls, and ate very little. Her mother became seriously concerned only when she realized Amy was not playing her records. On the fifth morning, Mrs. K. went into Amy's room and found her huddled in the corner of her closet, shaking violently and crying. She seemed not to hear her mother's questions, became more agitated, covered her head with a blanket, vomited, and was incontinent. When her parents tried to help her, she shrieked in terror and did not recognize them.

The family doctor consulted a psychiatrist who diagnosed Amy's condition as catatonic schizophrenia and recommended the state mental hospital, which was 100 miles away. The parents refused and Amy was hospitalized in a local general hospital where she was sedated. She was kept in bed with arm and leg restraints for fear she might harm herself and intravenous fluids were given for dehydration. She had frightening visual and auditory hallucinations whenever the sedation was reduced and was terrified of a crucifix on the wall. Either a member of the family or a nurse was in constant attendance, talking with her whenever she was awake. On the 16th day, Amy looked at her nurse, whispered, "I'm in the nut house," and begged to be allowed to go home.

Amy was sent home to recover after nearly a month in the hospital. Her withdrawal eased gradually but she remained depressed and listless for nearly six months. Then she began taking college courses at a slow pace and was able to continue without serious difficulty. One year after the psychotic episode, Amy married a fellow she met at college. She describes her illness as, "my crazy period," and has had no recurrence.

Amy's "crazy period" is an example of a self-limited psychotic episode in adolescence during which the patient was provided only supportive care. Had she been treated with psychotherapy, perhaps the meaning of the psychosis would be available for her greater self-understanding. Generalization from this example to other instances of schizophrenic collapse during adolescence should be made with the usual caution.

Few scholars or clinicians will deny the importance of both genetic and environmental influences. Clinicians and theoreticians have regarded the psychotic episode in adolescence, in contrast to an exacerbation of one of the genetically determined, chronic schizophrenic disorders, as a drastic retreat from the overwhelming stresses of adolescence. Treatment with psychotropic drugs to control the frightening symptoms is now quite standard and recovery following one episode is the more typical outcome.

It may be appropriate to consider R. D. Laing, one of the less conventional but more sensitive of the existential clinicians, who perceives the psychotic state to be a transitional, growth-potentiating but hellish experience from which the individual may emerge with greater understanding of self in the world *if* the individual is not irrevocably damaged by therapy. Laing (1967) believes ours is a society that methodically drives our children mad and that psychosis is an escape. He commented after working with 100 individuals diagnosed as schizophrenics:

> *Without exception,* the experience and behavior that gets labeled schizophrenic is *a special strategy that a person invents in order to live in an unlivable situation.* In his life situation the person has come to feel he is in an untenable position. He cannot make a move, or make no move, without being beset by contradictory and paradoxical pressures and demands, pushes and pulls, both internally for himself, and externally from those around him. He is, as it were, in a position of checkmate (p. 115).

SUMMARY

Two high school boys were talking and laughing as they were walking down a suburban street. Observed from a distance, first one and then the other of the boys would display a peculiar jerking motion of the head, something between a shrug and a rhythmical gesture, with just the suggestion of flamboyant defiance. It was an odd motion.

Casual observation over a period of weeks led to the conclusion that the gesture was very common among junior and senior high school boys, varying in vigor and grace, but following a quite uniform pattern: a quick jerking of the head upward and to one side, executed almost out of the boy's awareness.

It was the hair. Responsive to the invasion of the United States in the 1960s by British rock musical heroes who invariably wore their hair much longer than the prevailing style in this country, the boys of American suburbia were sporting long mops of hair that hung at mid-pupil level when at rest.

Those early longer hairstyles were barely collar length in the back but were heavy and full over the forehead. A quick reference to photos of the Beatles on their first trip to the United States will recall the era and the hairstyle. The endemic head-tossing gesture of adolescent boys was utilitarian. It cleared the visual field, but, like so many stylized, multidetermined actions, it became one of the signs of belonging, a mass communication among the young. Speculation that the hair-tossing gesture would become consolidated into a whole generation of men with an identical tic, whose origin would be lost in developmental history, never materialized. Other remnants of the period, however, have persisted and provide content for those who would understand the adolescent of today, reflecting on the fact that the youth of the sixties became the parents of today's adolescents.

Predictions of doom about the current generation of adolescents are as prevalent as expressions of indignation about their behavior. The cross-generational criticism continues. What became of the Beat generation, the Alienated and the Lost Generations, the Hippies, the Heads, the Jesus Freaks, and the reactionary neo-conservatives? They became older and sometimes wiser. They became a part of our complex, polyglot society. They sometimes learn to integrate the excitement, pain, and wonder of adolescence into adult life.

Only the surface has been touched in discussion of this most complex phase of human development. Considering the normal aspects of adolescence, we have outlined the predominant physical and psychosocial features of the "typical" youth, with full realization that people are unique and do not conform to any standard conceptualization of "The Adolescent." Presentation of some of the unfortunate variations beyond normal expectations was meant to bring into focus the differences between functional and dysfunctional adjustive patterns of behavior in preadolescent and adolescent individuals, including selected problems associated with genetic or developmental accident and the impact of physical disabilities on the adolescent.

Adolescence is a developmental period of vibrant growth, which like most human conditions that are linked to processes of change, carries both threat and promise. Given sensitivity to the characteristics of the period, nurses should enrich clinical experiences for both their young clients and themselves. An additional nuance is that understanding the dynamics of adolescence as a universal human experience can only lend depth to the clinician's understanding of the adult.

REFERENCES

Ackerman, N. J. The family with adolescents. In E. A. Carter & M. McGoldrick (Eds.), *The family life cycle.* New York: Gardner Press, 1980.

American Psychiatric Association. *Diagnostic and statistical manual of mental disorders* (3rd ed.). Washington, DC: APA, 1980.

Anthony, E. J. The behavior disorders of children. In P. H. Mussen (Ed.), *Carmichael's manual of child psychology II* (3rd ed.). New York: John Wiley & Sons, 1970.

Bakan, D. Adolescence in america: From idea to social fact. In C. J. Guards (Ed.), *The adolescent as individual.* New York: Harper & Row, 1975.

Bedrosian, R. C., & Beck, A. T. Cognitive aspects of suicidal behavior. *Suicide and Life Threatening Behavior,* 1979, *2,* 87–95.

Berger, M. M. (Ed.). *Beyond the double bind.* New York: Brunner/Mazel, 1978.

Berlin, I. N. Primary prevention. In I. N. Berlin & L. A. Stone (Eds.), *Basic handbook of child psychiatry,* Vol. IV. New York: Basic Books, 1979.

Blos, P. The child analyst looks at the young adolescent. *Daedalus,* 1971, *100*(4), 961–976.

Blos, P. *The adolescent passage.* New York: International Universities, 1979.

Capodanno, A. E., & Targum, S. D. Assessment of suicide risk: Some limitations in the prediction of infrequent events. *Journal of Psychosocial Nursing and Mental Health Services,* 1983, *21*(5), 11–14.

Crisp, A. H. *Anorexia nervosa: Let me be.* New York: Grune & Stratton, 1980.

De Luca, J. R. *Fourth special report to the U.S. Congress on alcohol and health from the Secretary of Health and Human Services, January, 1981.* Rockville, MD: U.S. Department of Health and Human Services. PHS, Alcohol, Drug Abuse, and Mental Health Administration, 1981.

Derezin, M. Inflammatory bowel disease. In R. L. Koretz (Ed.), *Practical gastroenterology.* New York: John Wiley & Sons, 1982.

Deutsch, H. *The psychology of women, Vol. 1. Girlhood.* London: Research Books, 1947.

Eisenberg, L. Introduction-preventive methods in psychiatry. In I. N. Berlin & L. A. Stone (Eds.), *Basic handbook of child psychiatry,* Vol. IV. New York: Basic Books, 1979.

Engel, G. Ulcerative colitis. In A. Lendner (Ed.), *Emotional factors in gastrointestinal illness.* New York: American Elsevier Company, 1973.

Erikson, E. H. *Childhood and society.* New York: W. W. Norton, 1950.

Erikson, E. *Identity, youth and crisis.* New York: W. W. Norton, 1968.

Freud, A. Adolescence. I. Adolescence in the psychiatry theory. *The Psychoanalytic Study of the Child,* 1958, *13,* 255–264.

Goldings, H. J. Normal development from ten to thirteen. In J. Noshpitz (Ed.), *Basic handbook of child psychiatry,* Vol. I. New York: Basic Books, 1979.

Haim, A. *Adolescent suicide.* New York: International Universities Press, 1974.

Hall, G. S. *Adolescence.* New York: Appleton, 1904.

Hendin, H. Growing up dead: Student suicide. In E. S. Schneidman (Ed.), *Suicidology: Contemporary developments.* New York: Grune & Stratton, 1976.

Inhelder, B., & Piaget, J. *The growth of logical thinking from childhood to adolescence.* New York: Basic Books, 1958.

Joint Commission on Mental Health of Children, Task Forces I, II, III. *Mental health: From infancy through adolescence.* New York: Harper & Row, 1973.

Kraft, S. Teen-age suicide becomes a devastating problem for U.S., Associated Press Release. *Salt Lake Tribune,* August 7, 1983.

Laing, R. D. *The politics of experience.* New York: Ballentine Books, 1967.

Lesse, S. Masked depression and depressive equivalents. In S. Arieti & H. K. H. Brodie (Eds.), *American handbook of psychiatry* (2nd ed.), Vol. VII, *Advances and new directions.* New York: Basic Books, 1981.

Lettieri, D. J., & Ludford, J. P. (Eds.). *Drug abuse and the American adolescent.* NIDA Research Monograph 38. Dept. of Health and Human Services, PHS, Alcohol, Drug Abuse, and Mental Health Administration. Rockville, MD: U.S. Government Printing Office, 1981.

Lidz, T. *The person.* New York: Basic Books, 1968.

Malmquist, C. Development from thirteen to sixteen years. In J. Noshpitz (Ed.), *Basic handbook of child psychiatry* Vol. I. New York: Basic Books, 1979.

Miller, J. R., & Janosik, E. H. *Family focused care.* New York: McGraw-Hill, 1980.

Minkoff, K., Bergman, E., Beck, A. T., & Beck, R. Hopelessness, depression and attempted suicide. *American Journal of Psychology,* 1973, *130*(4), 455–459.

Offer, D., & Offer, J. Four issues in the developmental psychology of adolescents. In J. G. Howells (Ed.), *Modern perspectives in adolescent psychiatry.* New York: Brunner/Mazel, 1971.

Otto, L. Antecedents and consequences of marital timing. In W. R. Burr, R. Hill, F. I. Nye, & I. L. Reiss, *Contemporary theories about the family.* Vol. II. New York: Free Press, 1979.

Pennington, R. (Ed.). Studies of adolescents and youth, report of Task Force III. In Joint Commission on Mental Health of Children, Task Forces I, II, III, *Mental health: From infancy through adolescence.* New York: Harper & Row, 1973.

Petersen, A. C., & Offer, D. Adolescent development: Sixteen to nineteen years. In J. Noshpitz (Ed.), *Basic handbook of child psychiatry* Vol. I. New York: Basic Books, 1979.

Piaget, J. The intellectual development of the adolescent. In A. H. Esman (Ed.), *The psychology of adolescence: Essential readings.* New York: International Universities Press, 1969.

Proefrock, D. W. Adolescence: Social fact and psychological concept. *Adolescence, 16*(64), 1981.

Proskauer, S., & Rolland, R. S. Youth who use drugs: Psychodynamic diagnosis and treatment planning. In S. Chess & A. Thomas (Eds.), *Annual progress in child psychiatry and child development, 1974.* New York: Brunner/Mazel, 1975.

Prugh, D. G., & Eckhardt, L. O. Psychophysiological disorders. In S. I. Harrison (Ed.), *Basic handbook of child psychiatry* Vol. III. New York: Basic Books, 1979.

Redl, F. Adolescents—Just how do they react? In G. Caplan & S. Lebovici (Eds.), *Adolescence: Psychosocial perspectives.* New York: Basic Books, 1969.

Rush, A. J. *Short-term psychotherapies for depression.* New York: Guilford Press, 1982.

Sandler, J., & Joffe, W. G. Notes on childhood depression. *International Journal of Psychoanalysis,* 1965, *46,* 88.

Shopper, M. Adolescent problems. In I. N. Berlin & L. A. Stone (Eds.), *Basic handbook of child psychiatry,* Vol. IV. New York: Basic Books, 1979.

Smart, M., & Smart, R. C. *Children: Development and relationships* (3rd ed.). New York: Macmillan, 1977.

Sullivan, H. S. *The interpersonal theory of psychiatry.* New York: W. W. Norton, 1953.

Tanner, J. M. *Growth at adolescence* (2nd ed.). Springfield, IL: Charles C. Thomas, 1962.

Tanner, J. M. Earlier maturation. *Scientific American,* 1968, *218,* 21–27.

Teicher, J. D. Children and suicide. In I. N. Berlin & L. A. Stone (Eds.), *Basic handbook of child psychiatry* Vol. IV. New York: Basic Books, 1979.

Toolan, J. M. Depression in adolescence. In J. G. Howells (Ed.), *Modern perspectives in adolescent psychiatry.* New York: Brunner/Mazel, 1971.

Wetzel, R. D. Hopelessness, depression and suicide intent. *Archives of General Psychology,* 1976, *33,* 1069–1073.

Young, H. B. The physiology of adolescence (including puberty and growth). In J. G. Howells (Ed.), *Modern perspectives in adolescent psychiatry.* New York: Brunner/Mazel, 1971.

BIBLIOGRAPHY

Arieti, S. *On schizophrenia, phobias, depression, psychotherapy, and the farther shores of psychiatry.* New York: Basic Books, 1978.

Bellak, L. (Ed.). *Disorders of the schizophrenic syndrome.* New York: Basic Books, 1979.

Bennett, G., Vourakis, C., & Woolf, D. S. (Eds.). *Substance abuse: Pharmacologic, developmental, and clinical perspectives.* New York: John Wiley & Sons, 1983.

Kastenbaum, C. J. The child at risk for major psychiatric illness. In S. Arieti & H. K. H. Brodie (Eds.), *American handbook of psychiatry* (2nd ed.), Vol. VII, *Advances and new directives.* New York: Basic Books, 1981.

Sullivan, H. S. *Conceptions of modern psychiatry.* New York: W. W. Norton, 1940.

CHAPTER 8

EARLY AND MIDDLE ADULTHOOD

Pamela G. Reed

A discussion of developmental issues during early and middle adulthood within a nursing framework will be presented in this chapter. The assumptions of a nursing framework and developmental models will be discussed first. Secondly, the developmental issues during early and middle adulthood will be presented. Finally, with this foundation, the sources of potential mental health problems and implications for nursing intervention will be explored.

THE NURSING PERSPECTIVE

Nursing conceptual models provide a framework for addressing the basic concepts of adult development and deriving implications for promoting adult mental health. While each nursing model offers its own unique perspective, there is a conceptual core that emerges from them to guide interpretations about adult development and mental health. This framework identifies five basic assumptions about human beings.

The first assumption acknowledges that the person is a whole entity. What seem to be parts of the human system, that is, biological or mental attributes, are more accurately attempts to describe some pattern observed about the whole person. Clinical manifestations of depression, for example, identify an observable problem of the total life of the individual, including physical, social, spiritual, emotional, and unknown dimensions. These dimensions have interacted in such a way as to produce a mental health problem.

Another assumption emphasizes ongoing interactions between person and environment. The importance of the context in health is evident in observations of the influence of family life, unemployment, or an ocean cruise on mental health. The continual interchange between person and environment precludes any notions about health as achievement of a steady state or equilibrium or as the absence of stress. Health is related to a dynamic process of creating possibilities, making choices, and deriving meaning from a given situation.

A third assumption describes a purposefulness and freedom in behavior. Behavior is a reflection of unconscious motivation and conscious choices. An individual can direct behaviors to effect personal or environmental changes as needed to promote mental health.

A fourth assumption identifies increasing complexity and diversity as correlates of human development. People, as individuals and as a group, increase in variability over the life span. Human potential does not "peak out" at some point in young adulthood and decline thereafter. Increasing complexity is an irreversible process that continues throughout adulthood.

A final assumption of nursing posits the existence of some innate potential for health and development. It is evident in the person's ability to reason, to feel, to be creative in a variety of situations and can be tapped as a resource for regaining or enhancing mental health. This resource is sometimes identified by the client, sometimes identified by the nurse for the client, and sometimes remains unaccounted for by both nurse and client.

Nursing is challenged to continue to uncover and facilitate human potentialities for mental health.

DEVELOPMENTAL MODELS

There are two developmental models that permeate interpretations about adult development and strongly influence clinical approaches to mental health care, namely the mechanistic and organismic models. A third, the dialectical or relational model, is emerging as a major framework and is particularly relevant to adult psychiatric mental health nursing.

Mechanistic Model

The mechanistic model depicts the human being as a closed, machine-like system, whose development is shaped by outside forces. The person, according to this framework, functions as reactive to, rather than interactive with, the environment. Direct cause-effect relationships are derived from this perspective and there is a focus on what "caused" a particular problem behavior. It is postulated that the source of human behavior is reducible to physical and chemical components and is best understood from this fundamental level. The person may be conceptualized as running out of energy during the aging process until death brings all to a halt. Finally, development is regarded as a bi-directional, linear process whereby skills and other behaviors are accumulated and lost in additive fashion over the life span.

Organismic Model

In contrast, the organismic view emphasizes the role of the person in development. Environmental and organismic factors both are influential in affecting change. The person is defined in human, holistic properties rather than mechanical properties. The parts of a human being are studied within the context of the whole. Development is a nonlinear and irreversible process, the goal of which is change and maturity. Development indicates the emergence of qualitatively different structures or characteristics in the organism such that backward movement is not possible.

Regression, as is traditionally understood, is not possible within this model. Losses that occur during aging in adulthood are better viewed in conjunction with the gains that accompany them. Losses and gains, or "de-differentiation and progression" (Werner, 1957, p. 139), are a rhythmic experience throughout life. Adults carry the vestiges of previous developmental levels and the precursors of future development. Thus, the adult who appears to be clinically "regressed" to an earlier stage is more appropriately described as still primarily at an adult level but also displaying vestiges of less differentiated levels.

Relational Model

The relational or dialectical model is emerging as one of the most useful perspectives of adult development (Baltes, Reese, & Lipsitt, 1980; Riegel, 1976). This model is similar to the organismic model but emphasizes the changes that occur as a result of ongoing interactions among events that are external and internal to the individual. Achievement of equilibrium and stable characteristics is not considered important to development. Developmental change occurs in reference to the conflicts and contradictions that arise between the individual and one or more of the following dimensions: inner-biological, individual-psychological, cultural-sociological, and outer-physical. Health is a continual process of integrating the asynchronies among these human dimensions. The significance of conflict in development has implications for understanding how emotional growth can emerge from a mental health problem.

The relational model of development is generally consistent with the nursing perspective. The person is viewed as an open system in continuous interaction with the environment. Although this model's delineation of the parts, for example, biological or psychological, is not entirely consistent with nursing models on the unitary nature of the person, the relational model aids in clarifying domains of assessment for nurses in adult mental health care practice. While the biological models have typically been given much emphasis in nursing in the past, the relational framework of adult development supports nursing's focus on the interactions among various human dimensions, including intrapersonal, familial, cultural, and environmental.

Life-Span Approach to Development

The word "development" as distinguished from "growth" describes qualitative change in the person over time without necessarily a change in size (Werner, 1948). Thus, although growth does not occur in adulthood to as great a degree as in childhood and adolescence, development continues throughout life. In addition, development implies not only change, but changes of "increasing differentiation and hierarchic integration," Werner's (1948) orthogenetic principle. In other words, it is characteristic for people to become increasingly specialized and organized as they develop. Both aspects are vital; an increase in specialization without organization becomes chaotic and disintegrative.

A life-span approach to adult development, then, acknowledges unlimited potential for development. In the past, the influence of biological growth models have limited perspectives about adults. However, the roles of both environmental and biological change have come to be regarded as significant factors in adult development. The individual is embedded within a society and a species; all three undergo development over time and interact in such a way as to ultimately influence the mental health of the individual. Thus, the basic concepts of adult development and implications for practice are understood in reference to a nursing perspective of health that incorporates relational principles of development and defines development as a lifelong process.

PHASES OF ADULTHOOD

Adulthood is a time of life that is more complex than any previous phase of development. In view of this, early and middle adulthood are divided into three phases, namely, early adulthood, middle adulthood I, and middle adulthood II (Stevenson, 1977). The approximate age span represented by these three adult phases is 20 to 70 years.

Early Adulthood

Early adulthood, estimated to span the years from age 20 to 30, is characterized by an increase in self-confidence and self-reliance, goal-directedness, and a motivation to achieve. There is also a burgeoning interdependence in relationships with parents. An increasingly secure self-identity facilitates the adult's ability for intimacy. The person is confronted with opportunities to make significant choices concerning career, relationships, life-style, parenthood, and political and philosophical ideologies. There is an interaction between the self-identity and the activity of making choices; a secure identity promotes appropriate decision making and, alternatively, the process of choosing clarifies and strengthens self-identity. The focus on personal identity, more typical in adolescence, becomes less significant as the relationship between self and society becomes more salient. Thus, the choices of young adulthood become a vehicle for realizing certain potentialities and for participating with the world (Levinson, Darrow, Klein, Levinson, & McKee, 1978).

The explorations that occur in early adulthood are stimulated by a predominant value for achievement (Lowenthal, Thurnher, & Chiriboga, 1975) and by what Levinson et al. (1978) identify as the "dream," a generalized vision of what one wants to become in life. The realization of this dream is affected by personal and environmental characteristics, particularly interpersonal resources.

Intimate Relationships

Establishing a marital relationship is a major event for most individuals in early adulthood. For some, choices may instead include a single life-style, homosexual relationships, or other forms of cohabitation without marriage. A secure partnership may be preceded by a series of trial relationships or by a short-lived marriage. The task of securing a love relationship is regarded as the central issue of young adulthood by Erikson (1963). He identifies this stage in terms of the crisis of establishing a sense of intimacy over a sense of isolation.

Intimacy in relationships is fostered by a mutual sharing of oneself, including experiences, ideas, values, goals, and physical expressions of love. Flexibility and complementarity of the dream of each partner are important factors. A "moratorium" phase may occur during which other facets of the adult's life, for example, relationship with parents or educational or career goals, may predominate and limit the capacity for intimacy. In summary, the development of intimacy in early adulthood is influenced by the security of self-identity, the existence of other commitments or preoccupations, and by the mutuality experienced with others.

Mentor Relationship

The mentor relationship is recognized as a particularly useful experience in facilitating achievement of career goals (Levinson et al., 1978; Sheehy, 1977). A mentor is someone who fosters development in a particular area by offering guidance, emotional support, and necessary opportunities. Although an employer, relative, teacher, or spouse can serve as a mentor, the relationship is characterized by its professional nature and a nonsexual intimacy. Although more men than women have had mentoring opportunities, it is expected that the experience will become increasingly available to women as more women enter and remain in career roles.

Career

Another significant issue of early adulthood is the identification of career interests and choice of a career. This phase of development is viewed as a trial work period during which enormous amounts of energy are expended in getting started in an occupation and evaluating it in reference to lifetime goals (Havighurst, 1982). Levinson et al. (1978) prefer the concept of "forming" rather than "choosing" a career in view of the possibility that the entire early adulthood phase may be spent in exploring, testing, and refining occupational endeavors. Factors that influence job selection include self-identity, sex role expectations, propinquity to the occupation, intelligence, financial resources, and motivation.

A task of early adulthood is to achieve a balance between a concern for achievement in the work environment and a sense of responsibility in love and family relationships. Some individuals may have multiple careers over a lifetime. The periods of disorganization that occur with the initiation of each new career can conflict with family relationships. Consistency between career pursuits and personal values is vital to adult development. The importance of the adult's career, whether it be housewife, engineer, househusband, or teacher, is a primary form of adult interaction with the environment and influences mental health (Havighurst, 1982; Livson, 1976; Stevenson, 1977).

Parenthood

Early adulthood is a time of decision making about potential parenthood and, for most, transition into that role. The experiences of parenthood facilitate resolution of the crisis of "generativity versus stagnation" (Erikson, 1963). Nurturing and guiding younger individuals provide generative experiences for the adult. These experiences ultimately benefit the child, adult, and society in general.

Gutmann (1975) conceptualizes parenthood as a central adult event in which individual satisfaction intersects with the need to perpetuate the species. He proposes that a potential conflict exists between current changes in sex role expectations and parenthood. His view is challenged, however, by Self (1975), who views the trend away from traditional sex roles of husband and wife as enhancing development of parent and child. The positive and negative influences of parenthood on adults are continuing to be a focus of research (Alpert & Richardson, 1980).

Regardless of the life-style of the parents, the first child is often an event of crisis proportion for the young adult. There is a sharp change in individual life-style and manner of relating to one's partner. New problems and sources of conflict, as well as joys, emerge and persist as the child grows and develops. Other unique problems and experiences exist for single parents. In addition, the choice against parenthood is becoming increasingly prevalent (Mussen, Conger, Kagan, & Geiwitz, 1979). Development of the individual and couple who do not have children may proceed differently from that presented in adult developmental models that typically include parenting as a major event.

Physical and Cognitive Abilities

Early adulthood is identified as a stage of peak biological and physiological functioning. Physical strength, endurance, speed, and coordination are at their greatest. Concerns about the body are usually not an issue and the choices that are made during this phase of development give little, if any, attention to physical limitations.

Cognitive development was regarded at one time as a process that concluded during early adulthood. However, increased attention has been given to the role of generational and environmental influences on cognition and longitudinal research has uncovered evidence that cognitive development continues throughout adulthood. Piaget (1972) himself has conceded to the possibility of the emergence of more differentiated mental structures in adulthood. Thus, early adulthood represents a phase when decision-making ability, creativity in problem solving, and an understanding of oneself in relation to the world are skills that have yet to become even more differentiated (Arlin, 1975; Birren, 1969; Labouvie-Vief, 1980; Schaie, 1977).

Middle Adulthood I

The first phase of middle adulthood is estimated to occur between the ages of 30 and 50 years. The transition into this phase from early adulthood begins as definitive choices in relationships and career are made. This may be a time of upheaval and turmoil as choices are finalized and alternatives are dismissed. The dream that was held in early adulthood is evaluated and revised to minimize discrepancies between past ideals and the actuality of the present situation and new goals. Middle adulthood I, then, is initiated as the person becomes relatively secure in commitments and "settles down" to responsibilities. The adult enters this phase with a repertoire of experience, self-knowledge, self-directedness, and an increasing ability to manage a variety of personal and societal responsibilities.

The first phase of middle adulthood is frequently referred to as the "prime of life," a time of productivity. Certain resources have been acquired and the adult can settle down and concentrate on making a contribution to society. Resources available include family life, a degree of financial stability, an established career, and association with a community of people. Neugarten (1968a) originated the term "executive processes" to describe the middle adult's problem-solving ability and heightened awareness of self as part of the larger context of family, work setting, and society. Although life becomes increasingly complex in this phase, the adult continues to display mastery in managing a variety of responsibilities.

The concept of responsibility characterizes middle adulthood I (Levinson et al., 1978; Schaie, 1977). Stevenson (1977) prefers the term "commitment" to responsibility because it emphasizes self-initiated choice in the adult's activities. There is a dual focus of responsibility or commitment; there are activities related to family members, both younger and older generations as well as the spouse, and there are activities associated with endeavors outside of the home setting. Earlier ideals of the dream have been converted into more practical goals of home ownership, job responsibilities, and childrearing. The adult continues to master the task of balancing emotional and physical investments between home and family commitments and career goals and responsibilities.

Family Relationships

Expressions of generativity become increasingly complex as children mature. The adult in middle adulthood I displays a capacity for nurturing the biological and social dimensions of the child in a manner that is unintrusive yet facilitative of the child's identity, sexuality, and budding independence. Midlife parents must transform their self-view from that of protector and caretaker of young children to that of "less powerful" facilitator of adolescent and young adult development (Colarusso & Nemiroff, 1981). In summary, during middle adulthood I, the person relinquishes mentor relationships and the exclusive focus on personal goals and becomes increasingly involved in rearing and teaching children and transmitting ideas to other generations.

The focus of relationships broadens to include friendships and social activities beyond the family and work settings. The eventual departure of children from the home presents the adult with opportunities for new ways of interacting with spouse and others and for viewing oneself without primary emphasis on the parental role. This change in family structure can have effects on the parents that range from distress to relief (Neugarten, 1979; Rubin, 1979).

The "empty nest" experience has typically been associated with the unemployed mother as one who is more likely to have invested her self-concept in her children. However, there is increasing evidence that the departure of children is welcomed by women (Chilman, 1968; Harkins, 1978; Lowenthal & Chiriboga, 1972), particularly among employed women. The "empty nest" phase of motherhood may become regarded less as an expected part of adult development as more women establish and maintain a career in young adulthood. Regardless, Livson (1976) found both life-styles of women, the traditional and the more independent, to be facilitative of development in midlife. Studies that indicate an increase in marital satisfaction in the postparental years suggest that any loss experienced when children leave home is outweighed by the advantages of postparental life. There is an increase in communication, spontaneity, and relaxation during this phase.

Children who have left home for educational or career endeavors may return home and confront the parent with new perspectives and friends. Often, though, this confrontation motivates the adult in some way toward new self-expectations and further development (Vaillant, 1977). In general, the adult has the capacity to shift emotional investments from one person to another and from one task to another as family relationships and responsibilities change. Peck (1968) identifies this as "emotional flexibility" and regards it as necessary in dealing with the complex relationships of middle adulthood. Middle adulthood entails the task of relating to several generations, including grandchildren, children, prospective in-laws, adult friends, and the adult's aging parents.

As the parent-child affiliation moves toward interdependence, the adult's relationship with elderly parents develops into a more complex form of interdependence termed "filial maturity" (Udry, 1971). Health or financial problems frequently add to the complexity of this relationship. The adult-elderly parent relationship is best characterized not by a reversal of parent-child roles, as it is too commonly conceived, but by a mutuality of respect and learning from each other (Troll, 1971).

Death of elderly parents affects the adult's self-perception. The adult becomes one of the oldest generations of the family and the next expected to die. The loss of a parent may contribute to greater valuing of remaining relationships with spouse and children. In middle adulthood, the awareness of mortality is balanced by a reaffirmation of life in renewed relationships with spouse, children, and grandchildren. The new role of grandparenthood offers the opportunity for sharing in generative activities, emotional fulfillment, and for a sense of continuity with the future.

Temporal Perspective

Sometime during the later part of middle adulthood I, the person undergoes a major transition in life perspective. This change may occur with the suddeness and intensity associated with a crisis, thus the term "midlife crisis," or it may occur as a more gradual transition. A primary feature of this transition phase is a change in time perspective wherein life is perceived less in terms of time-lived-since-birth and more in reference to time-left-until-death (Neugarten, 1968a, 1976). The change in temporal perspective may normally be accompanied by a sense that one is growing older more rapidly than others or by boredom in which there is a sense that time is standing still.

Although there are minimal physical changes during middle adulthood I, a decrease in physical endurance and attractiveness is anticipated. The slight graying of hair, slowed reactions, and changes in skin and muscle tone are bodily experiences that reinforce awareness of a limited life span. At a time when the adult is becoming increasingly aware of human mortality and physical change, the children are growing in physical vitality and their anticipation of the future.

Children may be integral in the middle-aged person's symbols of immortality. Lifton (1975, 1979) describes "symbolic immortality" as a universal experience, manifested in behaviors that provide a sense of continuity between life and death. Modes of expression include the biological and social modes. During middle adulthood, there is a regard for children as heirs of both biological and social characteristics of the parents (Neugarten, 1979).

Increased awareness of the inevitability of personal death influences a reevaluation of, and subsequent changes in, the values and goals first established in the dream of early adulthood. There is a heightened introspection, "interiority," in which the adult begins to explore the self and the meaning of life and death (Neugarten, 1972). This exploration continues into the next phase of adulthood as well. The adult experiences a sense of urgency and sheds meaningless goals and illusions of the past and focuses on effective use of energy and talents (Levinson et al., 1978; Livson, 1976, 1977). Choices are made in reference to what one wants to do rather than what one should do.

It is a time for the anticipation of retirement. An important task, and one easily overlooked, during middle adulthood is the nurturance of a second career or meaningful endeavor. This is done in realistic anticipation of retirement, decreased physical abilities, and the death of one's spouse, friends, and relatives. The change in temporal perspective, then, marks a time of giving up some ideas and endeavors and acquiring new perspectives about what is important in life. Integration of this new temporal perspective is facilitated by interpersonal resources, positive societal attitudes about aging, and by a secure self-identity.

Middle Adulthood II

The second phase of middle adulthood is identified by Stevenson (1977) as the "new middle years," and it spans the years from 50 to 70. It evolved in part out of the lengthening life span. During this period, there is a refinement and integration of many of the issues and events of earlier adult phases. This adult displays a markedly increased capacity for addressing the conflicts and contradictions in life. Introspection and personal philosophy emerge as tools in the adult's interactions with the environment. There is a shift from the "active mastery" of younger adulthood (Gutmann, 1975) to a mastery that appears less active but is better interpreted as directed toward more pragmatic issues of family, physical health, personal happiness, and a limited life span. There is a noticeable change in values from an emphasis on physical skills and strength to social relationships, social skills, and cognitive ability.

Physical Changes

A major task of middle adulthood is to integrate the physical changes associated with aging into the ongoing developmental process. Needless to say, these changes are integral to the adult's mental health. Some of the changes include a decrease in muscle size and strength, diminished bone mass and skin elasticity, losses in visual and hearing acuity, a reduction in cardiovascular efficiency, and changes in physical appearance that, by cultural standards, are less appealing.

A variety of physical symptoms may be associated with these climacteric changes. Among women, the physical and emotional problems have been attributed to changes in hormonal production and include feelings of anxiety and depression, headaches, and "hot flashes." Among men, the climacteric is proposed to occur over a longer period of time and less intensely than in women. A small percentage of men have been reported as experiencing symptoms similar to those of women owing to a rapid drop in hormone level (Ruebsaat & Hull, 1975). More typically, men may experience decreased sexual interest, slowed sexual response, and more frequent occurrences of impotence. Symptoms associated with the climacteric, however, are best understood within the context of societal, familial, and intrapersonal patterns, as well as specific biological changes (Colarusso & Nemiroff, 1981; Livson, 1976; Neugarten, 1976; Newman, 1979).

While the physical changes of middle adulthood II are commonly viewed as decremental, they can also be interpreted as facilitators of development in other dimensions of the adult's life. Life-span developmental theorists view the losses and gains that occur throughout life, including adulthood, as compatible with the developmental needs of each stage (Brent, 1978; Labouvie-Vief & Schell, 1982).

Peck (1968) outlines a developmental process in which adults integrate physical losses by learning to value wisdom and other pleasures that come with aging. Stevenson (1977) states that "if a person is growing emotionally and spiritually, he or she can accept the signs of physical deterioration, which may or may not include actual symptoms of acute or chronic disease" (p. 28). Finally, it is suggested that the physical changes associated with aging facilitate integration of personal mortality and assist the individual in the final developmental task of life—dying (Labouvie-Vief, 1980).

Sex Role Changes

Changes in sex role perception and activity occur in middle adulthood II. Women display a new sense of assertiveness and authority, while men exhibit more nurturant and affiliative behaviors. This shift in sex roles is interpreted as part of the process of integrating a polarity of behaviors and becoming more holistic or individuated (Jung, 1933; Levinson et al., 1978; Neugarten, 1976). The adult is becoming more aware of the entire spectrum of human potential, more cognizant of the uniqueness and commonalities of people, and more capable of interacting with the environment. "Socializing" replaces "sexualizing" as an emphasis in interpersonal relationships; appreciation of others is not limited by sex role stereotypes and expectations (Peck, 1968). Moreover, persons in this stage of development not only integrate gender-related differences but, because of their experiences in relating to three or more generations, acquire a strategic perspective of the life span.

Intellectual Dimension

Contrary to the myth that intelligence reaches a peak in young adulthood and declines thereafter, adult's possess enhanced abilities to reason, to understand the relativities and contradictions of life, and to derive meaningful patterns from a variety of problems and situations (Arlin, 1975; Labouvie-Vief, 1977, 1980; Riegel, 1973; Schaie, 1977; Sinnott, 1978). There may be a slowing in retrieval of information and speed of reacting to a problem and a diminishing focus on detail. However, these abilities are traded for the ability to assess the broader context of a problem, to perceive its consequences on the environment or future generations, and to make accurate judgments.

Age-related decline in intellectual abilities more likely reflects environmental, physical health, or motivational factors (Baltes & Willis, 1979; Birren, 1969; Labouvie-Vief & Schell, 1982) than inherent developmental factors. Research methodologies have been criticized for failure to account for cohort differences and environmental factors when drawing conclusions about the decline of intelligence in adulthood and aging (Baltes, Reese & Nesselroade, 1977; Schaie, 1970, 1978). A theory on "fluid" and "crystallized" intelligence has been proposed to explain the losses and gains in adulthood intelligence (Cattell, 1971; Horn, 1978), although this theory assumes a dualism between biophysical and mental attributes that is not consistent with a holistic perspective of human functioning. Intellectual ability in adulthood likely involves complex interactions between dimensions of both the person and the environment.

In later middle adulthood, there is the purposeful use of knowledge gained from past experiences in decision making and forming conceptions about reality (Neugarten, 1968b). This knowledge is enhanced by an acute awareness of the present context and pragmatic issues of a situation. A wisdom emerges out of this and provides a stability for younger generations (Brent, 1978). This stability provides a secure base of knowledge with which younger individuals can venture out, take risks, challenge and test existing knowledge, and make new discoveries. Thus, the wisdom of adults is a vital link to the discovery of new knowledge and progressive change in society.

A Final Dialectic

Gould (1972, 1975) has another interpretation of the stability of later middle adulthood that introduces more complexity into a perspective of this phase of adult development.

He describes this phase as one of "stability fraught with concern" (1975, p. 78). There is a stability in the adult's relationships with spouse, children, and friends and an increasing sense of acceptance about oneself and one's accomplishments. However, there remain unanswered some of the "big" questions in life that cause continuing concern, namely, purpose of life and meaning of illness and death. Increased leisure time, departure of children, and decreased physical activity have worked to set the stage for the adult's reflection on these issues. Interiority, initiated earlier in adulthood, is available as a tool for addressing these concerns and developing a unifying philosophy of life. In one sense, awareness of death can lead to a keener awareness of life. A broadened perspective of life and an increasing sense of completeness about one's own life, then, help the adult to accept death and to get on with living.

Development in middle adulthood II involves a dialectic process (Riegel, 1975), an interaction between polarities: past experience and perspectives of the future, philosophical and pragmatic concerns, physical and spiritual, young children and aged parents, stability and conflict, maleness and femaleness, social and interior, individual and contextual, life and death. This interaction can result in a synthesis of polarities and continued adult development or in problems that impede development. Implications for potential mental health problems can be derived from knowledge of the basic developmental issues of early and middle adulthood.

SOURCES OF POTENTIAL MENTAL HEALTH PROBLEMS

There is variation among individuals in the specific areas of life that contribute to mental health problems. Moreover, for any one individual, the potential for certain areas to become problematic varies over the life span. Two models of developmental events provide a basis for identifying adulthood issues that can pose mental health problems, the critical life events model and the timing-of-events model.

The critical life events model postulates that there are predictable normative life crises that are experienced by most adults. These "crises" require significant change in the adult's life pattern such that failure to affect the change can contribute to mental health problems. Healthy outcomes of the crisis are based on achieving a balance between the positive and negative aspects of the situation and a synthesis of polarities, for example, a balance between a sense of intimacy and isolation (Erikson, 1963).

The timing-of-events model emphasizes not the life event itself, but the time or life stage at which the event occurs. It is postulated that mental health is influenced by the individual's perception of whether the event occurs "on-time" or "off-time" in reference to an internalized time perspective. This perspective is based on a three-dimensional view of time, that is, chronological, social, and historical (Neugarten, 1972, 1976). In other words, expectations regarding the time in life when certain events will occur are based on the individual's chronological age, socially defined norms, and the historical era in which the person lives. The self-assessment that occurs in middle adulthood is intimately related to this time perspective. Moreover, Neugarten (1976) suggests that, as adults grow older, they become increasingly sensitive to the system of age expectations that operates in society. Unexpected events, or events perceived as "off-schedule," can contribute to the emergence of a mental health problem.

Both models attribute significance to the adult and the adult's perception of the environment or life context. Mental health problems can arise from among the many changes in certain life contexts. Life contexts that are particularly significant in adulthood are family, career, culture, and physical and temporal dimensions.

Interpersonal Relations and Family

There is, in early adulthood, the expectation that the person will find and choose a mate. While most are married, at least for the first time, by age 35, factors such as career or educational involvement, personal preference, immaturity, early divorce, or fear of rejection may work to prevent the young adult from establishing an intimate relationship. Failure to meet this expectation can contribute to feelings of anxiety, depression, fear of loneliness, and to premature decision making on marriage.

Expectations regarding the event of childbearing also present potential crises for the adult. The initial decision about whether or not to have children is becoming a major concern for some couples. Potential negative effects of this uncertainty on the marital dyad have yet to be studied.

Among those adults who do have children, children born "too early" impinge upon fulfillment of personal or marital goals. Children born "too late" can conflict with expectations for career mobility, travel, and retirement. Finally, infertility is an unexpected event that can threaten the adult's sexual identity and sense of generativity. Personal expectations, anticipations for the future, and the relationship with one's spouse must be redefined to integrate this issue.

Regardless of whether or not children arrive "on-time," the birth of the first child is an event that is impossible to anticipate fully. The suddeness and degree of change required in family life can threaten developing intimacy between the couple. Feelings of ambivalence arise as to whether it was the right time or the right decision to have a baby, despite the most faultless planning. The realities of childrearing contrast sharply with the media's image of parenthood, which veils such experiences as loss of privacy, loss of freedom, financial strain, interference with career or travel goals, increased worry, and physical exhaustion.

The birth of a disabled child is an unanticipated event that poses a major emotional crisis for the adult. Certain goals and fantasies have to be relinquished and new responsibilities incorporated. The adult may exhibit a variety of responses that can contribute to mental health problems. These include intense guilt and depression, an isolation of oneself and the child, denial of the disability and unrealistic plans for the child, or a perception of the disability as a defect in the adult.

The increasing independence of older children is problematical for some middle-aged adults. Mental health problems among women that have been associated with the eventual departure of children include a sense of meaninglessness and depression and a perception of the departure as a personal rejection. Departure of children, however, seems not to be the major precipitant of emotional crises so often associated with this stage of adult development. Rather, it is the period spent in anticipation of the departure before the actual event that may pose personal and family mental health difficulties (Livson, 1977; Lowenthal, 1975). Ambivalence experienced by both the child and parent about the child's departure from home may conflict with the adult's needs for further development of self and the marital relationship.

In the not-too-distant past, women typically gave up more than men did in adjusting to marriage. Societal norms encouraged women to assume a dependent role or to use the marriage to pursue childish needs (Livson, 1977). This fostered an unhappiness that related to a conflict between a deep resentment of the dependent role and a sense of enjoyment from the security that accompanied it. Nevertheless, these women were and still are left with a lack of resources, namely, a sense of individuality, personal interests, or career, that would promote self-esteem and confidence during critical family events such as the anticipated departure of children (Bernard, 1973). Bernard's research indicates that, in general, marriage is more beneficial to the mental health of men than of women. Married women, in comparison to single women and married men, were much more likely to have emotional disturbances such as depression and phobic tendencies.

Studies indicate that women around the age of 48 experience more emotional problems than either men at the same age or women of other ages (Livson, 1976; Lowenthal, 1975). This occurrence was particularly noticeable among nontraditional women. Nontraditional women or "independents" (Livson, 1976) were described as those who were ambitious, skeptical, and relied on their intellect to cope with the world, whereas the "traditionals" were more gregarious, nurturant, and employed somatization and repression to cope with anxiety. The depression, irritability, and conflict present in the independents' group were attributed to the conflict between life-style and personality. These women, however, were able to resolve the conflict within a few years and go on to new generative tasks.

In the postparental phase, both the husband and wife can experience mental health problems. A husband and wife who have not developed an intimate, mutually satisfying relationship separate from their values of each other as mother or father may fear being alone together once their children are grown. The two adults may have followed different paths of development, only to realize more clearly the incongruencies in the relationship once the children have left home (Troll, 1975).

The crossover in sex roles that occurs in later middle age may be an additional source of difficulty for the postparental couple. At a time when men experience stronger affiliative needs and desire for attention from their spouse, women may need to explore their increased interest in affairs external to the home. If the adult couple lacks understanding about the developmental changes occurring in each other, behaviors can be misinterpreted as disinterest, boredom in the marriage, or lack of affection.

Death of a spouse in middle adulthood is an event that is particularly relevant to the mental health of the surviving spouse. This event is rarely expected, despite the fact that half of all widows in the United States are under the age of 60 (Lopata, 1973). Death of one's spouse is ranked as the most stressful life event by Holmes and Rahe (1967). The first two years of widowhood are associated with significantly higher risks of mortality and morbidity (Carey, 1977; Clayton, 1974; Glick, Weiss, & Parkes, 1974; MacMahon & Pugh, 1965). Moreover, the younger widowed are at greater risk than the elderly widowed (Jacobs & Ostfeld, 1977), perhaps because widowhood is within the expectations of life events for older adults.

Another concern in middle adulthood is that of the welfare of elderly parents. Lieberman (1978) indicates that "parent-caring" is becoming a greater problem than marriage, parenthood, departure of children, or the climacteric. Parent-caring roles are usually not regarded positively by either the elderly parent or adult child and can contribute to anger and guilt, diminished self-esteem, and ongoing emotional stress.

The death of a parent can be emotionally traumatic in middle adulthood. Kastenbaum (1977) explains that society generally does not encourage grieving over the death of an elderly parent since it is viewed as timely and appropriate. However, it is often the adult's first personal experience with death of a significant other for which the adult has not prepared. Societal responses to the event can be perceived by the grieving adult as a denial of the significance of the loss or as abandonment in time of grief. In an attempt to resolve the grief, the adult may express increased dependency on children, spouse, and friends.

Death of the adult's parents brings the realization that the adult is among the next generation to die, according to the "pecking order of death" (Kastenbaum, 1977, p. 37). This sudden heightened awareness of the inevitability of death of oneself and other family members may threaten the sense of security and mastery over one's life or contribute to depression and increased risk of suicide. In addition, the adult may experience emotional conflict over feelings of both liberation and guilt associated with the parent's death. Thus, although the postparental phase of adulthood has been described as the "second honeymoon," it contains events that are potentially detrimental to the individual's mental health.

Career

The job represents a major form of interaction with the environment in adulthood. In addition to functioning as a source of financial support, a job often contributes to the needed sense of social participation and intimacy. For some adults, it is the primary source of contact with the outside world (Havighurst, 1982). The work setting provides an arena for sharing common goals, gaining self-esteem, and validating reality. A career also contributes to the adult's sense of generativity and, in so doing, is a means for creative self-expression and generation of ideas and solutions.

Because the career is significant to the achievement of adult developmental tasks, job-related problems can conflict with other life tasks and foster serious difficulties in mental health. Women have typically encountered conflict between the demands and personal goals of a chosen career and family responsibilities. Others may subordinate all other adulthood tasks to pursuit of success in a career. Anxiety associated with these issues can ultimately limit the adult's ability to derive satisfaction from either the work or home setting.

Cultural Norms

Changing cultural norms represent another potential source of conflict for adults as they engage in interactions with their environment. Person-environment interactions not only test and clarify self-identify but also introduce new conflicts. The stability and security of one's value system, which originated in the childhood era, may contrast sharply with the mores of a current and rapidly changing society.

Marriage and family life, in particular, have been the focus of much change in recent years. The increase in knowledge of sexual functioning and open communication on sexuality contrasts with the relative lack of knowledge and constricting views of sex roles and sexuality that existed during the present-day adult's earlier lifetime. Availability of birth control devices present new choices and expectations regarding expression of intimacy, fidelity, purpose of marriage, and children. A new focus on the value of human equality and personal growth has contributed to the increasing number of women who enter careers before or during childrearing and to new patterns of childrearing in which parental responsibility and authority are shared with outsiders. A devaluation of the housewife as the primary role for a person has taken place, along with increased expectations for both mother and father to assume roles of nurturer and provider. Potential emotional difficulties influenced by these emerging norms are compounded by a trend away from involvement of extended family in childrearing responsibilities. Finally, family arrangements in which the grandparent(s) live with the adult child (one-third of all families) can contribute to significant degrees of emotional tension. While there is negative social regard for nursing home arrangements, there are few alternatives available for dependent elderly parents.

Society has also embraced theoretical positions that emphasize the significance of early childhood experiences on health and development. This has served to increase anxiety and guilt among some parents who are in the throes of resolving conflicts between themselves and their aging parents and children. Parents may, as a result, blame themselves for a variety of problems experienced by their children.

An accelerated rate of social change creates a discontinuity between generations. Generational conflicts may occur because of these differences and the difficulty in discriminating between those principles that are meaningful and transferable for learning across generations and those that should be relinquished altogether.

Social norms reflect a greater tolerance of factors that are problematic for the establishment of intimacy and family life, namely, multiple sexual relationships, divorce, extramarital sexual relationships, and cohabitation. There is increasing acceptability and expectation for career mobility or major job changes in midlife in contrast to the work ethic of earlier years in which one provided family stability by choosing and abiding by a career until retirement. Thus, while these societal trends offer opportunities for enhancing mental health, conflicts between social and personal expectations can lead to disruptions in early and middle adulthood, particularly in reference to the degree that they challenge the adult's tasks related to intimacy and generativity.

Physical Changes

Although the physical changes of middle adulthood occur gradually, they may nonetheless pose threats to self-identity. Societal emphasis on youthful appearance and physical and sexual vigor convey a devaluation of the middle adult. Attitudes about aging and the increasing salience of death-related physical illnesses in middle adulthood accentuate the adult's sense of vulnerability. Attitudes about physical changes are generalized to cognitive capacity; opinions about the adult's declining ability to learn, which have been repeatedly disproved (Bayley, 1968; Labouvie-Vief & Schell, 1982; Owens, 1963; Schaie & Labouvie-Vief, 1974), continue to diminish the adult's perceptions of and interest in new opportunities.

It is estimated that 30% of all women seek medical help during this phase of life (Weideger, 1976), many of whom express concerns related to climacteric changes. The problems associated with the climacteric result from an interaction of physiological changes and attitudes about motherhood and aging. Livson (1977), for example, cites the pervasive double standard of aging by which older men appear more distinguished and older women are regarded as old.

Other behaviors may be evident in the middle-aged man or woman that indicate an inability to integrate the physical changes into a self-perspective. Attempts may be made to deny or compensate for perceived physical losses by engaging in excessive or inappropriate physical and social activity or displaying a neglect of hygiene and grooming. Extramarital sexual activity or worries about sex may be prominent. Middle-aged psychiatric patients rank sex as a concern to a considerably greater degree than nonpatients (Stein, Holzman, Karasu, & Charles, 1978). This experience was interpreted as an inability to integrate sexual activity into the self-concept.

The young adult is not without problems related to physical status. Because this person is regarded as being at the peak of physical abilities and stamina, there are sometimes unrealistic expectations of ability to endure physical or emotional stress. Young adults may overextend themselves at school, at work, or other activities and find themselves with such psychosomatic symptoms as ulcers, overeating, and other manifestations of unconscious efforts to cope.

Temporal Perspective

The characteristic change in temporal perspective during middle adulthood is accompanied by an increased awareness of the nearness of personal death. This normally stimulates healthy, introspective activity and reflection on the meaningfulness of life. However, there may instead be a self-indulgent, pessimistic attitude, rumination about petty annoyances and health concerns, and little regard for society (Gould, 1972). Some adults may express a pervasive depression or bitterness over missed experiences and the assumption that it is too late to make changes in life choices (Stein et al., 1978). Complaints of boredom, refusals to begin new projects, and a general distrust of the future operate as defenses against an awareness of personal mortality. Colarusso and Nemiroff (1981) state that their clinical experience indicates that the most problematic issue in midlife is clearly the increased awareness of time limitation and death.

The changing time perspective and cultural values about time underly many of the mental health problems associated with the changes in other dimensions of the adult's life, for example, career, physical health, and family. Adult temporality provides a beginning framework for interpreting pathology related to these various dimensions. Major life crises are associated with changes in temporal perspectives (Fitzpatrick, 1980). Concern about time was found to be greater among psychiatric patients than nonpatients (Stein et al., 1978). Thus, it is suggested that approaches to the prevention and treatment of disturbances in mental health in early and middle adulthood acknowledge the significance of developmental change in adult perspectives of time and death, as well as in other dimensions of the adult's life.

IMPLICATIONS FOR THE PSYCHIATRIC MENTAL HEALTH NURSE

Developmental events of early and middle adulthood play a pivotal role in mental health. These events bring new experiences and a number of significant life changes. Because of the increasing complexity of the adult's life and the variety of unanticipated changes that occur, middle adulthood is a time when people feel particularly out of control of their lives (Lowenthal et al., 1975). Thus, opportunities for enhancing development are accompanied by an increased risk to mental health. A developmental approach to nursing intervention transforms this risk into potentially healthy outcomes. Implications for intervention can be derived from this nursing perspective of adult health and development.

One major implication is in regard to *anticipatory intervention,* which facilitates the adult's sense of control and preparedness in life. There is therapeutic value in the ability to realistically anticipate and "rehearse" for major life events (Lowenthal, 1975; Neugarten, 1979; Peplau, 1975). Interventions that help adults to anticipate changes enhance their sense of mastery in the environment. The anticipatory perspective provides time for the adult to acquire information about the event, review feelings that possibly may arise, identify and evaluate potential solutions, and, if indicated, begin shifting emotional investments from certain people, objects, or goals to others.

A second implication for intervention is that of facilitating the adult's *sense of effectualness* during the life event. A requisite of this is a basic belief in the intrinsic human potential for ongoing development throughout the life span, regardless of age, emotional disorder, or other factors that may be perceived as detrimental to mental health. Conflicts and events that are initially perceived as obstacles to development and health are regarded instead as growth facilitators. Intervention primarily focuses not on elimination of symptoms but on purposeful use of the problem to promote mental health. Thus, within this developmental perspective, problems associated with changes in various life dimensions, for example, temporal, physical, or social changes, may be reinterpreted as usable in therapy to benefit mental health. For example, the increasing awareness of a limited life span can be used in counseling to stimulate selection and clarification of goals and efficient use of personal time and energy. It may also be used as a motivator for introspective activities and development of a "unifying philosophy" of life, a healthy characteristic of adulthood (Allport, 1968; Gould, 1972).

Chronically Mentally Ill Adults

Intervention with chronically mentally ill adults is particularly challenging. Repeated readmissions and failures to change behavior patterns contribute to a sense of inefficacy and frustration among nurses who work with these clients. Although these clients typically are not in the social mainstream experiencing developmental issues of others their age, they interact within a social environment which for better or worse influences their potential for mental health. A focus on identifying developmentally appropriate strategies to enhance client-environment interactions may prove to be a useful perspective for nursing intervention.

The timing of the onset of chronic mental disorders, that is, early adulthood, provides some understanding of the developmental needs of chronically mentally ill adults. Early adulthood marks an increase in expectations for societal involvement through marital, educational, and career activities. Adequate degrees of individuation, sexual identity, resolution of childhood losses, sense of self-esteem, social and coping skills, and a supportive environment are required. These developmental tools characteristically are absent in the lives of chronically mentally ill individuals; this is manifested in mental health problems. Interactions between the person's developmental deficits and environmental expectations of normality and responsibility contribute to chronic behavior patterns such as social isolation, mistrust, dependency, and identity confusion.

Nursing interventions can focus on providing developmental experiences that help the client to learn more positive ways to perceive self and interact with others. Developmental changes related to physiological, time perspective, or family dimensions that are anxiety producing may be addressed. Anticipatory guidance (Krauss, 1980) is a significant developmental approach with the chronically mentally ill, among whom "symptomatic exacerbation is the most common response" to unexpected change (p. 313). Other modes of therapy, such as occupational and medical, may be used to facilitate nursing interventions.

Modes of intervention can exacerbate mental health problems. Research suggests that interventions that present chronically mentally ill psychiatric outpatients with tasks that are too sophisticated for their developmental level are not effective (Slavinsky & Krauss, 1982). Alternatively, treatment programs that convey minimal if any expectations for development and use of social skills out in the community can foster chronicity (Krauss, 1980; Pasquali, Alesi, Arnold, & DeBasio, 1981; Strauss, 1981). Interventions that address only the alleviation of the most obvious pathology without facilitating achievement of basic developmental tasks set up the client for eventual failure and repeated admissions.

Intervention with chronically mentally ill adults is indeed a complex and challenging issue. These individuals need help in resolving developmental deficits at the same time that they are attempting to fulfill current adult-acquired responsibilities. A developmental perspective on interventions with the chronically mentally ill can provide new perspectives on an old yet prevalent mental health problem.

SUMMARY

Several implications have been explored in reference to a developmentally based approach to intervention for adult mental health. Early and middle adulthood mark a period of many changes. However, the potential for these events to contribute to mental health problems is based on the interactions between adult characteristics and environmental factors; mental health problems are not inevitable but arise out of a "probabalistic epigenesis" (Lerner, 1976) in which both the person and the life context influence mental health. The overall goal in intervention is that of facilitating adults' abilities to make choices and effect their environment in mental health-promoting ways (Danish & D'Augelli, 1980; Fozard

& Popkin, 1978). This cannot be done without an understanding of the conditions that foster development.

Thus, nursing intervention addresses those factors in the person that foster healthy interactions within a given life context. These factors include an anticipatory perspective, realistic expectations, a sense of effectualness, and a confidence in human potential expressed through temporal, intellectual, physical, and cultural dimensions. Knowledge of developmental principles and models, the significant events of adulthood, and the natural resources associated with healthy adult development are offered as a basis for intervention in adult mental health.

REFERENCES

Allport, G. W. *The person in psychology.* Boston: Beacon Press, 1968.

Alpert, J. L., & Richardson, M. S. Parenting. In L. W. Poon (Ed.), *Aging in the 1980's: Psychological issues.* Washington DC: American Psychological Association, 1980.

Arlin, P. K. Cognitive development in adulthood: A fifth stage? *Developmental Psychology,* 1975, *11,* 602–606.

Baltes, P. B., Reese, H. W., & Lipsitt, L. P. Life-span developmental psychology. *Annual Review of Psychology,* 1980, *31,* 65–110.

Baltes, P. B., Reese, H. W., & Nesselroade, J. R. *Life-span developmental psychology: Introduction to research methods.* Monterey: Brooks/Cole, 1977.

Baltes, P. B., & Willis, S. L. Life-span developmental psychology, cognitive functioning, and social policy. In M. W. Rilen (Ed.), *Aging from birth to death.* Boulder: Westview Press, 1979.

Bayley, N. Cognition and aging. In K. W. Schaie (Ed.), *Theory and methodology of research on aging.* Morgantown: West Virginia University Press, 1968.

Bernard, J. *The future of marriage.* New York: Bantam Books, 1973.

Birren, J. E. Age and decision strategies. In A. T. Welford & J. E. Birren (Eds.), *Interdisciplinary topics in gerontology* Vol. 4. Basel: S. Karger, 1969.

Brent, S. B. Individual specialization, collective adaptation, and rate of environmental change. *Human Development,* 1978, *21,* 374–387.

Carey, R. G. The widowed: A year later. *Journal of Counseling Psychology,* 1977, *24,* 125–131.

Cattell, R. B. *Abilities: Their structures, growth, and action.* Boston: Houghton Miffin, 1971.

Chilman, C. S. Families in development at mid-stage of the family life cycle. *Family Coordinator,* 1968, *17,* 306.

Clayton, P. J. Mortality and morbidity in the first year of widowhood. *Archives of General Psychiatry,* 1974, *30,* 747–750.

Colarusso, C. A., & Nemiroff, R. A. *Adult development.* New York: Plenum Press, 1981.

Danish, S. J., & D'Augelli, A. R. Promoting competence and enhancing development through life development intervention. In L. A. Boyd & J. C. Rosen (Eds.), *Primary prevention of psychopathology,* Vol. 4. Hanover: University of New England, 1980.

Erikson, E. H. *Childhood and society* (3rd ed.). New York: W. W. Norton & Co., 1963.

Fitzpatrick, J. J. Patient's perceptions of time: Current research. *International Nursing Review,* 1980, *27,* 148–153, 160.

Fozard, J. L., & Popkin, S. J. Optimizing adult development. *American Psychologist,* 1978, *33,* 975–989.

Glick, I. O., Weiss, R. S., & Parkes, C. M. *The first year of bereavement.* New York: John Wiley & Sons, 1974.

Gould, R. L. The phases of adult life: A study in developmental psychology. *American Journal of Psychiatry,* 1972, *129,* 33–43.

Gould, R. L. Adult life stages: Growth toward self-tolerance. *Psychology Today,* February, 1975, *8,* 74–78.

Gutmann, D. Parenthood: A key to the comparative study of the life cycle. In N. Datan & L. H. Ginsberg (Eds.), *Life-span developmental psychology: Normative life crises.* New York: Academic Press, 1975.

Harkins, E. B. Effects of empty nest transition on self report of psychological and physical well-being. *Journal of Marriage and the Family,* 1978, *40,* 549–558.

Havighurst, R. J. The world of work. In B. B. Wolman (Ed.), *Handbook of developmental psychology.* Englewood Cliffs, NJ: Prentice-Hall, 1982.

Holmes, T. H., & Rahe, R. H. The social readjustment rating scale. *Journal of Psychosomatic Research,* 1967, *2,* 213–218.

Horn, J. L. Human ability systems. In P. B. Baltes (Ed.), *Life-span development and behavior* Vol. 1. New York: Academic Press, 1978.

Jacobs, S., & Ostfeld, A. An epidemiological review of mortality and bereavement. *Psychosomatic Medicine,* 1977, *39,* 344–357.

Jung, C. G. *Modern man in search of a soul* (W. S. Dell and C. F. Baynes, Trans.). New York: Harcourt Brace Jovanovich, 1933.

Kastenbaum, R. J. Death and development through the life span. In H. Feifel (Ed.), *New meanings of death.* New York: McGraw-Hill, 1977.

Krauss, J. B. The chronic psychiatric patient in the community: A model of care. *Nursing Outlook,* 1980, *30,* 308–314.

Labouvie-Vief, G. Adult cognitive development: In search of alternative interpretations. *Merrill-Palmer Quarterly,* 1977, *23,* 227–263.

Labouvie-Vief, G. Adaptive dimensions of adult cognition. In N. Datan & N. Lohmann (Eds.), *Transitions of aging.* New York: Academic Press, 1980.

Labouvie-Vief, G., & Schell, D. A. Learning and memory in later life: A developmental view. In B. Wolman & G. Stricker (Eds.), *Handbook of developmental psychology.* Englewood Cliffs, NJ: Prentice-Hall, 1982.

Leiberman, G. L. Children of the elderly as natural helpers: Some demographic considerations. *American Journal of Community Psychology,* 1978, *6,* 489–498.

Lerner, R. M. *Concepts and theories of human development.* Menlo Park, CA: Addison-Wesley, 1976.

Levinson, D. J., Darrow, C. N., Klein, E. B., Levinson, M. H., & McKee, B. *The seasons of a man's life.* New York: Ballantine Books, 1978.

Lifton, R. J. On death and the continuity of life: A psychohistorical perspective. *OMEGA,* 1975, *6,* 143–157.

Lifton, R. J. *The broken connection.* New York: Simon and Schuster, 1979.

Livson, F. B. Patterns of personality development in middle-aged women: A longitudinal study. *International Journal of Aging and Human Development,* 1976, *7,* 107–115.

Livson, F. B. Coming out of the closet: Marriage and other crises of middle age. In L. E. Troll, J. Israel, & K. Israel (Eds.), *Looking ahead.* Englewood Cliffs, NJ: Prentice-Hall, 1977.

Lopata, H. Z. *Widowhood in an American city.* Cambridge: Schenkman, 1973.

Lowenthal, M. F. Psychosocial variation across the adult life course: Frontiers for research and policy. *The Gerontologist,* 1975, *15,* 6–12.

Lowenthal, M. F., & Chiriboga, D. Transition to the empty nest: Crisis, challenge, or relief? *Archives of General Psychiatry,* 1972, *26,* 8–14.

Lowenthal, M., Thurnher, M., & Chiriboga, D. *Four stages of life: A comparative study of women and men facing transitions.* San Francisco: Jossey-Bass, 1975.

MacMahon, B., & Pugh, T. F. Suicide in the widowed. *American Journal of Epidemiology,* 1965, *81,* 23–31.

Mussen, P. H., Conger, J. J., Kagan, J., & Geiwitz, J. *Psychological development: A life-span approach.* New York: Harper & Row, 1979.

Neugarten, B. L. Adult personality: Toward a psychology of the life cycle. In B. L. Neugarten (Ed.), *Middle age and aging.* Chicago: University of Chicago Press, 1968a.

Neugarten, B. L. The awareness of middle age. In B. L. Neugarten (Ed.), *Middle age and aging.* Chicago: University of Chicago Press, 1968b.

Neugarten, B. L. Personality and the aging process. *The Gerontologist,* 1972, Spring (Pt.1), 9–15.

Neugarten, B. L. Adaptation and the life cycle. *Counseling Psychologist,* 1976, *6,* 17–18.

Neugarten, B. L. Time, age and the life cycle. *The American Journal of Psychiatry,* 1979, *136,* 887–894.

Newman, M. *Theory development in nursing.* Philadelphia: F. A. Davis, 1979.

Owens, W. A. Age and mental abilities: A longitudinal study. *Genetic Psychology Monographs,* 1963, *48,* 3–54.

Pasquali, E. A., Alesi, E. G., Arnold, H. M., & DeBasio, N. *Mental health nursing: A bio-psycho-cultural approach.* St. Louis: The C. V. Mosby Co., 1981.

Peck, R. C. Psychological development in the second half of life. In B. L. Neugarten (Ed.), *Middle age and aging.* Chicago: The University of Chicago Press, 1968.

Peplau, H. Mid-life crises. *American Journal of Nursing,* 1975, *75,* 1761–1765.

Piaget, J. Intellectual evolution from adolescence to adulthood. *Human Development,* 1972, *16,* 1–12.

Riegel, K. F. Dialectical operations: The final period of cognitive development. *Human Development,* 1973, *16,* 346–370.

Riegel, K. F. Adult life crises: A dialectic interpretation of development. In N. Datan & L. H. Ginsberg (Eds.), *Life-span developmental psychology: Normative life crises.* New York: Academic Press, 1975.

Riegel, K. F. The dialectics of human development. *American Psychologist,* 1976, *31,* 689–700.

Rubin, L. *Women of a certain age: The midlife search for self.* New York: Harper & Row, 1979.

Ruebsaat, H. J., & Hull, R. *The male climacteric.* New York: Hawthorn Books, 1975.

Schaie, K. W. A reinterpretation of age-related changes in cognitive structure and functioning. In L. R. Goulet & P. B. Baltes (Eds.), *Life-span developmental psychology: Research and theory.* New York: Academic Press, 1970.

Schaie, K. W. Toward a stage theory of adult development. *International Journal of Aging and Human Development,* 1977, *8,* 129–138.

Schaie, K. W. External validity in the assessment of intellectual performance in adulthood. *Journal of Gerontology,* 1978, *33,* 695–701.

Schaie, K. W., & Labouvie-Vief, G. Generational versus ontogenetic components of change in adult cognitive behavior: A fourteen year cross-sequential study. *Developmental Psychology,* 1974, *10,* 305–320.

Self, P. A. The further evolution of the parental imperative. In N. Datan & L. H. Ginsberg (Eds.), *Life-span developmental psychology: Normative life crises.* New York: Academic Press, 1975.

Sheehy, G. *Passages: Predictable crises of adult life.* New York: Bantam Books, 1977.

Sinnott, J. D. *Adult intellectual development as social-cognitive growth: A model.* Paper presented at the 31st Annual Scientific Meeting of the Gerontological Society, November, 1978.

Slavinsky, A. T., & Krauss, J. B. Two approaches to the management of long-term psychiatric outpatients in the community. *Nursing Research,* 1982, *31,* 284–289.

Stein, S. P., Holzman, S., Karasu, T. B., & Charles, E. S. Mid-adult development and psychopathology. *American Journal of Psychiatry,* 1978, *135,* 676–681.

Stevenson, J. S. *Issues and crises during middlescence.* New York: Appleton-Century-Crofts, 1977.

Strauss, J. S. Schizophrenia in middle age. In J. G. Howells (Ed.), *Modern perspectives in the psychiatry of middle age.* New York: Brunner/Mazel, 1981.

Troll, L. E. The family of later life: A decade review. *Journal of Marriage and the Family,* 1971, *33,* 263–290.

Troll, L. E. *Early and middle adulthood: The best is yet to be—maybe.* Monterey: Brooks/Cole Publishing Co., 1975.

Udry, J. R. *The social context of marriage* (2nd ed.). Philadelphia: Lippincott, 1971.

Vaillant, G. E. *Adaptation to life.* Boston: Little, Brown, 1977.

Weideger, P. *Menstruation and menopause: The physiology and psychology, the myth and the reality.* New York: Knoff, 1976.

Werner, H. *Comparative psychology of mental development* (rev. ed.). New York: International Universities Press, 1948.

Werner, H. The concept of development from a comparative and organismic point of view. In D. Harris (Ed.), *The concept of development.* Minneapolis: University of Minnesota Press, 1957.

BIBLIOGRAPHY

Baltes, L. B., & Brim, O. G. *Life-span development and behavior* Vol. 3. New York: Academic Press, 1980.

Datan, N., & Reese, H. *Life-span developmental psychology: Dialectical perspectives of experimental research.* New York: Academic Press, 1977.

Golan, N. *Passing through transitions: A guide for practitioners.* New York: The Free Press, 1981.

Holland, J. L. *Making vocational choices: A theory of careers.* Englewood Cliffs, NJ: Prentice-Hall, 1973.

Lindemann, E. Symptomatology and management of acute grief. *American Journal of Psychiatry,* 1944, *101,* 141–148.

Schaie, K. W. Psychological changes from midlife to early old age: Implications for maintenance of mental health. *American Journal of Orthopsychiatry,* 1981, *51,* 199–218.

CHAPTER 9 OLD AGE

Shirley A. Smoyak

There *is* something new under the sun! Old people are getting older and there are more of them, proportionately and in actual numbers, than at any other time in history. Therefore, it is more important than ever to understand the aging process. This process is best understood when one keeps the following major points in mind:

1. People age in different ways because they belong to different social (ethnic, racial, religious, economic) groups, which are constantly changing.
2. Aging itself is never a fixed or immutable process. It is influenced by social change and the structures of social groups.
3. The changing ways in which people age are constantly reshaping society, both its structures and functions.

Younger people often succumb to the temptation to view old age and aging as rather stable and unexciting, if not dull and depressing. This chapter will attempt to challenge that view with evidence from recently reported research. Some people lead long, healthy, useful, satisfying, and fulfilling lives. Other people die early from illness and disease or live on in rather miserable ways, tortured by loneliness, disenchantment, or various frustrations. Still other people take a middle-of-the-road path of bearing with various forms of chronic ailments and complaints throughout their lives.

> We know that aging is not fully programmed by genetic dispositions or early childhood experiences, but is continually subject to social modification and change. We are beginning to understand *how* society influences the aging process; how the economic, cultural, and social aspects of society affect people's lives; how major changes in society (wars, depressions, inflation, energy shortages) influence the ways in which individuals grow up and grow old. (Riley, Abeles, & Teitelbaum, 1982, p. 11)

What is just beginning to be understood are the complex ways in which people, as they age, reshape society.

This chapter will discuss aging from an historical perspective and within the context of families. The interaction of social change, aging, and family relationships will be explored for effects on mental health in the elderly. Additionally, the physical changes of aging will be discussed, especially as these have implications for nursing assessment and psychotherapeutic drug use.

POSITIVE AGING

It is important to remember that only 5 percent of the elderly are institutionalized; the rest function in various living arrangements in communities. For the large majority, old age is a satisfying and fulfilling time.

Negative views of aging are formed when the norms of individual productivity and power are given central focus. On the other hand, when other values are brought into focus, the work ethic diminishes in importance. Older people tend to become more philosophical and more religious. They rethink what matters and what counts. Sometimes they wish that they had spent more time on human relationships and less on making and worrying about money.

Butler and Lewis (1982) define the major developmental task of old age as being able "to clarify, deepen, and find use for what one has already attained in a lifetime of learning and adapting. Older people must teach themselves to conserve their strength and resources when necessary and to adjust in the best sense to those changes and losses that occur as part of the aging experience" (pp. 25–26). Positive aging is more easily accomplished when there is relatively good physical health, societal supports, adequate finances, and a history of personality that engages others rather than puts others at a distance. Old age does not produce a personality change; it does, however, sharpen both good and poor features of interpersonal styles and approaches.

Butler and Lewis (1982) list six factors that positively influence an older person's relative position in any society. They are (1) ownership of property and control over the opportunities of the young, (2) command of strategic knowledge and skills, (3) strong religious and sacred traditions, (4) strong kinship and extended family bonds, (5) a less product-oriented society, and (6) high mutual dependence and reciprocal aids among members of the society. Old age and how it is experienced are determined by multiple factors at both the societal and individual levels—physical, emotional, and religious factors.

Examining closely what researchers have been studying and reporting in the journals and handbooks on aging, there is no doubt that the great majority of older people live independent and often productive lives even at advanced ages. Summarizing the social and behavioral studies on aging, Fiske (1980) reports:

> Despite the increased risk of organic brain damage with age, their susceptibility to other kinds of psychiatric impairment is probably not notably greater than that of younger people, except for depression, which increases very markedly with age. The lack of notable increase in other kinds of psychiatric impairment in the sixties and early seventies may have a twofold explanation: 'survival of the fittest' in the community . . . and the fact that some psychogenic disorders, including schizophrenia, 'burn themselves out' with advancing age. (p. 367)

INCREASED LONGEVITY

A person born in the United States in the middle of the 1800s could expect to reach and live into the fourth decade. Today, at birth, men can expect to reach age 70, and women age 77. Even at 65 years, life expectancy has increased since 1900 from 12 to 18 years for white women and from 12 to 14 years for white men (Brotman, 1981). These increased life expectancies have created family structures and relationships never before possible. Today, four or five generations can be alive at the same time and share births, marriages, separations, joys, and assorted crises. The three-generational family of nostalgia, often portrayed by artists and writers as typical of Americans, was largely myth until the last half of this century. Earlier, grandparents were simply not alive to participate in the ongoing family arrangements and rearrangements of patterns and norms.

Earlier, married couples could expect to be living together, after their last child left home, for only one or two years. Now, joint survival, after the leaving of this last child, has extended to 13 years and constitutes nearly one-third of married life (Glick, 1977). This postchildren period generally brings comparative economic well-being, even with factors such as inflation, fixed incomes, and retirement. Some of the effects of increasing longevity are offset because people are marrying later, having their first child later, and having to cope with the return of adult children (and grandchildren) when divorce splits up families.

The selection of age 65 to mark the beginning of old age was influenced by the social legislation of Otto von Bismarck in Germany in the 1880s; actually, Bismarck used age 70. That early legislation set the pattern for using 65 to determine not only the retirement point but also eligibility for various social services.

"Oldness," of course, cannot be determined by a number. There are both "young" 65-year-olds and "very old" 65-year-olds. One's state of mind, more than the calendar, determines age. In the United States, the fastest growing age segments of the population are the 75-plus and 85-plus groups (Butler & Lewis, 1982). This fact presents a dilemma to legislators, who are faced with planning for government support for this unexpectedly large number of people. In nursing homes, more than 40 percent of the residents are over 85.

By present projections, between the years 2020 and 2030, when the post-World War II baby boom are older adults, one in five, or 20 percent, of Americans will be over 65. Butler and Lewis (1982) suggest that this demographic revolution "should be seen as a triumph of survivorship rather than a cause for despair" (p. 6). What it means is that more and more people will have the opportunity to live out a full life cycle, rather than experiencing an end before retirement.

Survival rates for white people have always been better than for nonwhites, reflecting the impact of economic factors on health. Since the last census, however, the nonwhite groups are showing improved survival rates. For instance, the number of black older people has risen from 1.2 million in 1960 to 1.8 million in 1977; they now comprise 7.2 percent of the total black population of 25 million.

The significantly longer life expectancy of women produces an imbalance in the older years. There are more than three times as many widows as there are widowers. When older men outlive their wives, they have more options regarding remarriage. Older women have fewer choices and are looked upon negatively if they marry younger men. Older men, however, are approved of when they marry younger women.

Increased longevity, in one sense, can be thought of as a "health hazard." The older one gets, the more likely that certain body parts will wear down or malfunction. However, 81 percent of all old people move about on their own legs, requiring no special care (Butler & Lewis, 1982). Only 5 percent are confined to institutions for physical or emotional care. Yet, the tendency for young people is to think that this 5 percent is the norm for the older group. The healthy old are largely unnoticed. They blend into neighborhoods and shopping centers, with no one particularly noticing their increased numbers. They are visible in retirement communities and function very well there, but young people do not see this development for the most part. The stereotypes and myths about aging are spawned when attention is centered on the 5 percent who do need aid and who are impaired in various ways.

Chronological age is becoming an increasingly poor predictor of how people live. As longevity increases, the ways of living formerly reserved for younger people are being tried and successfully adapted by the elderly. For instance, an older couple may decide to "live together" for economic reasons and then find they really enjoy the new lifestyle. Older women may decide to ignore the gossip and date, and even marry, considerably younger men. Older people go back to school and pursue new degrees and second or third careers. Being a student, being in love, and experimenting with the right job are no longer the territorial domain of the young.

NUTRITION

Eating well cannot make one younger, unfortunately, but it can certainly serve as an effective preventive strategy. There is a new scientific interest in older people's diets and new information that clinicians should use in their planning and caring for older people.

Trabb (1983) reports that a geriatric nutrition scientist, Paul Griminger, has documented some of the changes that must be acknowledged and planned for as people age. Older people often eat less than they did when they were younger and so must obtain much the same nutrients from a smaller total diet. As they become less active, they burn fewer calories and need to adjust their intake. Appetites are also affected by medication and emotions.

Psychological, social, and financial conditions must be considered along with the nutritional information. Knowing what is best to eat is but one dimension. Older people also must have the necessary money to shop and the physical resources to do so. People who are grieving or depressed care little about food. Some older people who live in deteriorated neighborhoods in inner cities are afraid to go shopping for fear of physical harm.

Since kidney function deteriorates with age and since this function is needed for the excretion of the end products of protein metabolism it is actually wiser for the aged not to consume more protein than is necessary. Griminger (Trabb, 1983) recommends, for a 150-pound person, 55 grams of protein per day eaten, for example, as 4 ounces of fish or meat, 4 ounces of bread, and 1.5 ounces of cheese. He thinks that vitamin and mineral supplements are needed only for those whose diets are questionable.

His research also has documented the fact that people generally consume too much phosphorus and too little calcium. The latter has a direct impact on the degree to which osteoporosis becomes a problem. Moderate exercise and proper proportions of calcium and phosphorus are needed to improve bone density. The ideal calcium/phosphorus balance is one-to-one. This, however, is not easily achieved in a diet unless there are substantial amounts of milk products and green leafy vegetables. Most foods contain considerably more phosphorus than calcium, particularly meat and fish.

Contrary to popular belief, there is no evidence that elderly people, in general, lose their sense of taste to any marked extent, that they suffer from food allergies, or that they are more harmed by food additives than the general population. What they do lose is the incentive to eat when there are negative changes in their social environment.

Though nutritional needs and concerns are not usually within the realm of assessments and observations that psychiatric mental health nurses make, it is clear that they should be. Food is not just a biological necessity that produces physical well-being, it is part of the emotional climate of individuals and families. Families gather at mealtimes and use that opportunity for psychological refueling and energizing as well as getting caught up on individual news. At rituals and ceremonies of all kinds, including funerals, some food and drink are served. The earliest emotional memories are associated with food—mother's milk. When daily meals are eaten alone, the food certainly takes on a new meaning. For some it is overemphasized, and for others there is a loss of interest.

AGING AND FAMILIES IN TRANSITION

As Hareven (1982) has so succinctly put it, "through much of American history, the family has been seen as the linchpin of the social order and the basis for stable governance" (p. 446). The aging process is one that occurs within families. Changes in families—their structure, composition, rules of organization, and values—provide a useful perspective from which to understand aging and aging persons.

Families change more slowly than other institutions, yet there has always been the fear that the family is disintegrating. Every generation has produced writers who express their concerns about the family's demise and the breakdown of tradition. Industrialization and urbanization have been indicted as the causes of this family disorganization. However, many of these fears are built on the basis of myths rather than facts.

One myth, that there once was a golden age of family relations with three generations living happily together under one roof, was widely held. Recent research on the family in preindustrial America has dispelled this myth, showing that the "great extended families" that have become a part of the folklore were rarely in existence (Hareven, 1982). Nuclear families were the most common form of family living arrangement, although in the earlier centuries it was very likely that strangers, such as boarders and apprentices, were also there together with the parents and children. Grandparents rarely lived with their grandchildren. In 1920, the chance of a 10-year-old having two living grandparents was 40 percent; today it is 75 percent. In 1920, the chance of a 10-year-old having four living grandparents was 1.7 percent; today it is 8 percent (National Institute on Aging, 1972).

Industrialization did cause changes in how families function, although it did not destroy them as was feared. In the preindustrial period, families did everything that people needed within the family. Homes served as workshops, schools, hospitals, and asylums, as well as places where children were born and reared. Family and community were indistinguishably blended as the basic societal unit. Further, when all work was done within the family, there was no distinction between "family life" and "work life"; they were one and the same. With industrialization, many of the functions performed within families were transferred to agencies and institutions outside the family. Not only was work done outside, but education, religion, social welfare, and health care were given over to strangers. Thus, the family became a very specialized agency, performing the old functions of child-bearing and child-rearing, but now adding a new function, that of psychological refueling. Husbands and wives began to live by a new requirement—that they love each other. Our grandparents never were required to do that; they had only to be good economic providers and ensure that the children were raised properly.

The discovery of childhood as a distinct stage of life was closely tied to the emergence of the middle-class family in Europe and the United States in the early 19th century. Families became child-centered retreats. Children were no longer expected to join the workforce until the late teens. Mothers had many added requirements regarding the raising of these "at-home" children. "Tenderness, gentleness, affection, sweetness, and a comforting demeanor were all considered ideal characteristics for the domestic wife" (Hareven [quoting Aries], 1982, p. 454).

The relationships between husbands and wives, parents and children, and older kin were based upon shared values of support and assistance. Though three generations usually did not live under one roof, they often did help each other financially as well as in other supporting ways. There were operative social norms about families pulling together and aiding each other in crisis. Before crisis centers and mental health centers, problems were handled within families. The norm of family obligation was the very basis of survival. Family needs, not individual directions, were primary.

The major historical change in family values has been the change from the norm or ideal of collective family need to one of individualism. Individual priorities and preferences now can "come first." This has led to an exaggerated emphasis on emotional nurture, intimacy, psychological refueling, and privacy. The community is far less likely to be welcome within the family, now that it has become a haven for the performing of all these private duties. This liberation of people has had a severe price: the erosion of the resilience of the family and its ability to handle crises. Moreover, according to Hareven (1982), "it has contributed to a greater separation of family members and especially to the isolation of older people" (p. 456).

When family solidarity was the norm, an older person in crisis could count on a family member to come to his or her aid. This help could be expected not only for a grandparent, but also for an aunt, uncle, or cousin. The fact of the matter today, however, is that there are far more grandparents and aged aunts and uncles than ever before in history. Even if the individualism norm had not been born, it is questionable whether the increased numbers of elderly could have been handled, when in crisis, by their families.

Another widely held myth about the past is that the timing of family transitions was once more orderly and stable than it is today. The historical record, however, reveals precisely the opposite condition. Patterns of family timing, in the past, were far more complex, diverse, and less orderly than they are today. Family life-cycle shifts follow different patterns by class, race, and ethnicity.

In contrast to the past, most families see their children through to adulthood with both parents still alive as well as some grandparents. The adult children now are struggling with the need to develop new norms for their responsibility toward aged parents. Some authors have labelled people in their late forties to early sixties as the "trapped generation," those who are caught between the pressures of caring for, and financially supporting, both children (often in college) and aged parents. They wonder if there will be any time for personal enjoyment.

Since the possibility of a family pattern with four and even five generations alive at the same time never existed before, families have no norms or rules of organization to guide them through this new maze. Even when clinicians plot family members on a genogram when doing family therapy, establishing the family map for a five-generation living family can be very complicated. Such genograms will be even more complicated if members within the various generations continue to divorce and remarry at present rates. Since there is no apparent trend indicating that divorce will decrease, stepmothers, stepfathers, and the various half-siblings will continue to provide complexities and confusion regarding allegiances, alliances, and coalitions.

Women continue to outlive men to a considerable degree. This difference in the sexes produces still another new family reality. Daughters reach their late fifties before they lose their mothers. Today, the relationships between mothers and daughters are concentrated more in daughters' adult years than in their childhoods. It is not uncommon for 65-year-old daughters to still have living mothers and, of course, to be grandmothers themselves.

As stated previously, married couples today live together longer before being separated by death. This period typically brings comparative affluence, freedom from child-rearing concerns and pressures, and freedom for outside pursuits or careers. A new rhythm of retiring and unretiring and retiring again is being tried by couples. Widows are older. Since they are older, they are more likely to be bothered by a variety of physical problems.

The new norm of individualism forces a sometimes unwanted independence upon older married couples, and especially widows. Increasing proportions of people, particularly older widows, live alone. Though older people are not necessarily more lonely than the young, they do not always enjoy this style of living.

To some degree, living alone is offset by frequent visiting patterns. Various studies have shown that usually at least one or two adult children in a family live within easy commuting distance of their aged parents, sometimes less than a half-hour away. Further, the continuing rates of divorce produce an array of relatives such as present and past sons- and daughters-in-law, stepgrandchildren, and so on. When children have divorced, the in-laws often continue a very positive relationship. For instance, a divorced son-in-law may continue to see the grandparents of his children when he brings them to visit on holidays or weekends.

A common belief, now known to be a myth, is that people's beliefs, values, and competencies are set and formed in childhood. Sociologists are now describing lifelong socialization wherein adults continue to grow and to expand their capabilities. Learning abilities, once thought to peak in the early 20s and then decline, are now being shown to persist in later life (Riley et al., 1982). Researchers are finding that older persons respond positively to challenges in work and other social settings. Psychologists have shown that memory does not really decline, although some particular perceptive areas may be somewhat slower. Even nursing home residents, who had been ignored and allowed to sink to very damaging levels of anomie and despair, are being resocialized to enjoy a more meaningful life. Many strategies are being used to accomplish this resocialization or relearning, including bringing young children, pets, plants, and birds into the long-term care settings.

In other research, it has been demonstrated that people can change lifelong damaging habits, such as overeating, drinking too much, or failing to exercise (Riley et al., 1982). Positive health habits are being developed to avoid heart attacks and strokes.

Retirement

The interplay between aging and social change can be easily seen when retirement is the focus. Vast social changes (such as industrialization, social security programs, private pension plans, rising unemployment) have caused the mean retirement age to drop dramatically. Of the cohort of men reaching age 65 in 1900, about two-thirds were still counted in the workforce. By 1960, only one-third were working, and 20 years later only one-fifth of the age 65 male cohort were working (Rosenfeld & Brown, 1979). Not only are these men retiring earlier, but they are living longer after retiring, thus producing a marked impact on their income, leisure activities, social opportunities, health, and family patterns. For women, retirement is not yet a massive phenomenon. Married women, however, now have to develop new ways to cope with retired husbands who spend more time with them.

Social norms are affected by the fact that fewer older men continue to work. Laws and employment contracts are being changed. Social Security legislation in the 1930s built age 65 into its planning. What the appropriate age is, or should be, is undergoing great debate in Washington. In many places, mandatory retirement has been raised to 70. Some institutions or firms entirely ignore the retirement age question. A very vocal, younger, voting constituency is complaining bitterly about increased taxation that falls upon them under the current Social Security laws (Foner and Schwab, 1981). Butler and Lewis (1982) point out, however, that more attention should be paid by policy makers to the "dependency ratio" than the income maintenance and health costs of the burgeoning older population. The fact is that the proportional financial "burden" on the middle, working generations has really not changed very much at all because there are fewer children and youths today for these people to support. The total number of dependents for whom the middle group is financially responsible is actually dropping, at the moment, and will rise only slightly by 2025.

Mental Health and Families

At any age, mental health or illness can best be understood within the context of family systems. Mental health is linked to how families socialize their members for roles as adults in society, how they portray the value and meaning of life, how they handle departures from expected behavior, and how they deal with crisis and illness. The ethnic and religious backgrounds of families provide the direction for the rules of organization that they evolve and shape for themselves. These rules of organization that guide family life shift and change throughout the life-cycle of the family and the varying lifespans of its individual members. New nuclear families, with infants and children, organize themselves very differently from older families, wherein adults predominate. Since, for the first time in history, longevity is now becoming more and more the rule, families are faced with having no tradition to guide them as they evolve their rules for living. Families are facing the need to decide how to live as four and five generations. Such relatively simple things as where and how to spend holidays are much more complex when both grandparents and great-grandparents are in the picture. Parents have to stop and consider what to have their children call the "layers" of grandparents. Are all the older women "Nanny?" Should the oldest have a different title? Do they keep the title, or move up when the oldest dies? Such questions were never raised before. As Bengtson and Treas (1980) state, ". . . families provide a context of meaning for the changes associated with aging. In negotiating the uncharted career of old age, definitions of what is proper or inappropriate, usual or uncommon, valued or profane, are greatly influenced by family norms" (p. 400).

The fact that families are smaller today will continue to present dilemmas as older people increase in number. Aging parents, having raised fewer children, will have fewer descendants to call upon for help than in the past. Younger adults, having grown up in smaller families, have fewer brothers and sisters to help in the tasks of caring for aging parents. The norms of individualism and independence, new in this era, also add to the strain. Families will find themselves confronting the realities of decreasing human resources and increasing human needs to be met. It is far more likely that they will turn to agencies and institutions for help, whereas in the past the family rule might have been that "we care for our own at home."

The elderly are subjected to insults to their self-esteem, sometimes reaching depressive proportions, when they come to realize that they are no longer valued as they were when working or raising children. The pattern available in the past, of one child (most commonly a daughter) taking responsibility for aging parents, is often no longer a family option. More women today marry and have families of their own; if they remain single, they leave home and embark on careers. The aging parents, then, find that they have to take care of themselves. When one child was designated the caretaker, the issue of worth of the aged did not arise. Of course, the caretaker child had fewer options than her siblings. Today, it is very unlikely that such a child is designated and accepts this role. When siblings do discuss their obligations to parents, and divide the responsibility for caring, daughters still tend to be the "affective specialists," providing emotional support and nurturance, and sons still tend to be the "instrumental specialists," worrying about bills, mortgages, and bank accounts.

A bumper sticker that has attracted increasing attention states: "Mental illness is hereditary; you catch it from your kids." Increasing numbers of older adults are saying this as they contemplate a living arrangement with their children and grandchildren. Very often the noise and the chaos, where there are even a few children in the picture, act as a deterrent to the older generation's consideration of a move from a too-big house to some other arrangement. Another deterrent to the three-generation arrangement is the anticipated difficulty with two women in a kitchen. A woman in her eighties recently expressed her sentiments as, "my stroke has left me feeling very bad, but, if I moved in with them, I'd be both depressed and crazy. Depressed is all I can handle right now."

Territoriality and differing lifestyles prevent a more common occurrence of the three-generations-under-one-roof model. The elderly find that they do want to stay connected to the younger generations, but if they are physically able they tend to prefer to stay connected from a distance.

Transitions in old age, though they may not be technical causes of mental illness as defined in the DSM-III (American Psychiatric Association, 1980), do produce tensions and strains that then have sequelae of changes in psychic states, most commonly depression.

Bengtson and Treas (1980) list four crisis-producing events encountered by families with great regularity. These are (1) independence of children or the "empty nest" syndrome, (2) retirement from a paid job, (3) incapacitating illness requiring institutionalization, and (4) disruption of the family unit through death or divorce. Some families manage these transitions without outside help; others become so distraught or immobilized that they seek counseling.

MENTAL HEALTH AND AGING

Stereotypes held by health care providers can create dangerous situations for the elderly. When the helpers believe that illness and a general sense of not feeling well are normal concomitants of aging, they will not try very hard to get to the source of a difficulty being reported by an aged client. There is an often-repeated consciousness-raising story told about an older woman who had the necessary courage to counteract the negative expectations of her physician. She had been telling him of the pain she was having in her right knee. He had said to her, "Well, you'll just have to bear with it—learn to live with it." She replied, "Look, sir, my left knee is 84 years old too, and it is not bothering me at all!"

Instances of poor or half-hearted assessment and treatment are unfortunately all too common. Potentially treatable problems are sometimes ignored, and minor problems, which might be handled more naturally, are medicated to extreme degrees.

Zarit (1980) points out that older persons are rarely evaluated for reversible causes of dementia (those entities formerly referred to as "acute brain syndromes"). Clinicians who see many elderly patients in their practices sometimes are ignorant of distinctions between dementia and delirium. "Senility" is still appearing in charts and records. Depression is a frequently missed diagnosis. Sexual problems are often dismissed as being relatively unimportant (Wilson, 1984).

Precise data regarding the incidence and prevalence of psychiatric disorders among the elderly are nonexistent. Even estimates are difficult to make because of the lack of agreement on what criteria to use to denote impairment and the fact that community surveys have used different instruments and selection processes. Because of the variety of indicators that have been used (from self-reports to expertly executed diagnostic assessment), the estimations of prevalence vary widely. One summary of mental health surveys reported disorders as ranging from 45 per 1,000 persons to 308 per 1,000 (Zarit, 1980). Based on these studies, the estimate, then, is that no less than 2 percent and perhaps as many as 20 percent of aged persons are in need of mental health services.

Despite the extent of psychiatric impairment among the aged, they receive fewer mental health services than almost any other age group (Kramer, Taube, & Rednick, 1973). The one exception is very young children, who also are underserved in the mental health area. The elderly constitute more than 10 percent of the population, yet receive fewer than 2 percent of all services in communities. They fare slightly better in partial institutional care. In contrast to these low rates for community care, older persons represent a higher proportion of persons treated in state, county, and federal hospitals (Kramer et al., 1973). One side-effect of the current trend toward deinstitutionalizing the mentally ill is that older psychiatric patients are not admitted to psychiatric hospitals but instead find their way to nursing homes or other "long-term care" settings. Staff in nursing homes are generally ill-equipped to handle psychiatric behavior problems. The results of this maladaptation include patient abuse and high staff turnover.

A reason often offered for not actively treating older persons with psychological disorders is that the situation is hopeless and they cannot be helped. Zarit (1980) suggests tracing the roots of this negativity "to Freud, who cautioned his followers not to waste their time on the aged, because their defenses were too rigid" (p. 17). It is quite obvious, however, that one cannot possibly adapt to all the social, biological, and psychological changes going on in normal aging and be rigid; the rigidity was more in Freud's view than in the aged.

Some of the pessimism about treating the elderly stems from confusing chronic mental problems with disorders of old age. The earlier research on the aged mentally ill was done in state hospitals on populations who had been hospitalized many years. The samples, therefore, confounded the variables of chronicity and aging. There was no effort to identify aged populations of mentally ill with recent onsets of acute illness. The tendency is to see all illness as irreversible. The fact, however, is that chronic brain disorders affect only about 5 to 10 percent of the aged. Because the interest in aged mentally ill is so recent, the issues of whether the elderly benefit from standard psychological treatment, which groups of elderly have the best prognoses, or which groups respond best to treatment have not been raised systematically.

The attitudes of the aged themselves about care in mental health facilities contribute to their lack of service. Older people are wary of psychiatrists and anyone associated with psychiatry or "crazy people." They were socialized in times before the efforts to erase the stereotypes about the mentally ill had gained prominence. Reluctance to ask for help is common. Acknowledging problems is seen as synonymous with being weak.

At the moment, there are still relatively few professional people who are educated in the field of gerontology or who have sought those additional skills through continuing education. There is a widespread reluctance among the mental health professions to treat the elderly. Olshan (1983) recently documented the attitudes held by therapists leading to this reluctance. Therapists' own fears of aging, their stereotypes regarding aging, and hopelessness combined to produce an avoidance of older clients.

The medical model, applied to assessing psychopathology, has not lacked critics over the years. When dealing with aged people, all of the cautions that the critics have proclaimed should be heeded. Rather than looking for causes within individuals only, it is imperative to examine the environment. One cannot conclude "paranoia," if, in fact, children are discussing placing the aged person in a nursing home. Depression is rarely an entirely intrapsychic phenomenon. With the aged, the combined effects of losses, immobilities, and reduced biological functions must be considered. One's social network and changes within it contribute as much to how one feels about things as do physical changes in brain cells. Even for persons who actually have structural damage to the brain, the environment still continues to influence actions and feelings.

In order to be conversant with other providers in the mental health system, it would be well for the nurse to understand the logic used in classifying disorders in the DSM-III (American Psychiatric Association, 1980). Rather than inventing another system of terminology, the language used in DSM-III will suffice as a starting point. Additionally, texts such as Nathan and Harris (1975) or Zax and Cowen (1976) can be used for more definitive descriptions, including the distinctions between and among categories of illnesses and clusters of symptoms. Two basic processes can lead to the dysfunction of any body organ: (1) failure of metabolic processes to maintain adequate organ functioning or (2) death of a number of organ cells sufficient to impair functioning permanently. These two factors are, of course, related since the prolonged insufficiency would lead to death. In senile dementia, there is structural change and considerable cell death. Chief contributing causes are vascular disease and an Alzheimer's-type deterioration. In contrast, in acute brain syndromes (delirium), metabolic processes are being altered but reversal is still possible. As Zaret (1980) states, "the differential diagnosis of senile dementia from treatable illness is the most important skill in clinical practice with the aged" (p. 136). Nurses must learn to identify the cases where impairment is reversible and also must be able to distinguish dementia from normal changes in old age. These skills are being learned in graduate programs that specialize in aged populations, in continuing education workshops, and in a few baccalaureate programs.

With the present state of knowledge, there is still no definitive treatment to repair or to arrest the two major brain diseases of old age, senile dementia of the Alzheimer's type and multiinfarct dementia. However, nurses can be very helpful to patients and families in showing them how to adjust and modify the environment so as to reduce unnecessary stimuli and obstructions. Also, medication can be used to reduce agitation.

Nurses need to be aware of community resources that can be tapped by families. For instance, Butler and Lewis (1982), in a series of appendices, list organizations that serve the elderly (including those specific to Alzheimer's disease), government programs, and other resources. Since the time between listing and publishing is rather long, updated information for local areas needs to be obtained.

One of the benefits of aging, in regard to mental health, is that it is highly unlikely that one would become schizophrenic. It is rare to see a newly developed schizophrenic disorder in an older person. "Senile schizophrenia," or "paraphrenia" as it is called in England and on the Continent, are really more equivalent to what is called paranoia or paranoid state in the United States (Butler & Lewis, 1982). There are, of course, many older schizophrenics; some are still in state, county, and federal mental hospitals and others have been placed in programs following the trend to empty the large mental hospitals. Until the past decade, the back wards of mental hospitals contained large numbers of "chronic schizophrenics" who had lived there for more than half a century. These people usually did not exhibit the florid delusional systems and hallucinations that are symptomatic in younger groups. The term "burned-out schizophrenic" was used to describe the quieter, often withdrawn person. Since admissions to mental hospitals today are drastically reduced, it will be possible to study the long-term course of this illness in the community. The effects of institutionalization versus the disease process can be identified.

One major difference between the DSM-III and the previous edition was the elimination of the category "neurotic disorders." Now they are included under other categories, such as affective, anxiety, somatoform, dissociative, and psychosexual disorders. The old meaning of the term *neurosis* implied unconscious conflict producing overused defense mechanisms and personality changes. Some clinicians argue that the older category was more definitive for the kinds of symptoms and problems that have their onsets in old age, causing distortions in thinking, judgment, and general functioning. The International Classification of Diseases, published in 1979, still uses the older terminology (Butler & Lewis, 1982). Nurses who work with older clients will need to decide which set of descriptors is most useful to them.

Depression can occur at any time in life, but it is the most common emotional illness found among older people (Butler & Lewis, 1982). The bipolar disorders are more common in people under 30, whereas the unipolar depression is most common in older patients. The only difference between the two categories is that the unipolar type lacks the associated manic episode.

When a depression is less severe or less prolonged, it is called *cyclothymic* or *dysthymic* to distinguish it from the major depression. Depression varies from mild mood states, such as feeling blue or down, to the extremes of psychotic withdrawal or suicide. Depressive symptoms are often masked or missed because they are associated with other life events, such as deaths, major surgery, or economic changes. In those instances, the "feeling bad" is normal and expected; when too long a time is spent in grief and mourning, however, depression should be suspected. Depression is also often hidden under hypochondriasis or a lifestyle of complaining and expressed loneliness. Careful history-taking by an experienced interviewer is needed to determine the degree to which a depressive disorder exists. The contributions of social or situational factors and physiological and chemical factors need to be weighed carefully. Consultation with a psychopharmacologist yields a better treatment plan.

Chemicals in the brain play a decided role in regulating nervous system activity by their control messages. Two classes of such chemicals, important to affective disorders, have been identified: (1) the catecholamines, which include dopamine and norepinephrine, and (2) an indolamine, serotinin. Butler and Lewis (1982) summarize their effects as: "the catecholamine hypothesis suggests that the functional turnover of catecholamines is increased at specific central synapses in mania and decreased in depression. The indolamine hypothesis posits a deficit of serotinin turnover in both mania and depression, with a greater decrease of serotinin in depression" (p. 71). These chemical changes can be triggered by both external (exogenous) factors or by internal (endogenous) ones. In many instances, it is impossible to separate or determine accurately the exact contributions of external or internal factors to the onset of symptoms.

Though the chemical factors cannot be ignored, nurses would be wise to focus on the interpersonal and social network realities in each situation. Decreased self-regard and guilt are entities that need examination and intervention. Anger, in all its varieties, needs to be understood, grappled with, and dissipated. The contribution of drugs and poor health habits needs assessing. Eating poorly can cause electrolyte imbalances and associated mental changes.

Psychotherapeutic Drug Use in the Aged

Although people over 65 account for 11 percent of the total present U.S. population, they use a disproportionate amount of the prescribed and over-the-counter drugs. They use 25 percent of all drugs sold today. The most common drugs prescribed for the elderly are sedatives, hypnotics, oral hypoglycemics, oral diuretics, digoxin, and propoxyphene. The most common self-prescribed drugs are laxatives and the large variety of aspirin-containing or aspirinlike substances (Hollister, 1981). The elderly are very likely to be using more than one drug, since multiple symptoms and ailments are the norm.

The aged mentally ill, who are taking drugs to alleviate depression or other psychiatric symptoms, are at an increased risk for overdose and other untoward effects. Remarkably little reliable information is available about the kinetics of drugs in the elderly, yet adverse drug reactions occur seven times more often than in people 20 to 29 years old (Triggs & Nation, 1975). There are no definitive studies to guide the clinician in making judgments about the pharmacokinetic differences between the young and old. The articles that do attempt to address the subject generally are able to provide only the most general guidelines.

Most drug absorption is in the upper gastrointestinal tract, primarily in the small bowel. Most people assume that in the elderly, because of circulatory changes, this absorption is slowed down. This assumption, however, is not supported by research data. Decreased blood flow in the bowel can occur in congestive heart failure, but the effects on drug absorption are not clear. Failure of drugs to be effective can rarely be ascribed to inefficient absorption, nor toxicity to excessive absorption (Hollister, 1981).

Changing body composition in the elderly affects the distribution of certain drugs. From the mid to late seventies, there tends to be a decrease in total body weight but an increase in body fat, thus yielding a decrease in lean body mass. Also, water volume decreases to

18 percent of total body weight, compared with 25 percent for younger adults. A drug, such as ethanol or lithium, would be more highly concentrated given the decreased water volume. But lipid-soluble drugs would be diluted since there is more body fat. Furthermore, since the total number of neurons decreases with normal aging, any medication that affects the nervous system will have a therapeutic effect with a smaller dose as compared with younger individuals. For example, 8 mg of Demerol will result in approximately the same pain relief in a 65-year-old as 16 mg in a 20-year-old. This effect may be particularly true with mood-altering drugs since the neuron loss is disproportionately found in the frontal cerebral cortex in some aged individuals.

The kidney is especially vulnerable to the aging process, decreasing in size and functional capacity. Renal function in aged persons, measured by total blood flow, glomerular filtration rate or, tubular excretory capacity, may show declines of 40 to 50 percent (Hollister, 1981). Renal function is also affected by dehydration, hypotension, heart failure, and other physiological changes. Whereas most psychotropic drugs are eliminated by metabolism rather than excretion, lithium is an important exception. Since lithium is largely excreted by the kidney, doses in aged patients should be greatly reduced, certainly to less than 50 percent of the dose used with adults.

The results of various drug compliance studies show that people simply do not take what is prescribed for them by physicians (for instance, some estimates are that less than 40 percent of prescriptions written are ever filled) and, if they are, their dosage, frequency, and duration are often adjusted. More "lack of compliance" occurs with the elderly for a number of reasons. The poor elderly may not be able to afford what has been prescribed. Those who have difficulty with mobility may not be able to get to a pharmacy or shopping center easily. Those who are confused or forgetful may not take the drugs at all, the wrong amounts, or take all at once to "catch up" when they remember that the appointed time or times have passed. Overdoses of drugs such as Valium and Percodan are quite common since taking the drugs frequently interferes with memory and recall.

Given the physiological changes associated with normal aging for all elderly, and the mental changes for some elderly, considerable caution should be exercised when drugs are needed. Obviously, drugs should only be used when they are absolutely necessary. Nurses can provide a very valuable service to the elderly and their families by helping to assess the need for drugs and acting as interpreters for both the family and the physician. For instance, not all depressive states should be tranquilized or medicated away. Grief is a necessary experience and must be felt in order to be understood, integrated, and managed. To give drugs to the newly bereaved person impedes the grief and mourning process. Networks of support and expressions of sympathy and caring from family and friends are far more appropriate, safe, and useful than Mellaril or other antidepressive agents when the elderly have suffered losses.

The aging effects upon normal sleep include decrease in total sleep length, stage 4, and REM sleep, as well as increased irregularity of sleep patterns and sleep apnea. These changes are increased rather than abated when tranquilizers, antidepressants, and other "sleeping" medications are prescribed to treat insomnia and fatigue. Although these medications *can* help the aged person to fall asleep quicker, the aspects of sleep already altered by normal aging are affected even more by the medications. For example, sleep apnea is significantly increased in elderly taking these medications, presenting a potentially lethal problem for these individuals.

Regardless of why a nurse enters a home (family counseling, public health visit) he or she should give attention to medication cabinets, refrigerators, and any other place where drugs are kept. All drugs should be evaluated for current need and unnecessary ones eliminated. It is not at all unusual to find aged patients taking antipsychotic, antiparkinsonian, and antidepressant drugs all at once, together with medication for sleep. Stopping all medications related to the alteration of mood or behavior, and carefully observing the effect, is an excellent clinical strategy. Frequently, the elderly patient reports feeling fine for the first time in months or years.

When drugs are necessary, the following precautions should be taken. First, the form of the drug should be ingestible to the patient. Some people cannot swallow large capsules or pills. Liquids can spill if hands are not steady. Second, avoid suspension drugs; very often they are not shaken thoroughly. Third, be closely involved with the patient so that the physician will be more likely to try smaller initial doses. Close observation will document when the desired titration has been reached. Fourth, work with the physician and pharmacist to arrange the simplest of drug schedules. Daily dosages are possible with many of the commonly used drugs. Fifth, help the patient or family member to keep the treatment plan in clear focus by posting the drug schedule, in clearly typed or printed form, somewhere near the place where the medications are usually taken (kitchen, bathroom, or bedroom). Sixth, teach the most common side-effects and regularly monitor for their occurrence. Seventh, expect noncompliance and develop strategies to assess how much the patient has departed from the proposed plan. For instance, from time to time, count the number of pills remaining to see whether they match the number expected if the dosage had been followed exactly in the interim. Finally, periodically review the medication regimen with the patient and caregiver.

Suicide in the Aged

Suicide is one of the top 10 causes of death for all age groups in the United States. The highest suicide rate occurs in white men in their eighties. For women, the peak rate is in their middle fifties. Depression and suicide are related in all age groups but seem to be even more closely related in the elderly (Kastenbaum, 1983).

Identifying suicidal older patients requires interviewing skill since their messages may be clouded in expressions that appear expected or normal for older people. For instance, statements like, "Well, I'm the only one left now," or "I'll be the next to go," may not be noted as suicidal messages unless the listener carefully places them in context and searches out the intended meaning.

Some people have made many suicide attempts over the years or have discussed the possibility. Their families or friends may have become so accustomed to rescuing them or hearing their distress expressed that they miss the significant clue or message delivered by the older person. Faced with multiple losses and physical changes, they frequently act very quickly to exercise what they consider to be their only option, suicide. A very likely "interaction effect" occurs when the older person, expressing despair and voicing the suicide possibility, gets subtle validation of the choice from the younger person. Statements like, "I don't think I could handle that either," or "I don't know how you've managed to cope with all your troubles for so long," serve as validation of the choice or are heard as actual invitations.

Some clinicians believe that the "cries for help" are less common among the elderly. They believe that older persons contemplating suicide are less likely to announce their intentions and more quickly commit the act. Others disagree and insist that warning signs are still evident and readable.

Butler and Lewis (1982) point out that rational and philosophical decisions to end life are more common in old age. As people perceive themselves to be failing, the choice of being in charge of determining how the end will be becomes more and more attractive. "Older men, especially, may decide to kill themselves rather than leave their widows penniless from the cost of a long illness" (Butler & Lewis, 1982). News articles have documented the suicide plan sometimes carried out by married couples; some commit a double suicide and others carry out a combination of mercy killing and suicide of the other.

The most preventable suicides are those related to depression. Depressive reactions are very widespread in old age, including psychotic depressions, those depressions associated with lucid moments in the cerebral arteriosclerotic patient, and those usually labelled "situational," where there is loss, grief, and despair. Depression can emerge as an associate of guilt in instances where the person looks back over how he or she has lived and is overwhelmed by shame, remorse, and guilt. There are clues to the impending self-destruction when the person says things like, "How can my daughter ever forgive me for what I did to her?" or "I see now that my life is just one big hypocrisy."

Butler and Lewis (1982) note that "older people use all the usual methods of killing themselves: drugs, guns, hanging, and jumping off high places. . . . Suicide may also be accomplished 'subintentionally,' by the slower means of not eating, not taking medicines, drinking too much, delaying treatment, and taking risks physically" (p. 81). Of course, the longer processes of suicidal erosion or insults to one's health are not included in the suicide statistics. Long, drawn-out, destructive behavior is more difficult to intervene in because clinicians are reluctant to interfere with patients' rights. People can be involuntarily committed and treated if their self-destructive act has an immediacy to it, but the longer process cannot be legally managed.

Some older people unwittingly shorten their lives by poor nutritional patterns. Living alone, being unable to move about and shop easily, and having poor teeth often combine to produce lethal eating patterns. Too much salt and too little protein are deadly.

Kastenbaum (1983) cautions those who work with the elderly to explore, very carefully, the exact nature of physical complaints. The real issue for feeling poorly may be psychosocial losses not physical changes. Also, physical complaints may be maximized or minimized, depending on how hopeless or hopeful the person generally feels about life.

Emery (1981) encourages the use of cognitive therapy to intervene with both depression and suicidal directions. This approach is straightforward, easily learned, and a useful clinical tool for nurses who work with the elderly.

SUMMARY

Old age is a stage of human development plagued by myths and ignorance. This chapter has sought to dispel these beliefs by drawing from some of the latest research on the topic of aging. These data reveal that the phenomenon of aging in society is dynamic. If psychiatric mental health nurses are to work effectively with the elderly, they must adopt a perspective whereby they can view aging within a social/historical context and the elderly within their social/family context. The importance of a bio-psycho-social assessment for adequate care of the elderly has also been stressed.

REFERENCES

American Psychiatric Association. *Diagnostic and statistical manual of mental disorders* (3rd ed.). Washington, DC: American Psychiatric Association, 1980.

Bengtson, V., & Treas, J. The changing family context of mental health and aging. In J. Birren and R. Sloane (Eds.), *Handbook of mental health and aging.* Englewood Cliffs, NJ: Prentice-Hall, 1980.

Brotman, H. B. Every ninth American. In *Development in aging, 1980.* Annual Report of the Senate Special Committee on Aging, May. Washington, DC: U.S. Government Printing Office, 1981.

Butler, R., & Lewis, M. *Aging and mental health: Positive psychosocial and biomedical approaches* (3rd ed.). St. Louis: C. V. Mosby Co., 1982.

Emery, G. *A new beginning: How you can change your life through cognitive therapy.* New York: Simon & Schuster, 1981.

Fiske, M. Tasks and crises of the second half of life: The interrelationship of commitment, coping and adaptation. In J. Birren & R. B. Sloane (Eds.), *Handbook of mental health and aging.* Englewood Cliffs, NJ: Prentice-Hall, 1980.

Foner, A., & Schwab, K. *Aging and retirement.* Monterey, CA: Brooks/Cole Publishing Co., 1981.

Glick, P. C. Updating the life cycle of the family. *Journal of Marriage and the Family.* 1977, *39,* 5–13.

Hareven, T. American families in transition: Historical perspectives on change. In F. Walsh (Ed.), *Normal family processes.* New York: The Guilford Press, 1982.

Hollister, L. General principles of psychotherapeutic drug use in the aged. In T. Crook & G. Cohen (Eds.), *Physicians' handbook on psychotherapeutic drug use in the aged.* New Canaan, CT: NIMH and Mark Powley Associates, Inc., 1981.

Kastenbaum, R. Suicidality in the aged. In T. Crook & G. Cohen (Eds.), *Physicians' guide to the diagnosis and treatment of depression in the elderly.* New Canaan, CT: NIMH and Mark Powley Associates, Inc., 1983.

Kramer, M., Taube, A., & Rednick, R. Patterns of use of psychiatric facilities by the aged: Past, present and future. In C. Eisdorfer & M. Lawton (Eds.), *The psychology of adult development and aging.* Washington, DC: American Psychological Association, 1973.

Nathan, P., & Harris, S. *Psychopathology and society.* New York: McGraw-Hill, 1975.

National Institute on Aging. *Metropolitan Life Statistical Bulletin,* 1972, *53,* 8–10.

Olshan L. *A descriptive study of psychotherapists' beliefs and attitudes about the elderly.* Unpublished master's thesis, Rutgers, The State University of New Jersey, Newark, NJ, 1983.

Riley, M., Abeles, R., & Teitelbaum, M. *Aging from birth to death: Vol. II. Sociotemporal perspectives.* Boulder, CO: Westview Press, 1982.

Rosenfeld, C., & Brown, S. K. The labor force status of older workers. *Monthly Labor Review,* 1979, *102,* 12–18.

Trabb, H. Nutrition for the elderly. *MATRIX: Report on research at Rutgers.* New Brunswick, NJ: Rutgers, The State University of New Jersey, Spring, 1983.

Triggs, E. J., & Nation, R. L. Pharmacokinetics in the aged: A review. *Journal of Pharmacokinetic Biopharmacy,* 1975, *3,* 387–418.

Wilson, J. *Assessing sexuality needs of nursing home residents.* Unpublished master's thesis, Rutgers, The State University of New Jersey, Newark, NJ, 1984.

Zarit, S. *Aging and mental disorders.* New York: The Free Press, 1980.

Zax, M., & Cowen, E. *Abnormal psychology: Changing conceptions* (2nd ed.). New York: Holt, Rinehart and Winston, 1976.

BIBLIOGRAPHY

Beck, A., Rush, J., Shaw, B., & Emery, G. *Cognitive therapy of depression.* New York: Guilford Press, 1979.

Otten, J., & Shelley, F. *When your parents grow old.* New York: Funk and Wagnalls, 1976.

Ragan, P. *Aging parents.* Los Angeles: University of Southern California Press, 1979.

Schwartz, A. *Survival handbook for children of aging parents.* Chicago: Follett, 1977.

Silverstein, B., & Hyman, H. *You and your aging parent.* New York: Pantheon, 1976.

UNIT II

INTERVENTIONS

PART THREE CLINICAL ISSUES

The chapters in Part Three are included in Standards V Intervention, its substandards A through F, and Standard VI Evaluation of the *Standards of Psychiatric and Mental Health Nursing Practice* (American Nurses' Association, 1982). These standards provide guidelines for the nurse engaged in clinical practice.

Clinical practice is the common core in advanced psychiatric mental health nursing. The authors whose works are included in Part Three have not simply recorded those interventions they have found helpful or unsatisfactory. Rather, they have identified the conceptual frameworks within which they practice and the treatment issues these frameworks bring into focus. The six chapters that make up Part Three represent a variety of viewpoints but all exemplify the necessity and advantage of clinical work based upon theory.

Individual and group therapy with adults using a psychoanalytic framework is discussed in Chapter 10. Using this model, the stages and key concepts in therapy, the major defensive patterns of clients, and appropriate interventions are presented. Using the method of placing the client with the same therapist in both individual and group therapy, the advantages and disadvantages to both client and therapist when this approach is followed are discussed. In addition, the few treatment evaluation studies that have been performed by nurses are described and nurses are urged to publish their evaluations of treatment outcome to assist in documenting nursing's contribution to the care of the mentally ill.

In Chapter 11, individual and group therapy with adolescents from an integrated humanistic and behavioristic approach is discussed. Treatment of adolescents as requiring behavioral and educational components are identified and the rationale and manner in which assessment and treatment for the adolescent are different than for other age groups and how approaches used with other populations need to be adapted for effective adolescent treatment are presented. Appropriate treatment interventions are explained and the advantages and disadvantages of individual and group approaches to both the adolescent and the clinician are discussed. Throughout the chapter, it is stressed how the strengths of youth can be tapped to help them achieve their developmental tasks, increase their social skills and enhance their self-image.

In Chapter 12 are presented the rationale and process for individual and group play therapy with preschool and elementary school age children. The stages of therapy are presented as well as the significant issues involved in treatment with these age groups.

In Chapter 13, the theoretical concerns and aspects of family treatment including nursing's historical role in working with families and the current state of family therapy are discussed. The Circumplex Model is used in an effort to integrate common family concepts and provide a more coherent diagnostic system. The chapter also presents those treatment issues that are unique to specific family therapy models and those that seem to be common to all approaches together with suggested interventions are also presented. The conclusion is maintained that family therapy is a widely used and rapidly growing treatment modality and that there are many aspects of family treatment that have yet to be systematically evaluated and researched.

In Chapter 14 the principles of milieu treatment are discussed and related to establishing a therapeutic milieu with children, adolescents, and adults. Sources of the confusion that still prevail regarding the precise nature of milieu therapy are identified and the processes and issues inherent in this modality, such as the interaction between staff and patient behavior and staff/patient role issues, are presented. Finally, a case is made for the need for the psychiatric nursing administrator and clinical specialist to have clinical knowledge and management skills. The position is held that clinical and administrative interventions interact together to produce effective or ineffective milieu treatment.

In Chapter 15, the complex issue of pharmacotherapy in treating clients with emotional problems and the mentally ill is discussed, and the necessary pharmacological and medical information the clinical specialist requires to monitor the client's medication regimen and use it as an effective adjunct to interpersonal therapeutic intervention is identified. The principles of nursing intervention with patients receiving psychotropic medications are described and the hypothesized pharmacological action, desired medication effects, side effects and adverse effects of antipsychotic, mood-stabilizing and anxiolytic medications are presented. The special considerations required in using these drugs with children and the elderly are also discussed, as well as the overuse of these medications by women in our society. The chapter is focused on the opportunities for the clinical specialist to use her or his knowledge of the client and the medication to carry out effectively a nursing assessment and to plan, implement, and evaluate effective interpersonal interventions with clients and families.

Theory-based clinical practice and evaluation of the effectiveness of that practice is a clear necessity for the viability of psychiatric mental health nursing. Ongoing work to achieve that goal, although time consuming and difficult, indicates that progress is being made toward achieving a theory base more relevant to nursing practice and more comprehensively evaluated.

CHAPTER 10

PSYCHOANALYTICALLY ORIENTED INDIVIDUAL AND GROUP THERAPY WITH ADULTS

Suzanne Lego

Nurses began to practice psychotherapy in the 1950s. This role was initially inspired by Dr. Hildegard Peplau (1952), who wrote that the counseling role was a proper and important one for nurses. Many psychiatric nursing leaders did not agree, and controversy over this issue lasted for almost 20 years (Lego, 1980c).

Today, however, it is common for nurses prepared at the master's level to practice individual and group psychotherapy. This treatment occurs in inpatient settings, day hospitals, outpatient clinics, outreach programs, and more and more commonly in private practice. In this chapter, the qualifications of the nurse therapist and the goals and process of psychoanalytically oriented individual and group therapy with adults will be discussed. The stages in therapy and the major defensive patterns of clients are presented together with appropriate interventions. Finally, the need for evaluation of treatment outcome by nurses is supported as a means of documenting nursing's contribution to the care of the mentally ill.

QUALIFICATIONS OF THE NURSE PSYCHOTHERAPIST

Professional Qualifications

The nurse who practices psychotherapy is required by the American Nurses' Association (ANA, 1982a) to be qualified as a psychiatric and mental health nurse specialist. This criterion is best met by successfully completing the ANA requirements for certification as a Clinical Specialist in Psychiatric and Mental Health Nursing (ANA, 1982b). However, it is generally agreed that graduate students and nurses who have completed master's work and are undergoing supervision for certification may practice psychotherapy, since both groups are receiving supervision.

The Value of Theory

As a part of graduate preparation in psychiatric nursing, students are exposed to theories that are then integrated into clinical practice. Theories found to be important for the nurse psychotherapist include individual development, psychopathology, and theories of treatment.

An equally important part of the graduate program in psychiatric mental health nursing is a research orientation. As a psychotherapist, the nurse and client continually use an investigative approach to form hypotheses about the client's behavior and then examine data that either confirm or deny the hypothesis. For example, the nurse may note that the client complains of migraine headaches in situations where the client might be expected to be angry. This observation is presented in an investigative way, "I notice that you get these headaches when you might be angry. Do you suppose there is a connection?" The psychotherapist applys the same basic problem-solving approach, though not as rigorously, as is used in formal research.

The Value of Supervision

In supervision, the nurse reviews with a more experienced therapist, or with peers, the process of therapy between the nurse and the client. This may be done through process recordings, audio tape recordings, audiovisual tapes, observation through a two-way mirror, or even direct observation (as when the group supervisor sits in the group therapy session as a silent observer or co-leads the group). The purpose and process of clinical supervision is discussed in greater detail in Chapter 23.

Personal Qualifications

The Value of Personal Psychotherapy

Many believe that the clinical specialist who conducts psychotherapy functions best when personal psychotherapy is a part of the preparation as psychotherapist. Psychotherapy requires a close, intimate relationship over time with the client, who will present a wide range of irrational behaviors. This situation often touches off in the nurse a range of equally irrational thoughts and feelings. Personal psychotherapy helps nurses understand their own irrationalities so that they can avoid acting out and increase their useful, growth-promoting responses to clients. For example, the borderline client is apt to engender very strong, sometimes primitive reactions in nurses (Smith & Lego, 1984). Nurses who are familiar with their own primitive fears and conflicts will not be thrown by these feelings and will react calmly and constructively.

Important Personality Traits of the Nurse Psychotherapist

The practice of psychotherapy requires that the nurse possess certain traits, including

1. Patience: The ability to forego immediate gratification and endure the protracted time necessary for real change to take place.
2. Poise: "The ability to tackle concrete tasks without fanaticism but with vigor, keeping calm if there is no success" (Jaspers, cited in Chessick, 1974, p. 79). Restraint and balance in life are essential.
3. Open-mindness: The ability to put oneself "into every other man's place, listening to reason, entering into the rationality of the case, and boundlessly expanding (oneself) in ideas. It is resistance to sophisms, to the pressures of willful self-interest, and to accidental sensitivities. It is candor, understanding, accessibility and possibility . . . a disinclination to humiliate anyone, a courtesy in personal contact" (Jaspers, cited in Chessick, 1974, p. 79).
4. Alertness: The ability to see beyond the client's words to their subtle and complex implications. The ability to think abstractly is important.
5. Introspection: The ability to sense one's own irrationality in the therapy setting.
6. Authenticity: The ability to communicate one's feelings unambiguously.
7. Individuation: The ability to view and experience the client, over time, as a separate individual whom the therapist does not need and who need not need the therapist.

THEORETICAL APPROACHES

Nurse psychotherapists today employ a wide range of theoretical approaches. In 1980, a survey was conducted of the 52 listed graduate programs in psychiatric mental health nursing funded by the National Institute of Mental Health (Lego, 1980b). The purpose of the study was to learn what theories were used most often in teaching the practice of individual psychotherapy to students. The findings, with an 83% return, indicated that the psychoanalytical theories predominated. These included, in descending order of importance, interpersonal theory, ego psychology, Freudian theory, existential theory, and object relations theory.

Nonpsychoanalytical theories included systems, gestalt, Rogerian (Carl Rogers), transactional analysis, learning, Carkoffian, Bowen's, change, rational emotive, and social theories, including communication theory.

Nursing theories included those of Peplau, Johnson, Rogers, and Travelbee.

If these are the theories taught to graduate students in psychiatric mental health nursing, it is safe to say that nurses in practice employ a wide variety of theories and that the psychoanalytical theories predominate. Probable reasons for this emphasis include the following.

1. The psychoanalytical approaches are based on developmental theories; that is, those early happenings that are believed to play a part in the interpersonal problems clients have as adults. In most graduate programs, developmental theories are considered very important in treating psychiatric clients.
2. The nonpsychoanalytical approaches, for example, behavior modification, cognitive therapy, and rational-emotive therapy, are concerned not with what happened in the client's childhood but rather focus on the client in the present and on modifying current behavior. Nursing traditionally has favored a developmental approach over this approach.
3. Some of the nonpsychoanalytical approaches draw heavily on psychoanalytical or developmental approaches; for example, transactional analysis, gestalt therapy, and primal scream therapy. If nurses want to practice these therapies, it is helpful to be thoroughly familiar with the psychoanalytical theories.
4. Since psychoanalytically oriented therapies are widely practiced by the other mental health professions, the nurse who is not familiar with them will be at a disadvantage in communicating with colleagues.

Advantages and Disadvantages of the Psychoanalytical Approach

The major advantage of the psychoanalytical approach is that it is designed to be permanent by attacking the underlying problem rather than the symptoms or manifestations of the problem. To illustrate, if a client is fearful of leaving the house, the psychoanalytical approach would be to help the client identify the source of the fear. In the process, many underlying conflicts and feelings would be discussed and ultimately resolved.

A nonpsychoanalytical approach might be to use behavior modification to help the client become desensitized to leaving the house. The underlying problem would not be addressed. This approach leaves clients vulnerable to further, perhaps different, symptoms should they undergo stress that touches off the underlying problems. Symptoms aroused might be psychological or even physical. The connection between psychological and physical reactions has recently become clear in scientific circles, as well as in the popular media. The nurse is alerted to the possibility that underlying psychological problems can lead to a breakdown in the immune system leading to serious, even life-threatening illness. For this reason, it is important to treat underlying problems, not just symptoms, whenever possible.

There are a number of disadvantages to the psychoanalytical approach.

1. The therapist requires more intensive training than do therapists using other approaches. Such training often involves therapy for the therapist.
2. Psychoanalytical treatment usually takes longer than nonpsychoanalytical therapies and is, therefore, more expensive in time and money. However, psychoanalytical theory can be used effectively in crisis intervention and short-term therapy.
3. In clinical settings where "statistics" are important for funding, that is, where so many clients must be treated and discharged per month or year, psychoanalytical therapy is not practical, since it is difficult to tell initially just how long therapy will be necessary. One way this uncertainty may be handled is for the clinician to see the client for the allowed number of sessions using this approach. If more work is required, the client can be referred to another setting, a clinic or private practice, where the therapy can continue.

The remainder of this chapter will focus on the psychoanalytically oriented approach to individual and group psychotherapy.

ASSESSMENT AND DIAGNOSIS

If the psychiatric mental health clinical specialist is employed by an agency, the assessment of the client will take place in one or two "intake" interviews. Most agencies have intake forms or structured guides to aid the nurse in collecting the following data (Webster, 1984):

1. What is the client's reason for seeking treatment? How does he or she describe the problem?
2. What is the history of the current problem? When did it begin? What changes have occurred in the client's life recently that might account for increased stress? Has there been a change in the client's somatic functioning or mental status?
3. What is the client's past personal history? The nurse will ask the client to describe briefly what is known about experiences during infancy, childhood, adolescence, and adulthood using focused questions (Webster, 1984).
4. What is the client's medical history, including illness, surgery, and hospitalization? Does the client take any drugs and have there been significant side effects? Does the client have allergies?
5. What is the client's family history? Who constitutes the client's nuclear family, extended family, and family of origin? What is the client's sibling position? Is there a history of divorce, mental illness, hospitalization, alcoholism, suicide, child abuse, or sexual abuse?
6. What is the client's past psychiatric history? Has the client received any psychiatric treatment in the past? What kind? For how long?

Assessment of Current Status

In evaluating the client's current status, the nurse takes into consideration the following characteristics of the client (Webster, 1984):

1. Physical characteristics
2. Speech
3. Psychomotor activity
4. Mood
5. Affect
6. Perception
7. Orientation
8. Thought processes
9. Content of thought
10. Capacity for abstract thinking
11. Information and intelligence
12. Concentration
13. Memory
14. Judgment
15. Insight
16. Ego strengths

Diagnosis

Clinical agencies usually require the nurse to arrive at a diagnosis to be used in planning treatment. For this reason, and to maintain mutually respectful collaborative relationships with other mental health disciplines and to receive third-party reimbursement, it is imperative that the clinical specialist be familiar with the Diagnostic and Statistical Manual of Mental Disorders (DSM-III) (American Psychiatric Association, 1980). Diagnoses according to this classification system will then be understood by other members of the treatment team.

In nursing at large, there is a move toward a "nursing diagnosis" that is drawn from nursing theory and leads to theoretical nursing intervention. However, many psychiatric nurses question "the need for yet another unique psychiatric diagnostic or assessment system that is not systematically related to DSM III" (Williams, 1982). The American Nurses' Association is presently engaged in a five-year project to draw up a taxonomy of nursing diagnoses, some of which will be applicable to psychiatric clients.

Assessment in Private Practice

When the client is being seen in private practice, the assessment is often less formal and stylized. This occurs for several reasons. First, quite likely the assessment and treatment will be carried out by the same nurse, the private practitioner. Therefore, there is ample time to gather data and no need to fill out forms to pass on to another therapist who will carry out the therapy.

When data are collected over time, the nurse has the opportunity to see what the client considers to be important by noting in what order and with what emphasis information is offered. In one instance, a male client was seen with his wife and spoke almost exclusively of his mother, even making a slip and giving his mother's address rather than the address at which he and his wife resided.

A disadvantage of a formal, stylized intake interview with private clients who will be seen over time is that the nurse becomes established as a "data collector" in the first few sessions. It is then difficult for the client to assume responsibility for beginning the session and continuing to talk without direction from the nurse. The nurse can begin the client's first session by simply asking, "Why don't you begin by telling me what made you decide to call for an appointment?" Then, as the client talks, the nurse asks questions to clarify the material which the client presents.

The nurse in private practice will need to formulate a diagnosis even if no official forms are completed. This diagnosis provides a framework for the treatment to follow. For example, if the nurse decides the client is borderline, the interventions will differ from those directed at the neurotic or psychotic client. Frequently, the nurse will be required to fill out insurance forms. DSM-III nomenclature is often used for these purposes.

TREATMENT GOALS

Whether or not goals for the client's treatment are discussed depends on the theoretical framework of the nurse. Let us say the client comes to the nurse with the specific goal of wanting to drive a car without anxiety. If the nurse is a behavioralist, this goal will be set, and the nurse and client will take concrete, specific steps toward that goal.

However, in psychoanalytically oriented psychotherapy, the matter is more complex. In the example of driving a car, the nurse will begin to question and hypothesize about the meaning of the symptom. The nurse and client may agree over time that the client's fear of driving has to do with her aggression or a fear of separation. These underlying problems will then be discussed over several sessions, with only passing interest in the symptom. Frequently, the symptom disappears once therapy has begun and the underlying issues are addressed.

The Client's Goals

In psychoanalytically oriented therapy, it is generally *not* helpful to set specific goals for the following reasons (Lego, 1980a):

1. Clients do not always enter therapy for the reasons they state (and believe to be true).
2. Clients are often unable to formulate why they have come.
3. Clients often have very specific conscious goals that are for a time unobtainable owing to unconscious factors.
4. Goal setting implies a mechanical, problem-solving approach that can impede the process of exploring human experience.
5. Goal setting is antithetical to the natural process of developing ongoing intimate relationships, of which the client-therapist relationship is one.
6. Goal setting implies a kind of "closure" about life that is limiting in itself.

When the client presents specific goals to the psychoanalytically oriented nurse therapist, the nurse listens carefully, thinks about the meaning of the symptoms, and helps the client to clarify this meaning over time. The nurse points out that the symptom will probably decrease or disappear as the role it plays in the client's life becomes clear. It is important that this be done slowly and sensitively so the client does not think the therapist is saying, "It's all in your head!" or "That's not important—what's the *real* problem?" In other words, the nurse listens carefully, formulates hypotheses, sensitively draws out more information, and shares the hypotheses as the client becomes trusting and comfortable.

The Therapist's Goals

There are basic, overall goals for all clients in individual and group treatment. These goals (Wolberg, 1977) are to

1. Remove, modify, or retard existing symptoms.
2. Mediate disturbed patterns of behavior.
3. Promote positive personality growth and development.

ROLE OF THE THERAPIST

The therapist's role is to help the client to experience consciously those aspects of life that are unconscious or dissociated but which appear in the form of symptoms or unsatisfactory life patterns. This is done through the establishment of an intimate professional relationship between the client and nurse over time.

INDIVIDUAL THERAPY

The therapeutic relationship passes through successive phases, each with its own distinct characteristics.

The Introductory Phase

In the introductory phase, which may last several months, the client and therapist examine one another closely to assess the "boundaries" of the relationship. The therapist is alert to the problems of the client and his or her characteristic ways of handling them. At the same time, the client's strengths and attributes are being measured.

The client, in turn, is closely watching the nurse's ability to hear and understand what is being said. Both are aware of the other's ways of relating and are making the slight adjustments necessary to make each understood to the other. Once this method of communicating openly is established, the working phase of the relationship begins.

The Working Phase

In the working phase, the client comes to the session prepared to talk about what is bothersome that day. This discussion may include something that is currently happening, a memory of a past event or relationship, a dream, a fantasy, or thoughts or feelings about the therapist.

Anything the client brings up is considered "grist for the therapeutic mill." That is, all thoughts, feelings, dreams, and fantasies offer an entrée into the client's unconscious or dissociated experience. By talking about them, the client becomes aware of wishes, feelings, conflicts, and desires that may have been previously buried. Over time, this material fits into a general pattern that becomes clear to the nurse long before it is clear to the client by virtue of the fact that the nurse is an objective, though participant, observer. As the pattern becomes clear, the nurse helps the client to see how the pattern manifests itself.

For example, a client comes to the session with two dreams. The first is that she and her boyfriend are married and have a baby son. They learn that a natural disaster is about to occur. She calmly dresses her son while her "husband" does some other chores in preparation for their evacuation. In the second dream, she and her woman friend are shopping in a flea market. They find a nice jacket but it is pulled apart at the seams. The client shows her friend how easily it can be repaired and then worn.

In each dream, the client is taking a less than desirable situation and handling it in a calm, orderly, matter-of-fact way. Each dream involves cooperation with an "equal" partner. This client has been in therapy for some time and has made impressive progress. She is about to finish a doctoral dissertation, and having been divorced for two years, is involved in a new, satisfying intimate relationship. Nevertheless, she often feels overwhelmed by her increasingly obvious "adult" stance as a professional woman. In these dreams, she reassures herself that she can handle the stress she is experiencing, that she can be both helpful and helped without dire consequences.

The Termination Phase

In the termination phase of treatment, the relationship is ending. This is, ideally, through mutual agreement that the client has received maximum benefit from therapy. During this phase, the client usually relives past separations and looks optimistically to the future.

Key Concepts in Individual Therapy

In individual therapy, there are several concepts that are central to the process. These are content and process, transference and countertransference, resistance, acting out, and insight. Each will be considered separately.

Content and Process

The *content* of a therapy session includes all that is *said* and the *process* includes all that is *done.* For example, the process involves the sequence of topics, body language, voice level, and other nuances of communication.

An example of content and process occurred when a client explained to the nurse that he was not really wanted by his parents as he was born much too early in their marriage. His mother told him in later life that this was so and that she would have left her husband had it not been for her son. Later in the session he complained that he can never really enjoy his relationship with his lover, for he always feels a "burden," as though he's merely being tolerated by the lover. In content, both ideas are similar. Meanwhile, in the same session, the client behaved almost obsequiously with the therapist. He was careful to be polite and attentive and even brought some glue to the office to reset a small piece of molding that was separating from the wall.

In this example, it is clear how the content and the process are similar, and how they demonstrate the client's mode of being in the world. The nurse must be alert to ways in which clients *perform* in therapy the very problems they are describing in their lives. When these performances are observed, they are brought to the attention of the client and further explored.

Transference

Transference is the attribution to the therapist and to others of feelings, wishes, and conflicts originally felt toward parents or significant others (Lego, 1982). It is impossible for individual treatment to occur without transference. By virtue of the relationship where one person is dependent on the other for help, memories or images of the parent-child relationship occur. For some clients, this parallel is experienced from the start. For others, it is not perceived for some time. In any event, the success of the treatment depends on the ability of both client and therapist to see the areas in which the client distorts reality in line with past experience.

To illustrate, the client tells the nurse about a particularly difficult time she had being assertive with her thesis advisor. In describing their encounter, she bursts into tears and pounds the arms of the chair saying, "She makes me feel so inadequate and stupid! Just like my father did!" This is an obvious example of transference. A few minutes later she says, "When I told you about my meekness with Dr. ________ , you looked exasperated, as though I should be further along by now!" This, too, is an example of transference, for the client again believes the therapist holds the same high expectations for her that her father held.

When transference occurs, the nurse points it out to the client and explores the early relationship and ways in which it affects current relationships.

Countertransference

Countertransference occurs when the therapist experiences irrational, exaggerated, or unrealistic feelings toward the client based on the therapist's own past life or current conflicts. Countertransference may be either positive or negative. In positive countertransference, the nurse may overvalue the client and thus be blinded to important information about the client. In negative countertransference, the nurse may feel intense dislike, anger, or even contempt for the client.

When this situation occurs, two courses of action are important. The first is for the nurse to examine why this is occurring. In most cases, it will become evident that the client is in some way interfering with the nurse's narcissism or departing from some mode of being that the nurse considers important (Herron & Rouslin, 1982). The client just isn't acting "right" according to the nurse's system. It is important that the nurse have a therapist, supervisor, or colleague with whom to discuss these reactions. It is when countertransference occurs that the nurse's own personal psychotherapy or supervision is useful.

Following self-examination, the nurse investigates the possibility that the behavior exhibited by the client, which aroused such feelings in the nurse, might be used unconsciously by the client for just such a purpose. This behavior may represent a maladaptive pattern the client uses to keep people at a distance or to manipulate them.

For example, the nurse finds the client to be arrogant and manipulative. Offended by this behavior, the nurse tends to get into power struggles with the client. After discussing this in therapy or supervision, the nurse tells the client what the nurse experiences: "I find that we get into power struggles with each of us needing to convince the other of something. Do you find this happening in other situations?" The client may then be comfortable enough to discuss this attitude. It is very likely that when countertransference of this type occurs, it is not unique to the nurse-client relationship, but rather is common in all the client's relationships. If the client says, "You're the only person I ever struggle with," or "This must be your problem," then there is no point in pursuing the matter, for it would only start another power struggle.

Resistance

Resistance occurs when powerful, unconscious forces prevent clients from giving up defenses and distortions, often when the client is on the brink of insight or change (Lego, 1984). Resistance may take the form of lateness, missed sessions, a blocked or blank feeling in the session, "chatter" about other people or things that do not directly affect the client, or even a lack of progress.

When resistance occurs, the nurse immediately brings it to the client's attention to examine what is on the brink of being explored and to prevent further resistance or termination. An example occurred when a client said she was thinking of stopping therapy as she felt happy with her life. In recent sessions, she had been angry with the nurse for suggesting she was rather "clingy" with her husband and children. The rest of the session was spent exploring this idea and her fear of exhibiting anger at the therapist for suggesting she was a less than perfect wife and mother. In other words, the client was resisting facing her own anger and the fear of expressing her anger toward the therapist, who represented her mother.

Acting Out

Acting out occurs when the client relives or reproduces, through actions rather than words, the feelings, wishes, or conflicts operating unconsciously (Lego, 1982). Since these are the very conflicts that brought the client into therapy, it is expected that during the course of therapy, and within the context of this safe relationship, they will emerge. For example, a client who has spent a life of quiet resignation under the domination of another will frequently begin to act out anger in a blatant, rebellious way once therapy has begun.

Through acting out, the client "performs" openly and freely feelings or experiences that have previously been kept under wraps. As the acting out occurs, the client often experiences anxiety. This situation is partly caused by the new feelings that are emerging and partly because people react to the client differently based on new behavior.

An example of acting out occurred when Jane, a client raised by a domineering, hypercritical mother, took a new job. Her new supervisor had not wanted a woman from her discipline to be appointed to her job and believed Jane's salary was too high. A power struggle began at once. Jane reacted by doing all the negative things that would justify her supervisor's initial irrational dislike for her. She came late to work, dressed unprofessionally, filed her nails when she was supposed to be working, and in general "bugged" her boss. When her boss reacted accordingly with anger and resentment, Jane became outraged and experienced all the feelings toward her mother that she had repressed and suppressed. Once again, she was the helpless child, wronged by an uncaring and unsympathetic mother.

When acting out occurs, the nurse helps the client to figure out what is at the root of the behavior. What past experiences are involved in this current behavior? Once this has been thoroughly understood, the acting out loses its "kick" and becomes unnecessary.

Insight

Insight occurs when the client connects unconscious feelings, wishes, and conflicts to conscious behavior (Lego, 1982). The ultimate goal of individual therapy is for the client to gain insight. This does not simply mean that clients understand *why* they behave in a certain way. This kind of understanding is called "intellectual" insight and is often of no use in changing clients' behavior.

What does change both behavior and underlying feelings is "emotional" insight, that is, a truly emotional, experiential understanding of one's self. An example occurred when a client felt constantly angry at his wife and wanted to act out by punishing her for what he considered to be selfish, ungrateful behavior. When he realized not just intellectually but emotionally that he really loved his wife and was angry at her because she was at the moment doing things that *he* would like to do but could not, his anger disappeared.

The nurse's role in helping clients to achieve emotional insight is to poke and prod them to examine their *true* feelings apart from any facade or other defense they have erected to hide from the truth. This is not always easy for therapists, for they often do not know what lies beneath the facade and are to some extent "shooting in the dark." Obviously, there are no "true truths" and insight occurs only when an idea "feels" right to the client and when behavior then changes.

GROUP THERAPY

Goal

Group psychotherapy has been described elsewhere as

> a method of therapeutic intervention based on exploration and analyses of both individual and intrapsychic structures and the group process. As individuals interact in a group over time, they are able to observe their own and others' secret wishes, conflicts, and motivations. An understanding of these unconscious processes and the way they are acted upon with others can help clients to adopt more satisfying modes of interaction.(Lego, 1984)

Assessment

The ideal use of group psychotherapy is in conjunction with individual therapy. Once clients have established a relationship with the therapist in individual therapy, they may then be placed in group therapy as well.

At times, economic factors or shortage of therapists relative to number of clients dictate that group therapy be used alone, that is, not in conjunction with individual therapy. This situation has a severe disadvantage. Once clients enter a group, they begin to lose certain boundaries and inhibitions as the group consciousness takes over. This situation allows the client to experience and even act out thoughts and feelings previously kept in check. Often these thoughts and feelings cannot be handled totally within the group, and they spill over into individual sessions. For example, the client may be reacting strongly to another client but because another important issue is being discussed, he does not have a chance to bring it up. While his feelings are "fresh," he can discuss their source.

There is a school of thought that believes that "group matters" should be discussed only in group and that discussing them outside the group drains away the anxiety, making group interaction less potent. While this is true, the advantage of discussing these matters as soon as possible and in depth outweighs the disadvantage of draining feelings away from the group.

When the nurse sees the client in both individual and group therapy, the issue of "confidentiality" in individual sessions arises. It is best to communicate early that matters discussed in individual therapy should also be discussed in the group. This method is accomplished not by setting the rigid rule, "What is discussed *here* must be discussed in group," but rather by communicating this as these matters come up: "Why not bring this up in the group?" If the client protests that it is too personal, the nurse suggests, "But that's what group is for, to get personal." If the client shows an inability to bring up the matter, the nurse then brings it up in the group, within an appropriate context. For example, the client complains in individual therapy that he feels intimidated by John, a brusque group member. At some time when it appears this is happening in the group, the nurse says, "Is this the kind of thing John does that intimidates you?" Both clients will benefit from this kind of intervention. Clients soon learn and communicate to one another that "nothing is sacred" in individual therapy and that no boundaries need be made. In fact, sharp boundaries between individual and group therapy lead to pathological "collusions" between client and nurse that may be like unhealthy collusions in the client's original family.

The client does not always see the same therapist for both group and individual treatment. Clinical specialists should accept clients for group therapy who are seeing another therapist for individual therapy only when the philosophies and goals of both therapists are compatible. For example, if the group therapist takes an investigative, uncovering approach in group therapy and the client's individual therapist takes a supportive but repressive approach, the client becomes confused and therapy is not likely to succeed.

When clients are in individual therapy with someone other than the group therapist and are in a group with clients who see the group therapist for both, the client may feel like an "outsider." The clinical specialist should be alert to this "adopted child syndrome" and to the special transference and acting out. The client may complain, "You don't really understand me because you only see me here in group," to which the nurse might reply, "O.K., let's talk about what just happened here. Tell us how you felt." The transference may take the form of the client saying, "You like everyone else here better than you like me because they're all your clients." The nurse would encourage further discussion of this in the group, including an exploration of other times when the client has felt "left out." If the transference, resistance, or acting out are excessive, the client needs to be seen once by the group therapist for an individual session to discuss what is happening.

When the nurse is in a situation where only group therapy is offered to clients, a compromise is possible. Clients can be seen once a month by the nurse therapist in individual sessions, if the therapist sets aside ninety minutes per week. If there are eight clients in the group, two can be seen each week for 45 minutes each.

Certain clients are very difficult to treat in group and should therefore be seen only in individual treatment or in group when individual therapy is also ongoing and when the therapist is very experienced. These include the borderline client (Lego, 1979), the paranoid, and the hypochondriac.

In general, psychotic patients can benefit from group therapy, but should be treated in homogeneous groups. The same is true of alcoholics and drug addicted clients. Sociopathic clients are not appropriate for group psychotherapy as they are often disruptive to the group and are unable to relate in a way that is helpful to themselves. A rule of thumb in assessing clients for group is that if the client seems to have established a somewhat meaningful relationship with the nurse and with others, group therapy should prove useful in helping the client move further and faster.

In general, clients for group therapy should be over 20 and be placed in a heterogeneous group in terms of age, gender, diagnosis (except in the case of psychotic or addicted clients), and life-style. The more heterogeneous the group, the more opportunity for the emergence of transference. Variation in life-style also helps clients to recognize their own unconscious, unresolved conflicts. For example, gay men and women in a predominantly heterosexual group will help all the clients to recognize unresolved homosexual feelings.

Expectations and Limits

There are a number of expectations that the leader has of the clients in group but only one is voiced. This expectation is that clients attend every session or contact the leader personally when the client must be absent. The client is not simply to leave a message, but must contact the leader. The explanation given the client is that group therapy is cumulative and must be "taken every time" to be useful. The leader will try to discourage the absence when the client calls. This, too, can be told to the client in advance.

The other expectations are not shared in advance because the leader does not wish to establish a "Sunday school" environment in which the leader is the "teacher" who lays down the rules. Giving a number of rules to group members in advance tends to stifle spontaneity and promote a stylized, conforming group where clients do and say what is expected. Expectations that are not voiced in the beginning are that clients will be as open as possible, will not use physical violence, or discuss group members outside the group. Clients are also expected not to meet outside the group. If they do, they are expected to discuss these meetings in the group (Lego, 1982). This expectation does not apply to clients who live together on an inpatient unit or in a group home. Each expectation will be discussed separately.

Openness

It is very important for clients to be open and honest in group but to tell someone to be open is a little like saying, "Be spontaneous!" Instead, clients learn over time that openness is a norm of the group and is subtly rewarded by the others.

Physical Violence

It is obvious that clients might be very frightened to hear the nurse say that violence in group is forbidden. It may not have occurred to the client that violence was a possibility. When the nurse is alert to feelings and encourages their expression, physical violence does not occur.

Confidentiality

In a small community where most people are known to one another, confidentiality is an issue. However, the disadvantages of setting up a "school teacher" image and a rigid atmosphere outweigh the disadvantages of possible breakdown in confidentiality. When this does occur, the discussion over why it happened is often very valuable. For example, one group member, Mary, revealed to an outsider who knew Rose that Rose was having an extramarital affair. When this became known in the group, Rose was very angry at Mary. Mary, in an exploration of her behavior, came to the realization that she deeply resented Rose's affair because she felt envious of Rose's excitement over it and because her own father had often betrayed her mother (and her) in extramarital affairs. It soon becomes apparent to group members that confidentiality is a group norm.

Meetings Outside the Group

There are some groups where meetings outside are inevitable, as on inpatient units, and some where meetings are encouraged, as with "networking" groups of chronic patients. However, in outpatient groups, these meetings represent acting out and are often destructive to the group.

Acting out can occur as a result of members' secret wishes to be close to the leader. Another group member is the next best thing as they share the common bond of attachment to the leader. Acting out also occurs when members pair together to act out other earlier unresolved issues or to be certain, unconsciously, that they will always have a "friend" in the group should the going get rough.

When this pairing or subgrouping occurs, the leader must pursue an exploration of why it is occurring. As soon as it becomes evident that members are meeting outside the group, the nurse brings this up in the group. Rather than saying, "It's not a good idea to meet outside the group," the clinical specialist takes an investigative approach: "I notice that you, Mary, and you, Carol, leave the group together talking about dinner plans. Can we talk about what that means?" As the exploration continues, the nurse introduces the notion that subgrouping can occur for the reasons mentioned earlier. When the reasons have been thoroughly understood, the subgrouping stops. Again, it soon becomes apparent to new members that they are expected to interact in group only.

When the leader allows meetings outside the group for drinks, dinner, coffee, and so forth, one or all of the group members often leave the group. Clients are frequently in therapy because of problems of intimacy and problems relating to others. These problems quickly come up between clients during outside meetings and if they are not discussed and resolved in the group, they can lead to "bad feelings" and then termination.

Open Versus Closed Groups

In psychoanalytically oriented psychotherapy groups, open groups are far more useful than closed groups that begin, run for a specific number of sessions, and then end. Reasons for this belief include the fact that members are less likely to commit themselves wholeheartedly when they know the group is going to disband. In addition, members entering and leaving the group from time to time create a tension that is desirable and arouse earlier feelings of separation, abandonment, and sibling rivalry.

The Role of the Leader

The leader creates the group based on research and theory about psychotherapy groups. When preparing clients for group, the nurse needs to take the actions listed in Table 10.1 (Lego, 1984).

The role of the leader is to act as a stimulator to the natural group interaction, never

Table 10.1 Preparing Clients for Group Therapy

Nursing Action	*Theoretical Rationale*
1. All perspective members are seen at least once individually before admission to the group. (The more times they are seen, the better.)	A libidinal tie will develop between the client and nurse. This tie helps clients to remain in the group later when they become anxious.
2. Before entering the group, the client is not prepared for what happens in the group or who will be there. Only a general statement is made such as, "The group is a place to discuss feelings, problems, or reactions."	If the client knows a great deal about the group in advance, spontaneous reactions are lost to exploration. These spontaneous reactions are "grist for the therapeutic mill."
3. Group members are not told about new members before they appear.	Their spontaneous or irrational response to the new members is useful to explore. (For example, this may be reminiscent of the birth of a sibling.)

directing the group, but rather reacting to what is occurring naturally. The leader never does for the group what it can do for itself and speaks only when it is clear that others cannot yet do so. The leader prods and probes without ever taking over.

Stages of Group Development

Uncertainty Stage

The uncertainty stage lasts up to 20 sessions and is characterized by many demands on the leader. When interpetations or observations are voiced, group members take this to mean they should not continue to do what they are doing. Because of this belief, the leader must sometimes say that members need not stop their behavior, only explore its meaning. For example, the leader may point out competition only to have the involved parties say, "Oh, I'm sorry, I didn't mean to be so competitive!" The leader might then ask, "Who does she (the competitor) represent?" Table 10.2 describes behavior, examples, and interventions in the uncertainty stage (Lego, 1982).

Overaggressive Stage

In the overaggressive stage, the politeness and uncertainty has faded and regression, adaptation, and intimacy are in the future. As a defense against these three potential happenings, the group experiences a period of hostility, mainly expressed toward one another but sometimes felt (and not expressed) toward the leader. Group members are often afraid to get angry at the leader because of transference, that is, because the leader is seen as a parent. Table 10.3 shows behavior, examples, and leader intervention in the overaggressive stage (Lego, 1982).

Regression Stage

At this point in group development, earlier defenses are put aside and members experience pure anxiety, anger at more primitive sources, dependency, fear, longing, envy, jealousy, and other forms of pain. Members no longer feel the need to be in control (though there may still be unconscious resistance). Regression is no longer used as manipulation, but rather occurs spontaneously. Members are often surprised at the emotional reactions they experience when others regress. Members who regress are often surprised at the support they receive for they have previously believed that to lose control would be disastrous. In this phase, the leader comes to be seen as a resource person and as a human being (Lego, 1984).

Table 10.2 Behavior, Examples, and Leader Intervention in the Uncertainty Phase

Behavior	*Example*	*Leader Intervention*
Initial anxiety	Pacing the floor. Leaving and returning. Hallucinations and delusions. Excessive intellectualization. Organization of a "group plan."	Comment about the anxiety. Question what members fear happening in the group.
Demands on leader to explain purpose or provide structure	"Do we begin now?" "What is supposed to happen here?" "How does this work?"	Communicate to members that it is their group. ("Let's see how things go.")
Competition	Comparison among members, for example, of past group experience, past number of years of psychotherapy, knowledge of the leader.	Point out that competition is taking place, being careful to communicate that it is not wrong and should not necessarily stop just because it is noted.
Excessive politeness	Members feel anxious and angry about the lack of structure from the leader, but they are afraid to show this. Instead, they react with inappropriate kindness. To a monopolizer: "You certainly are talkative today."	Note the covert feeling and ask if it is present. ("Are you a little irritated by all that talking?") Encourage openness rather than politeness.
Silence	All members sit for five minutes staring at the floor or occasionally glancing at each other.	Comment on the silence. ("I guess everyone is afraid to start.") Comment on some nonverbal behavior. ("Mary, I notice you're staring at John. Do you wish he'd speak?")
Questions about the leader's personal life, qualifications, and competence	Member asks: "Are you a mother?"	"No. Are you afraid I won't know how to care for you because I'm not?"
	Member asks: "Are you an MD?"	"No. I'm a psychiatric nurse. Are you afraid I won't know enough to do things right?"
Avoidance of involvement in the group	Schizophrenic member talks to voices instead of other group members. Members intellectualize about their problems. Members adopt roles that were used in their families to reduce anxiety but which are not appropriate in the current group (for example, the buffoon, the boss, the incompetent person, the ingenue).	Comment that these are methods to avoid reacting emotionally to the current group. Explore why this is feared and avoided.
Strong, irrational reactions to the leader	The leader is seen as a "savior" with all the answers.	Explore why a "savior" is necessary.
	The leader is seen as using power to manipulate or humiliate members and as having a secret reason for every comment or move.	Explore the meaning of these ideas in the context of the members' lives.

SOURCE: Adapted from Lego, S. Group Psychotherapy, in J. Haber, A. M. Leach, S. M. Schudy, & B. F. Sideleau (Eds.), *Comprehensive psychiatric nursing* (2nd ed.) New York: McGraw-Hill, 1982.

Table 10.3 Behavior, Examples, and Leader Intervention in the Overaggressiveness Phase

Behavior	*Example*	*Leader Intervention*
Criticism of one another	One member who is very lonely but leads the life of the happy, sophisticated swinger is critical of another member whose isolation and loneliness are all too stark and evident.	Ask whether the "swinger" is reminded of herself by the isolated member. Explore their similarities and the resultant anxiety.
	One member becomes enraged when another acts stubborn and impenetrable.	Ask whether there was someone else in the member's life whom he could not "get through" to.
Anger at one another for using their own defenses in a clumsy way	One obsessional member begins sentences with "Please don't think I'm trying to be controlling but . . ." Another obsessional says "Don't warn us so obviously. It only calls our attention to the fact that you are!"	Point out the dynamic that people feel their own defenses should be used only in their own unique way and are spoiled or "exposed" if used "incorrectly."
Ganging up	One member who is secretly anxious about almost everything arrives late to group each week, giving various weak excuses. He refuses to acknowledge that he might have wanted to miss part of a session or that he may have wanted to stir everyone up.	Examine and explore both side of the process, why the member is so provocative, as well as why members cannot resist being provoked.
Hostility toward the leader	Clients distort the leader's behavior. ("You do nothing to help us.")	Accept their hostility in a nondefensive way. Avoid a win–lose approach. Weaknesses and eccentricities may be acknowledged freely. It is often a great relief to members to see that the leader is human and does not mind if this shows.
	Clients point out real eccentricities of the leader. ("You are too compulsive!")	

SOURCE: Adapted from Lego, S. Group psychotherapy. In J. Harber, A. M. Leach, S. M. Schudy, & B. F. Sideleau (Eds.), *Comprehensive psychiatric nursing,* (2nd ed.). New York: McGraw-Hill, 1982.

Adaptation Stage

Members in this phase accept one another in spite of their weaknesses and faults. As a result, defenses are lowered and in this atmosphere of acceptance members are able to explore their conflicts more openly. This mutual acceptance can be a disadvantage, as members may become "immune" to one another's neuroses. The leader must continue to "stir up the dust" and poke at members' defenses. Open-ended groups are advantageous at this stage as new members are occasionally admitted and bring a fresh perspective to old patterns (Lego, 1984).

Content and Process in Group Therapy

Just as in individual therapy, it is important for the clinical specialist to watch the subtle interplay between content and process in the group. Because of all the stimulation and the anxiety of having others in the room, the client will be more inclined in group than in individual therapy to act out individual dysfunctional behavior that is being described in content. For example, a male client, Ed, was complaining about how his wife bosses him around and undermines his self-confidence. Mary, a female, interrupted to ask a question. He replied, "Oh, I'm sorry, I guess I left that out. I'm no good at this business and I'm glad you stepped in and straightened me out." It was clear from this interaction that it is *Ed* who undermines *himself* and that probably he distorts the role his wife has in the process. The clinical specialist is alert to this interweaving between content and process and points it out only when no one else in the group does so.

Key Concepts in Group Therapy

As in individual therapy, the key concepts in group psychotherapy are transference, countertransference, resistance, and insight. Table 10.4 gives an example of each concept and an appropriate nursing intervention (Lego, 1984).

CASE EXAMPLE

To illustrate the key concepts of individual and group psychotherapy and nursing interventions, the following case example is presented.

History

Jan is a 60-year-old Jewish psychotherapist, married, and has two married children. Jan is a chronic helper, very much liked and admired by her friends and family, for she is always ready to help anyone in need; this helpfulness is unconsciously designed to meet her own dependency needs. Her children were slow to leave home and marry. Even now they come home frequently with the excuse that they must see their old dentists and doctors, having refused to find new doctors in the towns in which they live. Jan came into therapy because of dissatisfaction with her marriage and a wish to lead her life more in response to her own desires and less according to what is needed from her by those around her. Jan's husband is a passive-aggressive man who was recently indicted for failure to file his income tax for eight years. He was saved from a jail sentence by an articulate, impassioned letter Jan wrote to the judge.

Jan was raised in Brooklyn, New York. Her mother ruled the family with an iron hand, controlling and smothering Jan all her life. Her father was passive and hard of hearing.

Table 10.4 Concept, Example, and Intervention in Group Psychotherapy

Example of Concept	*Example of Intervention*
Transference The client says that the therapist prefers all the other members over her. In reality, this has never entered the therapist's mind, and on reflection she does not believe this to be true.	The leader asks the client what this is all about. As other members explore this with the client, it is learned that she had a "Cinderella" role in her large family. When the client's distortion is questioned by a group of people who do not believe the distortion, the client is able to view the situation more realistically.
Countertransference The therapist experiences the client as hostile, or very special, or inadequate and feels strongly about these attributes.	The leader explores silently or with a therapist, supervisor, or colleague what this is about. It is likely that the client does show some of these attributes and that these serve some neurotic purpose for the client. This should be explored openly in the group, for example, "Mary, you seem to be trying to control what happens here today." The strong emotional reaction of the leader to the client must be worked through by the leader, apart from the client.
Resistance The client begins to miss sessions or come late just after the birth of her first child. She tells the group that she is so happy at home with her husband and new baby that she hates to come to group and get all "stirred up" again.	The leader encourages a discussion of the resistance in the group. Most members enter into discussion because this is a familiar feeling. It is revealed that the client identifies with the new infant's own narcissism and omnipotence and is especially sensitive to the disruptions of this fantasy world that occur in group. This discussion continues for a few sessions and the resistance passes.
Acting Out A client secretly desires a close, special relationship with the therapist. Instead, she enters into an affair with a group member.	The leader brings this matter up in the group or encourages the members who are involved to do so. The meaning of the behavior is explored and analyzed by the group. As this is discussed, members become aware consciously of the real feelings, wishes, or conflicts that were previously only acted on without understanding of their meaning. The acting out loses its "kick" as understanding occurs, and the acting out stops.
Insight A client has been very angry at her husband whom she loves and admires. She is puzzled by the anger for she experiences him as loving and kind. She finds herself picking on him for no reason.	The client describes the situation in group, saying "I thought that marriage to a wonderful person would make my life complete. But it hasn't. He hasn't! He has let me down by not giving me total fulfillment!" As she tells this, she is very moved, as are all the group members. This insight into her irrational anger is further enhanced by continuing discussion of her experience.

SOURCE: Adapted from Lego, S. Group psychotherapy. In S. Lego (Ed.), *The American Handbook of Psychiatric Nursing.* Philadelphia: J. B. Lippincott, 1984.

He spent much of his life with his hearing aid turned off. When she married, it was to a man who could "stand up" to her mother. For Jan's husband, Steve, can be very aggressive and bombastic verbally, though this is clearly a defense against his feelings of inferiority and passivity. Jan often feels angry with him because of his passivity and lack of interest in anything but her and the children. She complains that his evenings are all spent asleep on the couch. On the other hand, he has a tendency to meddle in her affairs when his advice is not wanted or needed, much in the way her mother did. Jan was initially powerless to let him know how she felt about any of these behaviors, but since therapy she has been more direct with him and separate in her attempts to enjoy other areas of her life.

Transference

Jan's posture with the therapist initially was much as it was with her mother. She was the "good girl" often responding to suggestions or interpretations with the comment, "You know, you're right!" or "Yes, that's exactly it!" She almost never disagreed and never got angry even when pushed to examine aspects of her life and her behavior that were uncomfortable to face. Her behavior in group was cheerful and helpful to others.

However, after some time in therapy, she confessed to the group that she feared the therapist did not like the fact that she does short-term supportive therapy rather than the long-term therapy that the therapist practices. (The therapist had pointed out that she uses "support" with her clients to avoid their anger.) The group members asked why she thought this and Jan could only reply it was her "feeling." One member asked, "Are you sure this isn't the way your *mother* would feel, that you should do what *she* thought best rather than what *you* wanted?" Jan explored this idea and decided it was a possibility.

The group was helpful in pointing out times in group sessions when Jan deferred to them rather than being direct in expressing what she wanted. For example, a borderline client brought in some material she wanted Jan to read, including some glowing letters of reference about this client. Jan said, "Oh, thanks, I'll be sure to read these after group." When the therapist asked, "Are you *really* interested in reading these things?" Jan replied sheepishly, "Not really. But I think I *should* be interested and supportive."

As the therapy has progressed, Jan has become more direct and assertive. However, at times even this behavior appears to be in conformity to what she thinks the therapist and group expect. When this happens, it is pointed out, "Are you agreeing now just because you think we expect it?"

Countertransference

Because Jan is 15 years older than the therapist and is a therapist herself, there is the potential for the nurse to act with deference or to feel intimidated by Jan. In addition, her initial helpful, cheerful behavior could lead the therapist to respond in kind.

In group, the potential exists for the nurse to allow Jan to become a "cotherapist." Another potential countertransference reaction is toward Jan's tendency to move in and offer support to a client just when the client is becoming uncomfortable, working, and on the verge of insight. The therapist has to guard against becoming annoyed with Jan at times like this, realizing that this behavior of Jan's is useful to explore when the other client has finished.

Resistance

Just after a session in which the therapist pointed out that Jan tends to use "support" or "gimmicks" to prevent her clients getting angry at her or close to her, she came to a session saying that she was thinking of changing therapists. She said, "I know you believe in long-term therapy but I've been thinking of going to my supervisor for therapy. He tends to work 'faster.' But first I'm going to take a rest from all therapy." This decision was discussed in a number of successive sessions to determine what the client was attempting to avoid. In this case, it seemed that Jan feared becoming angry with the therapist, and perhaps closer. In addition, it seemed clear that Jan feared being herself in front of the therapist, that is, doing as *she* pleased within the context of the relationship. At the same time, she feared exploring the therapist's observation that she acts supportive with her clients to keep in their good graces. With both the clients and the therapist, Jan was attempting to hold on to her stylized way of reacting rather than a more human responsiveness that might lead to more feelings and to closeness.

In group, Jan brought up her desire to quit therapy. The group members made some of the same observations as the therapist had in individual sessions, but went further. One client said, "Maybe you're on the brink of seeing that you can be separate and your own person, while you are still in a close relationship with us, and that scares you. You want to run away before that becomes too clear." It was also pointed out that the group as a whole had been closer and that a few weeks earlier had agreed that they looked forward to sessions.

Acting Out

After one session of talking about wanting to quit therapy, Jan got in her car and prepared to drive down the driveway. It was icy and she impaled her car on the stone carriage steps next to the driveway. A tow truck had to be called to get her car out of the therapist's driveway.

In the next session, and in group, much joking ensued about Jan's ambivalence about leaving the therapist. It seemed that instead of saying, "I'm not sure I want to go," she dramatically, though unconsciously, acted this out. Both the therapist and group helped Jan explore her ambivalence.

Insight

During a period when Jan was talking in therapy about her resistance to therapy, she had this memory just before coming to an individual session: "I was in the shower this morning and I remembered a period when I was about 13. We had just moved back to New York and I didn't know any kids in the neighborhood. My mother and I had finished unpacking and setting up the new apartment and it was 'time' for me to go out and play. My mother urged me to go but I was afraid. I wanted to just stay home with her. Finally, my brother took me out and introduced me to his friend's sister and everything turned out fine. I made other friends and soon felt at home in the new neighborhood. But that feeling of not wanting to leave the house then was exactly the feeling I had this morning—not wanting to come here." She went on to say that she fears that therapy forces her out into the world "on her own." It is also possible that the new male therapist she sought was a fantasized replica of her brother who would help her out and make it all better.

In group that week she reached another insight. The borderline client mentioned earlier was saying how she *hated* group. The others were amused at how she needed to say this to cover her strong need for group. Jan said, "You know, Betty, you and I are alike. We both need so much, and act the opposite, you by acting angry all the time and me by acting helpful." Throughout the discussion, the therapist and group members listened carefully and validated those parts of the clients' experience that they had observed.

TERMINATION OF INDIVIDUAL AND GROUP THERAPY

Termination occurs ideally when both the clinical specialist and the client believe that the client has achieved maximum benefit. Freud once said that this happened when the client was able to "love and to work." Actually, these are good criteria for termination. Usually at this time, the client's symptoms are gone, self-esteem has improved, relationships are satisfying, as is time alone, and work is rewarding. The client is able to recognize areas that cannot be changed and accepts this fact.

However, termination is often not this ideal. Sometimes termination occurs because the nurse moves or changes jobs. This occurrence means that the client must face the reenactment of earlier painful separations. This can be a useful experience if the nurse is able to help the client to discuss openly all feelings toward the nurse, both negative and positive. Often these feelings are disguised or symbolically presented and the nurse must be especially sensitive to signs that the client is angry or sad about the termination. For example, a client who was being seen by a master's student who was about to graduate talked in her session about a city mayor who was about to run for the U.S. Senate: "He just used the city to promote his own career!" The student was able to interpret this as the client's anger at her "using" the client and then leaving.

Another kind of termination occurs when the client decides to terminate prematurely. When this situation happens, the clinical specialist works hard to help the client see the cause of the resistance. Almost always, the client is on the brink of change and is unconsciously frightened by the prospect. When clients cannot be dissuaded from terminating, the nurse simply encourages them to get in contact with the nurse if they decide to return to treatment.

For the client in a group, the group can be very helpful in all three kinds of termination. In the first type, the group helps the client to recognize progress made and areas that cannot be changed. In the second and third kinds of termination, members help the client to recognize feelings that may be hidden and unresolved.

EVALUATION

The client's progress in both individual and group psychotherapy is continually evaluated throughout the treatment. It is important for the clinical specialist to realize that symptom relief does not always mean progress in the true sense of the word.

Often the client feels relief from symptoms, anxiety, or depression almost immediately after beginning therapy. This is a kind of "honeymoon" effect that is a result of the client's having made a commitment to change. It also occurs because the client feels "understood" at last. The communication taking place in therapy is refreshingly "real," leading again to a feeling of relief and pleasure.

However, when clients begin to look at the part *they* play in their problems, the feeling of relief begins to change to one of anxiety. As it becomes evident that clients perpetuate problems through the use of defenses, they slowly begin to loosen the defenses and then to give them up. At the same time, they become vulnerable to many raw feelings that the defenses protected, such as anger, rage, anxiety, jealousy, envy, fear, and loneliness. At this point, clients often report feeling worse than ever, and in some cases even leave therapy. This demonstrates the paradox in evaluating psychotherapy: often when clients feel worse, it is a sign they are getting better.

This paradox may be one reason for the dearth of outcome studies of psychotherapy conducted by psychiatric nurses. A review of the psychiatric mental health nursing literature since 1975 reveals only three such studies. Carson and Huss (1979) studied 20 clients who were in one-to-one relationships with student nurses. One-half had prayer and interpersonal relationship therapy and one-half had interpersonal relationship therapy only. The group with prayer groups showed more improvement. It seems likely that the added interpersonal contact of the prayer group and possibly the enthusiasm of the "prayer nurses" had a beneficial effect on the clients.

Carter, Reed, and Reh (1975) studied the effect of home visits by two social workers and a nurse on child abusing and neglecting mothers. The mothers were divided into those receiving long-term, short-term, and no intervention. The mothers receiving long-term intervention showed significantly more change in their abusive behavior. Gelperin (1976) designed a study in which 21 clients were given increased hours with a nurse in a daily individual session. A control group received the usual care. The experimental group showed marked improvement.

As psychiatric mental health nurses continue to treat clients in individual and group psychotherapy, it becomes clearer that they have an important part to play in the improvement of mental health services. Outcome studies are one way in which they can demonstrate their contribution.

SUMMARY

Clinical specialists in psychiatric mental health nursing practice individual and group psychotherapy in a variety of settings. In both individual and group psychotherapy, the goal is to help clients to learn about the defensive patterns they use in response to unconscious anxiety, anger, fear, conflict, loneliness, envy, and jealousy. This learning takes place in the context of a professional yet intimate relationship with the clinical specialist and involves the gradual conscious experiencing of previously unconscious feelings. This experience is manifested in transference, countertransference, resistance, acting out, and insight.

Evaluation of the client's progress in therapy is ongoing. Yet there are few outcome studies of therapy offered by psychiatric mental health nurses. More such studies are necessary to help clinical specialists document their contribution to treatment of the mentally ill.

REFERENCES

American Nurses' Association, Division on Psychiatric and Mental Health Nursing Practice. *Standards of Psychiatric and Mental Health Nursing Practice.* Kansas City, MO: American Nurses' Association, 1982a.

American Nurses' Association, Certification Boards. *Take the Extra Step . . . Become a Certified Nurse*. Kansas City, MO: American Nurses' Association, 1982b.

American Psychiatric Association. *Diagnostic and statistical manual of mental disorders* (3rd ed.). Washington, DC: American Psychiatric Association, 1980.

Carson, V., & Huss, K. Prayer—An effective therapeutic and teaching tool. *Journal of Psychiatric Nursing,* 1979, *17,* 34.

Carter, B. D., Reed, R., & Reh, C. G. Mental health nursing intervention with child abusing and neglecting mothers. *Journal of Psychiatric Nursing and Mental Health Services,* 1975, *13,* 11.

Chessick, R. B. *Technique and practice of intensive psychotherapy.* New York: Jason Aronson, 1974.

Gelperin, E. A. Psychotherapeutic intervention by nurse clinical specialists. *Journal of Psychiatric Nursing,* 1976, *14,* 16.

Herron, W. G., & Rouslin, S. *Issues in psychotherapy.* Bowie, MD: Robert J. Brady Co., 1982.

Lego, S. Treatment of the acting out, borderline patient in private practice. *Clinical and scientific sessions—Nashville, 1979.* Kansas City, MO: American Nurses' Association, 1979.

Lego, S. Explicit goal setting: Is it appropriate in psychotherapy? *Proceedings of the Second Southeastern Regional Conference of Psychiatric/Mental Health Clinical Specialists.* Charleston, SC: 1980a.

Lego, S. *The nurse psychotherapist and the advanced nurse practitioner.* Presented at Perspectives in Psychiatric Care '80. Available on tape cassette, Teach 'Em, 160 E. Illinois St., Chicago, IL, 60611, 1980b.

Lego, S. The one-to-one nurse-patient relationship. *Perspectives in Psychiatric Care,* 1980c, *13,* 67.

Lego, S. Group psychotherapy. In J. Haber, A. M. Leach, S. M. Schudy, & B. F. Sideleau (Eds.), *Comprehensive psychiatric nursing* (2nd ed.). New York: McGraw-Hill, 1982.

Lego, S. Group psychotherapy. In S. Lego (Ed.), *American handbook of psychiatric nursing.* Philadelphia: J. B. Lippincott, 1984.

Peplau, H. E. *Interpersonal relations in nursing.* New York: Putnam's Sons, 1952.

Smith, M. C., & Lego, S. The client who is angry, manipulative, and self-destructive. In S. Lego (Ed.), *American handbook of psychiatric nursing.* Philadelphia: J. B. Lippincott, 1984.

Webster, M. Psychiatric nursing assessment. In S. Lego (Ed.), *American handbook of psychiatric nursing.* Philadelphia: J. B. Lippincott, 1984.

Williams, J. B. W., & Wilson, H. S. A psychiatric nursing perspective on DSM III. *Journal of Psychosocial Nursing,* 1982, *20,* 14.

Wolberg, L. R. *The technique of psychotherapy* (3rd ed.). New York: Grune & Stratton, 1977.

BIBLIOGRAPHY

O'Toole, A., & Morfka, V. Designing a clinical experience in psychiatric nursing for graduate students. In S. Lego (Ed.), *American handbook of psychiatric nursing.* Philadelphia: J. B. Lippincott, 1984.

CHAPTER 11

INDIVIDUAL AND GROUP THERAPY WITH ADOLESCENTS

Leona L. Eggert

This chapter is concerned with individual and small group therapeutic approaches for treating a range of behavioral and emotional problems experienced by adolescents. Two overall goals guide these approaches: to facilitate the adolescent in accomplishing the developmental tasks of the second decade of life and to provide assistance with behaviors indicating current difficulties with these tasks. Ultimately, the attainment of these goals means helping the adolescent to achieve individual, interpersonal, and social adequacy: necessary tools for a successful adult life (Greenberger & Sorensen, 1974).

SPECIAL ASPECTS OF WORKING WITH ADOLESCENTS

Nurses working with adolescents must first understand the normative aspects of their development (see Chapter 7). It is important to know the conflicts that confront the majority of adolescents. One must also view typical problems with a perspective that permits proper evaluation of the normative. This perspective comes from a clear understanding of what adolescence is like for the vast majority of youth. There is also a need to understand each adolescent as unique since many generalizations about the typical adolescent are based on limited data. Clinical views of normalcy often do not fit most youth. Research reveals that adolescence is not necessarily a turbulant time for the majority of youth (Dalis, 1981; Offer & Offer, 1975).

A sophisticated understanding of adolescents' age-typical behaviors and problems, based on current research, is also a prerequisite for working with the dynamics of adolescent development. This understanding is complicated by the wide range of behaviors and skills shown in early, middle, and late adolescence. Besides knowing which tasks are most relevant at each stage, it is also crucial to know the typical adolescent's coping "tools" at each stage.

Working with adolescents requires therapeutic communication with families since what occurs in therapy also affects the family and vice versa. Achieving independence includes a modification of relationship ties with the family. Regardless what form the pursuit for independence takes, frequently the family needs help in understanding and promoting adolescent development. The clinician working with adolescents needs to gain respect and confidence from both youth and parents. Being able to work effectively with the family is often as important to the adolescent's treatment as is the therapy with the adolescent. Clinicians must not inadvertently "replace" the family. Rather, they serve as a vital source of support, providing the structure within which adolescent self-identity can occur. When major conflicts or emotional and behavioral problems exist, most families desire involvement and assistance. Adolescents often need help in learning more effective ways of communicating with their parents.

Working with adolescents also means being able to work with school personnel. School is the adolescent's social world. Teenagers dominate this scene, spend the majority of their day and year in school with peers and teachers, and use this turf to build their own culture. A clinician helping an adolescent in therapy must, therefore, consider the impact of the school vis-à-vis the adolescent. Data gathered from school personnel are essential in making an accurate assessment. Moreover, communicating treatment goals and intervention strategies to school personnel is also critical for gaining necessary support and reinforcement of any behavioral changes the adolescent is attempting to achieve.

SPECIAL ATTITUDES AND QUALITIES OF THE CLINICIAN

Probably no group arouses such a range of feelings and behavioral responses in adults as do adolescents. Empirical findings suggest that there are attitudes and qualities necessary to be an effective helper with adolescents (Combs, 1968; Combs & Soper, 1963). Helpers perceived by adolescents as inspiring and effective believe youth are basically able, dependable, friendly, worthy, helpful, and internally motivated. Ineffective helpers seem to believe just the opposite. A strong positive correlation exists between acceptance of self and acceptance of others. Effective helpers identify with people and perceive themselves as trustworthy, adequate, wanted, and worthy. Effective helpers share no common set of methods and techniques of helping. Rather, methods used make the helper visible as a person. As one adolescent stated:

> I would like a therapist that really understood and cared for kids going through adolescence—who would try to make it easier by being patient, talking to them, not making them make hard decisions right away, but helping them go at their own pace until they understand who they are, what they like to do, and know what is expected of them. Adolescents really need someone to look up to, someone to talk to that knows what they are going through. (Notes From Teens, 1980)

A CONCEPTUAL FRAMEWORK FOR PRACTICE

Individual and group treatment with adolescents—grounded in a therapeutic relationship—is essentially behavioral and educational. It is designed to help young people learn, *for the first time in many cases,* methods and responses for coping with personal, interpersonal, or community-related problems. Common to most adolescents is the lack of a repertoire for responding successfully to the many new tasks facing them, tasks ranging from changing relations with family to mastery over their body and to communicating in intimate relations with the opposite sex. Adolescence is an ideal developmental period for learning healthy patterns of functioning in personal relationships, preventing the need for later amelioration or insight therapy. Individual and group work with adolescents can facilitate the developmental tasks of this age group by capitalizing on the importance of the development of the self, of peer group identification, and of the modification of ties with the family.

The overall conceptual framework for psychiatric mental health nursing practice with adolescents can be defined as a disciplined therapeutic and intellectual use of self while employing the nursing process. As clinicians, nurses ultimately use themselves as instruments in the therapeutic relationship that develops between nurse and adolescent. This requires special adaptations of nursing assessment, planning, and intervention and various tools, strategies, or problem-oriented theories in some treatment modality such as individual, group, family, or milieu therapy.

The overall purpose in this chapter is to provide a broad framework for individual and group work with adolescents. The chapter proceeds in four major sections. Special issues in adapting nursing assessment and care planning are discussed first. Next, principles and illustrations of care planning and nursing interventions using an interpersonal focus are presented followed by a description of group approaches. Selected issues of the therapeutic relationship are given special emphasis in both individual and small group work since the quality of the therapeutic relationship is more critical to treatment outcome during adolescence than in later life periods. Issues related to advancing the conceptual framework in clinical work with adolescents are revealed throughout each section. It would be impossible to cover all aspects of individual and group therapies for adolescents in depth. Instead, the chapter details those aspects that tend to present clinicians with the most difficulties. These include adolescent assessment, the therapeutic relationship, starting an adolescent group, and therapist role flexibility in encouraging problem expression and solution while setting sufficient limits. Generalizations, based on empirical evidence, are made. However, one needs to keep in mind that there are always exceptions to the rule.

NURSING ASSESSMENT AND DIAGNOSIS

The goal in nursing assessment is to identify and measure the degree of stress or vulnerability of the adolescent and behavioral responses or reactions to any existing stressors. The examining instruments are the clinician and particular assessment and interview guides. The process occurs primarily in an interaction between the clinician and adolescent. Interaction techniques depend on the clinician, the age of the adolescent, and the setting. Particular equipment, interview guides, or activities may be used to facilitate the adolescent's verbal and physical expressions.

Assessment is not easy. Conducting an interview with adolescents having adjustment reactions or emotional problems can be problematic. Influencing variables include (1) the clinician's own self-awareness, (2) what she or he introduces into the interaction, (3) the environment, and (4) most importantly, the adolescent. Outcomes are highly dependent on the clinician's competence in interviewing adolescents. Interpretations are especially critical; they are dependent on the clinician's knowledge and professional grasp of the wide spectrum of adolescent sociocultural behavior plus developmental and psychopathological phenomena. The following objectives are suggested as a helpful guide to assessment with adolescents and their parents:

1. To clarify the purpose of the assessment, introducing a psychosocial perspective of adolescence
2. To determine the areas and extent of deviation from the norm for others of the same age
3. To assess the chronicity of problems/concerns
4. To assess the adolescent's and family's strengths
5. To formulate hypotheses about possible contributing factors, past and present
6. To summarize the data and make a diagnosis
7. To negotiate priority concerns and the next steps (Duffy, 1974; Eggert, 1978; Group for the Advancement of Psychiatry, 1974; Kessler, 1966; Simmons, 1969)

Beginning the Assessment: Objective 1

Adolescents have special characteristics requiring adjustments in the clinician's thinking and approach. These include the adolescent's conflicting feelings about (1) having "problems" and accepting the need for an assessment, (2) establishing trust and rapport, and (3) confidentiality issues. Many initial difficulties such as reticence or distrust can be avoided by explaining how adolescents' concerns or problems are viewed psychosocially and how the need for assessment and treatment is presented.

Presenting a Psychosocial View of Problems

The perspective presented here is that problems are a normal part of everyone's life and can be solved rather than being abnormalities to be hidden. Youth with problems sometimes hurt themselves and others. Acknowledging this possibility is a sign of strength rather than admitting to an abnormality. Treatment consists of help in understanding the problem. Problems dissipate when the adolescent no longer needs to hurt self or others (Eggert, 1979b; Vorrath & Brendtro, 1974). This introduction serves as a leveling device that relieves guilt and misconceptions about emotional problems and their causes and, thus, facilitates problem solving.

Establishing Trust and Rapport

In the initial moments, it is essential to communicate the purpose of the assessment, what is entailed, and how the information will be used. The important principle is to promote an interaction with the adolescent, avoiding a monologue by the clinician. Questions should be sought and clarified, false impressions corrected, and anxiety reduced (Haverkamp, 1980; Sedgwick & Hildebrand, 1980; Simmons, 1969).

Frequently, the behavior of adolescents during an initial session is active opposition, suspicion, or nervousness related to the reasons for the referral and an anxiety about being labeled "defective" (Stein & Davis, 1982). Anxiety and fear of the unknown are best allayed by presenting information openly and frankly. Whatever the presenting problem or concern, it should warrant sensitive discussion. There should be no hidden agendas (Simmons, 1969).

The adolescent's typical distrust and suspicion in an initial interview should not be assumed to be pathological, but rather, as appropriate and expected (Vorrath & Brendtro, 1974). Forcing adolescents into communicating or inappropriately expecting openness is neither desirable nor therapeutic. It only serves to tear down an adolescent's defenses and does not lay the necessary foundation for present and future work. Additional principles on establishing the relationship are discussed more fully in the section on applying therapeutic use of self.

Dealing with Confidentiality Issues

Generally speaking, the same principles of confidentiality for working with adults apply to adolescents. Additionally, there is the need, by law, to communicate with family and other authorities under certain conditions if the adolescent is a minor. The clinician should promise adolescents confidentiality of interview content with the exception of suicide potentiality, child abuse, or other serious impending dangers to the adolescent or others in his or her life. More importantly, improved communication with the family and other authorities should be considered a treatment goal. Hence, when issues discussed need to be shared with the family, school personnel, or legal authorities, the clinician should first let the adolescent know and request his or her cooperation. In general, the choice becomes one of who will communicate the information: the clinician, the adolescent, or both. The goal is to help the adolescent communicate the material, whenever possible, with the family and significant others. This promotes the adolescent's struggle for independence and responsibility in problem expression and solution (Leyn, 1980). It also assures the adolescent of informed consent prior to disclosing any personal information (see also Davis, 1980; Haverkamp, 1980).

Determining Concerns and Strengths: Objectives 2, 3, and 4

After setting the stage and meeting the initial concerns of the adolescent, the clinician proceeds to determine the adolescent's problems, and their chronicity, and areas of strength. This assessment involves thorough observation and interviewing. It means gathering information about the following major topics:

1. Reasons for the assessment or referral
2. School, recreation, and interests
3. Ambitions, identifications, and plans for the future
4. Relationships with significant others
5. Concept of self and sense of identity
6. Additional discussion of presenting problem(s) and mental status review
7. General health and psychophysiologic status (Duffy, 1974; Eggert, 1978; Fagin, 1974; Howe, 1980; Simmons, 1969)

These topics are listed in rough temporal sequence for an interview. The sequence can be adapted to start with what the adolescent wishes, to his or her flow of talk, to what seems least threatening and intrusive, and to concerns most immediate.

Special tools and strategies for assessing adolescents are necessary. A real problem in completing a competent developmental assessment is the lack of a standardized tool for covering the basic topics mentioned above. Neither the tools used with children, for example, the play interview and the child mental status exam (Duffy, 1974; Goodman & Sours, 1967), nor those used with adults (Cohen & Harris, 1981) are wholly suitable for assessment with adolescents. To remedy this problem, the process and content of the child mental status examination was adapted in constructing the *Adolescent Development and Mental Status Assessment Tool* presented in Table 11.1. The tool takes into account the adolescent's need for action-oriented, concrete communication, for being an active participant in the assessment, and for variations in a face-to-face, sit-down conversation. Generally, it is best to ask the questions through participant observation (cf. Spradley, 1980).

Additionally, the "Significant Others" worksheet (Simon, Howe, & Kirschenbaum, 1972) is a variation sometimes used to assess the adolescent's relationships and degree of conflict with peers and parents. Additionally, Spradley's *The Ethnographic Interview* (1979) provides an excellent approach to understanding another's way of life. The point is that questions in the Adolescent Assessment Tool provide examples of ways to cover the basic topics.

Ideally, a complete developmental assessment includes adolescent psychosocial and developmental issues, a cognitive and academic assessment, a physical exam (including observations of sexual development), a neurological exam (see Patient Assessment, 1975, 1976), and a history within the family context. The clinician may not be the examiner for each component; if not, then data should be collected from alternate sources after obtaining parental consent for exchange of the information. There is no supplement for a complete, accurate history and assessment as the basis for effective diagnosis and planning treatment.

Interviewing the parents (or surrogates), alone or with the adolescent, is advisable to supplement the adolescent's personal history. This interview should include (1) the parents' main concerns about their child and the presenting problem; (2) the adolescent's personal history from his or her viewpoint; (3) the parents' marital history; (4) the parents' personal history especially related to their own adolescent development and their school, vocational,

Table 11.1 Adolescent Development and Mental Status Assessment Tool

Introduction

The purpose of this interview and questionnaire is to obtain a thorough developmental health inventory—to find out how you are progressing through your teenage years. It is strictly confidential except for a couple of questions which I will tell you about before you answer. I plan to use the information for ______. I hope you will answer all the questions you can and ask me any questions you have as we go along. I want this to be an opportunity for you to learn about yourself, besides being a time for me to get to know you.

Do you have any questions about the purpose of this assessment? About how the information will be used? Here's what the assessment will involve: ______. Do you have any questions?

We could start with ______, or, where would you like to begin?

Name

Your full name?
What do you like to be called?

Age

How old are you?
Date of birth?

Attitudes and ideas about assessment/reasons for referral

What are the reasons you know about for this referral (assessment)?
What kind of things did you think we would talk about?
How does that differ from what I've explained to you?

or

How does (name the problem) affect you at school? At home? Elsewhere?
How long has it been a problem for you? When did it first start?
How serious do you think the problem is—on a scale of 1 to 10?
Any medications or treatments required during school hours? Other times of the day? For how long now?
Your feelings about having this particular concern?

How do you regard your general health (or progress through teenage years)?
(a) generally in good health ______ (b) have minor troubles ______
(c) often have poor health (many problems) ______
How much does your health (problems) interfere with your school work?
(a) not at all ______ (b) a little bit ______ (c) a lot ______

School, recreation, and interests

What school do you attend? Grade?
What are your usual grades? Your best subject? Worst?
What kind of things do you like best about school? Least?
Have there been any changes in how you've done in school? During the last month? 6 months? Year(s)?
How do you compare your school life with the school life of the majority of the kids? With your friends?
Do you sign up for the same classes as your friends?
Would you take classes or go to school activities even if none of your friends will?
Do you participate in any athletics? ______ Which? ______
In any extracurricular activities? ______ Which? ______
What do you enjoy most in your free time? When alone? ______ When with your group? ______
Any favorite activities? ______ Your best? ______
What kind of things can you make? ______ Who usually helps you? ______
Do you save or collect anything? ______

Ambitions, identifications, and future plans

Thinking about your future, what would you like to do after high school?
What job or career are you considering? What are some other(s)?
Who would you like to be like? How come?
Do you think you take after your mother? Or father?
What is your mother's work? Your father's?
If you had three wishes for anything you wanted, what would your wishes be?
What would you do with a lot of money? What things would you buy?

Do you think you know what you want out of life?
Think about it now—what are three things that would be most important to you?

Relationships with significant others

1. **Peers:** (I would like to ask you next about your relationships with friends.)
   Do you have a best friend? What kinds of things do you do together?
   Do you have a special (boy)(girl) friend? Do you go steady (date someone exclusively)?
   How hard is it for you to make friends with boys? With girls?
   Do you stay overnight with your friends? How do you feel about talking with their parents?
   How hard is it for you to get into activities/games/parties?
   Overall, how do you think you get along with your peers?
   (a) great _____ (b) quite well _____ (c) so-so _____ (d) not so hot _____ (e) lots of problems _____
   Your feelings about that? Do you ever feel friendless?
   Can you (and do you) discuss your true feelings with your friend(s)?

2. **Family:**
   Who lives at home?
   What do you like most about your home?
   Do you have your own bedroom? Share with? _____
   How are you getting along with your family?

	Very Well	Quite Well	So-So	Not So Well	Badly
Father	( )	( )	( )	( )	( )
Mother	( )	( )	( )	( )	( )
Brother(s)	( )	( )	( )	( )	( )
Sister(s)	( )	( )	( )	( )	( )
Other relatives or others in the home	( )	( )	( )	( )	( )

   What worries do you have about anyone in your family? About any other person close to you?
   What are the things that could worry your parents about you?
   Can you and do you discuss your true feelings with your
   Mother _____ Father _____ Other(s) _____
   Are there some things where you and your parents don't see eye to eye? Major areas of disagreement?
   Your parent's actions that show they care for you and want to help you? That upset you?
   Things you do that make it hard for your parents to understand you/your actions?
   Things you do to try to bridge any gaps between you and your parents?
   Situations in which your parents are your best source of help to you with personal problems? In which they are not able to help? How come? Who could help you with these?

3. **Other authority figures:**
   How do you get along with your school teachers? ( )Very well ( )O.K. ( )So-So ( )Not so hot ( )Badly
   —With other authorities in your life? (e.g., employer, police, probation officer)
   What are some of the major areas of disagreement (conflict)?
   Do you get all the understanding you think you should?
   From family _____ From friends _____ From people at school _____
   What situations seem to result in hurt feelings/conflicts for you?

4. **Sociocultural adaptation and social awareness:**
   Do you prefer the company of (a) people your own age, (b) people in a different age group from your own?

Table 11.1 (*continued*)

Do you feel liked by most people who know you?
What is your cultural heritage? How do you think it affects you personally?
Do you feel pulled between the ways of (the majority culture) and the values of (the minority culture)?
What do you like/value most about your parents' way of life? Least?
What do you like/value most about your own or your peers' way of life? Least?
How important is your religion to you? Do you attend church regularly? What has your contact been with alcohol/drugs in your family? Outside your family?
Are alcohol or other drugs a problem in your family? How do you feel about that?
Is alcohol a problem for any of your friends? For you?
Would you even tell me if it was?

Self-image and sense of identity
What do you think about your physical development as a teenager?
(a) normal for your age (b) behind for your age (c) advanced for your age.
Your feelings/concerns about how you're developing physically?
What do you think about your height? (a) about right (b) too tall (c) too short.
Actual height ______
How about your weight? (a) about right (b) overweight (c) underweight. Actual weight ______
Do you have a driver's license? An allowance? A job?

Think about your life as a teenager. How do you feel about these various areas of your life?
Place an "x" on the following lines to represent what fits you.

The way I feel about myself most of the time is
Blah ______________________________ Great
In things I do, I usually expect to
Fail ______________________________ Succeed
About my body or image of myself, I'm feeling
Satisfied ______________________________ Dissatisfied
About school,
It's a bummer ______________________________ It's great
About my friends,
I tell them nothing ______________________________ I tell them everything
In relationships with the opposite sex, I'm
Doing great ______________________________ A complete flop
In my relationships with my parents, I'm feeling
Things are bad ______________________________ Everything is great
In dealing with my hangups, I'm feeling
Totally lost ______________________________ I manage just fine
If you could change something about yourself, what would that be? ______________

What do you feel you have already accomplished in becoming an adult?
Check those that apply and then rank the top three.

__Having good friendships with same-sex friends, and
__With opposite-sex friends
__Establishing my role as a young man/young women
__Learning about my body changes and feeling fit
__Becoming independent from my parents
__Preparing for marriage and family life
__Making a career choice and working toward it
__Developing my values and standards for living
__Developing intellectual and problem-solving skills
__Developing a good mental attitude
__Making a commitment to responsible citizenship
__Earning some money

Table 11.1 (*continued*)

Developing a sexual identity and making sexuality decisions is very important to teenagers. It is also an important part of any health evaluation.

With young women:

Let's start with your menstrual history. Age when menstrual periods began?
Any problems with periods? Do you have cramps?
Do you take any medications for cramps? Stay home during your periods?
Are your periods regular? Date of last period?
Do you feel you are developing like other girls your age?

With young men:

Many changes take place in your body, your thoughts, and your feelings as you grow during your teenage years.
Do you feel you are developing like other guys your age? Do you know that it's pretty normal for young men your age to have wet dreams? To deal with sexual desires by masturbating?

With both sexes:

Have you been wondering or questioning how to handle your feelings about being sexually mature?
What alternatives have you considered?
Are you sexually active now? Ever had intercourse (or sex)?
How many different partners?
Have you ever been pregnant? or Caused a girl to get pregnant?
Tell me what you know about contraceptives? About venereal disease symptoms?

How frequently do you find yourself affected by these moods or feelings?

	Never	Rarely	Monthly	Weekly	Daily
Shy	( )	( )	( )	( )	( )
Self-confident	( )	( )	( )	( )	( )
Mad/Angry	( )	( )	( )	( )	( )
Loved	( )	( )	( )	( )	( )
Bored	( )	( )	( )	( )	( )
Light-hearted	( )	( )	( )	( )	( )
Tense	( )	( )	( )	( )	( )
Capable	( )	( )	( )	( )	( )
Trusting	( )	( )	( )	( )	( )
Happy	( )	( )	( )	( )	( )
Lonely	( )	( )	( )	( )	( )
Indecisive	( )	( )	( )	( )	( )
Depressed	( )	( )	( )	( )	( )
Frustrated	( )	( )	( )	( )	( )
Easily hurt	( )	( )	( )	( )	( )
Hopeful	( )	( )	( )	( )	( )
Truthful	( )	( )	( )	( )	( )
Unfulfilled	( )	( )	( )	( )	( )
Other: ______	( )	( )	( )	( )	( )

What is the thing that you're most afraid of? ______
What else scares you sometimes? ______

Additional discussion of presenting problem(s) and mental status review

1. **Description**
   Onset: sudden vs. gradual Getting better or worse
   Predisposing factors: stress, illness, life-style changes, drugs, new foods, problems at school, etc.

Table 11.1 (*continued*)

Factors that aggravate and relieve What makes it better? What makes it worse?
Past treatment or assessments of the problem? What? Results?
Characteristics: (present status plus changes, including)
General appearance; Psychomotor behavior; Speech; Mood and affect; Thought content; Insight and Judgment; Sensorium functions (orientation, memory, attention span, fund of knowledge, past and recent memory, intellectual performance in relation to grade level)

2. **Associated symptoms** (review during next section and/or during physical or neurological exam) Most important: Ask, "what do you think is causing this problem?"
3. **Health education or information needs:**
What would you like to know about your health concern? Do you need any particular information?
How about special knowledge or skills to help you evaluate yourself or take care of yourself?
Do you need help in talking about your questions or concerns with your parents? Teachers? Doctor?
How about help with your friends and their understanding of your current problem?
Do you think you need, or would like, a referral to ______ (appropriate agency)?
Maybe you have some additional questions for me that you've been a little afraid to ask?

General health and development

1. **General:**

Do you often feel tired?
Do you like to get up in the morning?
Do some of your dreams ever scare you?
Do you have a good appetite?
Do you wake up more tired than when you went to bed?
How about going to sleep at night?
Tell me about a daydream you often have?
Tell me about what you usually eat in a day?

2. **Medical history:** Which of the following do you have now or have had in the past?

General:
- Insommnia
- Nightmares
- Waking during night
- Allergies/reactions
- Excessive sweating
- Insect bite or bee sting reactions

Head and Eyes:
- Headaches
- Dizzy spells
- Fainting
- Convulsion
- Loss of consciousness
- Brain concussion

Heart & Respiratory:
- Skipped heartbeats
- Chest pain
- Shortness of breath
- Wheezing/asthma
- Coughed up blood
- Pneumonia/bronchitis

Bone and Joint:
- Fractures
- Sprains
- Athletic injuries
- Backaches
- Painful bones or joints

Gastrointestinal:
- Stomachaces
- Constipation
- Diarrhea
- Nausea
- Bleeding from rectum
- Indigestion

Ears, Nose, and Throat:
- Earaches
- Ringing ears
- Hearing loss
- Nosebleeds
- Frequent colds
- Frequent sore throat

Gyn & Urinary Tract:
- Vaginal discharge
- Urinary infection
- Painful urination
- Blood in the urine

Skin:
- Eczema
- Acne
- Other skin rashes
- Hives

Have you ever thought there might be anything wrong with you or had questions about your health? What?

Table 11.1 *(continued)*

3. **Medications and drug use:** (insure confidentiality; explain why the truth is important for you to know)
Do you smoke cigarettes? How old were you when you started?
What medicines, vitamins, or tonics do you take regularly? ____________
When did you first use alcohol or other drugs? What and when?
If this room had all possible drugs in it, what would be your drug of choice? How come?
Drug most often used? Reasons? Pattern of use/changes?

Frequency of use of alcohol, marijuana, speed, cocaine, coffee, diet pills, barbiturates, tranquilizers, LSD, magic mushrooms, adrenal steroids, thyroid pills, birth control pills, allergy or cold pills, etc.
For each drug, ask if she or he has ever tried it? If so, ask about frequency of use:
tried once __, use a few times/year __, monthly __, every weekend __, daily __, if so, __times/daily?

What consequences have you experienced—blackouts, trouble with police, difficulty in controlling temper? trouble at home? hurting self or others? Trouble at school—skipping, loosing classes, failing?
How often have you tried to quit using ______? For how long have you been able to stick to it?

4. **Physical screening exam:**
Date of last exam? Examiner:
Findings:

5. **Neuro screening exam:**
Vision: Hearing
Cranial nerve functioning

6. **Academic testing:**
Specifiy tests:
Findings:

Psychological testing:
Specify tests:
Findings:

SOURCE: Developed by Leona L. Eggert.

medical, or psychological problems; (5) any family problems such as with other children or previous marriages; and (6) the parents' ideas about possible causes of their adolescent's problems and their views about priority concerns and various treatment methods. Identifying family issues related to the adolescent's problems are critical. The nurse is sometimes at a special advantage in being able to include a home visit to complete the interview.

Making a Diagnosis: Objectives 5 and 6

The clinician now analyzes and synthesizes the data collected and formulates hypotheses about possible contributing factors, past and present, to diagnose the adolescent's current status and concerns. The DSM-III system is a source of approved diagnoses of illness. Additionally, the Group for the Advancement of Psychiatry ([GAP] 1974) provides classification systems specific to emotionally disturbed children/adolescents. Working with adolescents includes knowledgeable use of both these systems.

While the DSM-III and GAP systems serve to classify disturbances and disorders, they involve precisely the kind of labeling that antagonizes the adolescent. Positive Peer Culture (PPC) recognizes this problem and suggests a standard, straightforward language that both adolescents and clinicians can use to identify and discuss problems (Vorrath & Brendtro, 1974). The taxonomy is easily understood and covers most difficulties youth experience:

General Problems: (1) low self-image, (2) inconsiderate of others, (3) inconsiderate of self.

Specific Problems: (4) authority problem, (5) misleads others, (6) easily misled, (7) aggravates others, (8) easily angered, (9) stealing, (10) alcohol or drug problem, (11) lying, (12) fronting (Vorrath & Brendtro, 1974, pp. 35–42). Descriptions of each problem and the indicators of their appearance once solved are particularly valuable.

It is beyond the scope of this chapter to discuss the pros and cons of multiple classification systems; however, it is important to use several frameworks for diagnosing the adolescent's concerns. For example, the DSM-III and/or a GAP typology to delineate major disturbances and the PPC list to identify general and specific problems can be used. If the nurse is seeking direct third-party reimbursement, then the DSM-III must be used for diagnostic formulations. Next, the behavioral symptoms organizer of Raths, Harmin, & Simon (1966) helps identify concerns of (1) unmet emotional needs, (2) cognitive functioning, and (3) values and attitudinal functioning (Eggert, 1978). As a global indicator, the clinician can use Offer's (1969; see also Offer & Offer, 1975) normal patterns of progress through adolescence: continuous growth, surgent growth, or tumultuous growth. Finally, to assess the ego-identity status, Erikson's (1964, 1968) theory as extended by Marcia's (1966, 1967; see also Marcia & Friedman, 1970) research findings can be used. Having analyzed the data in this manner, the clinician is now ready to make an informed diagnosis vis-à-vis: (1) normal adolescent development; (2) emotional, cognitive, and values conflicts; and (3) specific problems related to self-image and inconsiderateness of self or others. Additionally, a diagnosis may be made from symptoms indicating a transient or prolonged psychiatrically labeled disorder.

Negotiating Priority Concerns: Objective 7

The final step in assessment is summarizing and presenting the identified problems/strengths to the adolescent and family and negotiating the priority of concerns. The clinician should involve the adolescent in rank-ordering his or her concerns to set priorities for treatment. The family's rank-ordering is frequently determined and compared with that of the adolescent and the clinician. This step in negotiation helps to clarify the clinician's role vis-à-vis the family's role in the adolescent's treatment. The major task of the clinician is to help the adolescent in accomplishing his or her developmental tasks; the major task with the family is to assist their youth by supporting and facilitating his or her new behaviors and relationships. Moreover, negotiation helps the adolescent accept responsibility for his or her problems and strengths, helps the family determine their role, and prevents overcontrolling on the clinician's part.

NURSING CARE PLANNING

The assessment process ends with a negotiated list of priority concerns. Care planning begins with a negotiated agreement of the goals, type of treatment, and what will count as evidence of progress and successful outcomes. Therapeutic success is often dependent on consensus of these items among the adolescent, the family, and the clinician (Haley, 1976; Stein & Davis, 1982). Planning treatment approaches for adolescents involves a number of important steps: (1) selecting strategies for the specific diagnosed problem(s) and treatment goals, (2) establishing criteria for evaluating the selected approach(es) in meeting specified needs and problems, and (3) weighing the advantages and disadvantages of various treatment modalities for the specific adolescent.

Critical to therapeutic success with adolescents is selecting an appropriate treatment modality: individual, group, family, or milieu, among others. This chapter is limited to a discussion of individual and group modalities (see Chapters 13 and 14 for family and milieu modalities).

Choosing Individual and/or Group Therapy

It is important in negotiating therapy plans to determine the adolescent's motives before choosing individual and/or group work, since adolescents' behaviors in therapy frequently correspond with the motives they express. Deciding between individual and group treatment also means weighing each approach's advantages and disadvantages for both the adolescent and the clinician.

Advantages of Group Treatment for Adolescents

Groups can provide several important advantages to adolescents. Through the special interactions with peers in a safe, social group setting, adolescents become aware of the realities of their attitudes and actions. Frequently, they are more willing to discuss and solve problems with their peers than with adults. Finding out what "other kids think" is critical to adolescents, and group support enables them to work through developmental tasks or difficulties. A synthesis, from research evidence and empirical observations, reveals that adolescent group work (hereafter "AGW") is advantageous primarily because it facilitates the following characteristics.

Being both a giver and receiver of help: Personal growth can result from helping others in the group. Few adolescents enjoy or benefit from always being the recipient of help (Eggert, 1979a, b; Rosenstock & McLaughlin, 1982).

Exchanging ideas, opinions, feelings, and behaviors: Discovering that others also have the same fears, feelings of inadequacy, hatreds, doubts, or rejections can enhance the adolescent's comfort and esteem. Comparison opportunities and peer advice can help adolescents make behavior changes (Altshuler & Seidl, 1977; Berry, Demgen, Hardy, & Wicklund, 1982; Etters, 1975; Sewall, 1983; Siminerio, 1980; Williams, 1982).

Searching for and establishing self-identity: Individual differences discovered through social comparison can be reinforced as valuable sources of identity. Additionally, group novices may use experienced members as standards for judgment and models to emulate (Vorrath & Brendtro, 1974).

Expanding decision-making skills and alternative solutions: Adolescents can learn potential ways of solving problems and alternative ways of coping with situations not yet encountered by observing and participating in the decision making of others in the group (Eggert, 1979b, 1983; Mindek, 1974).

Learning and modifying social behaviors: The group setting provides a valuable opportunity for learning to express personal thoughts and feelings and for learning desirable behavioral responses to others' thoughts and feelings (Carruth, 1976; Eggert, 1979a; Scharer, 1979; Seigal, 1974).

Establishing new relationship ties: Groups can open possibilities for new relationships with those who are in the group. They can also promote a new network of additional ties, with potential rewards, through requests for help and information from other adolescent groups (Eggert, 1979b, 1983; Nicholas, 1969; see also Parks, 1982, for the value of "weak ties").

Advantages of Group Work for Clinicians

The group approach offers both diagnostic and treatment benefits to the clinical specialist as follows.

Direct observation of dynamic interpersonal processes: The "how," "when," "where," and the "ways" the adolescent communicates, responds, and makes decisions with his or her peers can be observed. The group provides a structured, yet realistic environment for diagnosing how an adolescent thinks, feels, and behaves within a social context.

Added treatment benefits: The group setting can "trap" self-defeating behaviors that members use interpersonally and can provide multiple avenues for support, insight, and identification. Conversely, in individual counseling, the clinician is usually the only support and feedback source.

Before concluding that group processes are a panacea for almost all adolescent concerns, several advantages of individual work merit consideration.

Advantages of Individual Treatment for the Adolescent

When the following features apply to the adolescent, usually individual therapy becomes the treatment modality of choice.

Harmful self-disclosure: Research on developing relationships indicates that ill-timed self-disclosure or disclosure of negative characteristics decreases attraction to and liking for the individual (Bochner, 1982; Goffman, 1959). These disclosures lead to norm violators being perceived as less mentally healthy (Berger, Gardner, Parks, Schulman, & Miller, 1976). Consequences for an adolescent who is too self-disclosing, particularly in the group's initial stages, can be more harmful than helpful.

Threatening group settings: Dashiff (1980) maintains that "an adolescent with poor ego strength and problems with capacity for thought, affect, perception, or reality-testing needs to be seen in individual therapy. Such a client will fear peer group settings unless they are oriented around activities" (p. 453).

Advantages of Individual Therapy for the Clinician

There are many more advantages of individual treatment for the clinician than for the adolescent, especially for clinicians inexperienced with adolescents and/or group approaches. The following reasons are often the clinician's basis for choosing individual therapy for an adolescent.

Behavior is easier to manage. In a one-to-one relationship, adolescents often require less discipline of volatile or other untoward behaviors than in groups. The excessive withdrawal of some adolescents or the aggression of others in a group requires sophisticated, humanistic approaches to disciplining adolescents in front of their peers.

Clinical competency requirements are less. Competencies required in group therapy are greater than for individual work (Gill & Barry, 1982). Individual, interpersonal, and group process variables require multiple attending skills (Allen, 1982; Bales, 1970). These skills are further complicated by the normal inconsistencies in adolescents' day-to-day behavior. Both discipline and process interventions require a greater flexibility in group leadership roles than does either individual therapy or adult group work.

Confidentiality is easier to control. While the clinician may guarantee confidentiality and keep this promise, one cannot always guarantee that adolescent group members will be as ethical, despite rules and members' promises to be so (Davis, 1980; Denkowski & Denkowski, 1982).

Many of the other disadvantages of adult group work, such as scheduling logistics, also apply to AGW. Group work with adolescents requires the clinician to be more alert, astute, flexible, and quicker in responding than does either individual adolescent therapy or adult group work.

In weighing the advantages and disadvantages, the benefits of AGW outweigh its disadvantages. Much growth and change can occur for adolescents in a group when the clinician is competent in planning the group treatment and in preventing potential hazards. Usual difficulties for clinicians result primarily from ill-planned group experiences or from naively assuming AGW is no different than group work with adults.

Thus far, discussion has covered adolescent assessment and has explored both general considerations of planning treatment and specific advantages and disadvantages of individual versus group treatment approaches. Principles of planning and intervention in individual therapy, followed by planning and interventions in adolescent group work, will now be discussed. The therapeutic relationship and clinician's role are given special emphasis in both sections because of their critical functions in process movement and therapy outcomes with adolescents.

PLANNING AND INTERVENTION IN INDIVIDUAL THERAPY

Nursing intervention requires the ability to implement specific planned interventions appropriate to the adolescent's identified needs. Also required is the ability to establish a therapeutic relationship and create a therapeutic environment while using a specific treatment modality. Each of these warrants further discussion.

Planning Individual Therapy for Diagnosed Problems

When the adolescent's concerns are identified in terms of recognizable symptoms, for example, within the major areas of unmet emotional needs, cognitive functioning, and values or attitudinal functioning as mentioned earlier, then specific interventions can help the adolescent resolve these concerns. Techniques vary for each set of symptoms. When working with unmet emotional and developmental needs, one is usually dealing with issues of independence, identity, and developmental tasks not previously accomplished, all of which frequently require some individual therapy. Dealing with cognitive difficulties means using concrete communication tools, games, or simulations. This approach often entails special education programs in school. Helping adolescents with values and attitudinal functioning usually involves value clarification strategies.

If the diagnosed problem is an acute or chronic depression, a psychological reaction to stress, an acute psychotic reaction, a recurrent crisis, or substance abuse, to name just a few examples, then the clinician may need to consult the literature for successful interventions specific to these problems. The reader is referred to the literature and to the volumes of Stein and Davis (1982) or Howe (1980).

Establishing the Therapeutic Relationship

A disciplined *therapeutic use of self* (hereafter TUS) is the foundation for any therapy with adolescents. The model is derived from clinical tests of the author's earlier work (Eggert, 1970). Two main components are essential in employing TUS: the human relations component and the action-oriented component. These two elements, one humanistic and the other behavioristic, integrate affective and cognitive domains in a working framework for both individual and group therapy. The combination of behavior modification or competency-based actions and the essential elements of humanistic psychology may seem strange to some and incompatible to others. However, the basis is both empirically grounded and based on a synthesis of most definitions of discipline: love, limits, and learning.

Specific requirements of the clinician are necessary to implement each component of the model; process goals and gains resulting from each component also differ. A brief description of the dimensions within each component and their functions follows.

The Human Relations Component of the Model

This component is characterized by a genuineness of self, expressed regard for the adolescent, and accurate empathy of the adolescent's current experiences and concerns. These concepts are based on the necessary therapeutic conditions for personal growth of Rogers, Gendlin, Kiesler, and Truax (1967).

Being genuine is particularly necessary in working with adolescents as they seem to have an uncanny sense of being able to detect a "phony." At the same time, because of their needs to be understood and regarded as an individual, both verbal and nonverbal expressions of warmth and empathy are essential.

Both helpful and nonhelpful levels of therapeutic use of self within the human relations component are presented in Table 11.2. Nonhelpful levels are operationalized at levels one and two. Conversely, helpful levels of these dimensions are operationalized at levels three to five. Thus, when clinicians are functioning at helpful levels of the human relations component, they are offering their own ideas, attitudes, and experiences *in accord with* the adolescent's needs and concerns.

Applying the principles of the human relations component has a critical and an exaggerated importance with adolescents. Teenagers seem to need much more concrete, consistent, sincere expressions of regard, acceptance, and empathy than do adults. Perhaps the best advice comes from youth themselves:

> To begin with, adolescents need a great deal of patience and understanding. They need to feel a sense of worth. They need a tremendous amount of understanding when it comes to themselves. What is really kind of depressing to me is the adolescent who cannot find a place in the world. They, too, maybe even much more so, need to feel important and recognized. (Notes from Teens, 1980)

The human relations component aids in establishing a therapeutic relationship based on trust and rapport. This component also is essential in maintaining the relationship and in helping teenagers fulfill affective objectives such as self-understanding, self-esteem, and developing values and ways of relating effectively with others.

The Action-Oriented Component of the Model

Dimensions of concrete communication, sensitive confrontation, and immediacy comprise the action-oriented or learning component of the model. Again, nonhelpful levels (one and two) and helpful levels (three to five) are operationalized in Table 11.2.

When clinicians are demonstrating concreteness, they are action oriented in their communication toward specific exploration and health teaching relevant to the adolescent's current feelings and concerns. When using confrontation, they are pointing out discrepancies in adolescents' behavior versus their expressed intentions in an appropriate, sensitive way that is attuned to their ability to accept and benefit from this feedback. Sensitive confrontation is also followed by helping adolescents exercise responsibility in decision making regarding their choice(s) of action. Finally, immediacy means that the clinician is actively attending to the here and now of what is going on between the adolescent and the clinician. When there is something getting in the way of growth or change, then it can be discussed in concrete, sensitive, and mutual problem-solving terms.

For adolescents, the gains of the action-oriented component are learning new social and

Table 11.2 The Dimensions of Therapeutic Use of Self: Facilitative and Nonfacilitative Behaviors
Part A: Dimensions of the Human Relations Component

	Level	*Genuineness/self Disclosure*	*Respect/nonpossessive Warmth*	*Accurate Empathy*
Nontherapeutic	I	Defensive Phony Lack of affect Withholding of self Elaborations about self are irrelevant	Rejecting (nonverbally and/or verbally) of feelings, experiences and/or potential of client Fills silence with own interests	Subtractive Dismisses problems and feelings No expressed awareness of content, meaning, or depth of client's experience or related feelings
	II	Rehearsed, professional facade Uninvolved Passive Use of many "techniques" that are incongruent with self	Mechanical, passive, or possessive caring Judgmental of client's person Caring expressed in "cliches"	Subtractive Awareness of only obvious meaning and feelings; reflects these; offers pat solutions
Minimally facilitative	III	Congruent nonverbal and verbal cues but noncommittal Not phony or defensive Techniques "fit" the person of the helper	Nonverbal & verbal behavior demonstrates caring (although may be conditional) Open body posture Warm nonverbal and verbal expressions	Interchangable nonverbal and verbal response (intensity of client feelings and helper response are mutual) Reflects accurately all obvious meaning and content of client's message
	IV	Freely and completely congruent Nondestructive sharing of self (although may be hesitant) Sharing in accord with client's needs	Verbal and nonverbal prizing, valuing of client Nonjudgmental of client's person Expecting, encouraging client's best	Searching Paraphrased responses and behavior indicates accurate understanding of full content, meaning, and depth of client feelings even though not fully verbalized by the client
Maximally therapeutic	V	Freely and deeply being true self Completely spontaneous sharing in accord with client needs Responses used constructively and relevantly (both positive and negative)	Freely expresses (nonverbally and verbally) deep respect for client Committed to client's value as a person Reinforces strengths	Additive Same as level four, but also, response adds to client's understanding of feelings, experiences Able to express deep awareness

Table 11.2 *(continued)*
Part B: Dimensions of the Action-Oriented Component

Level	*Concreteness (For personally relevant material)*	*Sensitive Confrontation*	*Immediacy*
I	Vague Anonymous Highly intellectual Abstract No personal relevance Interaction kept on a superficial basis	Ignores client discrepancies—remains silent or changes subject Starts interaction with threatening topic and/or threatening tone (Effect: client withdraws or becomes hostile)	Ignores communications dealing with the nurse-client relationship—remains silent or changes subject
II	Personally relevant material discussed vaguely, abstractly Encourages verbalization/detailing of inappropriate or irrelevant material	Destructive (harsh) confrontation of discrepancies in client's behavior (for example, ideal self vs. real self, insight vs. actions) Uninvolved following confrontation (Effect: client defensive)	Disregards client's messages that are related to the nurse Talks about client's feelings for nurses in general
III	Vacillates Hesitant Sometimes guides discussion into personally relevant material in specific, concrete terms, through questioning, paraphrasing	Does not disregard discrepancies Gets involved with client during and following confrontation Confrontation raises questions only (Effect: Client accepting of confrontation/feedback)	Open to interpretation of client's expression of what is going on in here and now of nurse-client relationship, but does not extend these
IV	Enables feelings, experiences to be discussed specifically Hesitates on emotionally laden material	Discrepancies attended to directly and sensitively Confrontation delivered in question form or as tentative conclusions open for discussion (Effect: client responds by self-examination)	Attempts to relate client's expression of immediacy to self in an open but cautious, tentative manner
V	Enables discussion of feelings, experiences in specific, concrete, direct fluent terms, regardless of emotional content	Same as level four with attuned perceptiveness Confrontation direct yet sensitive Explicit and sufficient in quantity (Effect: Client freed to engage in more fruitful or less destructive behavior)	Direct, explicit, nonhesitant discussion and interpretation of the nurse-client relationship, of inherent feelings.

SOURCE: © Leona L. Eggert, September 1974, Revised 1980.

coping skills, gaining self-insight, and achieving behavioral growth and change. Many adolescents behave more responsibly when they know how. Current unacceptable responses stem as much from a lack of knowledge or social skills as from maladaptive personalities or psychological processes (Eggert, 1979a, b, 1983; Stein & Davis, 1982).

Both the human relations component and the action-oriented component constitute an eclectic model designed to help adolescents with feelings, values, thoughts, and desired behavioral action. While the dimensions of both components are identified as separate constructs for purposes of discussing and measuring TUS, in practice they are employed in an integrated fashion. Thus, when higher levels of the action-oriented constructs are being employed, higher levels of the human relations constructs are also necessary.

Applying Therapeutic Use of Self in Phases of Therapy

It is helpful to think about nursing interventions in relation to the various stages in the helping process. In the initial phase of the relationship, only the human relations component and the concreteness dimension of the action-oriented component are applied. Minimal therapeutic levels (level three) characterize the initiation phase of the relationship. Once trust and rapport are established, levels three, four, and five on all dimensions are used interchangeably in concert with the adolescent's tolerance and needs.

Of special concern during the working phase is the need to work through conflicts. Here, helpful levels of sensitive confrontation are required. Transference-countertransference issues may also become relevant now, and, thus, higher levels of the immediacy dimension may be necessary.

Also during the working phase of therapy, content-specific interventions become necessary; variations of basic therapy approaches are used to deal with specific issues such as depression, suicidal behavior, physical disorders, poor communication with parents, running away behaviors, teenage pregnancy, or substance abuse, to name but a few. Interventions can be based on either current theories of etiology (directed at elimination of causative factors) and/or applicable research findings regarding elimination or reduction in symptomatology (Haber, Leach, Schudy, & Sideleau, 1982; Howe, 1980; Stein & Davis, 1982). These interventions require higher levels of concreteness and sensitive confrontation because they embody problem-solving steps specific to the concern at hand.

Throughout the individual therapy, the challenge for the clinical specialist is to understand the responsibilities in the therapeutic relationship and the skills needing further mastery to be more effective with adolescents and their parents. Improvement of these skills is clearly and predominantly based on behavioral practice. Progress and current functioning can be measured using videotape recordings of actual sessions and can be correlated with client process movement and outcomes.

Creating a Therapeutic Environment

Specific tools and strategies can aid the practitioner in applying the human relations component of therapeutic use of self. For example, adolescents frequently cannot respond to questions like "How do you feel about that?" simply because they lack the appropriate vocabulary. A concrete list of "typical feelings" can help adolescents identify their current feelings in a situation. The clinician can also ask them to check likely feelings of others (such as a parent) in the situation, thereby facilitating them in empathy training.

Clinicians' own self-awareness is essential for responding with genuineness and warmth to an adolescent. Understanding the particular adolescent with whom they are working is also vital. No one can be "perfect" in all these dimensions. Some clinicians maintain personal analysis is necessary preparation. Others believe personal therapy is neither practical nor always essential. Effective functioning in the human relations component can be enhanced through practice, for example, by rehearsing therapeutic responses to anticipated expressions from adolescents: anger, affection, or seductive behavior, as well as the host of personal questions they invariably ask. Empathy for adolescents in general can be enhanced by conscious efforts to understand their culture, their way of speaking, and their typical feelings (see also Dalis, 1981).

Certain specific tools and strategies can aid the practitioner in applying the action-oriented component of therapeutic use of self. Some examples include (1) personal objectives and guides to goal attainment, (2) individual contracts and action plans, and (3) the use of communication as a treatment tool, saying what clinicians mean, meaning what they say, and teaching the adolescent likewise. Lauver, Holiman, and Kazama (1982) analyzed the common rhetoric of counselors and therapists and found it included both "a rhetoric of caring and a rhetoric of warfare" (p. 99). Descriptors of clients are often warlike: on the defensive, counter-controlling, aggressive, directly resistant, or manipulative. These concepts are descriptive of a transactional friction between two or more persons; they evoke an adversary image, the client as enemy, sabotaging clinicians' psychotherapeutic efforts. They are also incongruent with the philosophic message of "I care" and can contribute "confusion, mistrust, and the seeds of alienation to any relationship" (Lauver et al., 1982, p. 99).

With adolescents, clinicians need to abandon this rhetoric of warfare for action language; otherwise they are covertly, if not overtly, reinforcing an image of adults as enemies. Action language is embodied in the dimensions of concreteness and sensitive confrontation. For example, in resolving a conflict, clinicians need to explore what part and how much of the problem is caused by the adolescent, how much by the parents, and how much by the clinician. Abstract concepts like passive-aggression require identification and description in concrete behavioral terms. Illegal or embarrassing behaviors need to be discussed in a relaxed manner. Perceptions need to be verbalized so the adolescent can react and respond. Thereby, the clinicians demonstrates confidence in addressing the adolescent and the issues that are often threatening. In turn, adolescents can then discuss, explore, problem solve, and take action.

Some special interpersonal communication issues typically encountered in working with adolescents require indepth variations of basic empathy and communication skills. These include working with the adolescent with limited verbal skills, with the gifted or highly articulate adolescent, or with the adolescent with lability of affect. Clinicians need to review the literature and extend themselves to find creative ways to match the therapeutic approach with the adolescent's manner of understanding and style of learning.

PLANNING AND INTERVENTION IN ADOLESCENT GROUPS

When selecting group work as the treatment modality of choice, particularly when working with adolescents, care planning is critical. Special concerns include (1) therapeutic use of self in group work, (2) planning the leadership role of the clinician, (3) planning evaluation criteria, and (4) starting an adolescent group and selecting group members. Many of the principles apply equally in individual therapy; however, planning for a group experience entails added dimensions. The basic principle illustrated throughout is that having a plan as well as backup plans permits flexibility, considers likely consequences, and, thus, prevents most potential hazards or fiascos.

Employing Therapeutic Use of Self in Adolescent Group Work

Many authors writing about adolescent group work (AGW) emphasize the helpfulness of a permissive counseling situation. This view is incomplete at best; at worst, it is naive. While the humanistic component of TUS is essential, the concreteness and disciplinary action, characteristic of the action-oriented component of TUS, are frequently necessary when working with adolescents (cf. Fink & Eyde, 1983; Walshe-Brennan, 1976). A synthesis of the pragmatics of implementing the TUS model in group work with adolescents is presented in Table 11.3.

Effective group leaders use the action-oriented dimensions of TUS to integrate process and task orientations, balancing the need for both with the group's purposes and needs (cf. Gill & Barry, 1982; Nicholas, 1969; Scheidel & Crowell, 1979). Fiedler's (1978; see also Fiedler, Chemers, & Mahar, 1976) contingency theory of leadership emphasizes the lack of success of applying any one leadership style to all group situations. The personality of the leader, leader-member relations, task structure, and position power all interact, and the situation determines the success of a task-oriented or an interaction-oriented leader. His findings support the need for leadership skills in both dimensions.

Table 11.3 Therapeutic Use of Self in Adolescent Group Work: A Synthesis

The Leader Does	*The Leader Does Not*
Become involved with the group	Present self as detached, passive, too nondirective
Express caring, concern, understanding	Communicate in cold, intellectual style, or fear presenting self as warm and caring
Exude confidence and competence, relating with diplomacy and sensitivity	Relate in ingratiating, condescending, or authoritarian manner
Become knowledgeable in youths' cultural, ethnic, and colloquial ways of speaking to understand their meanings	Adopt their subcultural language or profanity trying to be "one of them"
Exhibit behavior with youth that is "beyond reproach" functioning as a strong, positive, maturely behaving adult person	Become "one of the kids," or become involved in their "horse-play"
Enjoy working with youth	Dislike working with youth
Believe in youths' capacity for positive change	Communicate a lack of faith in youth or undermine their potential
Believe that people have a responsibility to each other and to keeping commitments	Behave selfishly or break commitments or promises
Work to develop positive group strength and inspire confidence in self and others	Encourage dependence or "hero worship" from youth
Set limits effectively and discipline when necessary, responding decisively with firmness	Ignore infractions of group rules or norms; does not struggle with youth on one's own issues of authority
Use private communication to discipline group members or challenge them regarding their participation	Encourage private, confidential communication with individuals isolating them from the group in this way; or undermine group effectiveness by functioning as an individual therapist
Gain trust of both youth and adult staff	Permit youth to draw one into taking sides against staff coworkers
Work cooperatively with other staff coworkers	Undermine staff coworkers
Accept supervision but exercise own judgment and initiative	Become overly dependent or require continuous approval and positive feedback

Effectiveness in AGW means having a communication repertoire that blends task-oriented and socioemotional dimensions. A verbal behavior highly suitable for this is the question. It can focus the process and task of the group, for example, "What reasons do we have for accepting this argument?" or "Why do you suppose Jane takes this position?" Vorrath and Brendtro (1974) point out that if group members are all talking at once and miss a perceptive comment by one member, the leader need only ask if the group heard Ronald's comment. The advantages of being a question-asking leader with adolescents are twofold: questions are nonauthoritarian messages, and they inspire young people to learn by answering them instead of being told what to do.

It is critical that the group leader's nonverbal and verbal communication be congruent. Adolescents seem to rely heavily on assumptions made by reading nonverbal glances and gestures. They rarely clarify these assumptions. For adolescents, actions speak much louder than words.

Planning the Leadership Role

The clinician needs to take on a central leadership role in AGW to insure the development of a positive peer group experience (Betz, Wilbur, & Roberts-Wilbur, 1981).

Group work with adolescents requires great role flexibility and a broad repertoire of related activities. What often works best is the active role of a helpful teacher or "coach" rather than the usual reflective or interpretive therapist role (Gill & Barry, 1982; Haley, 1976).

Vorrath and Brendtro (1974) claim the most difficult therapist role with adolescents is encouraging problem expression and solution while preventing chaos by setting sufficient limits. Their identification of proper/improper staff roles and hazards to new and veteran staff is some of the most insightful work on the topic and is summarized below. The role descriptions can apply in individual therapy as well.

Proper and Improper Staff Roles

Proper staff roles enhance movement toward independence and responsibility. These roles include (1) motivating youth to build a concerned group; (2) reversing responsibility, teaching youth to assume responsibility for one another; and (3) guiding and redirecting the group to resolve problems.

Improper staff roles generally function to take over for the adolescent, preventing movement toward independence and responsibility. These roles include (1) overnurturing youth, keeping them in a dependent role; (2) overcontrolling to instill obedience; and (3) assuming the group's responsibility by handling all problems.

Hazards to New and Veteran Staff

The novice in AGW is subject to three major hazards: (1) becoming "one of them"—overidentifying with youth to win acceptance and then losing the adult role; (2) avoiding uncomfortable group interactions or escaping difficult topics; and (3) losing the initiative and, thus, spending most of their energy putting out fires.

Veteran staff or clinicians assuming AGW is no different from group work with adults are also subject to particular pitfalls. These problems include (1) overconfidence or carelessness, (2) underinvolvement assuming the group can run itself, and (3) experimenting with "hybrid" approaches once the novelty of proven methods wears off (Vorrath & Brendtro, 1974).

Research evidence and the conventional wisdom of many clinicians familiar with AGW support Vorrath and Brendtro's (1974) findings (Bruce, 1974; Duffey, 1979; Eggert, 1979b;

Fagin, 1974; Igoe, 1980; King & Strawn, 1980; Nicholas, 1969; Stogdill, 1974; Turner, 1978). Basically, the permissive role, advocated by many in the literature, is not appropriate for most AGW. A role that deals with the dialectic of discipline and love is needed.

Planning Evaluation Criteria

Planning AGW includes considering evaluation criteria—what will count as evidence of growth. Nicholas (1969) identified some realistic expectations the clinician can have of adolescent group members. Identifying their participation as objectives within five general areas makes this a useful tool for evaluating group member progress. Frequently, the clinician can give adolescents the member evaluation criteria, listed below, so they can measure their own individual progress and/or the group progress (see also Paritzky & Magoon, 1982).

1. *Accepting responsibility for group task accomplishment.* Evidence: Suggests ideas; gives information, facts, and relevant personal experiences; tests and examines ideas for validity; discovers the relatedness among own and others' ideas; and helps in summarizing and pulling together loose ends in the discussion or activity.
2. *Communicating socially with more comfort in the group.* Evidence: Verbalizes appropriate self-disclosures; interest in other group members; sensitive, constructive feedback in response to others. Nonverbally displays more relaxed eye contact with the speaker; comfort with short periods of silence; decreased behaviors such as nervous laughter, continual body movements, withdrawal, or playing with hair or hands.
3. *Developing sensitive relationships with group members.* Evidence: Listens while others talk; encourages and accepts others' contributions; develops empathy for others; relieves tension when appropriate.
4. *Increasing effectiveness in working through conflicts.* Evidence: Clarifies conflict situations; helps to identify possible alternatives and outcomes; estimates consequences of outcomes for self and others; and chooses to act on alternatives having more desirable and successful outcomes for both self and others.
5. *Demonstrating an improved self-image.* Evidence: More socially poised, relaxed, and self-assured; participates more frequently and with more originality; looks more to self and less to others for evaluation, approval, behavioral standards, and decisions or choices. Less defensive, expresses more self-awareness and acceptance of thoughts, feelings, and behaviors (Nicholas, 1969, pp. 20–22).

What can we realistically expect of adolescents in groups differs from what can be expected of adults. Many of the above behaviors require teaching. This is accomplished better by example than by precept. Additionally, the clinician needs to match expectations with what can realistically be accomplished in each group phase. One can expect the adolescent to understand the basic ideas of what the group is all about during the immediate phase. However, acting on a sense of responsibility for self and others and demonstrating an improved self-image comes in the late phase of the group (cf. Brandes & Gardner, 1973).

Starting an Adolescent Group

Getting off to a good start with a group of adolescents is critical to successful process and outcomes; careful planning helps insure this goal. The checklist in Table 11.4 provides

Table 11.4 Checklist for Planning Adolescent Groups

Why are you establishing this particular group? What is the overall goal or your motive?

__To facilitate self-awareness, enhance self-esteem
__To promote accomplishment of some developmental task
__To provide opportunities for adolescents' decision making or solving of common problems
__To supplement individual counseling for participants
__To provide for contact with a larger group of students
__To provide a therapeutic milieu experience
__To promote community action directed toward factors adversely affecting adolescents
__To accomplish some professional goal or motive
__Other: ____________________

What are the specific objectives for this group?

__Primary prevention or health teaching related to ____________________
__Intervention or treatment related to ____________________
__Rehabilitation aims directed toward ____________________

What will be the formal elements of the sessions?

These will vary with the nature and purposes of the group.

1. Who will you invite to join the group?
__Adolescents, __Parents, __Staff members?
__Both sexes, __Females only, __Males only? Why?[a] ____________________
__Age range: __________ Why? ____________________
__Voluntary participation or __A contracted requirement of treatment?[b]
__Similar concerns or __Similar level of concerns?

2. What size will your group be?[c] Number of adolescents__, Parents__, Others__.

3. How will you schedule your group sessions?[d]
Time: ____________________
Place: ____________________
Frequency: ____________________
Duration: ____________________
Projected starting date: __________
Schedule for individual interviews with potential group members: ____________________

What will you cover in an individual interview with each potential group member?

__Explain the purpose of the group
__Explain the basis on which the potential member is being invited to participate
__Share the names or the similar concerns of other prospective group members
__Explore with each his or her feelings and opinions about group participation
__Identify with each the goals he or she has in mind if he or she chooses to join the group
__Discuss possible methods the group might use to achieve these goals
__Ask each member to come prepared to share a little about him- or herself and his or her goals for the group experience
__Establish with each the best options for time and place for the group meetings
__Indicate when you will get back in touch with them, know the time, place, and the date of the first group session

How will you answer the following anticipated questions from adolescents?

__Why should I consider joining this group?
__Who else will be in the group?
__Who decides which members will be in the group?
__How do you know which kids have common problems?
__What will you expect kids to do in the group?
__What do you do in the group?
__What can kids say in the group?
__I'm worried about discussing personal problems in the group?
__Can I bring my close friends, parents, or anyone else to the group? Why not?
__Can I really trust the other members of the group with my problems?
__How will we decide things in the group?
__Where does the group meet?
__Do I have to come each time?
__Now that the group has met three times, can I bring my boyfriend/girlfriend next time?

Table 11.4 (*continued*)

__What will you tell my parents about what goes on in the group?
__Others: ______________________________

The Final Planning

1. Deciding on group membership.
__How will each potential member be affected by the group?
__How will each potential member affect the group?

2. How will you create an environment where group members will feel free to talk and participate, that is, how will you provide for each member's investment in the group?
__Each member will be encouraged to talk, to hear his or her own voice, and to listen when others are talking
__Each member will be encouraged to demonstrate his or her support for each member's contribution by discussing what was said and providing constructive feedback
__The group as a whole will cooperatively define its goals and work toward their achievement
__The leader(s) will not begin by monopolizing the conversation, but rather, will facilitate involvement of all members
__Leaders may have to come prepared to share alternatives and suggest various methods of achieving the goals identified by the group
__The group's task work and team work are of equal value; having each member achieve group goals is as important as keeping relationships harmonious among group members

3. Deciding on the objectives for the first few meetings to get the group off to a good start.
This is dependent on the nature and purposes of the group and the characteristics of the participants.
__Clarifying with the group how and for what reasons it will operate
__Clarifying the clinician's participation and role
__Clarifying the norms and expectations of group members' participation (See ground rules below)
__Creating a climate within which goals may be achieved
__Moving toward productive group functioning
__Other:

4. How will you structure the first meeting?
This is dependent on the nature and purposes of the group and group member needs and characteristics.
__Objectives: What are they specifically? ______________________________
____
__Content: Introductions, Purposes, Norms, etc.? ______________________________
____
__Activities: Which ones will be used for each content area?
____
____
____

SOURCE: Developed by Leona L. Eggert.

[a] Younger adolescents are often more comfortable with the same sex; older adolescents profit from mixed groups. In addition, Vorrath & Brendtro (1974) claim that delinquent "gang" groups should be of the same sex.

[b] Whenever possible, making participation voluntary for the adolescents is preferrable. Making group treatment a requirement introduces an element of coercion: then the clinician faces problems of motivating and persuading members of the potential benefits of full participation in the group process.

[c] More mature, better adjusted adolescents can cope with larger groups, that is, eight to ten or more members. Otherwise, I suggest five to seven members. Generally, the following occurs in small versus large groups:

Smaller Groups (5–10)	*Larger Groups* (12–15+)
More member participation	Leader will talk more
More member involvement	Members will feel more inhibited, threatened
More feeling of belonging	More frustration, less cohesiveness
Process movement may be faster	Process movement takes longer

[d] Generally, I schedule a primary prevention discussion group once weekly for an hour; however, any therapy group requiring behavior changes such as a "quit smoking" group may meet several times per week or even daily, from one-half to one hour each session. Thus, decisions of how frequently the group meets and for how long should be contingent on the therapeutic goals and purposes and how much support the group members will need to accomplish these goals.

a way of clarifying and coordinating key issues in starting an adolescent group (cf. Betz et al., 1981; Duffey, 1979; Landreth & Berg, 1979). It is meant to be suggestive and could also be used, with minor modifications, to plan individual therapy.

Besides determining the rationale and structural elements for the group, the selection process is critical in AGW: How adolescents are grouped can make the difference between a success and a "flop." Wide disparities in age and range of problems do not work well. What seems to work better is to match the needs of the adolescents with the overall group goal and the selection criteria (Brandes & Gardner, 1973; VanDyck, 1980). Another dimension crucial to the selection process and in getting off to a good start is having a brief interview with each potential group member. Frequently, when working with a new coleader, rehearsing aspects of working together helps coordinate and clarify leadership goals, behaviors, and key issues involved in structuring the group.

Considering ground rules is also critical for creating a positive peer group environment and providing for each member's investment in the group. Suggested rules include establishing (1) who belongs to the group, (2) expected behaviors for talking and listening, (3) how decisions are made and problems solved, (4) what constitutes confidentiality, (5) expected member behavior, and (6) group leader behavior and responsibilities (Christen & McKinnon, 1977; Gendlin & Beebe, 1968). The clinician can introduce a "draft" of the ground rules during the first meeting as a way to negotiate norms and expectations. The rules often work to teach adolescents appropriate group interaction and group decision making. They usually prevent many problems that would otherwise require much disciplining "after the fact."

Probably some of the most important principles to juxtapose in AGW are the individual vs. the group; stability vs. flexibility; and overall goals with continued group process assessments. Experience indicates that every group is different and no prescribed approach fits all groups.

One notable application of the TUS model was in a peer counseling program. It is presented as an example of the positive effects that can occur for youth when they are taught to be natural helpers for their peers (but see also Alpert & Rosenfield, 1981; Carruth, 1976; Pearson, 1983; Seigal, 1974; Vorrath & Brendtro, 1974).

Peer Counseling: A Group Intervention Approach

The peer counseling program was developed and empirically validated by the author and coleader; we worked with six separate groups over two years (Eggert, 1979b). Evidence exists that peer counseling works in helping adolescents learn to help themselves and others with the problems they face, whether drug abuse, running away from home, interpersonal relationships with the opposite sex, personal anxieties about school and family, or the everyday worries of coping with adolescence. Typical statements indicate adolescents see as most valuable learning:

> Where people can go when they need help. Sources that are around when you need help. It's given me a better understanding of problem solving for myself as well as others.
>
> What to say when somebody needs help, where to send them, that's the main thing. I always felt like I could be no help because I would just sit and listen and wouldn't know what to say.

Typical of what the adolescents thought most effective was

> Enacting real life problem situations. The whole group working to find alternatives and consequences was good. The role playing, and after, the comments and suggestions of the group—the way we practiced in small groups and then went over the good and bad points. That helped me learn a lot.

Peer counseling seems very promising both as a primary and secondary treatment modality. It provided an opportunity to use those valuable, informal adolescent channels of communication and offered form and substance to the unfocused idealism of the teenager's desire to help a friend. It also provided a vehicle to clarify values and make overt the process of personal problem solving and decision making, exploring and choosing alternatives. It further allowed exploration of behaviors, feelings, and needed personal changes with a group of teenagers over time. This type of experience was valuable because it occurred without the teenagers needing to see themselves as "clients" in a counseling process. The peer counseling program not only provided for growth and development of those who were active participants, but also offered significant benefits to a whole network of their peers.

A primary challenge in the program was to bridge the gap between the helpful peer group experience and continued growth and development in family and community life. Youth who gained new skills in the group, who surmounted problems, who made significant behavioral changes in a positive direction, were immensely beneficial to others needing help. But the ultimate test of this and other similar programs is to subject them to controlled study. Little is currently known of the long-range effect on youth who participate. Many of the claims made warrant validation. Studies should include exploration of the effects of different adult leadership styles with particular youth groups and investigations of how and why particular methods seem to work with some youth and for some concerns and not others. These are but a few of many questions and challenges for research.

SUMMARY

Adolescent psychiatric mental health nursing practice is characterized by responses to the developmental and sociocultural needs of young people 10–20 years old. Their maturation occurs within the family for the most part and, to a large extent, within a school setting. A major focus of prevention and therapy involves facilitating successful accomplishment of adolescent developmental tasks and, thus, promoting psychosocial maturity. This requires particular competencies: knowledge of "normal" developmental processes and the ability to recognize unhealthy deviations; skill in individual, small group, or other treatment modalities; and the ability to incorporate the family and school systems into treatment. Throughout this chapter it was demonstrated, in several ways, how important planning and specific skills are in working with teenagers both as individuals and in group treatment.

In the section on the clinician's role and therapeutic use of self, principles of human relations were combined with principles of learning to enhance the mental health teaching and rehabilitation role of the clinician. Adaptations of the basic model, combined with problem-oriented interventions, can help adolescents with unmet emotional needs, difficulties in cognitive functioning, and concerns related to exploring various values or specific problems.

Finally, in the section on group treatment approaches and in the peer counseling example, an intervention and rehabilitation model was described. This model enabled youth to help each other with a range of concerns from common adolescent anxieties to avoiding substance abuse.

A common theme throughout the chapter was that the strengths of youth can be tapped. Opportunities exist for helping them achieve their developmental tasks, increase their social skills, and enhance their self-image. Individual and group work methods support and provide these learning opportunities for youth. Group approaches, especially, have the potential for strengthening the old or creating a new network of supportive resources for the adolescent members. In both approaches, the clinician needs to be responsible, caring, firm but fair, and a human being whom youth can come to know and from whom they can learn. Also necessary is being able to work within the context of both the adolescent's family and school since these are the primary systems in which youth must achieve self-identity and social responsibility.

REFERENCES

Allen, E. E. Multiple attending in therapy groups. *Personnel and Guidance Journal,* 1982, *60,* 318–320.

Alpert, J. L., & Rosenfield, S. Consultation and the introduction of social problem-solving groups in schools. *Personnel and Guidance Journal,* 1981, *60,* 37–40.

Altshuler, A., & Seidl, A. H. Teen meetings: A way to help adolescents cope with hospitalization. *Maternal Child Nursing,* 1977, *2,* 348–353.

Bales, R. *Personality and interpersonal behavior.* New York: Holt, Rinehart & Winston, 1970.

Berger, C. R., Gardner, R. R., Parks, M. R., Schulman, L., & Miller, G. R. Interpersonal epistemology and interpersonal communication. In G. R. Miller (Ed.), *Explorations in interpersonal communication.* Beverly Hills: Sage, 1976.

Berry, J., Demgen, M., Hardy, R., & Wicklund, C. Implementing eliminating self-defeating behavior theory in group home treatment. *Personnel and Guidance Journal,* 1982, *60,* 571–573.

Betz, R. L., Wilbur, M. P., & Roberts-Wilbur, J. A structural blueprint for group facilitators: Three group modalities. *Personnel and Guidance Journal,* 1981, *60,* 31–36.

Bochner, A. P. On the efficacy of openness in close relationships. In M. Burgoon (Ed.), *Communication Yearbook 5,* New Brunswick, NJ: Transaction Books, 1982.

Brandes, N. S., & Gardner, M. L. (Eds.). *Group therapy for the adolescent.* New York: Jason Aronson, 1973.

Bruce, S. J. Adolescence: Delinquent or distressed? In C. M. Fagin (Ed.), *Child and adolescent psychiatric nursing.* St. Louis: C. V. Mosby, 1974.

Carruth, B. F. Modifying behavior through social learning. *American Journal of Nursing,* 1976, *6,* 1804–1806.

Christen, W. L., & McKinnon, B. E. Opportunity hall: A place for dropouts—truants—kickouts. *Personnel and Guidance Journal,* 1977, *55,* 605–607.

Cohen, S., & Harris, E. Mental status assessment. *American Journal of Nursing,* 1981, *81,* 1493.

Combs, A. *The helping relationship.* Paper presented at Washington State Personnel and Guidance Association, Port Angeles, Washington, 1968.

Combs, A., & Soper, D. W. The perceptual organization of effective counselors. *Journal of Counseling Psychology,* 1963, *10,* 222–226.

Dalis, G. T. On the level: A new TV series for and about teenagers. *Health Education,* 1981, *12,* 13–15.

Dashiff, C. J. Adolescents in mental health counseling centers. In J. Howe (Ed.), *Nursing care of adolescents.* New York: McGraw-Hill, 1980.

Davis, K. L. Is confidentiality in group counseling realistic? *Personnel and Guidance Journal,* 1980, *59,* 197–201.

Denkowski, K. M., & Denkowski, G. C. Client-counselor confidentiality: An update of rationale, legal status, and implications. *Personnel and Guidance Journal,* 1982, *60,* 371–376.

Duffey, M. Factors contributing to the development of a cohesive adolescent psychotherapy group. *Journal of Psychosocial Nursing,* 1979, *17,* 21–24.

Duffy, J. C. *Child psychiatry.* New York: Medical Examination Publishers, 1974.

Eggert, L. L. *A theoretical model of nursing as a helping relationship: Synthesis and development.* Unpublished master's thesis, University of Washington, Seattle, 1970.

Eggert, L. L. The therapeutic process with adolescents experiencing psychosocial stress. In D. C. Longo & R. A. Williams (Eds.), *Clinical practice in psychosocial nursing: Assessment and intervention.* New York: Appleton-Century-Crofts, 1978.

Eggert, L. L. *Adolescent sexuality: Decisions and outcomes.* Paper presented at the Fourth Annual Sexuality Workshop, Marion County Health Department, Salem, Oregon, 1979a.

Eggert, L. L. *A peer counseling program: The model and an evaluation of how it works.* Research report for the King County Drug Commission, Seattle, Washington, 1979b.

Eggert, L. L. *The effects of structured approaches on small group decision making processes and outcomes.* Unpublished field study in progress, University of Washington, Seattle, 1983.

Erikson, E. H. *Childhood and society* (2nd ed.). New York: Norton, 1964.

Erikson, E. H. *Identity: Youth and crisis.* New York: Norton, 1968.

Etters, L. E. Adolescent retardates in a therapy group. *American Journal of Nursing,* 1975, *75,* 1174–1175.

Fagin, C. M. Aspects of therapeutic intervention with adolescents. In C. M. Fagin (Ed.), *Child and adolescent psychiatric nursing.* St. Louis: C. V. Mosby, 1974.

Fiedler, F. E. Recent developments in research on the contingency model. In L. Berkowitz (Ed.), *Group processes.* New York: Academic Press, 1978.

Fiedler, F. E., Chemers, M. M., & Mahar, L. *Improving leadership effectiveness: The leader match concept.* New York: Wiley, 1976.

Fink, A. H., & Eyde, D. R. *Don't do that! and other counseling strategies for the chronically disruptive.* Ann Arbor, MI: University of Michigan (ERIC/CAPS Document Reproduction Service), 1983.

Gendlin, E. T., & Beebe, J. III. An experiential approach to group therapy. *Journal of Research and Development in Education,* 1968, *1,* 19–29.

Gill, S. J., & Barry, R. A. Group-focused counseling: Classifying the essential skills. *Personnel and Guidance Journal,* 1982, *60,* 302–305.

Goffman, E. *The presentation of self in everyday life.* New York: Doubleday, 1959.

Goodman, J. D., & Sours, J. A. *The child mental status examination.* New York: Basic Books, 1967.

Greenberger, E., & Sorensen, A. Toward a concept of psychosocial maturity. *Journal of Youth and Adolescence,* 1974, *3,* 329–358.

Group for the Advancement of Psychiatry (GAP). *Psychopathological disorders in childhood.* New York: Jason Aaronson, 1974.

Haber, J., Leach, A. M., Schudy, S. M., & Sideleau, B. F. (Eds.). *Comprehensive psychiatric nursing* (2nd ed.). New York: McGraw-Hill, 1982.

Haley, J. *Problem-solving therapy: New strategies for effective family therapy.* San Francisco: Jossey-Bass, 1976.

Haverkamp, L. F. The health assessment. In J. Howe (Ed.), *Nursing care of adolescents.* New York: McGraw-Hill, 1980.

Howe, J. *Nursing care of adolescents.* New York: McGraw-Hill, 1980.

Igoe, J. B. School health programs. In J. Howe (Ed.), *Nursing care of adolescents.* New York: McGraw-Hill, 1980.

Kessler, J. *Psychopathology of childhood.* Englewood Cliffs, NJ: Prentice-Hall, 1966.

King, R. B., & Strawn, S. M. The adolescent in a rehabilitation setting. In J. Howe, (Ed.), *Nursing care of adolescents.* New York: McGraw-Hill, 1980.

Landreth, G. L., & Berg, R. C. Overcoming initial group-leader anxiety: Skills plus experience. *Personnel and Guidance Journal,* 1979, *58,* 65–66.

Lauver, P. J., Holiman, M. A., & Kazama, S. W. Counseling as battleground: Client as enemy. *Personnel and Guidance Journal,* 1982, *61,* 99–101.

Leyn, R. B. The nurse-adolescent relationship. In J. Howe (Ed.), *Nursing care of adolescents.* New York: McGraw-Hill, 1980.

Marcia, J. Development and validation of ego-identity status. *Journal of Personality and Social Psychology,* 1966, *34,* 551.

Marcia, J. Ego-identity status: Relationship to change in self-esteem, general adjustment, maladjustment, and authoritarianism. *Journal of Personality and Social Psychology,* 1967, *35,* 118.

Marcia, J., & Friedman, M. L. Ego-identity status in college women. *Journal of Personality and Social Psychology,* 1970, *38,* 249.

Mindek, L. Sex education on a psychiatric unit. *American Journal of Nursing,* 1974, *74,* 1856–1858.

Nicholas, L. J. *The counselor and the group process.* Bellevue, WA: Bellevue Public Schools Publication ASICO129/9370, 1969.

Notes from teens: On what would make adolescence easier. L. Eggert (Ed.), Unpublished collection, 1980.

Offer, D. *The psychological world of the teen-ager.* New York: Basic Books, 1969.

Offer, D., & Offer, J. Three developmental routes through normal male adolescence. In S. Feinstein & P. Fiovacchini (Eds.), *Adolescent psychiatry, Vol. IV: Developmental and clinical studies.* New York: Jason Aronson, 1975.

Paritzky, R. S., & Magoon, T. M. Goal attainment scaling models for assessing group counseling. *Personnel and Guidance Journal,* 1982, *60,* 381–384.

Parks, M. R. Ideology in interpersonal communication: Off the couch and into the world. In M. Burgoon (Ed.), *Communication Yearbook 5,* New Brunswick, NJ: Transaction Books, 1982.

Patient assessment: Neurological examination, parts I and II. *American Journal of Nursing,* 1975, *75,* 1511, 2037.

Patient assessment: Neurological examination, part III. *American Journal of Nursing,* 1976, *76,* 609.

Pearson, R. E. Support groups: A conceptualization. *Personnel and Guidance Journal,* 1983, *61,* 361–364.

Raths, L. E., Harmin, M., & Simon, S. B. *Values and teaching.* Columbus, OH: Chas. E Merrill, 1966.

Rogers, C. R., Gendlin, E., Kiesler, D., & Truax, C. (Eds.). *The therapeutic relationship and its impact.* Madison: University of Wisconsin Press, 1967.

Rosenstock, H. A., & McLaughlin, M. Positive group efficacy in adolescent treatment. *Journal of Clinical Psychiatry,* 1982, *43,* 58–61.

Scharer, K. M. Helping disturbed children change their passive-aggressive behavior through milieu therapy. *American Nurses' Association Publication* (NP-59), 1979, 275–292.

Scheidel, T. M., & Crowell, L. *Discussing and deciding: A desk book for group leaders and members.* New York: Macmillan, 1979.

Sedgwick, R., & Hildebrand, S. The adolescent at risk: Crisis, the delicate balance. In J. Howe (Ed.), *Nursing care of adolescents.* New York: McGraw-Hill, 1980.

Seigal, M. A. Los Angeles teen challenge: A resocialization program for drug abusers. *Journal of Psychiatric Nursing,* 1974, *12,* 21–24.

Sewall, K. S. Peer-group reality therapy for the pregnant adolescent. *Maternal Child Nursing,* 1983, *8,* 76–79.

Siminerio, L. M. Establishment of a diabetes youth group. *Diabetes Education,* 1980, *6,* 22–23.

Simmons, J. E. *Psychiatric examination of children.* Philadelphia: Lea & Febiger, 1969.

Simon, S. B., Howe, L. W., & Kirschenbaum, H. *Values clarification.* New York: Hart, 1972.

Spradley, J. P. *The ethnographic interview.* New York: Holt, Rinehart & Winston, 1979.

Spradley, J. P. *Participant observation.* New York: Holt, Rinehart & Winston, 1980.

Stein, M. D., & Davis, J. K. *Therapies for adolescents.* San Francisco: Jossey-Bass, 1982.

Stogdill, R. M. *Handbook of leadership: A survey of theory and research.* New York: Free Press, 1974.

Turner, J. Nursing in the adolescent service: A different role. *Journal of Adolescence,* 1978, *1,* 14–15.

VanDyck, B. J. An analysis of selection criteria for short-term group counseling clients. *Personnel and Guidance Journal,* 1980, *59,* 226–230.

Vorrath, H. H., & Brendtro, L. K. *Positive peer culture.* Chicago: Aldine, 1974.

Walshe-Brennan, K. S. Teenage violence in psychiatric wards. *Nursing Mirror,* 1976, *143,* 63–64.

Williams, M. Anorexia nervosa—milieu therapy of young adolescents. *Australian Nurses Journal,* 1982, *11,* 38–40.

BIBLIOGRAPHY

Cook, T. D., & Campbell, D. R. *Quasi-experimentation.* Boston: Houghton Mifflin, 1979.

Hamm, B. H., & Brodt, D. GUTS: Teaching assertiveness skills by simulation and gaming. *Nursing Research,* 1982, *31,* 246.

Heppner, P. P., & Dixon, D. N. A review of the interpersonal influence process in counseling. *Personnel and Guidance Journal,* 1981, *59,* 542–550.

Igoe, J. B. Health counseling and teaching. In J. Howe (Ed.), *Nursing care of adolescents.* New York: McGraw-Hill, 1980.

Krivatsy-O'Hara, S., Reed, P., & Davenport, J. Group counseling with potential high school dropouts. *Personnel and Guidance Journal,* 1978, *57,* 510–511.

CHAPTER 12

INDIVIDUAL AND GROUP PLAY THERAPY

Deane L. Critchley

Child psychiatric nursing emerged as a specialty requiring advanced knowledge and skills following the National Mental Health Act of 1946. This act was the impetus for graduate education in nursing. The resulting graduate programs in child psychiatric nursing, though few, prepare their graduates to function effectively in varied practice settings using multiple treatment modalities.

One of the more popular treatment methods with children is the use of behavioral techniques and behavior modification in particular. This approach is based on the knowledge that behavior that is rewarded is likely to be repeated. Developmentally, behavior that is desired in a child is usually spontaneously praised or rewarded by adults. When behaviors that are rewarding to an individual child are identified, these same behaviors can then be used as reinforcers for desired behaviors. This approach has proven effective in working with children with a variety of emotional and behavioral problems (McNamara, 1979).

This chapter does not focus on this particular treatment modality because it is an approach easily learned and already widely used by nurses. Its effective use does not require special qualities of the nurse or thorough understanding of the developmental and psychopathological processes that are major contributors to the problems of children, especially those children experiencing chronic physical illness, emotional problems, or mental disorder. Effective use of behavioral techniques requires only that the target behavior is objectively defined, the behavioral techniques are systematically applied, and careful observations and measurements are recorded.

Milieu therapy is another widely used treatment approach with children. It is used in therapeutic day treatment, residential treatment, or in psychiatric hospitalization. The principles of milieu treatment for both adults and children are discussed by Maurin in Chapter 14.

This chapter will be concerned with the use of individual and group psychotherapy with children. This approach, often called play therapy, can be used in working with children either on an outpatient, day treatment, or inpatient basis. The therapeutic knowledge and techniques used in individual and group play therapy require the same skills: empathetic awareness and self-knowledge, which are invaluable in establishing psychotherapeutic relationships with children in a variety of clinical situations.

Individual and group play therapy will be discussed in terms of stages, process, and rationale for types of therapist interventions. Important issues in child treatment such as limit setting, sexual behavior by the child in therapy, resistance, and other process issues will be discussed.

ASSESSMENT AND TREATMENT

Initial Assessment

Before undertaking any preventive or interventive work with a child, the nurse needs to evaluate the strengths and deficits in the child's past and current functioning. An evaluation requires information from the immediate and extended family, the child's pediatrician, and teachers. Permission must be obtained from both the parents and the child, when appropriate, to make such inquiries. An assessment needs to include a thorough developmental, social, and health history and the report of a recent physical examination. The evaluation necessarily needs to include some type of structured and unstructured observation and interaction with the child as in a mental status examination (Critchley, 1979). The information obtained and the DSM-III diagnosis need to be incorporated into a nursing diagnostic formulation with an appropriate treatment plan designating goals and interventions.

The most useful framework in which the above data can be understood is derived from ego psychology, more recent object relations theory, and nursing diagnosis. Because of the complexity of mental illness and the multiplicity of factors involved, work with any given child will involve a number of nursing diagnoses or identified problems. The length and extensiveness of the evaluation process is directly related to the severity of the child's disturbance.

The Bayley Scales of Infant Development are a valuable tool in assessing a young child's sensorimotor, cognitive, and psychological development. The therapist role for both child and family usually involves both therapeutic and educative aspects. Many parents need help in learning to parent more effectively. The troubles of both parents and child usually require therapeutic intervention by the clinical specialist.

Treatment Goals

Goals and interventions for a particular child need to be individualized. There are, however, broad treatment goals for work with mentally ill children. These goals involve assisting the child with new learning regarding self and environment; helping both child and family to explore new expectations, roles, and relationships; and assisting the child through restoring adaptive functions and remediating maladaptive aspects of functioning. To achieve these goals generally requires intervention in several areas, depending on the child's strengths and deficits. Usually, alteration in the child's pathology, especially ego functioning; alteration in the child's social adaptation and school functioning; and alteration in intrafamily functioning are required.

Table 12.1 illustrates typical problems experienced by mentally ill children and their families as well as possible goals and interventions to achieve the goals. Using clearly specified goals and nursing assessments and evaluation of the effectiveness of intervention provides both more validity and reliability.

SIGNIFICANCE OF PLAY

During this century, the importance of play in human development has been deliberated. Play is the vehicle by which the child masters the environment and his own impulses and increases his adaptive behavior. Play is the precursor of discovery, creativity, and invention. As the child's form of communication, it is worthy of careful observation and research. The role of play in psychomotor development, cognitive development, and the expression

Table 12.1 Nursing Assessment and Intervention Guide for Child and Family

Problem Behavior/Nursing Assessment	*Goal*	*Intervention*
Unsatisfying interpersonal relationships with family/peers	Child interacts age appropriately with a family member/peer for a measurable period of time	Assist child to learn appropriate social skills through: a. therapeutic play/activity group b. individual therapy c. modified school activities
Negative self-concept	Can identify own abilities realistically	Provide opportunities for success Provide frequent encouragement and reward
Specific learning disabilities (e.g., verbal processing)	Will respond to increasingly complex verbal directions/requests with a specified degree of accuracy (e.g., 60–80%)	Provide small segments of interactions based on understanding and reaction to verbal behavior Provide behavioral cues to assist in understanding verbal behavior
Significant developmental lag (e.g., deficient perceptual motor skills, poor large muscle coordination)	Evaluation is completed and recommendation acted upon by family Child is able to successfully engage in some age-appropriate activity involving large muscle coordination which he/she was previously unable to do	Provide referral for necessary evaluation (e.g., sensory motor, neurological) Provide activities and rewards for participating in skill building activities appropriate to child's current abilities (e.g., swimming, bike riding, soccer)
Self-destructive behaviors (e.g., head banging, biting self, etc.)	Diminish/eliminate self-destructive behaviors	Identify situations/stimuli that precipitate such behavior Attempt to prevent behavior via decision, redirection, reassurance, interrupt behavior as soon as it begins Provide more satisfying behaviors for child, rhythmical movements with adult (e.g., rocking, swinging) Provide protection so child can not hurt self (helmet, gentle restraint)
Withdrawn and isolated behavior	Child tolerates/seeks out contact with another person on a measurable basis	Provide frequent low key approaches to child Reward any of the child's responses to such approaches with something acceptable to the child (e.g., food, objects) Always couple and try to replace other rewards with a social reward
Excessive anger and blaming within the family focusing on the mentally ill child	Family members are able to identify sources of guilt/blame Decrease in expressions of	Provide family meetings in order to discuss family members feelings and attitudes Provide acceptance and sup-

Table 12.1 *(continued)*

	anger and blame towards the child	port of feelings expressed Help family members identify more appropriate coping behaviors
Inadequate knowledge/understanding of child development and child's needs	Parents can identify their child's developmental and emotional needs in relation to basic stages and principles of development	Assist parents with anticipatory developmental guidance Refer to parent education classes Provide guidance for appropriate parent-infant interactions
Inability to meet child's needs due to inadequate parenting skills	Parents can demonstrate effective parenting skills with their infant	Provide opportunities for effective parenting Provide reinforcement for effective parenting
Inability to meet child's needs to tolerate child's behavior as a result of unresolved internal conflicts	Parents are able to recognize a need and respond appropriately	Provide psychotherapy/counseling to deal with these issues Assist parents in finding repite care for their child
Inconsistency in responding to child's behavior	Parents can identify inconsistencies	Assist parents in identifying inconsistencies in their behaviors and possible sources for such behavior
	Parents can identify expectations for their child	Assist parents in identifying clear expectations and limits for their child
	Parents can follow through with established expectations and limits	Assist parents to follow through with established expectations and limits

of inner feelings and fantasies is well recognized. Play therapy has become an effective mode of treating the troubled child.

Play is the language of the child; the language of inner processes, the unconscious, and the ego functions. Adults talk; children play. Table 12.2 provides an overview of play according to developmental stages.

Meaning of Play

Many theorists have discussed play in terms of its symbolic meaning, structures and process, developmental and therapeutic aspects, and as a measure of assessing progress (Erikson, 1950, 1972; A. Freud, 1965; Klein, 1955; Lorenz, 1972; Peller, 1954; Piaget, 1962; Woltmann, 1955). Many of the original articles on these topics were reprinted in Haworth's *Child Psychotherapy* (1964), which provides a representative selection of different approaches to child psychotherapy. Much of the discussion on play therapy will draw on these sources.

Therapeutic Use of Play

> If he [Tom Sawyer] had been a great and wise philosopher, like the writer of this book, he would now have comprehended that Work consists of whatever a body is *obliged* to do [emphasis added], and that Play consists of whatever a body is not obliged to do.
>
> Mark Twain (1876, p. 29.)

Table 12.2 Developmental Stages and Aspects of Play

Age	*Psychosexual Stage (Freud)*	*Psychosocial Stage (Erikson)*	*Cognitive Stage (Piaget)*	*Typical Fears*	*Developmental Problems*	*Stage of Play*	*Social Aspect of Play*	*Play Materials*	*Psychotherapeutic Gains of Play*
0–1½	Oral	Basic trust vs. mistrust	Sensorimotor	The dark Strangers Being alone Sudden noise Loss of support	Autism Depression Extreme stranger anxiety Feeding and sleeping problems Pica	Body movement Imagery Exploratory	Solitary	Variations on use of body parts	Increased body skills and mastery Learns to actively search for gratification
1½–3	Anal	Autonomy vs. shame and doubt	Symbolic	Separation Desertion Sudden movements	Symbiosis Negativism, temper tantrums Toilet training disturbances Sleep disturbances, night terrors Bedtime rituals Shyness and withdrawal		Solitary or with single adult Use of people as objects Parallel play	Parental play with dolls, stuffed animals, other children, peek-a-boo, block play	Ability to bear delay, frustration Acts out rage, anxiety in play Ability to develop lasting object relations Release through fantasy play

Table 12.2 (*continued*)

Age	*Psychosexual Stage (Freud)*	*Psychosocial Stage (Erikson)*	*Cognitive Stage (Piaget)*	*Typical Fears*	*Developmental Problems*	*Stage of Play*	*Social Aspect of Play*	*Play Materials*	*Psychotherapeutic Gains of Play*
3–5½	Genital Oedipal	Initiative vs. guilt	Intentive representational	Animals Injury Imaginary creatures	Phobias Speech problems Disturbances in elimination Anxiety states Food rituals School problems	Fantasy	Early coplay Shares fantasy Either solitary or social activity Peer cooperation	More elaborate doll play Drawing Finger paints Clay, Water Hand puppets Imaginative play with props, emblems "Dress-up clothes"	Preparation for adult roles and skills Adventure accomplishment Acts out family rivalry issues Peer identification Release through fantasy play
5½–10	Latency	Industry vs. inferiority	Concrete operational	School failure Ridicule Loss of possessions Disfigurement Disease Death	Learning problems Psychoneurosis Personality disorders Tics Pervasive developmental disorders Predelinquent patterns	Games Same sex gangs	Organized coplay Shared fantasy Peer competition	Organized games, team, board, mutual story telling, hobbies, checkers Individual and group projects Psychotherapeutic games	Loosens family ties Gratifying experiences as follower and leader Rapid ego growth Consolidation of ego defenses

Play is an important psychotherapeutic tool in work with preschool- and elementary school-aged children. Klein (1955) and Anna Freud were its earliest exponents. They believed that the child's free play was like the adult's free association. They identified the inner processes in the minds of children through observation of their play.

Today, with greater understanding of the world of childhood, the ideas of Freud and Klein appear somewhat obvious and logical. The therapist needs to display understanding and nonintrusiveness to gain admission into the child's world of play. The therapist who tries to force entry or interpret too quickly often is turned away. When one is able to interact with the child according to Axline's principles (1947), that is, to be warm, friendly, accepting, patient, tolerant of the child's expression of feelings, and respectful of the child, then one is able to demonstrate that he or she can be a useful ally to the child in reducing or alleviating anxiety. Coercion in play therapy as Twain so correctly points out creates obligated play, which no longer is play.

PLAY THERAPY

It is beyond the scope of this chapter to examine each of the predominant schools of child therapy. The reader's knowledge of these major approaches is assumed. Instead, this section will examine the more commonly employed interventions used in therapy of children in each developmental stage from preschool through elementary school. In addition, specific aspects of the content and process of therapy with children and their families will be discussed.

Axline's Principles of Treatment

Although the specifics of the therapeutic approach will vary with the child's age and developmental level, Axline's eight principles of treatment are as appropriate today as when they were first presented (Axline, 1947). The principles provide guidelines appropriate for the child therapist of any discipline. They include: child therapist of any discipline. They include:

1. Establishing as quickly as possible a warm, friendly relationship to promote a positive rapport between therapist and child
2. Accepting the child exactly as he is
3. Providing a relationship that is conducive to the child expressing feelings completely
4. Recognizing the child's expressed feelings and reflecting them back in such a manner that the child gains insight into his behavior
5. Accepting the child's ability to solve his own problems if given the opportunity (It is the child's responsibility to make choices and initiate change.)
6. Following the child's lead at all times and making no attempt to direct or lead the child
7. Realizing that therapy is a gradual process and should not be hurried
8. Setting limits only to provide a sense of reality and security for the child and to help him recognize his responsibility in the relationship

Since Axline published her work, the abused and neglected child who has a severe character disorder or prepsychotic disturbance has been seen in increasing numbers. Axline worked primarily with neurotic children. Due to the increased numbers of abused and neglected children an additional principle can be suggested:

9. The abused and neglected child usually requires more time to establish a relationship. These children often need the use of food as rewards to feel cared about. They also require firm limits to contain their anger and hostility toward adults.

As one works with children of different ages, it becomes apparent that following the Axline guidelines requires flexibility.

Setting

Play therapy can occur in a variety of settings. It may take place on a pediatric unit with toys brought by the therapist or in a regular office where the therapist's concerns with not dirtying the carpet or furniture may interfere with attentiveness to the child's behavior. To minimize these hazards, a special playroom set aside for play therapy works best for both therapist and child. Use of the same setting promotes the child's familiarity and comfort and leads to free expression of feelings. Inevitably children ask, "Do other kids come here? What do they do here? Do you play with them, too?" These questions clearly indicate the room's symbolic significance to them.

For some children, the playroom may be one of the few stable settings in their lives. For most children, it represents a safe place where a very special relationship with an adult they have grown to trust and respect can occur and where the child is free to express feelings, secure about their confidentiality. The room and toys may be shared with others; however, the child comes to feel that their relationship is very special and unique.

Toys

Though the contents of the playroom may vary, there are certain considerations to be kept in mind. The toys should lend themselves to free expression and creativity. There should be toys that match the child's developmental level, in addition to toys that allow for both previously learned and more advanced behaviors. Generally, more simple and versatile toys permit greater fantasy play.

Typically, playroom equipment includes:

1. Paper, crayons, watercolors, brushes, and fingerpaints are probably the most versatile and widely used of all the play materials. They can be used in many different ways to express the child's moods and thoughts.
2. Clay, or, generally, the easier-to-handle Play-doh, provides the child with the opportunity for sensual enjoyment and sensorimotor and three-dimensional expression.
3. Hand puppets seem to lend themselves to safe expression of strong emotions in words and action.
4. Water is an option that is frequently used by preschool children and is attractive to children who are obsessive-compulsive or autistic.
5. Dolls are used the most symbolically of all the toys by the child. A family doll set is generally useful in that the child's play with it will illustrate the family life-style and family conflicts and alliances. A large doll and baby bottle permit regressive play and are particularly useful when the child is feeling rivalry with a sibling. Anatomically correct dolls are helpful in working with sexually abused children.

6. Doll houses represent the child's perception of home and family and provide a setting for playing out the child's or family conflicts.
7. Toy telephones are a widely accepted symbol of communication. Children will often use the toy telephone to carry on fantasy conversations with significant figures in their lives and to discuss feelings they cannot express directly.
8. Guns are another optional toy. The aggression and destruction they symbolize can also be played out with tinker toys or a finger.
9. Blocks for building can be helpful.
10. Transportation items (toy cars, trucks, etc.) are often included.

Initial Session

The first session with a child is a most important experience for both child and therapist. The child is brought to a strange place, usually for reasons unclear to the child, introduced, and expected to remain alone with a strange adult. Erikson (1964) sensitively speculates on how a child might feel and react in such a situation. The therapist's sensitivity in perceiving and responding to the child's feelings sets the stage for and begins establishing the parameters of the child-therapist relationship.

One can learn a great deal about a child in the initial session. For instance, factors such as the child's and parents' approach to the situation, whether the child is oblivious or reluctant to leave the parent, the toys the child chooses or avoids, and the nonverbal and verbal response to the therapist begin to provide a picture of the child. The picture will include thoughts about the child's sense of competence, curiosity, degree of separation anxiety and interpersonal skills, to name only a few. Prior to meeting with the child, the nurse will need to have thought out how to deal with one or more of the following issues that will probably arise. Typical issues include difficulty in separating parent and child, the child's hesitancy or refusal to accompany the therapist, or whether or how to explain the purpose of the visit to the child or answer the questions put about why the child is coming. To respond appropriately, the nurse must keep in mind the developmentally appropriate behaviors for the child. Being clearly aware of the usual fantasies, conflicts, and play patterns of the developmental period permits one to differentiate more precisely behaviors that represent stage-specific conflicts from those that indicate psychopathology. Even within the norm there are individual differences. A single area of difficulty does not necessarily mean the child is disturbed. Finally, it is important to remember, especially since it is the initial session, that repeated observations of the child are necessary to provide sufficient information for an adequate assessment.

Setting Limits

The issue of limit setting in play therapy raises numerous questions and basic philosophical differences among therapists. Most would agree that children need to be stopped from hurting themselves, the therapist, or destroying property wantonly. Other questions arise. Should limits be set in advance or only as they are needed? Should situations be structured in order to avoid limits? Is it possible to have too many limits? What attitude, tone of voice, or behavior helps set limits nonpunitively? There are many ways to state a limit against shooting at the therapist with a dart gun and each would convey a different attitude. The following statements exemplify such differences: "I can't let you do that," "There's a rule you can't do that," "You must not do that," or "You can shoot at the target, but not at me." Again, once a limit has been set, what if the child defies it? Should the child ever be removed from the playroom? These are only a few of the difficult questions each therapist must find answers to in order to maintain a therapeutic relationship with the child.

Keeping the following questions in mind is helpful when looking for guidelines to understanding the child's aggressiveness. Why is the child "testing limits?" What is the meaning of the aggressive behavior to the child? What are the feelings being expressed? What other feelings are being triggered by the behavior? What is the child's reaction to being "limited?" How can the child be helped to understand the feelings he is experiencing? And how is the therapist handling her or his own feelings during the interaction?

Careful observation of the antecedent play leading to aggression and subsequent to the aggressive behavior gives the therapist clues. Does the child relax and become constructively playful, or attempt to "make up" or make peace with the therapist, or fear retaliation, or feel guilty, or continue with ever increasing aggressiveness?

While Schiffer's (1952) permissiveness and Moustakas' (1953) more strict limit setting represent both ends of the continuum of therapist positions on the subject, there is little research to support either position. It does seem reasonable that in therapy, as in other areas in life, children need a clear definition of acceptable and unacceptable behavior.

Purpose

Ginott (1959) identified a rationale for the use of limits in individual and group play therapy.

1. Limit setting encourages symbolic expression of wishes and feelings that might otherwise be expressed in destructive ways, leading to fear of retaliation. Sexual and aggressive feelings can be played out with dolls, puppets, paints, or through talk. These same feelings would be frightening or bring punishment if acted out with people.
2. Limit setting permits the therapist to maintain an empathic and accepting attitude toward the child. In the face of therapist-directed aggression, rapid limit setting reduces therapist anxiety and anger. Setting limits creates security for both child and therapist. Ginott makes the point that limit setting or therapeutic controls always apply to behavior but not to verbalization. The child needs the freedom to express his feelings and fantasies verbally and through play.
3. Limit setting ensures the physical safety of child and therapist. Responsible adults cannot allow children to engage in behaviors that are unsafe such as hanging out of windows or throwing darts at the therapist.
4. Limit setting assists in strengthening a child's ego controls. Many impulsive children require the therapist to bolster their deficient ego and superego controls. By accepting the child's feelings expressed in play or words and preventing unacceptable behavior, the therapist demonstrates how such feelings can be nondestructively expressed and reinforces realistic controls of behavior.
5. Some limit setting occurs to reinforce legally, ethically, or socially acceptable behaviors. Children may not sexually play with each other or deliberately defecate or urinate in the playroom in part because these behaviors are socially unacceptable. A child may use "off color" language in the playroom but may not yell obscenities out the window or with staff outside the playroom.
6. Finally, limits are also set for economic reasons. Toys and materials should not be destroyed needlessly. No matter who is stocking the playroom, an agency or the therapist, budgets are limited.

Process of Limit Setting

Limits need to be stated in a friendly but firm manner. They need to be presented nonpunitively and stated clearly and firmly for a specific behavior. "Walls are not for painting." Other more appropriate alternatives are offered to the child; "This paper is fine for painting." The child's feelings are recognized and expression of them is facilitated. "I can tell you really want to paint that wall." And, finally, if the child indicates resentment at the limit set, expression of those feelings is also facilitated; "You don't like it that you can't paint on the walls." It is important to phrase limits in ways that do not lessen the child's self-respect. That is, "Time is up for today," is a more neutral statement than "Your time is up, you must leave now."

One often can set limits nonverbally so that it is even less an issue for the child. If a child is tapping the window with a mallet, one can simply give her/him the pounding board. Time limits are also necessary. Children need time to prepare for the end of the session, so a five-minute and a one-minute reminder are helpful. When the time is up, this fact should be stated clearly and adhered to consistently. Children who have difficulty separating may balk, but usually even they will gain security from limits that are predictable and consistent.

Timing

Many therapists believe that limits are best not mentioned until they are needed. To begin therapy with a list of rules and prohibitions for behaviors that may never occur seems unnecessary and can also serve to further inhibit an already overly inhibited child or act as a challenge to aggressive children.

"Breaking" the Limits

Despite the above discussion, what does one do when a child does break the rules? The difficulty such infractions create for therapists is perhaps illustrated by their reluctance to discuss it. The literature on the subject is scanty. Few writers, even those who emphasize the importance of limits, discuss specifically how to deal with such situations. What does one do when the child attempts to engage in a physical battle with the therapist? Some therapists (Bixler, 1949; Moustakas, 1953) suggest that, after an initial warning, the therapist should end the session and send the child from the playroom. Other writers (Ginott, 1959) object to making the child leave the playroom. This approach not only indicates rejection of the child, it also dramatically reinforces the child's belief that he or she can defeat the therapist. It is frightening to feel that no one can help the child control his or her behavior. The therapist needs to be prepared to stop any possible physical attack with nonpunitive physical restraint. Therapists who are prepared to quickly employ such restraint rarely need to do so. Ordinarily, firm verbal interdiction of behavior and clearly stated alternatives that the therapist might use if the behavior continues halt the impulsive behavior. Limit setting can be instrumental in establishing a safe, secure, yet accepting environment for the child. Without limits, an atmosphere conducive to effective therapy would be impossible.

Issues in Therapy

The therapist needs to be attentive to the child's verbal and nonverbal behavior. Early in therapy, the child asks the therapist numerous, seemingly irrelevant questions. For example, "Who broke this crayon?" is not simply a request for information. This or similar questions are most likely disguised versions of "What happened to the kid who broke the crayon?"

If the therapist understands this as the real question, then most likely the response will be something such as, "Sometimes things get broken, that happens." A response like this gives the child the information that children do not have to be extra careful or specially good here and that the therapist does not get angry easily even over broken toys. By responding to the hidden meanings of the child's questions, the therapist conveys an understanding of the child's curiosity, fears, and wishes and helps present a clear picture of both the therapist and the structure of therapy.

Therapist Language

The therapist needs to use language that is both simple and at the child's developmental level. Making interpretations or identifying the symbolic meaning of an act only turns the child off. It is best to follow the child's lead. When a girl points to the mother doll and says, "She hates the girl," it is better to respond in the character created with "She hates her" rather than to say "Mother hates you." One waits for the child to identify the characters and objects in play.

To Play or Not To Play

There is a controversy among child therapists about whether or not the therapist should participate with the child in play and games. Children often try to engage the therapist in their fantasy play or involve him or her in board games, tic-tac-toe, or checkers. Some therapists believe that therapy is inhibited when the therapist assumes an assigned role. Each role the therapist assumes requires self-examination of the feelings aroused by playing the role. Not playing with the child ensures that the session is strictly centered on the child.

Therapists who believe in playing with children recognize that many children have usually not had enjoyable play experiences and pleasure with adults so that the therapist serves as a role model for them. The child needs interaction with a friendly participant as part of engaging her or him in treatment. Erikson's (1940) principle that the therapist does not intervene in the child's play by gesture or interpretation except to facilitate it or to reduce rising anxiety that would lead to play disruption provides a meaningful guideline for therapists. It would be appropriate for the therapist to engage in an activity with a child to facilitate therapy. For example, the therapist may use a storytelling technique and begin a story that symbolizes some of the significant issues the child is dealing with in therapy and expect the child to continue the story. Berlin (1977) discusses the use of checkers as a means of communication with children who find it difficult to play or talk.

Do's and Don'ts

DRESS. Both therapist and child need to wear comfortable clothes that are easily cared for and appropriate to playroom activities. Overdressing focuses on cleanliness and may be used unconsciously to inhibit "messy" play with paints and clay as smearing and sensual pleasure may be frightening.

GIFTS. Gifts are also a controversial issue. Some therapists refuse all gifts such as gum or candy from children and refrain from offering gifts as well. Others will accept small gifts offered by the child such as a picture made during the session and will also provide children with gifts in the form of snacks or treats. Therapists must decide on an approach consistent with their own treatment philosophy. Once decided, they need to be consistent with themselves and the children about the policy and the rationale for it.

PERSONAL QUESTIONS. At times, a child may quiz the therapist asking very direct personal questions. Therapists do not need to provide children with their life histories. It is usually sufficient to acknowledge the child's curiosity and interest in the therapist. If pressed, the therapists' responses to specific questions should be truthful, short, and, if possible, general.

CLEANING THE PLAYROOM. Therapists may question whether or not a child needs to pick up toys at the end of the session. The answer to the question largely depends on the needs of the child and the therapist's treatment philosophy. For an overly neat, compulsive child, it may be best to encourage leaving the playroom sometimes in disarray in order to support greater freedom of expression in the child. With a rebellious child, picking up the toys can become a battle and nontherapeutic, so one might not bring up the issue. Having other children pick up part of the play materials may help to underscore the end of the session and a return to those behaviors expected in reality. The sharing of the cleaning up may provide a new adult model for the child. This issue is best dealt with on an individual basis.

Types of Play Therapy

There are some special types of play therapy for dealing with specific psychopathology and therapeutic problems in children. Among these are structured play therapy as described by Levy (1939), Solomon (1955), and Hambridge (1955); using games to involve nonverbal or resistive children, as discussed by Loomis (1957), Gardner (1974, 1979), and Berlin (1977); and using drawings and children's art productions as described by Naumberg (1973) and others.

Crisis intervention and brief therapy both require active therapist participation to structure the child's activities in sessions. A more focused approach is used to help children work through recently experienced crises such as a death in the family, divorce, and severe physical illness in the child, sibling, or parents. Jernberg's book *Theraplay* (1979) presents a detailed discussion of structured play therapy.

Structured play therapy techniques are used to deal with crises and emergent situations. The stage is set by the therapist so that the crisis a child experiences around the birth of a sibling can be enacted in play. Having a mother and a baby doll out in the playroom with no other toys in sight usually focuses the child's play so that eventually the feelings aroused about the new arrival come out. Repetitive playing out facilitates both release of feelings and mastery of conflicts by the child.

Another common crisis in which structured play therapy is particularly beneficial is in preparing a child for hospitalization or traumatic procedures such as surgery. Utilizing both real and facsimiles of necessary implements and dolls, the child can enact the situation. Repetitive reenactments of such themes permit the child to deal with conflicts and anxieties about threats to body integrity, pain, passivity, powerlessness, and punishment. There have been numerous discussions in the nursing literature by nurses who have worked with physically ill children in this manner. Petrillo's work is one of the earliest in this vein (Petrillo & Sanger, 1972).

PROCESS IN PLAY THERAPY

The process of play therapy can only be learned experientially through the therapeutic relationship with the child and careful supervision of the clinical issues that arise during the course of treatment. This section will focus on significant issues that frequently arise and need consideration and resolution in order to facilitate the treatment process.

Developmental Aspects of Play

In play therapy, one of the treatment goals is to facilitate the child's reaching a level of development appropriate for his or her age and abilities. A disturbed child may become "stuck" at a particular stage or level or may return to previously learned and then outgrown behaviors. During therapy, such a child's progress can be assessed by the extent to which he or she relives or "outgrows" earlier stages or behaviors and moves to a more age-appropriate level. In order to facilitate this forward movement, the therapist needs to be attentive not only to the child's emotional needs but also to his or her developmental needs for sensory-tactile and spatial exploration, motor muscular movement, and cognitive stimulation. During therapy, opportunities are provided for the child to explore objects tactilely and through taste, smell, sight, and hearing.

The more severe the child's illness, the more apt is exploration to be limited to the tactile sphere. A child's progress in therapy is usually reflected in the increasing use and self-confidence in using other senses and in acquiring new skills. These same senses are important in facilitating the child's ego development during therapy. Young children seeking their own body boundaries and capacities may need to squeeze themselves into cabinets, jump off tables, or pick up heavy chairs. Though these behaviors may have other meanings, the therapist needs to be alert to the possibility that the child is exploring new sensations and refining skills that will enhance his or her sense of competence and body image. After the initial opportunities for facilitated exploration are experienced in the playroom, the child then is more free to seek out other opportunities outside the playroom.

Play as Conflict Expression

Freud's observation of the young child's play with a toy tied to a string by throwing it away and pulling it back again may have been the first attempt to look at play symbolically and diagnostically (Freud, 1922). Freud interpreted from his knowledge of the child's life and ordinary behaviors that the child was reenacting through play the inner conflict aroused by his mother's disappearances and returns.

Play as a Diagnostic Aid

A mentally ill child's play differs from that of an emotionally healthy child in many clearly defined ways. The differences in the approach to play, the behavior toward others during play, and the feelings expressed in play are all significant variables. A child's play may indicate both the type and severity of the illness experienced.

The four-year-old autistic child may sit in one place spinning an object, refusing to be moved, not talking, and ignoring everyone. The four-year-old neurotic child may be tentative in play and speech, fearful of adults, and engage in safer repetitive drawings that adults accept. The normal four-year-old may be in constant motion, exploring the world, curious about people, and demanding to know "why" certain events or things occur.

The child's play can be studied in relation to the materials chosen for play and the nature and type of play in which the child engages. Questions to be addressed include whether the play is spontaneous, lively, and free or solemn and inhibited. Is the play appropriate to the child's developmental level, more typical of a younger child, or even oversophisticated and adultlike? Does the child use the play materials constructively or destructively? Does the child exhibit appropriately focused concentration and attention span, or is the play restricted and confined to certain objects or activities, or within a brief period does the child handle all of the toys and focus on none? Does the child's play show fantasy and symbolism, or is it repetitive and constricted as in arranging objects in neat patterns? How does the child relate to the adult in the situation? These queries help the therapist understand the nature of the child's problem and give clues to the underlying conflict.

Resistance

It is assumed that the reader is familiar with the concept of resistance. This discussion will focus on the unique aspects of the process in working with children. Resistance is used to refer to the many and varied ways the child avoids becoming involved in treatment.

Resistance usually becomes apparent in the initial or early sessions with a child. Resistance is usually an expression of conflict about destructive impulses that must not be made known to others. It may be well established even before the child and therapist meet. Markowitz (1959) discusses possible reasons for resistance especially at the beginning of treatment. For example, the child is often, if not actually unaware as sometimes happens, unconvinced of the need for treatment. Realistically, a child is smaller and weaker than and dependent on the adult. The child is afraid of adults to some extent. The child's own difficulty in impulse control and perhaps painful past experiences contribute to the fear. Children frequently believe the therapist can "read their minds," which to their way of magical thinking only makes them more fearful of having their hostile, destructive thoughts revealed. Anna Freud (1946) describes permanent defense phenomena in children, defensive processes that have become dissociated from their original source and remain as permanent character traits. She believes that body rigidity, stiffness, a fixed smile, and contemptuous or arrogant behavior are often examples of this phenomenon and represent a form of resistance against the expression of impulses. Most therapists agree that premature interpretation of the resistance is frightening to the child and only heightens the resistance. Sugar (1974) points out that attention should be given first to the most easily accessible levels of resistance. What is in awareness and troublesome needs to be dealt with first, before proceeding to those resistances out of awareness. Missed appointments by older children may certainly be a form of resistance. With younger children, missed appointments are more likely to be the result of parental resistance.

Common Forms of Resistance Seen in Children

Most children enter treatment at their parents' insistence. A child prefers to live in the present, prefers to act rather than to ruminate, and prefers to externalize rather than internalize the source of problems.

The child may often fear that the need to see a therapist means the child is "bad," "stupid," or "crazy." However, children are also afraid to discuss these fears, as they might discover that others think they are awful as well. Therefore, therapists need to verbalize the possibility of such fears and allay the anxiety with most, if not all, children they see.

A child who is chronically angry often directs the anger felt towards the parents at the therapist partially in an attempt to avoid treatment. Behaviors used can include excessive use of silences, shrugs, or "I don't know" in response to therapist overtures.

Overcompliance with the therapist's suggestions may also serve as resistance. The child who ingratiatingly complies may be seeking to avoid anxiety-provoking interactions with adults and to ensure the therapist's positive regard.

A child often feels that criticizing his or her parents to the therapist is both disloyal and unsafe. It is helpful to enlist the parents' help in encouraging the child that he can reveal his feelings with no fear of repercussions. This fear also makes the issue of confidentiality for the child of all ages a major issue.

A child who has been abused or neglected usually anticipates similar treatment from all adults including the therapist. With such children, the major treatment goal may be to help them experience a nurturing and concerned relationship with an adult that helps the child to develop a new sense of trust with adults.

Resistance in children may also be an attempt to express their independence and to deny their dependency needs and feelings of helplessness. Usually, tremendous ambivalence is present and the child's behavior may both express refusal to participate and a wish to be made to come. Therapists need to be attentive to such expressions of ambivalence. The positive aspects of the relationship must be used to keep the child in treatment.

Transference and Countertransference

Issues of transference and countertransference that occur in work with children are not frequently discussed in the literature. Transference refers to the projection onto the therapist by the child of attitudes experienced with parent figures. Countertransference refers to the therapist's reaction to the child's behaviors with unconscious feelings from past experiences. Both concepts are critical to therapeutic work with children. Their negative manifestations may not only interfere with therapeutic progress but could also result in disruption of treatment if not recognized and resolved. Positive feelings need to be recognized in order to be used judiciously to promote a therapeutic outcome.

Anna Freud (1946) believes that transference in children is different from that in adults because the child is still usually living with and emotionally tied to the parents. Thus, transference in the classical sense does not occur in children. Fraiberg (1962) points out that the therapist inevitably shares with the parents the child's feelings toward them of affection, dependence, and aggression. The child then projects upon the therapist both covertly and overtly the attitudes, expectations, and feelings aroused in the child by experiences with parents.

Common Expressions of Transference and Countertransference in Children

Preschool children are generally brought for psychiatric treatment because of problems with attachment, trust or separation—individuation. Such problems may result in withdrawn, needy children who are generally apathetic or who are angry, oppositional, and destructive. These children are frequently enuretic or encopretic. Both types of children generally evoke countertransference feelings in the therapist that may be expressed as retaliatory anger, disgust, and withdrawal. The following is a clinical illustration:

> Louise was a six-year-old girl who suffered from grand mal seizures as a result of brain damage from an illness in infancy. The resulting guilt of the mother contributed to severe marital problems, divorce, and a severely disturbed mother-child relationship in which the child used her seizures to control her mother's life and protect herself from the necessity of growing up and assuming responsibility for her own behavior. Louise was an obstinate, negativistic child who was expelled from a first grade special education class because of her noisy disobedience and refusal to attempt any classroom work. During a session in which Louise was angry at the therapist, she said, "You just wait, I'll make myself dizzy until I have a seizure and then you'll be sorry." The therapist replied that she would be sorry if Louise did that, since she knew having a seizure scared Louise and made her tired and sleepy afterwards. The therapist added that she thought it would make Louise feel better if she would say her feelings instead

of trying to make herself have a seizure. Mad feelings, sad feelings, even scary feelings would be less scary once she could talk about them. Louise said nothing but engaged the therapist in play with the doll family in which the mother doll was always leaving the children alone, locking them out of the house or in their room for minor infractions. The play portrayed the child's projected anger at being expected to behave more age-appropriately. All adults were seen as rejecting and depriving when they expected more age-appropriate behaviors of her, thus threatening her avoidance of growth and independence.

The behaviors of very ill or psychotic children, such as hostility, destructiveness, and very infantile and bizarre behaviors, tend to arouse anxiety and occasionally even fear in the therapist. The repetitive, seemingly meaningless, ritualistic behavior and the oppositional attitudes to every adult approach of the psychotic child serves to control the situation. The child's behavior can also be enraging and produce feelings of helplessness that result in withdrawal or rejection by the therapist. Therapists need to explore these feelings as possible derivatives of early childhood feelings about being controlled or powerless. Once the origins of such feelings are identified, the therapist can be more attentive to the child and understand the need to produce such feelings in adults in order for the child to protect his or her own sense of vulnerability (Berlin, in press).

Children who are experiencing intense feelings of rivalry with the same-sex parent for the opposite parent often come to treatment because of fears, nightmares, and generally high levels of anxiety. The child in the midst of experiencing the family romance often projects onto the therapist both the hostile and the seductive behavior they may have experienced from their parents.

There is little in the literature about the feelings aroused in the therapist by a child's seductive behavior. Though some of the therapist's reaction may be due to unresolved past sexual conflicts, some aspects may be due to the adultlike quality of the child's sexual behavior (Berlin, in press; Christ, 1973; Yandell, 1973). Awareness of such responses in oneself is critical to being able to assess their meaning from the therapist's past and thus to identify the possible meanings to the child and help children with their conflicts.

Constricted, repressed parents may confuse sensually gratifying behavior with sexuality. Therapists may also make the same mistake. In doing so, the child's seeking of cuddling-closeness may be prevented. Recognition of the child's needs permits the therapist to offer the nurturance and closeness the child is seeking.

Self-stimulating behavior from the child often elicits either retaliation or paralysis from the parent. Masturbation in our society has usually been characterized as a forbidden activity. A child masturbating in the playroom makes us acutely aware of our own residual conflicts from our childhood about such behavior. Awareness of our own conflicting feelings permits therapists to recognize the developmental aspects of the behavior. In a toddler, it may be a search for previously not experienced warmth and physical comfort and in a preschool child a focus for self-satisfaction and pleasure (Berlin, in press).

Other therapists focus on transference as an integral part of the therapeutic alliance. The therapist's supportive stance reinforces the child's ego functions and reality testing while communicating an understanding of the child's feelings. A therapeutic alliance is essential in order for the child to trust the therapist. It enables the therapist to be effectively supportive during periods of resistance and negative transference.

Countertransference feelings are common in working with children. Only close attention on the therapist's part permits such feelings to be used as data about the child's developmental needs and problems rather than having them detrimentally affect therapeutic work. To accomplish this goal, child psychotherapists require clinical supervision, consultation, and/or personal therapy to resolve the personal issues that affect their clinical work.

Dealing with the child's projected feelings is inevitable in working with children. Understanding of both transference and countertransference issues is critical to psychotherapeutic work with children.

Reflections and Interpretations

Depending on one's position as a nondirective or dynamic therapist, either reflection of feelings or interpretative statements is considered to be the most important tool of treatment. Reflection usually precedes interpretation. Haworth (1964) points out that to the child the difference of emphasis or meaning is probably less obvious than either school would like to admit.

Whereas all therapists recognize that the content of the play is important in conveying the child's message, it is the attitudes and emotions expressed in the play that should be the focus of the therapist's attention. This skill is perhaps one of the most difficult for a therapist to learn. Many have noted that, in work with children, significant material will reoccur until the therapist has recognized the cues, provided he or she has done nothing to discourage its expression (Colm, 1951; Ross, 1959). Most agree that the more data the therapist has understood from the child's play, the more chance for accuracy in the interpretation but, even more importantly, the more likely the child will be to accept its accuracy.

Nondirective therapists are more concerned with accurately reflecting the feeling tone expressed in the activity that then communicates an empathetic understanding to the child.

Erikson (1940) points out that a critical aspect of symbolic play occurs when the child begins to remember previously forgotten conflicted feelings. Emergence of such intense feelings often brings about a disruption in the child's play behavior. According to Erikson, these situations are in fact therapeutic crises. If handled empathetically and effectively by the therapist, the child acquires insight; if handled poorly (i.e., not recognized), the child's resistance is intensified and therapeutic progress may be halted.

Termination

Many issues need to be considered concerning the timing and process of termination. Who should make the decision to terminate, the child or the therapist? Should parents be involved in the decision and if so when? Should termination be final once planned for or should it be gradual with increasing intervals between sessions? What feelings are the therapist, child, and family likely to experience at ending treatment? What if the child "regresses" as termination approaches? Does this mean the child is not ready to leave? How should such behaviors at this time be handled by the therapist?

One may regard termination of treatment for the child as an opportunity to deal with those feelings that are troublesome to all of us. Learning to deal in a healthy fashion with endings is a necessary component of living.

In most settings where children are seen, community mental health centers or private practices, children can be seen for only a limited period of time. It is generally necessary to limit treatment to meeting the treatment goals originally established. In the settings mentioned, therapy is usually ego supportive, which may mean that the treatment is terminated even though the child has not achieved insight into or mastery of most underlying conflicts.

The child and family need to be prepared for the end of treatment as far in advance as possible. The child needs to be involved with the decision and help reflect on the original reasons for treatment and whether these reasons continue to make treatment necessary. Depending on the age and development of the child, the date of termination can be set by the therapist or by mutual agreement with the child. The reasons and time for termination require repeated discussion. The therapist's continued interest in the child after ending treatment needs to be emphasized. Letters and phone calls may be helpful. If therapy is ended because the family is moving or has financial troubles or illness, the child needs preparation for the termination and an evaluation of the progress made during treatment.

The child's developmental stage and concept of the future determine how far in advance preparation for termination needs to begin. Very young children with short memory spans need at least two to four sessions to deal with the process. The therapist's communication of interest in the child's future and willingness to see the child again if the need arises is reassuring.

Emotional reactions to ending the relationship are inevitable. Children need the opportunity to work through, with therapist help, the conflicting feelings aroused by termination. Children may on the one hand assert that they wish to come for the rest of their lives or may abruptly state that, "This is my last time." The ambivalence expressed in these behaviors is typical but also indicates the child's attempt to resolve the ambivalence by taking control. A concrete plan mutually decided upon about the number of sessions left and what still needs to be worked on helps the child assume control and diminishes anxiety. Often the anxiety about ending is expressed in a recurrence of the behaviors that had originally led to treatment. The reappearance of earlier behaviors is common at this time and not an indication to continue treatment; usually such behaviors validate the importance of the therapeutic relationship for the child. The therapist's clarity about the progress made helps the child gently face the fears of ending the relationship and being on his own.

If therapy has been successful, children have gained more confidence in their abilities to think and act independently. They are usually anxious to do so and to move on in their lives and relationships. Termination of the relationship represents both the end of the old and the beginning of the new for the child. Successfully dealing with this termination provides a model for the child in future relationships.

WORK WITH THE FAMILY

Although this chapter focuses primarily on work with the child in individual and group treatment, it is clear that improvement is determined by the behavioral changes that occur in "real life" rather than in the therapeutic setting alone. Most child therapists agree that, to achieve any long-term therapeutic gains, the child's family must be involved in the treatment process.

Families usually function as units and the behaviors, pathology, and strengths of their individual members affect all the other members. Family conflicts can create and maintain pathology. Conflict resolution is necessary to reduce or extinguish pathology. Even though therapeutic progress has been achieved with a child, return to an unchanged family situation greatly increases the probability of recurring psychopathology.

Approaches to Working with Families

A number of modalities have evolved to engage families of children in treatment. Family therapy may well be the treatment of choice in most instances (Critchley, 1982b). Family therapy is discussed in detail in Chapter 13. However, in many instances there may be other therapeutic approaches that are more appropriate and less threatening. If significant family members refuse to participate in treatment, or one or both parents suffer from severe mental illness or psychophysiological disorders, or the family is extremely disorganized and chaotic, or skilled family therapists are not available, other approaches with the family need to be tried (Critchley, 1982a).

Other modalities include individual and couple therapy. Parent education and counseling are often appropriate for the families described above. Supportive parent groups are valuable for families with severely mentally ill or physically ill members where sharing common problems can reduce the sense of isolation and the intense guilt and anger these families feel.

Work with the family accomplishes several purposes: first, it prepares the child and family for treatment; second, it helps the parents to deal with conflicts that result in or affect the child's psychopathology; third, it helps the parents deal with their own problems that contribute to the child's illness and make it difficult for them to be aware of the child's developmental needs and of how to assist in resolving the child's problems. Finally, in some instances parents will need help to accept their child's need for foster care or relinquishment.

No matter what the therapeutic goal is for the child, parent collaboration is a necessary ingredient for successful child therapy. Many parents fear involvement in treatment. Frequently, these fears arise from an understandable apprehension of the unknown, especially of possible changes in the equilibrium within themselves and their families. However, most parents wish to do what is best for their child. Before they are able actively to be helpful to their child, they need assistance and support to change a poor self-image as a parent and to be able to meet some of their own previously unmet needs.

Task-Oriented Approach

Work with the family as part of the child's treatment is usually different from family therapy because it is more directive and task-oriented. With infants and young children, the parents' inability to facilitate the child's play and exploration may result in a frozen, apathetic, or very angry, defiant child. Parents can be helped to recognize their child's developmental needs as well as their own conflicts around such issues as play and mastery. Encouraging parents to be more playful with their children can be aided by the use of one-way mirrors and ear microphones. Parents can then observe the therapist and be observed, directed, and encouraged in their efforts to play with their child.

Videotaping may also help the parents to recognize their frozen, inhibited, and monotonous tone of voice. They can then practice other ways of interacting with their child. Parents will often use the therapist as a role model in play, imitating the therapist's exaggerated affect and expression of feelings until they are more free to express their own feelings in play.

Focusing parental awareness on the child's needs and their own critical part in meeting these needs characterizes task-oriented work with families. This type of family intervention focuses not on family problems and pathology but on learning new behaviors for interaction with the child. For some parents this is an impossible task, for others carrying out tasks and finding that they can alter the child's behavior produces immense satisfaction and motivation to continue.

A related focus in task-oriented work with parents is on parental interactions that seriously affect their child's self-concept and behavior. For example, if parents are passive and helplessly accepting of their child's encopresis rather than expressing firm and clear expectations, this will be an issue in work with the parents. Parents are helped to be more firm and clear, and this response changes not only the child's behavior but also parental attitudes toward each other. They can express greater self-expectations and expectations of the spouse.

This focused, task-oriented approach to work with parents is in part determined by the particular problems of the child that reflect parental behaviors that can be modified.

GROUP THERAPY

Play group therapy for children was first carried out by Slavson in 1934. Today, those clinicians who use play group therapy generally use developmental ego psychology as their theoretical orientation. Despite having been in existence for almost 50 years, play group therapy is still not widely used nor is it generally well understood. Frequent questions include the differences and similarities between group activity and group psychotherapy, benefits of individual versus play group therapy, indications and contraindications for group psychotherapy, and issues of transference and countertransference in groups.

Preparation

Children need to be prepared for group therapy as one would prepare a child for individual treatment. In language appropriate to the child's capacity to understand, he can be told that children come to the group because they are sad, have worries, feel unhappy, get mad easily, or have troublesome feelings towards themselves or others. Even a preschool child can understand such an explantation. An honest explanation rather than telling the child the group is for playing games is far more conducive to trust and openness.

Types of Groups

Several different types of group therapy have evolved since Slavson's original work. Table 12.3 indicates the different types and characteristics and the most appropriate age groups for each type.

The group therapy experience described by Slavson requires considerable space and extensive equipment. Most settings are limited in both areas, so Slavson's original technique has been modified to include more restricted types of activities and more use of discussions or interviews both individually and as a group. With young children, the play activities are the therapeutic modality. As children grow older, verbal interchange and discussion are used as the mode for therapy and the activities primarily are for release of tension and anxiety.

Group Size and Length of Sessions

Group size depends on the ages of the children and their presenting problems. The younger the child, the smaller the group needs to be. Groups with children with poor impulse control also require fewer members. Group sessions for children can last from 45 minutes to two hours. Preschool children's short attention span limits the useful length of a session. Administrative constraints may only permit 50- to 60-minute sessions. Sessions are usually held weekly, although twice-a-week groups are common. Despite statements to the contrary, group therapy is not the answer to treating more children in less time. Any group requires time for trust and relationships to develop. Additional time is required of the therapist besides the actual time in sessions in order to maintain contact with parents, teachers, and absent children and for clinically recording the sessions. Cotherapists can be helpful in understanding and dealing with the greater number and complexity of interventions required.

Table 12.3 Ages, Size, and Characteristic Types of Group Psychotherapy for Children

Age Range	*Group Size*	*Type*	*Goals*	*Characteristics*
Preschool	4–6	Play group therapy	Normalizing feelings expressed Socialization Positive interactions with peers and adults	Structured by therapist Age-appropriate Doll-play house equipment, (furniture, dishes, etc.) "Dress-up" clothes, hats, shoes Graphic materials (clay, sand, water, paint) Minimal reflections and interpretations
6–9	5–8	Therapeutic play group	Provides corrective life experiences	Structured by children and therapist Age-appropriate
9–11	6–8	Activity group therapy	Acts out conflicts and trial resolutions via group play and verbalization Positive interactions with peers and adults	Minature toys and animals Outlets for aggression (hand puppets, "Bo Bo," punching figure, plastic knives and guns, etc.) Minimal reflection and interpretation
9–11	5–8	Activity-interview group psychotherapy	Expression of conflicts both in play and verbally Group support for expression of conflict and trial resolution Develop acceptance/insight into problems	Structured by children and therapist Arts and crafts, group activities, games, board and team games Active reflection and interpretation by therapist and encouraging this from group members

Selection and Screening

Slavson and Shiffer (1975) have stated that the effectiveness of group therapy with children is a direct result of the care taken in selecting and grouping children correctly. Group balance is a goal to be strived for at all times. They indicate that the children who benefit the most from activity group therapy are those with behavior disorders, neurotic traits, and mild neuroses and schizoid personalities. They believe that children who are negativistic, lack minimal impulse control, or are immature and regressive are inappropriate for group therapy. MacLennan (1977) describes the types of children for whom he believes activity group therapy to be most helpful. They include children with problems in ego development, specifically such problems as defiance, aggressiveness, ego constriction, overdependency, withdrawal, and poor social skills. He further states that totally self-absorbed children and those who experience major regression in unstructured settings are poor candidates for group psychotherapy. Sugar (1974) believes that only those children who have the ability to use play or language to express their conflicts and fantasies and who can profit from interpretations will benefit from group psychotherapy. Generally, group therapists tend to agree that the most suitable children for interpretative groups are those with behavior disorders in the neurotic range or those with psychosomatic disorders, neurotic symptoms, inhibitions, and sexual problems, all of which are responsive to verbalization. Schiffer (1969) identified preschool children who are hostile, destructive, compulsive, and narcissistic as being poor candidates for play group therapy.

Selection and screening of children for a group therapy experience is based on the child's developmental level, ego growth, capacity for object relations, and peer grouping.

Phases of Group Development

Child therapy groups have definite phases of development. The phases described are for latency age groups, but apply to other age groups with appropriate modification.

Initial Phase

During the initial or introductory phase, the focus is on having children get to know each other. This period is also called the preparatory or preaffiliation phase. There tends to be many approach-avoidance behaviors among children in this phase.

Therapeutic Phase

Gradually, subgroups appear in which the play activities occur. Initially during this phase, the drop-out rate may be the highest because competition is strong and the risks of self-disclosure, intimacy, rejection, and hurt are the greatest. Early detection of the anxiety by the therapist permits him or her to provide reassurance and physical comfort and to separate the hostile, angry child briefly from the group. These interventions may reduce the drop-out rate.

Gradually, as the children develop peer relations, greater personal involvement in the group occurs with greater sharing and more satisfying relationships. Much of the play is symbolic, reflecting both individual and group conflicts. This phase develops more quickly with latency-age groups due to the affinity of this age group for gangs and enthusiasm for peer group play.

Differentiation Phase

By this time, the children are developing greater autonomy and increased freedom in expressing individual feelings. Children will cooperate and work on common problems and age-appropriate developmental conflicts in the group during this period.

Termination Phase

Children indicate behaviorally and verbally the reduction in their original problems and their readiness to leave the group. The group can be helpful and supportive in assisting individual members to identify behavioral changes that have occurred and to evaluate the group therapy experience. This phase is helpful to all members in dealing with issues of separation and loss. Both departure and entry of children in the group must be dealt with in order for children to work through these issues. Departures of the therapist for reasons of vacation, illness, or for other reasons need to be dealt with before and after the absence as it reactivates the issues of parental separation and loss.

Individual Therapists Versus Cotherapists

There are both advantages and disadvantages to single versus cotherapists with children's groups. Because of the nature of children's groups and the activity level involved, it is often helpful to have more than one therapist to supervise and be attentive to the group process. Most children in group treatment deal at some time with family issues and conflicts. Having a male and a female as cotherapists can facilitate this process. However, unless the therapists have been able to develop an effective working relationship and are jointly supervised, difficulties may occur. Rivalry, dominance-submission patterns, and recreating parental conflicts are only a few of the issues needing to be dealt with by the therapists. Attention needs to be given to the same processes in group treatment as in individual child treatment.

Group Issues

Resistance is a major issue in child treatment as previously discussed. Some clinicians believe group treatment may minimize its occurrence. Groups have the potential of reducing the child's fear and suspicion at the beginning because of the presence of other children. Slavson and Schiffer (1975) point out that young children do not seem to have the difficulties with groups that adolescents and adults do. They speculate that this is due to the younger child's lessened concern with what is right and proper, permissible and taboo. Manifestations of positive and negative transference and countertransference are important in group work as well. Since the therapist remains relatively passive and permissive in activity group therapy, mostly positive transference is elicited that facilitates the formation of a therapeutic alliance. In activity-interview group therapy, the therapist is less passive, makes more interpretations and is thus more likely to elicit negative transference. Both activities and interviews focus on eliciting responsive reactions in the child.

Countertransference issues in child group work have been discussed especially in working with groups of acting-out aggressive children (Schreiber, 1969). Again, Slavson and Schiffer (1975) emphasize that therapist neutrality in maintaining emotional objectivity is critical. This level is difficult to achieve, but, when not accomplished, jealousy, rivalry, and competition among the group members become major issues. Rivalry may be intensified if the group therapist sees one or more children individually outside the group. Unless the therapist can see all the children individually as well as in the group, it is generally better to have the children seen individually by another therapist. The rationale for this decision involves the intensity of sibling rivalry as a common phenomenon in childhood, which is exacerbated by any perceived favoritism by the therapist. Because children are more open in displaying emotion, both positive and negative, it is important that the therapist neither solicit nor reject the behaviors on the basis of his or her own needs and conflicts.

The beginning child group therapist often feels exposed and vulnerable. It is crucial that group therapists receive support through clinical supervision and institutional acceptance. Without such support, many group therapists become frustrated and decide group therapy is not for them.

EVALUATION OF TREATMENT

If the therapeutic relationship moves through discernable stages that coincide with the child's progress, then it would seem that objective criteria could be developed to measure such progress, for example, by measuring a child's current functioning in treatment compared with behaviors displayed at the beginning of treatment. Naturally, every therapist uses some sort of evaluative criteria and process for individual children but very little research has dealt with this issue.

Issues that still need to be addressed in both individual and group treatment of children include the following:

1. Regardless of the type of treatment evaluated, the therapeutic results need to be evaluated comparably. Without such comparability, a determination of which treatment approach is more effective cannot be made.
2. Perhaps a more important issue is to be able to identify with some precision which categories of mental illness respond best to which type of treatment.
3. The evaluation process needs to be objective and well controlled and not designed to confirm the investigator's preconceived ideas.

The three points presented are important in the evaluation of any treatment regardless of whether it concerns adults or children. However, in evaluating treatment of children, there is an additional variable that is more troublesome than with adults. As Fish (1964) notes, since children are developing organisms, one needs to be able to differentiate the results of treatment from the results of development and "growing up." To do this, sound data are required on both normal development and the natural history of psychiatric illnesses. Additionally, children are very responsive to changes in their environments. So both environmental and individual factors need to be identified and appropriately dealt with in any research designed to evaluate aspects of treatment. Some epidemiological studies have found that often childhood psychiatric disturbance is relatively situation-specific (Rutter, Tizard, & Whitmore, 1970). Other studies have shown that treatment gains achieved in a therapeutic setting do not transfer to the home setting (Lovaas, Koegel, Simmons, & Long, 1973; Weissberg, Coeston, Rupkin, Cowen, Davidson, de Apodaca, & McKim, 1981).

Goals of Treatment

The promotion of normal development is increasingly seen as an essential treatment goal. There are limited efforts reported about measuring the effectiveness of child treatment to accomplish this goal (Furman, 1980). There have also been limited efforts to evaluate treatment in its ability to foster a child's autonomy and self-reliance (Rutter, Yule, Berger, & Hersov, 1977). One study attempted to determine what was therapeutically necessary to ensure that generalization of gains occurred (Wahler, Berland, & Coe, 1979).

Determining the persistence of the improvement gained by children through treatment is another means to gauge its effectiveness. Some studies have indicated that, though children made progress during treatment, the longer-term outcome was no different than that of the no-treatment control group (Kent & O'Leary, 1976). In other cases, treatment efforts deteriorated over time (Rutter & Giller, 1982). However, other studies have found that the treatment gains increased over time, being greater after an extended period than they were initially (Kolvin, Garside, Nicol, Macmillan, Wolstenholm, & Leitch, 1981; Wright, Moelis, & Pollack, 1976). One explanation given was that the treatment was effective in altering the child's environment or in increasing skills in coping with it. However, though plausible, this explanation remains basically unconfirmed.

One interesting finding is that shorter-term–focused child therapy with specific aims has been found to be more effective in both individual and group treatment than the traditional long-term, open-ended psychotherapeutic approaches (Kolvin et al., 1981; Reid & Shyne, 1969). One possible explanation is that short-term treatment often has as its goal developmental gains in cognitive, social, and ego development. These areas lend themselves to measurement that can be done at the beginning and end of treatment.

Evaluation of Overall Treatment Effects

In looking at empirical findings regarding the overall efficacy of child therapy, most researchers have concluded that it is without measurable beneficial effect (Levitt, 1971; Shephard, Oppenheim, & Mitchell, 1971). More recently, better data from better quality studies have become available. As a result, more recent reviews have drawn positive though still tentative conclusions from the data (Howlin, 1981; Kolvin et al., 1981; Lask & Mathew, 1979). Their findings indicate that some psychological therapies can and do alter children's maladaptive behavior in positive ways. Though these findings are reassuring to those of us involved in clinical work, they are still far too general and tentative in nature to be of much use in terms of practical guidance. The findings refute the overgeneralization that clinical interventions with children are totally without effect. Further evaluations of the effects of child therapy are essential, but such studies need to focus far more specifically on types of interventions used and outcomes achieved.

SUMMARY

Clinical nurse specialists provide individual and group play therapy in a variety of settings. This chapter discussed the knowledge and skills required to work with preschool- and elementary school-aged children using these modalities. Both individual and group play therapy were discussed in terms of their characteristics, stages, processes, and criteria for screening assessment and selection. Significant therapeutic issues with children such as limit setting, resistance, transference and countertransference, and sexual behavior by the child in the playroom were explored. The importance of working with parents was discussed and therapeutic, educative, and task-oriented approaches were described. Controversies regarding the therapist's participation in the child/children's play, accepting or giving gifts, or whether or not the child/children should put their toys away were presented.

Finally, treatment evaluation studies were discussed in terms of their contradictory and inconclusive findings. The state of the art in both child treatment and research indicates that studies are needed that are conceptually and methodologically more refined to evaluate specific interventions and their outcomes.

REFERENCES

Axline, V. *Play therapy: The inner dynamics of childhood.* Boston: Houghton Mifflin, 1947.

Berlin, I. Communication as a means of communication in therapy with children and adolescents. In

P. F. Ostwald (Ed.), *Communication and social interaction.* New York: Grune & Stratton, 1977.

Berlin, I. Transference and countertransference issues in the playroom. *Journal of the American Academy of Child Psychiatry,* in press.

Bixler, R. Limits on therapy. *Journal of Consulting Psychology,* 1949, *13,* 1–11.

Christ, A. Sexual countertransference problems with a psychotic child. In S. A. Szurek & I. N. Berlin (Eds.), *Clinical studies in childhood psychoses.* New York: Brunner/Mazel, 1973.

Colm, H. Play as a means of communication between child and adult—Three cases. *Journal of Child Psychiatry,* 1951, *2,* 100–112.

Critchley, D. Mental status examinations with children and adolescents: A developmental approach. *Nursing Clinics of North America,* 1979, *14*(3), 429–441.

Critchley, D. A developmental perspective for treatment of families with young children. In I. Clements & D. Buchanan (Eds.), *Family therapy: A nursing perspective.* New York: Wiley, 1982a.

Critchley, D. Therapeutic group work with abused preschool children. *Perspectives in Psychiatric Care,* 1982, *20,* 79–85. (b)

Erikson, E. Studies in the interpretation of play: I. Clinical observation of play disruption in young children. *Genetic Psychology Monographs,* 1940, *22,* 557–671.

Erikson, E. *Childhood and society* (2nd ed.). New York: W. W. Norton, 1950.

Erikson, E. The initial session and its alternatives. In M. Haworth (Ed.), *Child psychotherapy.* New York: Basic Books, 1964.

Erikson, E. Play and actuality. In M. Piers (Ed.), *Play and development.* New York: W. W. Norton, 1972.

Fish, B. Evaluation of psychiatric therapies in children. In P. Hoch & J. Zubin (Eds.), *The evaluation of psychiatric treatment.* New York: Grune & Stratton, 1964.

Fraiberg, S. Technical aspects of the analysis of a child with a severe behavior disorder. *Journal of the American Psychoanalytic Association,* 1962, *10,* 338–367.

Freud, A. *The ego and the mechanisms of defense.* New York: International Universities Press, 1946.

Freud, A. *Normality and pathology in childhood: Assessments of development.* New York: International Universities Press, 1965.

Freud, S. *Beyond the pleasure principle.* London: Hogarth Press, 1922.

Furman, W. Promoting social development: Developmental implications for treatment. In B. Lahey & A. Kazdin (Eds.), *Advances in clinical child psychology* (Vol. 3). New York: Plenum Press, 1980.

Gardner, R. Dramatized storytelling in child psychotherapy. *Acta Paedopsychiatrica,* 1974, *41*(3), 110–116.

Gardner, R. Helping children cooperate in therapy. In S. Harrison (Ed.), *Basic handbook of child psychiatry* (Vol. III). New York: Basic Books, 1979.

Ginott, H. The theory and practice of therapeutic intervention in child treatment. *Journal of Consulting Psychology,* 1959, *23,* 160–166.

Hambridge, G. Structured play therapy. Symposium, 1954. Therapeutic play techniques. *American Journal of Orthopsychiatry,* 1955, *25,* 601–617.

Haworth, M. (Ed.). *Child psychotherapy.* New York: Basic Books, 1964.

Howlin, P. The effectiveness of operant language training with autistic children. *Journal of Autism and Developmental Disorders,* 1981, *11,* 89–106.

Jernberg, A. *Theraplay.* San Francisco: Jossey-Bass, 1979.

Kent, R., & O'Leary, K. A controlled evaluation of behavior modification with conduct problem children. *Journal of Consulting and Clinical Psychology,* 1976, *44,* 586–596.

Klein, M. The psychoanalytic play technique. *American Journal of Orthopsychiatry,* 1955, *25,* 223–237.

Kolvin, I., Garside, R., Nicol, A., Macmillan, A., Wolstenholm, F., & Leitch, I. *Help starts here: The maladjusted child in the ordinary school.* London: Tavistock, 1981.

Lask, B., & Matthew, D. Childhood asthma: A controlled trial of family psychotherapy. *Archives of Disease in Childhood,* 1979, *54,* 116–119.

Levitt, E. Research on psychotherapy with children. In A. Bergin & S. Garfield (Eds.), *Handbook of psychotherapy and behavior change* (1st ed.). New York: Wiley, 1971.

Levy, D. Trends in therapy: Release therapy. *American Journal of Orthopsychiatry,* 1939, *9,* 713–736.

Loomis, E. The use of checkers in handling certain resistances in child analysis. *Journal of American Psychoanalytic Association,* 1957, *5,* 130–135.

Lorenz, K. The emnity between generations and its probable ethological causes. In M. Piers (Ed.), *Play and development.* New York: Norton, 1972.

Lovaas, O., Koegel, R., Simmons, J., & Long, J. Some generalization and follow-up measures on autistic children in behavior therapy. *Journal of Applied Behavior Analysis,* 1973, *6,* 131–165.

MacLennan, B. Modification of activity group therapy for children. *International Journal of Group Psychotherapy,* 1977, *27,* 85–96.

Markowitz, J. The nature of the child's initial resistances to psychotherapy. *Social Work,* 1959, *4,* 46–51.

McNamara, J. R. (Ed.). *Behavioral approaches to medicine.* New York: Plenum Press, 1979.

Moustakas, C. *Children in play therapy.* New York: McGraw-Hill, 1953.

Naumberg, M. *An introduction to art therapy: Studies of the "free" art expression of behavior problem children and adolescents as a means of diagnosis and therapy.* New York: Teachers College Press, 1973.

Peller, L. Libidinal phases, ego development and play. *Psychoanalytic Study of the Child,* 1954, *9,* 178–198.

Petrillo, M., & Sanger, S. *Emotional care of hospitalized children.* Philadelphia: J. B. Lippincott, 1972.

Piaget, J. The stages of intellectual development of the child. *Bulletin of the Menninger Clinic,* 1962, *26,* 120–128.

Reid, W., & Shyne, A. *Brief and extended casework.* New York: Columbia University Press, 1969.

Ross, A. *The practice of clinical psychology.* New York: Grune & Stratton, 1959.

Rutter, M., & Giller, H. *Juvenile delinquency: Trends and perspectives.* New York: Penguin, 1982.

Rutter, M., Tizard, J., & Whitmore, K. *Education, health and behavior.* London: Longmans, 1970.

Rutter, M., Yule, W., Berger, M., & Hersov, L. *An evaluation of a behavioral approach to the treatment of autistic children.* London: Department of Health and Social Security, 1977.

Schiffer, M. Permissiveness versus sanction in activity group therapy. *International Journal of Group Psychotherapy,* 1952, *2,* 255–261.

Schiffer, M. *The therapeutic play group.* New York: Grune & Stratton, 1969.

Schreiber, S. Some special forms of aggressiveness in activity group therapy and their impact on the therapist. *Smith College Studies in Social Work,* 1969, *39,* 138–146.

Shepherd, M., Oppenheim, B., & Mitchell, S. *Childhood behavior and mental health.* London: University of London Press, 1971.

Slavson, S., & Schiffer, M. *Group psychotherapies for children: A textbook.* New York: International Universities Press, 1975.

Solomon, J. Play technique and the integrative process. Symposium, 1954. Therapeutic play techniques. *American Journal of Orthopsychiatry,* 1955, *25,* 591–600.

Sugar, M. Interpretative group psychotherapy with latency children. *Journal of American Academy of Child Psychiatry,* 1974, *13,* 648–666.

Twain, M. *The adventures of Tom Sawyer* (special ed.). New York: Heritage Press, 1876.

Wahler, R., Berland, R., & Coe, T. Generalization processes in child behavior change. In B. Lahey & A. Kazdin (Eds.), *Advances in clinical child psychology* (Vol. 2). New York: Plenum, 1979.

Weissberg, R., Gesten, E., Rupkin, B., Cowen, E., Davidson, E., de Apodaca, R., & McKim, B. Evaluation of a social problem-solving training program for suburban and inner-city third-grade children. *Journal of Consulting and Clinical Psychology,* 1981, *59,* 251–261.

Woltmann, A. G. Concepts of play therapy. *American Journal of Orthopsychiatry,* 1955, *25,* 771–783.

Wright, D., Moelis, I., & Pollack, L. The outcome of individual child psychotherapy: Increments at follow-up. *Journal of Child Psychology and Psychiatry,* 1976, *17,* 275–285.

Yandell, W. Therapeutic problems related to the expression of sexual drives in children. In S. Szurek & I. Berlin (Eds.), *Clinical studies in childhood psychoses.* New York: Brunner/Mazel, 1973.

BIBLIOGRAPHY

Abramowitz, C. The effectiveness of group psychotherapy with children. *Archives of General Psychiatry,* 1976, *33,* 320–325.

American Nurses' Association. *Standards of psychiatric and mental health nursing practice.* Kansas City, Mo; ANA, 1982.

Berlin, I., & Critchley, D. The work of play for parents of schizophrenic children. *Child Psychiatry and Human Development,* 1982, *13,* 111–119.

Colm, H. A field theory approach to transference and its particular application to children. *Psychiatry,* 1955, *18,* 329–352.

Critchley, D. Nursing intervention with disturbed latency age children. In C. Fagin (Ed.), *Nursing in child psychiatry.* St. Louis: C. V. Mosby, 1972.

Critchley, D. The child as patient: Assessing effects of family stress and disruption on the mental health of the child. *Perspectives in Psychiatric Care,* 1981, *19,* 144–155.

Critchley, D. Interventions with disorganized families of disturbed children. *Issues in Mental Health Nursing,* 1982, *4,* 199–215.

Fagin, C. *Nursing in child psychiatry.* St. Louis, C. V. Mosby, 1972.

Fagin, C. *Readings in child and adolescent psychiatric nursing.* St. Louis: C. V. Mosby, 1974.

Fraiberg, S., Shapiro, V., & Cherniss, D. Treatment modalities. In S. Fraiberg (Ed.), *Clinical studies in infant mental health: The first year of life.* New York: Basic Books, 1980.

Freud, A. *The psychoanalytical treatment of the child.* London: Imago, 1946.

Joint Commission on Mental Health of Children. *Crisis in child mental health challenge for the 1970s.* New York: Harper & Row, 1970.

Kraft, I. Child and adolescent group psychotherapy. In H. Kaplan & B. Sadock (Eds.), *Comprehensive group psychotherapy.* Baltimore: Williams & Wilkins, 1983.

Kraft, I. Group therapy. In S. Harrison (Ed.), *Basic handbook of child psychiatry* (Vol. III). New York: Basic Books, 1979.

Psychopathological disorders in childhood: Theoretical considerations and a proposed classification. New York: Group for the Advancement of Psychiatry, 1966.

Rutter, M. Psychological therapies in child psychiatry: Issues and prospects. *Psychological Medicine,* 1982, *12,* 723–740.

Schiffer, M. Activity-interview group psychotherapy: Theory, principles and practice. *International Journal of Group Psychotherapy,* 1977, *27,* 377–388.

Swanson, F. *Psychotherapists and children: A Procedural guide.* New York: Pittman, 1970.

The Task Force on Nomenclature and Statistics. *Diagnostic and Statistical Manual of Mental Disorders* (DSM-III) (3rd ed.). Washington, DC: American Psychiatric Association, 1980.

Wesner, D., Dowling, J., & Johnson, F. What is maternal infant interaction? The role of infant psychotherapy. *Psychiatry,* 1982, *45,* 407–415.

CHAPTER 13 FAMILY APPROACHES

Judith T. Maurin
Imelda W. Clements

Treatment of the family as a whole has become an important modality for psychiatric mental health nurses. Even when working with individual clients, nurses usually express the importance of understanding that individual's social/family context. However, there are many theoretical perspectives within which family relationships can be conceptualized. Each perspective has its unique problems on which there is an extensive literature.

This chapter will consider theoretical concerns and aspects of treatment that family therapists need to consider regardless of their own particular orientation. The first section includes a brief summary of nursing's historical role with families and the current state of family therapy. Second, the Circumplex Model will be discussed as an attempt to integrate the many discrete concepts that have been used to discuss and describe families. Finally, selected pragmatic issues that are common concerns among family therapists will be explored.

HISTORY

Nursing's Role With Families

As Smoyak stated, "In one sense, nurses have worked with families since nursing began—giving care and comfort to family members, first in homes and, later, in institutions, hospitals, or outpatient clinics" (1975a, p. 38). However, Smoyak's review of the literature from 1946 to 1974 revealed an evolution over the years in the way nurses wrote about what they had to offer in their care of families, and presumably this reflected the way they worked with families. First, nurses saw their role as family life educators, giving information about such areas as normal child nutrition, growth, and development and offering help and suggestions when there were deviations from the norm in the way of illness or developmental problems. Beginning about 1952, the literature revealed that nurses were beginning to assume a liaison function with families, preparing them for the discharge of their mentally ill member and visiting them on follow-up. Finally, since 1962, psychiatric mental health nurses are writing about their family therapy work with families.

Nurses have relied heavily on a systems perspective (Smoyak, 1975b) but have also learned from the various therapeutic perspectives (such as Psychoanalytic, Communication, and Structural) either as a result of their graduate education or as a result of personal selection. The eclecticism is evident in a recent text by Clements and Buchanan (1982). Only recently have the nursing models available been deliberatively applied to the family (Clements and Roberts, 1983).

Family Therapy

The family therapy field has been called the " 'melting pot' of therapists" (Olsen, Russell, & Sprenkle, 1980a, p. 973) because the field has attracted individuals from many diverse professional and academic backgrounds. A unifying characteristic has been an emphasis on treating problems within a relationship context. Of singular importance to this field has been the work of Von Bertalanffy (1969). Whereas psychotherapists became aware, during the late 1940s and early 1950s, that families were having an effect on their patients' pathology, General System Theory as explained by Von Bertalanffy provided the integrating framework needed to accommodate the rich array of variables and relationships that accompanied the family focus. There seems to be no end to the list of presenting problems that have been conceptualized as a signal of family system distress for which family therapy has been prescribed.

Olsen et al. (1980a) reviewed the field of marital and family therapy during the 1970s and found the following four characteristics. First, there has been a mushrooming of interest as indicated by the numbers of books, articles, and journals on the topic and by membership in the two national associations, The American Association for Marriage and Family Therapy and American Family Therapy Association. Second, there has been the development of distinct schools of therapy and specific therapeutic techniques. While most schools rely on a system orientation, each has important differences in their basic assumptions about how change occurs, the goals of treatment, and the role of the therapist. Third, they found a wealth of concepts, often redundant, that have been generated related to marital and family dynamics. Fourth, there is evidence of an ongoing interest in evaluation research. While there are still many problems with this research (Gurman & Kniskern, 1978b), the quality and quantity of outcome research is improving.

A result of the growth in this field, both in terms of the number of schools and range of presenting problems treated, is increased attention to theoretical tasks. While a majority of therapists admit to being eclectic, the problems of eclecticism are recognized (Liddle, 1982). In an effort to understand the similarities and differences among therapeutic schools, several classification schemes have been proposed (for example, L'Abate, Frey, & Wagner, 1982). There is also increasing interest in being able to specify which mode of therapy is most effective for which group of clients presenting which sorts of problems.

This search for a match of an appropriate method for a specific problem has led researchers back to the dilemma of how to conceptualize the problem. An alternative to focusing on presenting symptoms is to focus on types of family systems. Olson, Russell, & Sprenkle (1980b) provide an example in which four families with the same presenting symptom (alcoholism) were found to be a different type of family system when assessed in terms of cohesion and adaptability. One would expect that in spite of the common presenting problem, the therapeutic task would have to be different for each of these families. If the family system is disengaged, with significant "cutoffs," the therapeutic task will be viewed differently than in a connected, but rigid, family system even though the presenting problem may be alcoholism. This approach points to the importance of being able to make a system diagnosis prior to intervention.

Clarkin and Glick (1982) identify the need for a family typology but cite a practical issue that discourages the abandonment of the presenting problem focus for a family typology focus. That practical issue is funding. First, programs are funded to combat specific presenting problems that can generate political interest (such as drug abuse or autism). Second, those situations of greatest interest to family therapists, such as marital problems or parent-child problems, are found in the DSM-III under *Conditions Not Attributable to a Mental Disorder* (American Psychiatric Association, 1980). Third-party insurers are becoming increasingly reluctant to fund treatments that are not specified for the amelioration of a specific mental disorder.

The prevalence and potentials for inconsistency in an eclectic approach to family therapy has led Liddle (1982) to urge that family therapists engage in an Epistemological Declaration. This is an "idiosyncratic statement of what we know and how we know it, what and how we think, and what and how we make the clinical decisions we do" (p. 247). This statement is aided by answering the questions listed in Table 13.1 that comprise Liddle's Ideological Checkup.

Finally, while some argue that it is premature (Liddle, 1982), others are calling for the development of a theoretical model(s) that would begin to integrate the numerous concepts in the field. One such model, the Circumplex Model, will be discussed below. This model is important to consider because it achieves the inclusion of ideas represented in the concepts of numerous authors and because it also offers a typology of family systems that have implications for both research and practice.

CIRCUMPLEX MODEL

The Circumplex Model is a theoretical model developed by Olson, Sprenkle, & Russell, 1979; see also Olson, Russell, & Sprenkle, 1983), in an effort to integrate the recurring concepts and principles found in the family literature and provide a framework that could be used by clinicians to make a more systematic diagnosis of family systems. With a meaningful diagnosis, theory-based treatment goals would be possible. The model does not specify therapeutic techniques to achieve these goals, however. Olson and coworkers (1979, 1983) argue that techniques are, for the most part, atheoretical. Therapists can select any technique with which they are familiar and skilled and that they judge will achieve the treatment goal.

Their review and conceptual analysis of the family and family therapy literature yielded a clustering of concepts along three dimensions: family cohesion, adaptability, and communication. The first two dimensions contain four levels. Combining these dimensions into the four parts shown in Figure 13.1 results in a taxonomy of 16 distinct types of marital and family systems. While all 16 are theoretically possible, it is assumed that some types are more common than others.

Table 13.1 Ideological Checkup

Definitions
- What is your view of the definition and nature of therapy?
- What are your basic assumptions about people and their contexts?

Goals
- What should be the goals of therapy?
- Who should determine them?
- Should they be overtly defined, and if so how precisely?

Therapist behavior
- What is the role and function of the therapist?
- What mechanisms permit or force change?

Dysfunction/normative behavior
- What is your theory of pathology; of normative family functioning?
- What is the unit of the problem?
- What is the role of the past vis-à-vis the present in relation to why problems exist in a family

Evaluation
- How should a therapist evaluate his or her work?

SOURCE: Liddle, H. A. On the problems of eclecticism: A call for epistemologic clarification and human-scale theories. *Family Process,* 1982, *21*(2):248.

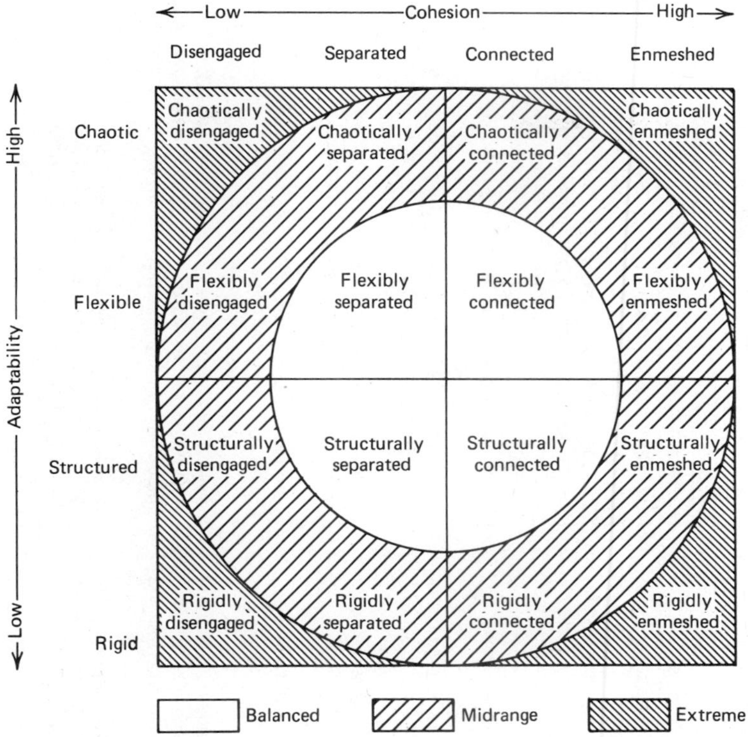

Figure 13.1 Circumplex model of sixteen types of marital and family systems. (From Olson, D. H., et al., Circumplex model of marital and family systems: VI. Theoretical update. *Family Process,* 1983, *22,* p. 71.

Family cohesion is the emotional bonding that members have toward one another. It has to do with the degree of separateness or connectedness of individuals within the family system. The four levels of this dimension are disengaged, separated, connected, and enmeshed, which represent very low to very high cohesion, respectively. The central two levels are where individuals experience a balance in their independence from and connection to their families. It is hypothesized that these central levels make for optimal family functioning. Table 13.2 contains the specific concepts or variables that can be assessed to diagnose and measure the family cohesion dimension.

Family adaptability has to do with the extent to which the family system can be flexible and change. It is the ability to change the power structure, role relationships, and relationship rules of a marital or family system in response to situational and developmental stress. There are four levels of adaptability: rigid, structured, flexible, and chaotic, which represent a very low to very high range of adaptability, respectively. Once again, the central levels of adaptability are hypothesized to be the most conducive to family functioning. Table 13.3 contains the concepts or variables that can be assessed to diagnose and measure the family adaptability dimension.

The family communication dimension is different from the first two in that it is a facilitating dimension. "Positive communication skills (that is, empathy, reflective listening, supportive

Table 13.2 Family Cohesion Dimension: Interrelated Concepts

	Disengaged (*Very low*)	*Separated* (*Low to moderate*)	*Connected* (*Moderate to high*)	*Enmeshed* (*Very high*)
Independence	High independence of family members	Moderate independence of family members	Moderate dependence of family members	High dependence of family members
Family boundaries	Open external boundaries; closed internal boundaries; rigid generational boundaries	Semi-open external and internal boundaries; clear generational boundaries	Semi-open external boundaries; open internal boundaries; clear generational boundaries	Closed external boundaries. Blurred internal boundaries. Blurred generational boundaries
Coalitions	Weak coalitions; usually a family scapegoat	Marital coalition clear	Marital coalition strong	Parent-child coalitions
Time	Time apart from family maximized (physically and/or emotionally)	Time alone and together is important	Time together is important. Time alone permitted for approved reasons	Time together maximized; little time alone permitted
Space	Separate space both physically and emotionally is maximized	Private space maintained; some family space	Family space maximized; private space minimized	Little or no private space at home
Friends	Mainly individual friends seen alone; few family friends	Some individual friends; some family friends	Some individual friends; scheduled activities with couple and family friends	Limited individual friends; mainly couple or family friends seen together
Decision making	Primarily individual decisions	Most decisions are individually based; able to make joint decisions on family issues	Individual decisions are shared. Most decisions made with family in mind	All decisions, both personal and relationship must be made by family
Interests and recreation	Primarily individual activities done without family; family not involved	Some spontaneous family activities; individual activities supported	Some scheduled family activities; family involved in individual interests	Most or all activities and interests must be shared with family

SOURCE: Olson, D. H., Sprenkle, D. H., & Russell, C. S. Circumplex model of marital and family systems: I. Cohesion and adaptability dimensions, family types, and clinical applications. *Family Process,* 1979, *18,* 21.

Table 13.3 Family Adaptability Dimensions: Interrelated Concepts

	Assertiveness	*Control*	*Discipline*	*Negotiation*	*Roles*	*Rules*	*System Feedback*
Chaotic (very high)	Passive and aggressive styles	No leadership	Laisse-faire Very lenient	Endless negotiation Poor problem solving	Dramatic rule shifts	Dramatic rule shifts Many implicit rules Few explicit rules Arbitrarily enforced rules	Primarily positive loops Few negative loops
Flexible	Generally assertive	Equalitarian with fluid changes	Democratic Unpredictable consequences	Good negotiation Good problem solving	Role making and sharing Fluid change of roles	Some rule changes More implicit rules Rules often enforced	More positive than negative loops
Structured	Generally assertive	Democratic with stable leader	Democratic Predictable consequences	Structured negotiations Good problem solving	Some role sharing	Few rule changes More explicit than implicit rules Rules usually enforced	More negative than positive loops
Rigid (very low)	Passive or aggressive styles	Authoritarian leadership	Autocratic Overly strict	Limited negotiations Poor problem solving	Role rigidity Stereotyped roles	Rigid rules; many explicit rules Few implicit rules Strictly enforced rules	Primarily negative loops Few positive loops

SOURCE: Olson, D. H., Sprenkle, D. H., & Russell, C. S. Circumplex model of marital and family systems: I. Cohesion and adaptability dimensions, family types, and clinical applications. *Family Process*, 1979, *18*, 22.

comments) enable couples and families to share with each other their changing needs and preferences as they relate to cohesion and adaptability. Negative communication skills (that is, double messages, double binds, criticism) minimize the ability of a couple or family members to share their feelings and, thereby, restrict their movement on these dimensions" (Olson et al., 1983, p. 71).

Family types in the central circle of Figure 13.1 (Flexibly Separated, Flexibly Connected, Structurally Separated, and Structurally Connected) reflect balanced levels of the adaptability and cohesion dimensions and are thought to be most functional for individual and family development. None of these four types is designated as "the ideal," however.

The four types in the outer circle of Figure 13.1 (Chaotically Disengaged, Chaotically Enmeshed, Rigidly Enmeshed, and Rigidly Disengaged) reflect extreme levels of the adaptability and cohesion dimensions and are seen as least functional to individual and family development. Because the extreme behaviors are exaggerated but continuous with functional behavior, this model accounts for the frequent observation that "normal" families display some of the same behaviors, albeit limited, as that found in clinical families described as dysfunctional.

The insight gained by the use of the Circumplex Model becomes apparent in the following case study. A psychiatric liason consult was requested by the nursing staff on an orthopedic unit for a young man with multiple injuries because his physicians and nurses believed him to be ready for discharge, but discharge plans consistently fell through. They suspected that he sabotaged them each time.

Steve was a 26-year-old man who had sustained multiple injuries in an automobile accident. While he no longer needed hospital care, he would need considerable assistance at home because of pins and casts on both lower extremities and one upper extremity. Steve was married to Ruth and lived in a second floor apartment which they shared since their marriage eight months ago. They identified their discharge choices as (1) returning to their apartment, which would mean limited mobility for Steve, because of the stairs, and complete dependence on Ruth or (2) temporarily moving in with Steve's family, who had a large, single story house. Also, because Steve's family was large and multigenerational, many people could share in seeing to his needs. Since Ruth's parents lived in another state and in a small single family dwelling, living with Ruth's parents was ruled out.

Exploration of the family systems of Steve's and Ruth's families of origin revealed the following. Steve's family would be characterized as Connected and Rigid. Roles were stereotyped and rigidly defined with the father exerting authoritarian leadership. Family activities together were very important, although personal time was permitted for approved reasons. Ruth, on the other hand, came from a Separated and Flexible family system. Roles were negotiated with considerable sharing of tasks, and personal time and space were valued in addition to family time.

Steve and Ruth were in the early stage of their marriage where they were in the process of defining their family system. They had developed a Connected and Structured family system. While Steve tended to have more power to make decisions in the relationship, Ruth tolerated this role as long as his leadership was democratic. Steve had clear ideas about family sex roles but was able to do some role sharing. Both valued their time and activities together and believed togetherness should take priority over independent activities. The administration of the Family Cohesion and Adaptability Evaluation Scales (FACES II) (Olson et al., 1983) revealed their differences in expectations about "family life" and provided an opportunity to problem solve about the situation.

Both Steve and Ruth agreed that accepting the resources of Steve's parents was objectively the best solution. The problem, however, was that Steve had violated Ruth's expectation that he be a democratic leader by consulting with his father on his own and arranging for this move. Secondly, Ruth feared that their separateness as a couple would be threatened if they joined this extended family. With the issues now identified, they were able to plan for certain arrangements that would give them separate space as a couple in Steve's family's house. They also learned the importance of communicating about these issues and gained practice with the nurse's support.

A summary of the relationships proposed among these major concepts and family functioning have been clearly presented as a list of seven hypotheses derived from the Circumplex Model. These hypotheses are the following:

I. Couples/families with balanced (two central levels) cohesion and adaptability will generally function more adequately across the family life cycle than those at the extremes of these dimensions.

II. Balanced family types have a larger behavioral repertoire and are more able to change compared with extreme family types.

III. If the normative expectations of a couple or family support behaviors extreme on one or both of the Circumplex dimensions, they will function well as long as all family members accept these expectations.

IV. Couples and families will function most adequately if there is a high level of congruence between the perceived and ideal descriptions for all family members.

V. Balanced couples/families will tend to have more positive communication skills than extreme families.

VI. Positive communication skills will enable balanced couples/families to change their levels of cohesion and adaptability more easily than those at the extremes.

VII. To deal with situational stress and developmental changes across the family life cycle, balanced families will change their cohesion and adaptability, whereas extreme families will resist change over time. (Olson et al., 1983, pp. 73–74)

A particular strength of the model is that it accounts for the effect of normative expectations and cultural bias (hypotheses III and IV). Also, it is based on an assumption that families not only can change, but that functioning families are likely to change as the situation and stage of the family life cycle require. Thus, even an extreme family type may not be dysfunctional for a family during a particular stage of the life cycle. These assumptions were empirically supported in a large, cross-sectional study of normal families across the life cycle (Olson et al., 1983). Clinically, however, it is suggested that therapists try to move a couple or family only *one* level on one or both dimensions. Too dramatic a change is likely to produce family resistance or a dramatic shift to the opposite extreme (Olsen et al., 1979, p. 23).

Accompanying this theoretical work has been a research program to test and validate the model that has lent empirical support. Summaries of this research can be found in Russell (1979) and Olson et al. (1980b). In the process of needing to operationalize family cohesion and adaptability for purposes of research, FACES II has been developed. FACES is an acronym for Family Cohesion and Adaptability Evaluation Scales, a 30-item, self-report scale with high levels of reliability and validity (Olson et al., 1983). Because it is short and easy to administer, it can be used for clinical assessment and for research. The Circumplex Model is promising for theory-based assessment and goal formulation and is worthy of further study by nurses working with families.

SELECTED ISSUES IN FAMILY THERAPY

As stated previously, nurse family therapists espouse a variety of perspectives on family therapy (Bowen, Structural, Communication, and so forth). Each of these schools provide the therapist with implicit and explicit guidelines for decision making in the assessment preceeding and the conduct of family therapy. Kolevzon & Green (1983) found that family therapists trained within a specific model of family therapy (Bowenian, Communication, or Strategic) were significantly different in terms of their belief and action systems than therapists trained in either of the other two schools. Gurman (1978) found that therapists from different perspectives were in relative disagreement about the ultimate goals of marital and family therapy.

> The major parameters on which the four approaches [Psychoanalytic, Bowenite, Communications, and Behavioral] appear to go their separate ways not surprisingly involve those that reflect the importance, or lack thereof, attributed to the impact of conjoint treatment on (1) each spouse's *and* the dyad's relationships outside their two-person subsystem; (2) the impact of treatment on characterological traits, conflicts and mechanisms for handling *intra*personal conflict, and vice versa; and (3) the establishment of a functional and adaptive balance between affect and cognition, or feelings and rational thinking.
>
> (Gurman, 1978, p. 544)

While there are many issues that are meaningfully discussed only within a specific theoretical perspective, there are a variety of pragmatic issues that are of common concern to all therapists regardless of their theoretical orientation and that impact on the therapeutic outcome. Such questions as when is family therapy indicated; who should take part, for example, young children; how can reluctant family members be engaged; where should therapy be conducted; should a therapist work with a cotherapist; and how can rapport be established with the *whole* family must be addressed by family therapists. Many of these issues are inadequately explored in the literature. However, the following discussion will identify what guidance can be gleaned from the experience of others as shared in the literature.

When Is Marital/Family Therapy Indicated

Family therapy appears to be as effective as individual therapy for a wide range of presenting problems. It is not yet possible, however, to specify which type of family treatment is best for which presenting problem. This issue clearly needs to be addressed; however, no one "school" of marital or family therapy has been demonstrated to be effective with a wide range of presenting problems (Olsen et al, 1980a; Kniskern & Gurman, 1981).

Broderick (1983) recommends marital or family therapy when relationship conflict appears to contribute to an individual's symptoms. Genthner & Veldkamp (1977) advise the family therapist to assess how personally responsible each member is for the performance of family tasks and family identity. They indicate that families that assume an attitude of responsibility but lack problem-solving skills are responsive to short-term family therapy aimed at improving problem-solving skills during a period of severe stress. However, families inclined to use scapegoating and blaming external persons and to assuming responsibility only part of the time usually need more long-term support to change these destructive patterns.

When the problem is in the marital relationship, marital therapy is clearly superior to individual therapy (Olsen et al., 1980a; Kniskern & Gurman, 1981). However, family therapy research has yet to explore whether family therapy is more effective with relationship-centered problems, such as an adolescent's separation from the family, than with problems less clearly relationship centered, such as depression or anxiety. Of course, as Lebow (1981) points out, "The rating of how family-centered a problem would be can be expected to vary with the orientation of the rater, creating low reliabilities" (p. 169).

Deterioration during marital and family therapy has been documented, although poorly. Gurman & Kniskern's (1978a) review of the literature suggested that 5–10% of patients or marital or family relationships worsened as the result of marital/family therapy. While they state that this rate is consistent with that reported for other modalities, a most interesting finding was an association between negative therapeutic change and therapist behavior.

> In summary, the available evidence points to a composite picture of deterioration in marital-family therapy being facilitated by a therapist with poor relationship skills who directly attacks "loaded" issues and family members' defenses very early in treatment, fails to intervene in or interpret intra-family confrontation in ongoing treatment, and does little to structure and guide the opening of therapy or to support family members. Such a style is even more likely to be counter-therapeutic with patients who have weak ego-defenses or feel threatened by the nature or very fact of being in treatment. Therapist factors alone are unlikely to account for all negative family therapy effects, since at times some couples and families are likely to worsen because of their own internal structure and/or by virtue of the very fact of being in treatment (e.g., probable self-disclosure and confrontation, problem identification). . . . The interaction of a structurally brittle family and an unskilled or insensitive therapist further heightens the chances of deteriorative therapeutic processes and effects. Still, the therapist seems clearly to occupy a central role in most negative treatment outcomes.
>
> (Gurman and Kniskern, 1978a, p. 14)

Guidance from the literature suggests that marital/family therapy is indicated when the problem is a relationship problem and marital therapy is the choice when the problem is most appropriately kept within the couple relationship. However, more research is needed to determine which presenting problems are relationship problems and which are not.

Which Family Members Should Participate

Having decided that marital or family therapy is indicated, who should participate? While there is little research on the subject, the consensus seems to be that if the problem is in the marital relationship, at least both spouses should participate. Furthermore, if the topics to be discussed are those not usually or comfortably shared with children, the children should be excluded. This approach both frees the spouses to discuss more openly and draws clear generational boundaries.

If the problem is focused on one of the children, at least all members of the nuclear family, or all persons living in the household, should attend. Many realistic barriers prevent achieving this ideal; for example, divorce, physical separation, and resistance.

If the problem concerns an adult family member who is an identified patient, the initial assessment phase should also include all persons living in the household and others who may be known to be involved in the problem. An exception is the advice by Stanton & Todd (1981) that for problems of drug abuse it is more important to convene the identified patient and his or her family of origin rather than his or her spouse.

Engaging Family Members in Therapy

Broderick (1983) states that bringing one's problems to a third party takes a great deal of personal courage. It is no wonder, then, that the process of convening all family members important to the therapeutic task is one that takes some special attention and investment of energy on the part of the therapist. Teismann (1980) and Stanton & Todd (1981) have provided a particularly thorough discussion of the issues and offer practical suggestions. This section will draw heavily on their work.

Fathers have been observed to be the most difficult family member to engage, and yet they are reported to be pivotal in recruiting other family members for therapy (Berg & Rosenblum, 1977) and promoting the continuation of the family in therapy (L'Abate, 1975; Shapiro & Budman, 1973; Slipp, Ellis, & Kressel, 1974). The approach recommended toward fathers displaying resistance is similar to that recommended for any resistant family member and takes into account an awareness of the personal courage needed to enter therapy. Individuals need to be approached with a nonblaming, nonpejorative reason for treatment. The rationale may be framed in a way that increases the attractiveness of participation; for example, (1) by reassuring them of their importance to gaining an understanding of the situation in the family and the power they hold to sabotage therapy; (2) reducing the threat by suggesting a role of information-giver or accuracy-checker until they are ready for full participation; or (3) reducing fear of the unknown by providing a copy of an article from a lay magazine that described family therapy or providing a referral to a former client who has agreed to share his or her experience of family therapy with others.

If increasing the attractiveness of participation fails, the therapist may need to resort to attempting to decrease the attractiveness of nonparticipation. This can be done by pointing out that without their participation, their point of view will not be represented. Another point would be that they can expect changes to result from therapy and without participating they will not have input into deciding those changes. Brehm (1976) cautions, however, that this approach threatens individuals' sense of freedom and, in such a situation, individuals act to regain the threatened freedom whether it is personally beneficial or not. Clearly, the former strategy is preferable.

There is concensus in the literature that the sooner family members are contacted to participate in therapy, the more likely they are to become engaged. It is often difficult to bring others in after therapy has begun. Therefore, when a therapist has received the initial contact about a problem (often by phone), he or she needs to gain as complete a description as possible of the presenting problem or identified patient, the household membership, and family and/or extrafamilial networks involved with the presenting problem. Ideally, the therapist should assess in the initial contact whether he or she needs to see just the person making the request or the whole household or family for the first appointment. Teismann (1980) recommends following this conversation with a letter,

> specifying the negotiated appointment time, agency phone number, fee structure, confidentiality agreement, name of the therapist, and the names of those who are to attend the initial session. The letter concludes with the directive that the letter be posted in a conspicuous place (e.g., refrigerator door) for all family members to read and that any concern arising from the letter be phoned to the therapist at least 48 hours prior to the initial session. (p. 394)

While there is consensus that the task of convening the family or couple for therapy is of central importance, there is some disagreement about whose task this ought to be. Stanton & Todd (1981), working with drug abusers, state very clearly that the therapist must directly contact at least both parents prior to the first session and that the chances for successful family recruitment increase if the therapist does the recruiting. Teismann (1980) believes that this is first a family task. The therapist may help the motivated family members consider ways to engage all of the family, but this is an opportunity for the family to exercise its own resources to affect change. Teismann is willing to give the task to the therapist if the family fails, but cautions that this carries the risk of being a highly visible therapeutic failure if the therapist also fails or of fostering the belief that the therapist, not the family, affects change if he or she is successful.

In spite of the best of efforts, there are times when an incomplete contingent appears for the initial session. Napier & Whitaker (1978) believe that treatment should be postponed in such a case until the requested composition is achieved. Most authors are not that adamant. Other options include retracing the convening steps, referring the motivated client to an individual therapist, granting a private session, or treating the unconvened family systemically through that subgroup motivated to participate. (For an example of an unconvened family treated systemically through the individual motivated for therapy, see "The Profile of Mary Donovan, Alcoholic" in Chapter 20.) All options have consequences that need to be deliberately considered in the decision making.

Sometimes the problem is such that the therapist has recourse to networks that will participate in enforcing the family's participation in therapy. Enforcement may range from the threat of prosecution, hospitalization, discharge, or expulsion. However, both Teismann (1980) and Seabury (1976) discuss the difficulty of developing a working relationship with such involuntary clients.

Office or Home Session

Another under-researched question is, what are the consequences of convening the family for therapy in the home or office? It is our impression that nurses are more comfortable meeting families in the home than are therapists from other disciplines. The clinical material found in both Smoyak (1975b) and Clements & Buchanan (1982) provide evidence that nurse family therapists go to clients' homes. But why? In this era of cost accountability, it is important to be able to specify when a visit to the home is therapeutically indicated and when one could be just as effective in the office.

There are times when a home visit appears warranted. Stanton & Todd (1981) and Teismann (1980) both recommend going to the home when one or more family members are resistant to becoming engaged in family therapy. Going to the home enables the therapist to present him- or herself in a trustworthy, nonthreatening manner in an environment in which the family can feel in control. Thus, the home is a place where it is easier to gather reluctant family members. Second, it is hard to deny that the home is a rich arena for the assessment phase of family therapy (Fagin, 1970). The opportunity to witness the family in the context in which they live and interact can provide valuable insights. Third, it is common experience that families suffering from a collapse of their executive function (the ability to organize necessary activities of daily living) are most effectively seen in the home, at least until this function is once again operative. The therapist can most effectively help them mobilize when all are present in the setting where the tasks to be done are so obvious. Also, under these conditions, the parents are often powerless to assure that all the children in the family (especially adolescents) will attend an office session. Finally, there are many instances where care of a family takes the nurse to the home for more than family therapy, but it is meaningful to meet with the family in conjunction with that visit. For example, the nurse may be providing hospice care to one family member and meet with all family members to help them deal with family issues that emerge during such a family life stage.

No cautions against family therapy in the home were noted in the literature. However, surely the fact that therapists recognize that families have a territorial advantage in the home makes it likely that there are times when this becomes problematic. Fagin (1970) states that the therapist's role changes in the home. "Regardless of the purpose of the visit, the therapist is in the position of guest or visitor" (p. 2). Clearly, this issue is an area where nurses need to gather data systematically and share their experiences.

Individual or Cotherapy

Another pragmatic decision that family therapists need to make is whether they will work alone or with a cotherapist. Cotherapy is said to have certain unique advantages. First, there is the benefit of having one therapist in the observing role while the other is engaged in interaction with the family. Second, a variety of transactions become available with cotherapists: they can intentionally use their similarities and differences to interact differentially with the family; therapist B is available to form a supporting alliance with a family member who views with hostility the supporting alliance developed (or developing) between therapist A and another family member; and finally, the therapists can model a cooperative relationship.

However, the literature does not provide empirical evidence for the superiority of cotherapy (Kniskern & Gurman, 1981), and Hannum (1980) offers two cautions. First, cotherapy necessitates a mature, open, often playful relationship between two therapists who know one another's style of therapy. Without such a relationship, tension can arise and effective implementation of cotherapeutic transactions is unlikely. Second, he cautioned against pairing experienced and inexperienced therapists for the purpose of training. Gurman (1975a,b) and Rice, Fey, & Kepecs (1972) report that the inexperienced therapists frequently have difficulty participating creatively because of feelings of lesser status and competence, and a pattern of competition is fostered. Hannum recommends matching cotherapists on level of experience and placing the supervisor behind a one-way mirror.

Establishing Rapport

It is a basic principle of psychotherapy, regardless of the modality, that nothing constructive is likely to happen unless effective rapport is established between therapist and client. When the client unit is composed of more than one individual, this caveat presents some special problems to the therapist. The task of establishing rapport with a couple or family requires a noncritical acceptance of the clients' behaviors, perceptions, and feelings and unconditional support of each client as a person (Broderick, 1983).

It probably should go without saying that if one is striving to convey noncritical acceptance, one must avoid blaming messages. Yet the frequency with which authors warn against blaming messages suggests that this is easier said than done.

Smoyak (1975b, p. 6) uses the systems perspective and systems analogies of the problem to conduct "no fault" therapy. Redefining the situation from an individual's problem to a family problem is a strategy many use to avoid blame laying. Yet Terkelsen (1983) points out that the therapist can still fall into the trap of blaming even when the problem has been defined as a family problem. He argues that the sociogenic models with which many therapists approach families with a schizophrenic member almost assures a therapeutic misalliance. The message of blame is usually covert but can be communicated by showing less interest and concern for the impact of the illness on the family than the family on the maintenance of symptomatic behavior. A therapist using analogies needs to examine them to see if they are communicating an interrelationship among parts or difficulty in one part being caused by the others.

Stanton & Todd (1981), working with the problem of drug abuse, recommend placing primary focus on helping the index patient rather than the family, but they too stress a nonblaming stance. They approach the family with the rationale that the index patient needs their help to solve this problem. Thus, it appears that approaching family therapy acknowledging that the index patient has a problem, or defining the problem as the family's, neither assures a no fault stance nor prohibits it. Achieving and communicating noncritical acceptance is something all therapists must work toward regardless of their theoretical perspective.

Communicating support of each individual in the therapeutic situation is achieved by what Broderick calls the "principle of symmetricality" (1983, p. 24). Each individual must feel equally accepted and supported and must feel that the therapist has maintained neutrality.

It is very easy to break neutrality and initiate an alliance with one member or another. When the therapist invites one member to comment on the relationship or statement of other members, the therapist appears to be allied to that person at that time. Expressing a judgment, whether approval or disapproval, allies the therapist with one member or subgroup. Using symmetry (spatial, temporal, or moral) can help the therapist overcome the establishment of ineffective alliances.

Using spatial symmetry, the therapist can sit in a position facing the family and equidistant from the members or shift his or her position or orientation toward a member being distanced by the verbal exchange of the moment. A cotherapist can also aid symmetry by supporting the distanced member. Temporal symmetry is achieved by passing the podium back and forth, asking member after member to express their point of view. Moral symmetry refers again to the nonblaming message. It entails looking for two sides to every question and the likelihood that there is hurt on both.

Other threats to neutrality and the establishment of rapport that are as important in family treatment as in other forms of therapy are the processes of transference and countertransference. The availability of clinical supervision will help in the identification and intervention with these problems. However, if unsuccessful, the therapist must be ready to refer the family to another therapist less biased about the issue in question or more acceptable to the family members.

Finally, especially problematic for the couple or family therapist is the family secret when he or she is drawn into the awareness context by the secret-holder. Karpel (1980) summarizes the consequences of the therapist being drawn into a secret. First, the therapist acquires important information, yet she or he is unable to use it openly. Second, the therapist becomes susceptible to the same feelings of guilt and anxiety that accompany holding a family secret. Third, the therapist has entered an alliance with the secret-holder(s) and is in a more difficult position to operate effectively in the interests of the whole couple or family. Ethically, by colluding with the secret-holder to deceive the unaware members, the therapist's trustworthiness is endangered. Finally, like any other secret-holder, the therapist runs the risk of an unanticipated and destructive disclosure of the secret. The dilemma in managing secrets in treatment is that the therapist's need to know is in conflict with his or her need to maintain trustworthiness.

Some therapists make it a point to avoid ever seeing one member of the treatment unit in private to avoid the sharing of secrets. Another approach is to tell family members very early in treatment that the presence of family secrets is not unusual, involve them in a discussion of the dangers and problems of special confidences, and ask them how *they* would like the therapist to handle this should it arise in the course of their work together (Karpel, 1980). Of course, should they choose to sanction such confidences, the therapist will have to inform them that such an arrangement may become unworkable, in which case the therapist would tell them so and they would have to choose between disclosure and termination.

The therapist can also use a flexible, gradual approach to disclosure should he or she find him- or herself having been dragged into the awareness context without warning. In this case, the therapist insists that for ethical and practical reasons the secret must be revealed, but the circumstances and timing may be negotiated. Depending on what is most helpful in the situation, the therapist can offer the support of his or her presence or permit the family member to reveal the secret in private or in a session without the children. Both Karpel (1980) and Broderick (1983) caution against forcing a disclosure despite the wishes of the secret-holder.

Clearly, this issue of confidentiality is something that must be anticipated by the therapist and discussed with the client system. Broderick (1983) states that marital and family therapists must also be knowledgeable about the laws of their state, which sometimes require the reporting of certain information.

As is apparent from the above, there are many dangers to rapport and the achieving of neutrality. However, what is important is what is communicated by the therapist's total behavior during the session (Selvini, Boscolo, Cecchin, & Prata 1980). The therapist will appear to be supportive of one after another member as the result of specific therapeutic strategies. It is the overall message that is crucial.

Goal Setting

As discussed above, the goals thought to be appropriate for marital/family therapy are influenced by the therapist's theoretical perspective. However, there is considerable agreement in the literature that if therapy is to be effective, the therapist and family must agree on the goals for treatment. This is also consistent with Standard IV (American Nurses' Association, 1982) that therapists need to collaborate with their clients for mutual goal setting.

While family-therapist goal congruity is a frequently discussed issue, it is obvious from the above that arriving at a "family goal" for treatment is not unproblematic either. Therefore, the early phase of therapy with a family includes not only assessment but also an exploration and negotiation between and among the therapist and family members regarding the acceptable goal of treatment.

In an effort to be clear and explicit about goals, many therapists use a contract. The precision and formality of these contracts vary considerably, however. Some are verbally stated goal statements. Others are written and are in behavioral terms. Seabury (1976) warns that contracts can be viewed too rigidly and used punitively, however. There is a need to distinguish between the contract being broken because its terms were unrealistic or broken as a test of its limits and to determine when negative sanctions should be applied and when it should be renegotiated.

Also, in the quest for precision of goal statements, therapists should not be limited to finite tasks easier to formulate and evaluate. Bowers (1980) discusses finite and continuous tasks. Finite tasks are clear-cut goals that are either accomplished or not (such as finding a job). Continuous tasks are ongoing and usually process oriented (such as checking out one's perceptions of the other's opinion). These latter tasks are frequently important behavior changes that facilitate new modes of family interaction.

Bowers (1980) also states that contracts express an agreed upon exchange between two parties. Therefore, the family is entitled to know what to expect of the nurse as well. For example, what kind of access will they have to the nurse between sessions should uncertainties or questions arise? Bowers recommends that such access not be prohibited unless problems arise that necessitate limits.

While defining goals is a difficult therapeutic task, it is essential for purposive work in therapy and for the evaluation of outcomes.

SUMMARY

In its relatively short history, the family approach to psychiatric mental health problems has had an important impact on the way nurses understand those problems. This reorientation has prompted considerable epistomological questioning which is ongoing. For that very reason, it is an exciting, substantive area.

Psychiatric mental health nurses have found the family approach to mental health problems compatible with the nursing perspective and so have added the modality of family therapy to their repertoire. There are many issues in the conduct of family therapy that have yet to be systematically described and researched, however. This chapter has surveyed a number of those issues.

REFERENCES

American Nurses' Association. *Standards of psychiatric and mental health nursing practice.* Kansas City, Mo: American Nurses' Association, 1982.

American Psychiatric Association. *Diagnostic and statistical manual of mental disorders* (3rd ed.). Washington DC: American Psychiatric Association, 1980.

Berg, B., & Rosenblum, N. Fathers in family therapy: A survey of family therapists. *Journal of Marriage and Family Counseling,* 1977, *3,* 85–91.

Bowers, J. E. Planning the therapeutic process with the family. In J. R. Miller & E. H. Janosik (Eds.), *Family focused care.* New York: McGraw-Hill, 1980.

Brehm, S. *The application of social psychology to clinical practice.* Washington, DC: Hemisphere, 1976.

Broderick, C. B. *The therapeutic triangle.* Beverly Hills: Sage Publications, 1983.

Clarkin, J. F., & Glick, I. D. Recent developments in family therapy: A review. *Hospital and Community Psychiatry,* 1982, *33,* 550–556.

Clements, I. W., & Buchanan, D. M. (Eds.). *Family therapy: A nursing perspective.* New York: John Wiley and Sons, 1982.

Clements, I. W., & Roberts, F. (Eds.). *Theoretical approaches to family health.* New York: John Wiley and Sons, 1983.

Fagin, C. M. *Family-centered nursing in community psychiatry.* Philadelphia: F. A. Davis Company, 1970.

Genthner, R., & Veldkamp, L. A scale for assessing family dysfunction-function. *International Journal of Family Counseling,* 1977, *5,* 79–85.

Gurman, A. S. Attitude change in marital cotherapy. *Journal of Family Counseling,* 1975, *2,* 50–54.(a)

Gurman, A. S. Couples' facilitative communication skills as a dimension of marital therapy outcome. *Journal of Marriage and Family Counseling,* 1975, *1,* 163–174.(b)

Gurman, A. Contemporary marital therapies: A critique and comparative analysis of psychoanalytic, behavioral, and systems theory approaches. In T. Paolina & B. McCrady (Eds.), *Marriage and marital therapy.* New York: Brunner Mazel, 1978.

Gurman, A. S., & Kniskern, D. P. Deterioration in marital and family therapy: Empirical, clinical, and conceptual issues. *Family Process,* 1978, *17,* 3–20.(a)

Gurman, A. S., & Kniskern, D. P. Technolatry, methodolatry, and the results of family therapy. *Family Process,* 1978, *17,* 275–281.(b)

Hannum, J. W. Some cotherapy techniques with families. *Family Process,* 1980, *19,* 161–168.

Karpel, M. A. Family secrets: I Conceptual and ethical issues in the relational context. II Ethical and practical considerations in therapeutic management. *Family Process,* 1980, *19,* 295–306.

Kniskern, D. P., & Gurman, A. S. Advances and prospects for family therapy research. In J. P. Vincent (Ed.), *Advances in family intervention, assessment and theory* (Vol. 2). Greenwich, CT: J. A. I. Press, Inc., 1981.

Kolevzon, M. S., & Green, R. G. Practice and training in family therapy: A known group study. *Family Process,* 1983, *22,* 179–190.

L'Abate, L. Pathogenic role rigidity in fathers: Some observations. *Journal of Marriage and Family Counseling,* 1975, *1,* 69–79.

L'Abate, L., Frey, J., & Wagner, V. Toward a classification of family therapy theories: Further elaborations and implications of the E-R-A-Aw-C model. *Family Therapy,* 1982, *9,* 251–262.

Lebow, J. Issues in the assessment of outcome in family therapy. *Family Process,* 1981, *20,* 167–188.

Liddle, H. A. On the problems of eclecticism: A call for epistemologic clarification and human-scale theories. *Family Process,* 1982, *21,* 243–250.

Napier, A., & Whitaker, C. *The family crucible.* New York: Harper & Row, 1978.

Olsen, D. H., Russell, C. S., & Sprenkle, D. H. Marital and family therapy: A decade review. *Journal of Marriage and the Family,* 1980, *42,* 973–993.(a)

Olsen, D. H., Russell, C. S., & Sprenkle, D. H. Circumplex model of marital and family systems II: Emperical studies and clinical intervention. In J. P. Vincent (Ed.), *Advances in family intervention, assessment and theory* (Vol. 1). Greenwich, CT: J. A. I. Press, 1980b.

Olson, D. H., Russell, C. S., & Sprenkle, D. H. Circumplex model of marital and family systems: VI. Theoretical update. *Family Process,* 1983, *22,* 69–97.

Olson, D. H., Sprenkle, D. H., & Russell, C. S. Circumplex model of marital and family systems: I. Cohesion and adaptability dimensions, family types, and clinical applications. *Family Process,* 1979, *18,* 3–28.

Rice, D. G., Fey, W. F., & Kepecs, J. G. Therapist experience and "style" as factors in co-therapy. *Family Process,* 1972, *11,* 1–12.

Russell, C. S. Circumplex model of marital and family systems: III. Empirical evaluation with families. *Family Process,* 1979, *18,* 29–45.

Seabury, B. A. The contract: Uses, abuses, and limitations. *Social Work,* 1976, *21,* 16–21.

Selvini, M. P., Boscolo, L., Cecchin, G., & Prata, G. Hypothesizing-circularity-neutrality: Three guidelines for the conductor of the session. *Family Process,* 1980, *19,* 3–12.

Shapiro, R. J., & Budman, S. H. Defection, termination and continuation in family and individual therapy. *Family Process,* 1973, *12,* 55–67.

Slipp, S., Ellis, S., & Kressel, K. Factors associated with engagement in family therapy. *Family Process,* 1974, *13,* 413–427.

Smoyak, S. Family therapy. In F. L. Huey (Ed.), *Psychiatric nursing 1946 to 1974: A report on the state of the art.* New York: American Journal of Nursing Co., 1975a.

Smoyak, S. (Ed.). *The psychiatric nurse as a family therapist.* New York: John Wiley and Sons, 1975b.

Stanton, M. D., & Todd, T. C. Engaging "resistant" families in treatment. *Family Process,* 1981, *20,* 261–294.

Teismann, M. W. Convening strategies in family therapy. *Family Process,* 1980, *19,* 393–400.

Terkelsen, K. G. Schizophrenia and the family: II. Adverse effects of family therapy. *Family Process,* 1983, *22,* 191–200.

Von Bertalanffy, L. *General system theory* (rev. ed.). New York: George Braziller, 1969.

BIBLIOGRAPHY

Jones, S. *Family therapy: A comparison of approaches.* Bowie, MD: Robert J. Brady Co., 1980.

Olson, D. H., McCubbin, H. I., Barnes, H., Larsen, A., Muxen, M., & Wilson, M. *Families: What makes them work.* Beverly Hills: Sage Publications, 1983.

CHAPTER 14 TREATMENT THROUGH THE MILIEU

Judith T. Maurin

Milieu treatment is a concept that fluctuates in its level of acceptance as other competing treatment emphases come and go. The past 15 years have seen a marked deemphasis on the importance of the hospital social environment as the community mental health and family therapy movements have cast doubt on the long-term importance of inpatient treatment. Yet inpatient treatment shows no sign of disappearing, and it is inconsistent with a nursing framework to assume that any hospitalization experience is neutral. Therefore, it is important to consider the dynamics that have been documented to accompany psychiatric hospitalization.

Even during its height of acceptability, milieu treatment has been problematic. There has been confusion over just what it is, and it has been difficult to implement. This chapter will begin with a brief history of milieu therapy and a discussion of the sources of conceptual confusion regarding it. Most of the chapter, however, will be devoted to a discussion of the dynamics important to this form of treatment. The processes and issues among team members, the reciprocal relationship between staff and patient behavior, and staff/patient role issues in milieu treatment will be explored. The similarities and differences between milieu treatment principles for the adult as compared to the child and adolescent will also be discussed. Finally, the implications of these insights for psychiatric nursing administration and psychiatric nursing specialist practice will be suggested.

HISTORY OF MILIEU TREATMENT

The idea that the immediate psychosocial environment in which psychiatric patients function is an important aspect of the treatment process is not new. Most trace the roots of this philosophy in the United States to the Moral Treatment approach brought from England by the Quakers in the early 1800s. However, Hollander (1981) cautions one not to overemphasize the parallels between nineteenth century moral treatment and modern milieu therapies. Moral Treatment conceptualized a humane living environment drawing on the Quaker's ideas of a well-ordered family: the appropriate authority and responsibility of parents (staff) toward their children (the patients). It encompassed removing the patient from his or her home to an asylum where the staff emphasized humane care, meaningful activities, and regular exercise in a calm retreat, preferably in the country.

Moral Treatment as a dominant treatment ideology was short-lived, however. In the 1840s, in combination with the huge influx of immigrant poor settling in the large cities, a humanitarian reform movement to transfer large numbers of insane paupers from jails to asylums, and a value shift which placed new hope for the insane in "scientific medicine" based on neurophysiology, the asylum changed markedly. Facilities enlarged, services deteriorated, and treatment relied increasingly on physician-ordered physical interventions. However, during the last four decades, interest in the effects of the treatment environment has resurfaced (Magaro, Gripp, & McDowell, 1978; Wolf, 1977).

CONFUSION OVER THE TERM

The confusion concerning milieu therapy is that there is no consistency in its definition in the literature. There are many different ways to integrate psychiatric hospital policies, social structure, and treatment modalities, which comprise the environment, into a broad treatment program. For example, early in the twentieth century, a number of psychoanalysts developed a type of milieu therapy that called for prescribed staff attitudes (Menninger, 1936) and specific activities and staff interactions individualized for each patient based on the psychoanalyst's understanding of the patient's unconscious needs (Bettelheim & Sylvester, 1948; Fromm-Reichman, 1947). Later, Maxwell Jones (1953) developed another type of milieu therapy called the Therapeutic Community, which was a significant departure from the milieu therapy that had gone before. It called for active responsibility on the part of the patient for his or her own treatment and the treatment of others, with nurses and physicians functioning as role models and catalysts for healthful behavior. Today, the ideas of democratization and active patient participation in treatment contributed by Jones are integral but troublesome components of the current, widely accepted understanding of what milieu therapy means.

The absence of a clear definition or precise identification of procedures that comprise the milieu approach has been attributed to several factors. Rossi and Filstead (1973) list the following: (1) failure to define precisely the specific aspects of the procedure; (2) the vague relationship between the concepts of "therapeutic community" and "milieu therapy"; (3) the overriding clinical interest in pharmacotherapy; and (4) the fact that few clinicians recognize the importance of social forces in group treatment setting. Magaro et al. (1978) add the lack of empirical research that would contribute to the clarification of relevant and irrelevant variables, and Rasinski, Rozensky, and Pasulka (1980) cite the absence of a theoretical framework within which a milieu approach could be grounded.

The milieu approach does bear a compatibility with the theoretical positions of the Interpersonal Theory of Psychiatry of Sullivan (1953) and the Symbolic Interaction Perspective from sociology (Blumer, 1969). The authors of these theoretical positions propose that it is through the individual's social interaction with others that the self is formed. The difficulty in trying to use theoretical positions such as these as a guide for building a therapeutic milieu is that they still can provide only a limited understanding of the relationship between group processes and intrapersonal dynamics. They do not suggest prescriptions of interactions for specific results.

In the absence of theoretically grounded and empirically supported treatment approaches for psychiatric illness, Magaro et al. (1978) argue that dominant therapy systems come and go according to the dominant cultural standard of the "good man" that the professional converts into a technology of helping.

In an effort to emerge from this morass of conceptual confusion, Rasinski et al. (1980) propose that milieu therapy be viewed within a conceptual framework of process variables, content variables, time variables, and outcome. *Process variables* are interpersonal, intrapersonnel, or transactional characteristics and the overall atmosphere of the unit that permits or impedes therapeutic encounters between and among patients and staff. *Content variables* include the specific procedures and activities that make up the treatment program of a unit: structured activities (group therapy, patient government, or open medical records); unstructured activities (time alone or unstructured time with patients and staff); specific content issues addressed therapeutically (mania, low self-esteem, or inadequate social skills); and specific treatment regimes (medication or individual therapy). *Time variables* include length of stay, amount of treatment time, and when, in the sequence from admission to discharge, a process or content variable occurs. Finally, *outcome* is the general result of treatment.

Rasinski et al. (1980) see milieu therapy as a generic approach. It is "the organizing therapeutic force of the treatment environment brought about by the specific interplay of process, content, and time variables of the unit and utilizing those variables as its tools and techniques" (p. 20). Different types of milieu therapy result from modifying the above variables. Thus, the Attitude Prescription of Menninger and the Therapeutic Community of Jones can be understood as different types of milieu therapy. Attending to these variables and their interaction may sensitize the clinician to dimensions of the environment that impact on patients and on which patients in turn have an effect. The variables may also provide an analytical scheme from which to observe the interrelationship among variables and outcome. It is unlikely that one approach will prove effective for all psychiatric patients. Yet to date, with few exceptions (Bjork, Steinberg, Lindenmayer, & Pardes, 1977), the milieu therapy literature largely ignores the individual differences among patients and the ramification of these differences on and for milieu therapy.

CONTRADICTIONS IN MILIEU TREATMENT

The difficulty in implementing a therapeutic milieu for the treatment of psychiatric patients stems first from the structural contradictions inherent in the situation. These contradictions exist in (1) the definition of patient and illness in the medical model versus the definition of staff and patient roles in milieu therapy and (2) the treatment versus social control functions assigned to psychiatric institutions by our broader society.

Medical Model Versus Milieu Model

The medical model assumes a role relationship between physician and patient that was first clearly articulated by Parsons (1951). He identified that the role expectation for a patient in the medical model included (1) exemption from normal social role responsibilities, (2) an inability to get well without help, (3) an obligation to want to "get well," and (4) the obligation to seek and cooperate with competent help (the physician). In contrast to the patient's helplessness is the physician's professional, technical competence and the responsibility to "do everything possible." Contrasted with the patient's emotional involvement in the situation is the physician's affectively neutral stance and the obligation to render help regardless of individual characteristics of the patient. These expectations for patient and physician roles clearly run counter to the relationships expected in the more democratized therapeutic milieu.

The characteristic elements of a democratized therapeutic milieu approach include (1) the patient is an active agent of treatment rather than passive; (2) the authority pyramid between staff and patients is flattened with an effort to share authority with patients; (3) distinctions among disciplines are minimized, with efforts to share authority and roles; and (4) open, adult communication between and among staff and patients is essential (Rossi & Filstead, 1973; Skinner, 1979). These elements representing democratization of the treatment environment have become assumed components when one speaks of milieu therapy for adults today. However, it is important to interject that not all forms of milieu therapy embody these characteristics. Menninger's Attitude Prescription attempted to achieve a specific, therapeutic environment for each patient, but the psychoanalyst was clearly the authority who knew better than other staff, and certainly better than the patient, what the patient's needs were. Based on this understanding, the psychoanalyst prescribed the approach that should be taken in interaction with the patient. Such a form of milieu therapy is far more compatible with the medical model than the Therapeutic Community.

Treatment Versus Social Control

Finally, one must acknowledge that society has delegated a social control function to psychiatric institutions in addition to a treatment function. It is expected that the mentally ill will be treated humanely, but also that society will be protected from those whose social behavior is unacceptable to that society.

Hoffman and Singer (1977) argue that the inherent incompatibility of the medical model and the therapeutic community results in antitherapeutic mixed messages to patients. They conclude that for this reason a true therapeutic community has a chance to develop only outside the hospital setting. However, even outside the hospital, staff carry the assumptions and understandings of their education and must still face the social mandate for social control. Most mental health professionals are familiar with the frequent community objection to a therapeutic community being located in a particular neighborhood. Even outside of the hospital, a therapeutic community must confront numerous social forces that attempt to limit the treatment prerogatives of staff.

While no one appears to have an answer to the contradictions and problems inherent in a therapeutic milieu, a first step toward coping with them is to understand the processes and issues that become problematic as one attempts to establish a therapeutic milieu.

PROCESSES AND ISSUES AMONG TEAM MEMBERS

Negotiation of Team Role Functioning

As an illustration of team role negotiation in action, consider the following vignette.

The team is gathered for their regularly scheduled conference. One of the staff nurses begins the conference, saying with unmistakable anger in her voice, "Tomorrow is the trip to the fair which has been planned for some time. I want to know how many team members we can expect to accompany us this time. The last trip was dumped on the nursing staff, and we don't have enough nurses scheduled tomorrow to cover the unit and handle the trip alone too."

After a short, uncomfortable pause, a couple of the psychiatric residents explain that they have clients coming in for follow-up. There was just no other time to schedule them. The social worker explains that that afternoon is when she has a standing appointment to supervise two graduate students in their group experience.

The head nurse, also angry, reminds the team that on this unit an indispensable part of treatment is the role modeling of staff and staff-patient interactions around normal activities of daily living. It is important that all team members see patients interacting in more normal environments, as that is part of the treatment program and will provide grist for later therapy sessions.

Finally, after an emotionally charged conference, an interdisciplinary group is designated to accompany patients to the fair the next day.

Such an exchange could have been overheard on an adult or children's unit around the issue of meals or preparing children for bed. It could have involved any activity of daily living. Sometimes the confrontation is prompted by a disturbing incident, for example, a child having become dangerously out of control at bedtime the night before. Often, however, the confrontation appears to be sprung "spontaneously" on the team. What was going on? Why did it feel so awful and so important to everyone there? Why was everyone so emotionally involved in the exchange?

The Importance of Ideology

Most units have a predominant ideology that has consequences for what is done to and for patients and who does what kinds of work. Ideology in this context means a shared or collective set of psychiatric ideas about the etiology and treatment of mental illness (Strauss, Schatzman, Bucker, Ehrlick, & Sabshin, 1964). Given similar patients and institutional conditions, persons with different ideological positions will operate differently. On a unit where somatic therapies and the hospital experience as a respite during which treatment is administered are believed in, an exchange such as in the vignette above would not have taken place. Team members would not likely be pressed into service for anything as "frivolous" as a trip to the fair. The kinds of negotiations that can be struck regarding who does what is limited, in part, by the dominant ideology of the unit (or the ideology of those with the most power on the unit).

Negotiating Tasks

How can one understand what was taking place in the vignette? Strauss et al. (1964) argue that team organization on a psychiatric unit emerged from a process of negotiation about which tasks should be performed by whom. Because ideology involves conceptions of treatment and, therefore, implies the tasks necessary to effect treatment, the selection and negotiation about tasks is an integral part of ideological discussion. The question of who should carry out particular tasks is inseparable from the team's discussion of treatment ideologies and the defining of necessary tasks to effect this treatment. When Strauss and his colleagues studied psychiatric institutions, they identified the following kinds of interactions through which an organization of teamwork emerged:

1. *Task-Claiming*: A team member lays claim to an area of competence and particular associated tasks that may be either new for his or her profession or traditional rights.
2. *Task-Proffering*: A particular area of endeavor is offered to other team members.
3. *Task-Discovery:* Like task-claiming, a team member assumes a task. However, it tends not to have the intense initial investment in the task as when task-claiming. Instead, task-discovery tends to occur as team members become aware of loose ends or unanticipated consequences of teamwork that should be handled.
4. *Task-Stripping*: One or more team members attempt to deny another's claim to a particular task on the grounds that it is inappropriate (Strauss et al., 1964).

Each of the above interactions initiates a series of responses. In the aforementioned vignette, the team had behaviorally proffered the supervision of planned outings to the nursing staff. Exclusive responsibility for this task was rejected by the nursing staff, who countered by proffering to share the task with all team members. After some argument, the team agreed to tolerate this distribution of tasks. However, it should not be expected that the issue is settled.

The Importance of Professional Identities

The reason that task distribution is not settled so easily is that team members come to the setting with professional identities that include understandings about the direct therapeutic roles they are prepared to play. As these mental health professionals stake out claims to share in the treatment process, and team members either accept or reject these claims, the professionals experience an acceptance or rejection of their professional identities as well. The reason that the exchange in the vignette feels so awkward to the participants, and is so charged with emotion, is that professional identities are deeply involved both in what team members seek for themselves and in their response to others.

The selection of tasks to be claimed, rejected, or proffered is obviously not random. Certain tasks are more widely acknowledged to be associated with direct therapeutic roles (for example, the "therapies"—group, family, play, and so on). Typically, and in spite of milieu therapy ideology, tasks associated with activities of daily living are less valued, their role in therapeutic change less clear.

The organization of teamwork on each unit is continually negotiated around the tasks to be performed using the rhetoric of treatment ideologies either implicitly or explicitly. The head nurse's appeal to the ideology of the therapeutic milieu in her proferring to share responsibility for the trip to the fair with other team members was important. Tying task distribution to a treatment ideology both provides a justification and rationale for the task distribution, while the accepted task distribution in turn validates the team's continued acceptance of the treatment ideology. The stakes in these negotiations are high because the consequences are not just reasonable work loads, but validation or rejection of a valued professional identity.

Divergent Treatment Ideologies

The discussion thus far has implied that all the core mental health professionals on a team hold a consensus about what ought to be done to or for patients. Such an assumption could not be further from reality. Ideological commitments are built into professional training. While students are learning clinical skills, they are also acquiring convictions about what is basic to treatment and what is proper treatment. Again, it would be too simplistic to suggest that ideological differences fall along disciplinary lines. The psychologist whose work is dynamically informed has as little base of understanding with his or her behavior modifying colleague as a nurse taught to see the "identified patient" as a symptom of family distress. The consequence of these conflicting perspectives among mental health professionals is more than a difficulty in constructing a treatment plan toward which all can work in a concerted effort. Ideological convictions generate their own morality so that treatment issues are anything but objective differences of professional opinion.

The most obvious example of this phenomenon frequently involves the suggestion that electroshock treatment (EST) be used on a unit. Some staff will argue that it is cruel to withhold a procedure that can offer the patient relief from the torture of his depression. Others will argue that such a method is medieval and in fact renders the patient inaccessible to real therapy as a result of the confusion following EST. The choice of terms (cruel, torture) are value-ladened terms heard in many a team meeting. They are indications of the moral judgements inherent in the respective positions. Ideologies provide the practitioner with a framework within which to judge specific treatments practiced by self and/or others. As Strauss et al. (1964) stated, "only a thin line divided efficacy and 'rightness' " (p. 365).

Coordination of Teamwork

Even on units that value the sharing of tasks among team members, some division of labor will emerge. First, it is simply not workable for everyone to be responsible for everything. Even if the division is not based on strictly disciplinary lines, some staff will be more skilled or find more satisfaction doing some tasks over others. Second, the division may be influenced by outside standards and/or policies. Whatever the factors contributing toward the division of labor, it presents the team with the problem of integrating all aspects of a program toward a common treatment goal for patients. On a children's unit that may mean coordination among the teachers, the cottage or unit staff, the family therapist, and the recreation therapist. On an adult unit it may mean communication between the individual therapist, the unit staff, or simply between the unit staff working days and evenings. While there is no magic solution for effecting the kind of singleness of purpose thought to be in the patient's best interest, it is impossible without communication between and among staff.

It should be taken for granted that patient-centered communication will occur *routinely.* This means, first, constituting a team based on the numbers of staff interacting with this patient. Some patients will use more services than others, and their "team" will be correspondingly larger. Second, the task during team conferences is to develop a treatment plan and articulate how the principle in the plan will be operationalized in the various contributing programs. Translating abstract principles into day-to-day behaviors is never easy. Some discussion about how various staff in the classroom and on the unit could help an adolescent "assume increased responsibility for his behavior," is important. It is crucial to clarify what this means to respective staff as well as provide anticipatory guidance to those who will have to implement the treatment principle. Finally, team conferences must happen routinely, and not be called only as problems arise. In the case of the latter, team members usually respond defensively because they have no established working relationships. Even in the best of circumstances, however, team members must be on the lookout for hidden agendas, precipitated by the status strategies and ideological differences addressed above, which can stalemate teamwork. The most effective strategy in such situations is to stop and do some group processing. As will be argued later, staff differences are less consequential when they are overt.

RECIPROCITY BETWEEN STAFF AND PATIENT BEHAVIOR

It is imperative that milieu therapists conceptualize their field of interest very broadly to incorporate not just single patients, but the interaction between and among patients and the interaction between and among staff and patients as well. While research into the explanation of these processes is disappointingly sparse, there is documentation in the literature of the reciprocal consequences of patient and others' behavior. These relationships will be discussed in order of social system complexity beginning with a focal patient and ending with the consequences of staff issues for patient behavior.

Therapeutic Use of Self

First, considering a focal patient, psychiatric mental health nursing knowledge has long included the principle that behavior has meaning, and the nurse's response to that behavior can either reinforce or alter it (Peplau, 1962). As such, the nurse is directed to assess not only verbal messages but also behavior patterns. The nurse's behavior patterns vis-à-vis the patient can be therapeutic or detrimental for the patient's recovery. The strategy of behaviorally presenting oneself as a trustworthy person in the beginning of a relationship is a familiar example of a behavior pattern believed to be therapeutic (Schwartz & Shockley, 1956). Likewise, "mutual withdrawal" is an equally classic example of the detrimental consequences of a nurse's behavior pattern for a patient (Tudor, 1952). The potency of interpersonal relationships is part of the discipline's knowledge base. While milieu therapy admittedly demands more than the dyadic focus, the dyadic interpersonal understanding is basic knowledge that ought to inform nursing practice in a therapeutic milieu.

Nurse/Patient Relationship Within a Treatment Unit

The Problem of the Special Patient

Evidence that what goes on within a nurse-patient relationship can affect the whole unit and vise versa can be found in the discussions of the "special patient." Stanton and Schwartz (1954) documented this phenomenon in a psychiatric institution. This example is worth discussion because of the conflict it can generate.

As an illustration of a problematic special patient, consider the following case study.

Bob is a 28-year-old, married, unemployed man hospitalized for the third time with the diagnosis of schizophrenia. Upon admission, he exhibited symptoms of auditory hallucinations. He was also verbally loud and abusive toward his wife, making her fear for her safety and precipitating the hospitalization. Upon hospitalization, however, he functioned well. Yet he resisted the staff's efforts for job placement in preparation for discharge and presented behavior that staff interpreted as being comfortable in the hospital and unwilling to work at therapy.

Sue, a psychiatric nurse clinical specialist working on this unit, had become interested in Bob during a previous hospitalization and began to work with him in a one-to-one relationship. One-to-one relationships were not unheard of on this unit but were not provided for each patient. During this relationship, Sue assessed that while Bob did not have a high school diploma, he appeared bright; he had very low self-esteem which he attempted to mask with a carefree demeanor; he had poor individuation which was threatened in relationships with his mother and his wife; and finally, his resistance to job placement indicated fear that such situations would reveal his inability to read and result in ridicule. Sue's treatment plan included strategies to strengthen his sense of identity and his self-esteem. Among other things, Sue encouraged and facilitated Bob's enrollment in an adult education program for persons preparing to take the General Education Diploma (GED).

The evening of his second hospital day, Bob became very angry with staff because he insisted on a pass to attend the adult education class. He was refused the pass because the unit policy did not permit a patient a pass without a team discussion. Bob ended up spending the night in seclusion and on extra medication.

The next morning there was a very angry exchange between Sue and the rest of the team. The team was of the opinion that Bob's out-of-control behavior the night before was evidence that he was not ready for a pass. Sue argued that the team never had understood or liked Bob. Two consecutive absenses would result in his being dropped from the class. The team knew the work she had been doing with Bob and the importance of his working toward the GED. Mindless adherence to rules is antitherapeutic. Why hadn't she been called if they had a question? Last night could have been avoided. The team in turn told Sue she was over-involved with this patient and could not see his need for limits on his manipulative behavior.

How can one understand the above? Certainly many requests for exceptions to rules or individualized considerations result in accommodation. What happened here?

When Special Requests Become Problematic

Using Stanton and Schwartz's work (1954) four factors can be cited that predispose unique treatment to be problematic. First, unique treatment is more likely to be a problem if the request comes from the patient than if the need is identified by staff. Staff initiation fits the accepted norm of health care provider as expert. Furthermore, staff-initiated action becomes an anticipated part of the work flow and is incorporated into the functioning routine. Patient requests may be unanticipated by staff and experienced as burdensome interruptions in the flow of work to be done.

Second, when the unique treatment given a patient is something in limited supply, it is more likely to be problematic. One of the most precious commodities in a treatment setting is the time and interest of personnel.

Third, unique treatment tends to become a problem when the special consideration given by one staff member has consequences for other staff. The consequence is sometimes added work: unavailability of a staff member while spending extra time with a patient may mean others must pick up extra tasks or the time and effort required to justify hospital routine when others deny an exception. A second consequence is the direct or implied message from the patient and/or his special staff person that those who do not provide the unique treatment compare unfavorably with those who do. Staff are likely to respond with guilt and/or anger to such messages. Every work group, including a hospital staff, evolves a norm regarding how much and what kind of work is reasonable. When a member violates that norm, repercussions will be felt by the group. Finally, unique treatment tends to be problematic when it triggers the expression or resurfacing of an unresolved staff issue.

The consequence of a disagreement over the legitimacy of the unique treatment, as demonstrated in the vignette above, is an interference in the cooperative, supportive team relationship that is likely to spill into other situations and make the work place decidedly unpleasant. Not infrequently, the situation is complicated by the inability to communicate about the disagreement openly between the principal parties. Everyone seems to be talking about the problem, but complaints tend to be discussed with third parties. A second consequence is that negative feelings may become fixed on the patient, interfering with the team's ability to respond to the patient therapeutically.

The situation in the above vignette may involve a commitment to differing treatment ideologies. While the special treatment that was clearly debated among staff was the issue of the pass, there is sufficient evidence to suggest that the one-to-one relationship may have been special treatment as well. In the absence of consensus over the acceptability of the one-to-one relationship, numerous peripheral issues loom in their importance.

Intervention Strategies

While resolution of the above problem is admittedly difficult, there are certain strategies to be recommended.

1. The team must be brought together to address the problem openly. Resolution is impossible under a condition of closed communication among the principal parties.
2. In addressing the problem, there are certain patient-focused and treatment-focused questions to keep in front of the group: Is the special treatment negatively affecting other patient's care? Is the patient being promised more than the institution can deliver? Is the special treatment beneficial to the patient? Is the team disagreement negatively affecting the patient's care and, if so, how?
3. The patient's advocate must evaluate the possibility that his or her behavior is contributing to the team division. This would be facilitated by regular clinical supervision. Sometimes the primary therapist is giving the message, "Hands off, this is my special project. Only I understand this patient," and then becoming angry when other staff respond to that

message. Supervision could help anticipate situations like the one in the vignette. Using the clinical specialist's knowledge of the patient acquired in a long-term relationship, supervision would help identify issues important to communicate in a pre-admission conference.

4. The team leader can facilitate profitable discussion by the way in which the problem is framed for discussion. While staff process is an integral part of this problem and thus important to uncover, the purpose of doing so is to understand the consequence of that process for patient care and not to assign blame.
5. The team leader must be prepared to decide the treatment issue if staff are unable to do so. Furthermore, the effectiveness of the decision should be evaluated at a predetermined future date. Once again, the reevaluation should be in terms of the outcome for the patient and any other patients affected. It is unreasonable to expect that team members will change how they feel toward the patient or that they will change their treatment ideology. It is expected, however, that these feelings will cease to interfere with the implementation of a plan of care based on the assessment of patient needs.

Hidden Staff Disagreement

Imbedded in the discussion above was the "hidden staff disagreement" that became a hidden agenda in staff interaction. This factor is important to discuss in its own right because it has been associated in the literature with symptoms of agitation, pathological excitement, and paranoia on the part of individual patients (Bradshaw, 1972; Stanton & Schwartz, 1954). Stanton and Schwartz are attributed with having brought the phenomenon to attention. The patients involved characteristically were the center of a disagreement about management, frequently involving a disagreement about diagnosis as well, and the disagreement was covert. Also noted was the immediate subsiding of patient symptoms coinciding with solution to the staff disagreement. Solution may occur "(1) by the patient's being moved to another ward, under different authorities, (2) by withdrawal of one or both of the authorities, or (3) by the authorities' beginning to discuss their differences seriously and directly with each other" (Stanton & Schwartz, 1954, p. 353).

This phenomenon of acute agitation associated with covert disagreement between at least two authorities having control over a particular patient and the rapid subsiding of that agitation when the disagreement is resolved or made overt is fascinating to consider. Bradshaw (1972) states, "One may presume that there are subtle cues to which the schizophrenic patient is particularly sensitive, but the exact mechanisms in relation to the Stanton-Schwartz phenomenon remain to be elucidated" (p. 22).

While the phenomenon still remains to be researched, there is a striking parallel between it and the double bind believed to play a role in the family life experience of schizophrenic patients (Bateson, Jackson, Haley, & Weakland, 1956). The conflicting primary and secondary injunctions in the hidden staff disagreement are represented by the two authorities from whom the patient appears unable to escape. As in a double bind, the disagreement is covert. When the disagreement becomes overt or the patient is released from one of the authorities, the interpersonal field is altered significantly and the symptoms disappear. Stanton and Schwartz (1954) suggest that patients who respond in this way to hidden staff disagreements are different from other schizophrenic patients on a unit. They observed that these patients tended to move toward any disturbance rather than withdraw. The significance of this observation, as well as the phenomenon itself, needs to be further explored.

Staff Morale and Patient Behavior

The final logical extension of the reciprocity between staff and patient behavior, both in terms of extent of pathology and involvement of the social network, is the phenomenon of a collective disturbance associated with the breakdown of morale or the lack of integration within the staff (Boyd, Kagels, & Greenblatt, 1954; Caudill, 1958; Crabtree & Levinson, 1980; Miller, 1957; Stanton & Schwartz, 1954). On any psychiatric unit, there will be some periods when for days things seem to go from bad to worse. One can feel the tension when stepping onto the unit. While one patient may be the center of attention, there is a general increase in level of disturbance and agitation among the patient group as a whole. At just the time that patient needs are most demanding, there seems to be fewer staff available, and those available appear to be repeatedly responding to crises in an isolated uncoordinated manner. For staff, the experience is chaos and each new shift is approached with dread.

Crabtree and Levinson (1980) see the collective disturbance as one cycle in an oscillation of tension that is an inevitable outgrowth of a ward culture that permits sufficient interaction and acting out to provide opportunities for therapeutic confrontation. In such a ward culture, the cycles arise from fluctuations in relationship patterns among patients and staff. The goal is to manage these cycles optimally rather than try to repress them altogether. To achieve this stage, they found that each cycle calls for different modes of leadership, usually provided by different staff members.

Stanton and Schwartz (1954) associated this phenomenon with a particular social field. They suggested an association between collective disturbance and the quality and quantity of participation in work accompanying low morale. They identified three levels of participation in work: Collaborative Role Performance, Cooperative Role Performance, and Disintegrative Role Performance. They argue that the morale associated with these levels of role performance range from high to low, respectively, and that the Cooperative Level is the modal category among staff.

The value of elucidating the behaviors accompanying the varying levels of morale is that intervention points become evident. Of special note is that during the early phase of Disintegrative Role Performance, key staff withdraw and communication channels become blocked. This withdrawal of staff has been observed by most who have discussed the collective disturbance. It may be the nursing supervisor or head nurse who finds many compelling reasons to be off the unit. The chief resident may become unusually busy with his or her outpatient clients. As a result, unit staff feel deserted. At the same time, just when open communication is most essential, customary communication channels are blocked. Team meetings are cancelled because everyone is too busy. Written avenues of communication either go unused or become cryptic and stereotyped. This occurrence suggests the point at which intervention strategies can be aimed resulting in a changed social field. With the return of key staff and the reestablishing of communication, the problem can hopefully be identified, but probably more important, the ability to count on one another can be restored with an accompanying return of a sense of support and corresponding changes in specific behavior.

The foregoing discussion of staff and staff-patient processes are not exhaustive. However, they serve to make the point that "disturbed" patient behavior is neither random nor explanable solely by the patient's psychopathology. The patient's behavior is influenced both positively and negatively by the behavior of his care-givers in ways that are still inadequately understood.

STAFF-PATIENT ROLE ISSUES

The Nature and Extent of Patient Participation

Practically every program that calls itself a Therapeutic Community for adults and/or adolescents uses the technique of regular community meetings or patient government. The community meeting is attended by all patients and usually all staff and is conducted for the purpose of discussing issues of concern to the community. As a cornerstone of the therapeutic community, this strategy bears discussion, for it exemplifies most of the dilemmas that plague the therapeutic community: the dilemma of staff responsibility and accountability versus patient participation as reflected in decision making, limit setting, and confidentiality. This dilemma is intensified on today's short-term units characterized by a wide spectrum of patients and a patient group whose composition is continually changing.

The purpose of the community meeting stated above is deceptively simple. To operationalize that purpose one must decide: What issues of concern are community concerns? Who is the community leader? What does it mean for staff and patient roles when there is the desire for patients to participate in their treatment? What is the difference between a community meeting and patient government?

The literature is replete with examples that suggest that many treatment teams are uncertain and ambivalent about how much and what kind of responsibility should be exercised by staff and by patients with the result that both approach the community meeting with a mixture of apprehension, annoyance, and apathy (Abramczuk, 1972; Kisch, Kroll, Gross, & Carey, 1981; Klein, 1981).

Once again, the answer to successfully incorporating a community meeting into the treatment program of a unit means giving consideration to the characteristics of the patients, their behavior patterns and needs; the length of patient stay; the skills and knowledge of the staff; and the treatment goal of the unit. Russakoff and Oldham (1982) describe specific structural and technical parameters of the community meeting that they have found to meet the situational needs of a short-term unit that admits a heterogenous group of acutely disturbed patients. Their description clarifies the many decisions to be made about a community meeting. As the authors point out, the structure can be loosened if there is a significant shift to healthier patients on the unit.

The *structural aspects* of the community meeting include (1) Duration. There must be sufficent time to permit meaningful discussion of issues but it cannot last beyond the endurance of substantially disturbed patient. Forty-five minutes is recommended. (2) Seating arrangements. The leader should sit so that he or she can be seen by all. Staff members arrange to sit next to potentially disruptive patients to help control antisocial impulses. (3) Attendance. All patients are expected to attend. All nurses, therapists, relevant activity-therapy staff, and ward administrators are expected to attend. Others are invited when there are special issues. (4) Leader. The leader is a staff member or trainee who has been identified beforehand and will serve as leader for a designated period of time. Formal training and supervision of the staff who run these meetings is important.

The *technical aspects* of the community meeting include (1) The leader introduces him or herself, reviews the structure and function of the meeting, indicates when it well begin and end, and whether smoking is allowed. (2) Begin with a roll call or attendance of both staff and patients. Explanations ought to be provided to account for those absent, because the absence of a member can have a significant effect on the group. Staff need to assess if the explanation has been sufficient (Benton, 1980). (3) New community members (staff, trainees, patients) are introduced. New patients are not asked to explain why they have come to the hospital, however, as such a question is embarrassing to a new person in such a large group. (4) An agenda is openly created by soliciting agenda items from the group. The leader makes the order of priority, however, aiming to maintain a supportive beginning and ending. (5) Since the focus of the meeting is on issues of concern to the entire community, all relevant information about the issue should be presented publicly. (6) An issue should be brought to closure before moving on to another topic. This step does not mean a premature decision need be made. Closure might be, "We cannot suggest a solution to this problem without discussing it with dietary. I will ask that the dietician attend tomorrow's community meeting." (7) The dynamics of separation are especially important for psychotic inpatients; therefore, careful attention should be paid to patients being admitted or discharged.

The above structure and technique described by Russakoff and Oldham (1982) is clearly a community meeting and not patient government. Many aspects of the above could be modified if the patient group were less disturbed and/or the group experienced less client turnover. Mechanisms for selection of a patient leader could be provided. Limit-setting on disruptive behavior within the group could be shared with the patient group. Certain aspects of the day's activities could be the sole prerogative of patient decision making (Jacobs, 1977). As there is no best milieu, there is no one answer to whether or not a unit should have patient government or to the kind of community meeting to institute. These decisions must be deliberately made based on the needs and strengths of the patient population.

The One-to-One Relationship in the Community

The one-to-one relationship does not enjoy unquestionable acceptance within milieu therapy. Some staff believe that it runs counter to the philosophy of the therapeutic community, perhaps a reaction to the philosophy that only individual therapy "counts." Others fear that it will foster dependency (Paine, 1981). There is also the fear that the individual therapist will come to identify exclusively with the perspective of the patient. The individual therapist and other team members see the patient in different settings and different relationships where different aspects of the patient become evident. Each team member may become convinced that only he or she knows the "real" patient, resulting in a conflict similar to that described earlier in discussion of the "special patient." Such need not be the case, however.

One-to-one relationships can be successfully incorporated into a therapeutic community if the team is supportive of the individual therapist, as well as the work this person is to do with the patient, and the therapist, in turn, supports the roles, norms, and importance of the community (Carser, 1982; Druck, 1982). This can be accomplished by the therapist refusing to see the patient when a milieu group is in session, encouraging the patient to bring up issues in the appropriate group, and demonstrating a valuing of community activities by inquiring about the patient's participation. The team can be supportive of the therapist by keeping to the schedule of activities so that clients can make their appointments with therapists on time without being forced to choose between the therapist and other team members; communicating openly about the patient with the therapist in the spirit that only through such sharing will a full, coherent picture of the patient emerge and being sensitive to the possibility that a therapist may have difficulty in the relationship with a patient at times. During such times, the therapist, too, may need special help and support.

MILIEU TREATMENT OF CHILDREN AND ADOLESCENTS

It is perhaps unfortunate that milieu therapists dealing with adults, adolescents, and children share so little of the same literature. It is striking how many milieu issues are similar across these three age groups. Equally striking are the points on which there is divergence. The similarities include (1) concern for the effect of staff attitudes, conflicts, and triangulation on individual patients and the group as a whole (Krug, 1952; Martin, 1977); (2) continual struggle to find the proper balance between limits, boundaries or discipline and participation, and freedom or space to grow (Martin, 1977; Redl, 1959a); (3) evidence that a process of negotation about work tasks and their importance exists among staff whereby status and identities are created and maintained (Critchley & Berlin, 1979; Krug, 1952); (4) the importance of clear, unambiguous communication between and among staff and patients (Puskar, 1981); and (5) the opinion that ward atmosphere, milieu activities, and the overall experience for patients are correlated in some meaningful way with the therapeutic outcome.

Providing Security

The points on which child and adolescent milieus diverge in emphasis from milieus of adults provide subjects for discussion for those who deal with adults. First, meeting dependency and security needs in order that more developmentally mature skills may be nurtured is an accepted principle underlying work with disturbed children and adolescents (Krug, 1952; Rossman & Knesper, 1976). In fact, the milieu is seen as crucial in this important task.

> This process whereby the relationship between the child and an adult becomes therapeutic is stated as a third principle of psychotherapy: within the security of the therapeutic relationship the child's emotional development is recapitulated in a new, corrective manner for meeting his needs for both dependency and growth. . . . All children first gain security with adults by receiving concrete tangible evidence of acceptance through physical activities and care. . . . Through the daily experiences residential workers have many opportunities to demonstrate to the child these concrete evidences of acceptance. As a result these children sometimes develop their first meaningful relationship in residence rather than in individual therapy. (Krug, 1952, p. 696)

To further protect this sense of security and acceptance, a division of labor is recommended between the individual therapist and other team members. While all are encouraged to adopt a style of thinking that assumes that the child's behavior has communicative value, an understandable meaning, and a fundamental logic emanating from the child's view of himself and others, team members are encouraged to reserve interpretive comments and exploration of unconscious conflicts for individual therapy. There is the concern that in the presence of multiple therapists, the child or teenager may feel psychologically assaulted (Krug, 1952; Rossman, 1979).

The Life Space Interview

While the interpretation and stimulation of painful unconscious conflicts is left to the individual therapist, unit staff take advantage of everyday issues and experiences and convert them into therapeutic experiences through "life space interviewing" (Redl, 1959b). The life space interview is a form of crisis intervention on the spot for those moments of stress in everyday living that are impossible to avoid. It may also be an opportunity for clinical exploitation of a life event when something central to the incident relates to a therapeutic goal for the child. Any such event becomes a signal to whatever staff person happens to be present and part of the event to then and there intervene with an interview. The interview may be with a single child or a group. The interview is about what has just happened, what it feels like, what it means. Sometimes, with a very upset child, two people might dialogue between them about the event while the child is held and contained.

Program Considerations

In keeping with the notion that the overall setting is a basic treatment modality, a great deal of careful thought has gone into the ingredients of the milieu. What has emerged is a major emphasis on programming. "It [programming] deals with the structuring of time and the prescribing of activity for the individual's life and for the group's life, and it depends on an accurate reading of individual and group dynamics in terms of needs and potentialities" (Noshpitz, 1975, p. 643). In assessing each child, a multiaxial developmental framework is recommended to evaluate such areas as cognitive functioning, relationships with peers and adults, sensorimotor, ego functioning, and physical development. Based on this multidisciplinary evaluation, the team collaboratively plans the child's treatment around his or her individual developmental capacities and needs (Berlin, 1978; Whittaker, 1975). This approach means unit programming must provide for individual and small therapy groups, education and sensorimotor remediation, recreation including large muscle sports and fine muscle crafts, social interactive time to include both adult-oriented and peer group-structured moments, and solo contemplative time. Through programming, time is structured to provide a rhythm to the events of the week (with the work-school quality of the weekdays and the relaxation-recreation quality of the weekend) and of the day which the children can count on and grow within (Berlin, 1980; Critchley & Berlin, 1979; Noshpitz, 1975).

The above is not meant to imply that interdisciplinary team functioning is any easier for teams working with children and adolescents than for teams working with adults. All the interdisciplinary processes and conflict issues discussed earlier are evident.

The Role of Parents

Finally, hospitalization of a disturbed child is a decision not made lightly. It usually occurs only when the problems that the child and parents have in living together have reached such an impasse that progress cannot be made in treatment without the separation. While most professionals who work with disturbed children see the parents as intimately involved in the problems of the child, programs vary widely in the relationship they prefer vis-à-vis the parents. Some prefer that the parents permit the center to take over the child's life completely (Bettelheim, 1950). Others require that while the child receives treatment in the residence program, the parents receive treatment apart from the child (Krug, 1952). There is increasing concern, however, that traditional residential treatment of children increases parents' guilt and thus enhances the parental rejection that often accompanies the physical separation of the child and his parents (Christ & Wagner, 1965). Therefore, it is recommended that a basic purpose of residential programs for troubled children should be to function as a family support system, recognizing the parents as troubled and hurt human beings whose trouble with their child has only reinforced their feelings of doubt about their adequacy (Whittaker, 1975). Critchley and Berlin (1981) describe a program that encouraged parent participation in the milieu of psychotic children so that (1) staff could role model more effective parenting behavior toward the child; (2) parents could observe and practice more nurturant and more effective limit-setting behaviors; and (3) through these means reduce the helplessness and promote feelings of competence, effectiveness, and, finally, playfulness and spontaneity in all family members.

Prior to the child's acceptance into the program, a mutually agreed upon treatment contract is developed that includes planned, weekly participation of both parents in the milieu. Second, a parent liaison is assigned from the staff. This is the parents' contact person. The parent liaison plans the goals and purposes of each parents' program participation with the team, taking into consideration the parents' expressed needs and interests. This person then works with the parents to plan their participation. Finally, the parent liaison provides on-the-spot assistance and support, as well as role modeling for the parents' ways of interacting with their own and other children during parental involvement in the program. At these times, the parents require very active assistance and support, for a psychotic child's behavior can be frustrating and anger provoking and the parents already feel helpless and incompetent in relation to it.

IMPLICATIONS FOR NURSING ADMINISTRATION

There is a debate in nursing today as to how best to prepare individuals for nursing administrative positions. Should clinical knowledge or administrative/management skills be emphasized in their preparation? It is undeniable that the management of health care organizations has become increasingly complex as these organizations have become more complex and subject to increasing external forces. However, the nursing administrator of psychiatric mental health services first needs clinical knowledge and then administrative skills. This opinion is based on the belief that administrative decisions must be made with an understanding of the work done in psychiatric institutions and an appreciation for the relationship between staff attitudes and behavior and patient behavior and clinical progress. Administrative decisions can significantly affect staff attitudes and behavior.

To the clinically uninformed, psychiatric nursing in a therapeutic milieu looks simple enough: staff and patients talk a great deal, in pairs and groups; some staff may play volleyball with a group of patients; others may help a patient with his or her hygiene. Much of it appears unskilled. Beneath the surface of such mundane activities is, however, the demanding and challenging aspect of the work. It tends to reawaken any unresolved emotional problems. There is the need to handle situations immediately at all hours, and because patients and staff see each other in many different contexts, there is always the need to decide on what level to respond in each situation. Sometimes behavior must be taken literally while at other times behavior must be understood as a symptom and responded to accordingly. Such sensitivity during interaction is physically and emotionally fatiguing and demands both self-awareness and a solid knowledge base.

Decisions about levels of nursing positions budgeted, staffing patterns, resource allocation, and appointment and evaluation of personnel cannot help but be influenced by one's conception of the work to be done. As a result of these decisions, administrators mold organizational design.

Previously, Stanton and Schwartz's (1954) argument for a relationship between staff behavior associated with low morale and an increase in disturbed patient behavior was presented. Their concept of low morale appears closely related to the current concept of burnout (although they were discussing a group phenomenon and burnout usually refers to an individual phenomenon). Nevertheless, Cherniss (1980a,b) argues that organizational design (the normative structure, the power structure, and the role structure) can either promote or discourage job stress and burnout.

The psychiatric nursing administrator is not only important in his or her part in creating and maintaining a given organizational design, however. The relationship between the supervisor and the worker is thought to be important in its own right as an influence on the level of job stress and coping in human service settings.

Cherniss and Egnatios (1978) note that supervision in human services usually serves two different functions. First, it is a mechanism of administrative control whereby the supervisor monitors and evaluates the work of subordinates and ensures conformity to organizational policies and rules. However, it is usually intended that the supervisor will serve a professional development function as well, offering support, learning, and professional growth. There is often the expectation that supervisors will help the worker to understand and constructively manage his or her emotional responses to situations that arise in the work. Some settings try to divide the administrative and professional development functions between two distinct positions. However, in many settings these functions are combined in one role, especially in administrative positions lower in the hierarchy, such as head nurse.

Effective supervision is a skill, the key to which is sensitivity and responsiveness to the needs and competencies of individual staff members. Cherniss' (1980a) summary of the research of effective supervision suggested that it includes finding the right combination of support and autonomy for staff members. Support may take the form of direct suggestions and/or emotional support as they come to terms with their feelings and perceptions. However, this needs to be coupled with the room to think through difficult problems on their own and experience growth and mastery.

IMPLICATIONS FOR THE PSYCHIATRIC NURSE SPECIALIST

The specific implications of the above will depend on the organizational role assumed by the psychiatric mental health nurse specialist. His or her advanced knowledge and skills enable the nurse to contribute to the milieu in many ways: provide clinical supervision to other staff to assist them to identify their own conflicts and difficulties; participate in treatment planning for individual patients; participate in program planning for the unit as a whole; serve as a role model for being a milieu team member and for the therapeutic use of everyday milieu events; and identify clinical nursing problems for research. If the nurse specialist role on a unit is limited to coming as an individual or group therapist, the milieu is deprived of his or her expertise and other nursing staff are given the message that these other therapies are more important.

Whether the clinical specialist is organizationally a part of the milieu team or a resource person to the unit, the larger group processes must be taken into account. They must also be better understood. Milieu issues and dynamics need to be more thoroughly described and researched. Clinical specialists need a way of characterizing differences among milieus and the impact these differences have on different patients. They need an understanding of the processes and dynamics inherent in residential treatment and how to best influence them. No better argument could be made for this need than Stanton's comment regarding milieu therapy.

> I do not take milieu therapy for granted. I do take for granted that the milieu has major effects on the patients—but I fear I often expect them to be unfavorable effects. Nearly everyone working in a hospital must for his own self-respect give lip service to milieu therapy (remember continued treatment?). But lip service does not necessarily mean therapy. Therapy is a planned, theoretically-based conscious procedure or technique aimed at certain more or less well-defined goals which comprise improvement. It must be undertaken with reasonable consistency, and

with interest in and self-critical evaluation of its course and integrity. These are not easy to come by in any hospital. (1963, p. 353)

SUMMARY

This chapter was focused on the dynamics of staff-patient interaction that are likely to become troublesome issues during hospitalization for psychiatric treatment. The similarities and differences between milieu treatment principles related to adult versus child and adolescent populations were explored. Finally, implications for psychiatric mental health nursing administration and specialist practice were suggested.

REFERENCES

Abramczuk, J. The type of leadership and the topics of discussion in a large open group: Observations on community meetings. *International Journal of Social Psychiatry,* 1972, *18,* 53–60.

Bateson, G., Jackson, D., Haley, J., & Weakland, J. H. Towards a theory of schizophrenia. *Behavioral Science,* 1956, *1,* 251–264.

Benton, D. W. The significance of the absent member in milieu therapy. *Perspectives in Psychiatric Care,* 1980, *18,* 21–25.

Berlin, I. N. Developmental issues in the psychiatric hospitalization of children. *American Journal of Psychiatry,* 1978, *135,* 1044–1048.

Berlin, I. N. Opportunities in adolescence to rectify developmental failures. In S. C. Feinstein, P. K. Geovacchini, J. G. Looney, A. Z. Schwartzberg, & A. D. Sorosky (Eds.), *Adolescent psychiatry: Developmental and clinical studies* (Vol. 8). Chicago: University of Chicago, 1980.

Bettelheim, B. *Love is not enough.* New York: Free Press, 1950.

Bettelheim, B., & Sylvester, E. A therapeutic milieu. *American Journal of Orthopsychiatry,* 1948, *18,* 191–206.

Bjork, D., Steinberg, M., Lindenmayer, J. P., & Pardes, H. Mania and milieu: Treatment of manics in a therapeutic community. *Hospital and Community Psychiatry,* 1977, *28,* 431–436.

Blumer, H. *Symbolic interactionism: Perspective and method.* Englewood Cliffs, NJ: Prentice-Hall, 1969.

Boyd, R. W., Kagels, S. S., & Greenblatt, M. Outbreak of gang destructive behavior on a psychiatric ward. *Journal of Nervous and Mental Disease,* 1954, *120,* 338–342.

Bradshaw, W. H. The coffee-pot affair: An episode in the life of a therapeutic community. *Hospital and Community Psychiatry,* 1972, *23,* 17–22.

Carser, D. L. Primary nursing in the milieu. *Journal of Psychosocial Nursing and Mental Health Services,* 1982, *19,* 35–41.

Caudill, W. *The psychiatric hospital as a small society.* Cambridge, MA: Harvard University Press, 1958.

Cherniss, C. *Staff burnout: Job stress in the human services.* Beverly Hills, CA: Sage Publications, 1980a.

Cherniss, C. Human service programs as work organizations: Using organizational design to improve staff motivation and effectiveness. In R. H. Price & P. Politser (Eds.), *Evaluation and action in the social environment.* New York: Academic Press, 1980b.

Cherniss, C., & Egnatios, E. Clinical supervision in community mental health. *Social Work,* 1978, *23,* 219–223.

Christ, A. E., & Wagner, N. N. Iatrogenic factors in residential treatment: The psychiatric team's contribution to continued psychopathology. *American Journal of Orthopsychiatry,* 1965, *35,* 253–254.

Crabtree, L. H., & Levinson, D. F. Recurrent large-group phenomena: Studies of an adolescent therapeutic community. *Adolescent Psychiatry,* 1980, *8,* 512–528.

Critchley, D. L., & Berlin, I. N. Day treatment of young psychotic children and their parents: Interdisciplinary issues and problems. *Child Psychiatry and Human Development,* 1979, *9,* 227–237.

Critchley, D. L., & Berlin, I. N. Parent participation in milieu treatment of young psychotic children. *American Journal of Orthopsychiatry,* 1981, *51,* 149–155.

Druck, A. The role of the psychoanalytically oriented psychotherapist within a therapeutic community. *Psychiatry,* 1982, *45,* 45–49.

Fromm-Reichman, F. Problems of therapeutic management in a psychoanalytic hospital. *Psychoanalytic Quarterly,* 1947, *16,* 325–356.

Hoffman, I., & Singer, P. R. The incompatibility of the medical model and the therapeutic community. *Social Science and Medicine,* 1977, *11,* 421–425.

Hollander, R. Moral treatment and the therapeutic community. *Psychiatric Quarterly,* 1981, *53,* 132–138.

Jacobs, M. Promoting responsibility and mutual concern through a modified form of patient government. *Journal of Psychiatric Nursing and Mental Health Services,* 1977, *15,* 30–34.

Jones, M. *The therapeutic community.* New York: Basic Books, 1953.

Kisch, J., Kroll, J., Gross, R., & Carey, K. In-patient community meetings: problems and purposes. *British Journal of Medical Psychology,* 1981, *54,* 35–40.

Klein, R. H. The patient-staff community meeting: A tea party with the mad hatter. *International Journal of Group Psychotherapy,* 1981, *31,* 205–222.

Krug, O. The application of principles of child psychotherapy in residential treatment. *American Journal of Psychiatry,* 1952, *108,* 695–700.

Magaro, P. A., Gripp, R., & McDowell, D. J. *The mental health industry: A cultural phenomenon.* New York: John Wiley, 1978.

Martin, D. N. Disruptive behavior and staff attitudes at the St. Charles Youth Treatment Center. *Journal of Child Psychology and Psychiatry,* 1977, *18,* 221–228.

Menninger, W. C. Psychiatric hospital therapy designed to meet unconscious needs. *American Journal of Psychiatry,* 1936, *93,* 347–360.

Miller, D. The etiology of an outbreak of delinquence in a group of hospitalized adolescents. In M. Greenblatt, D. J. Levinson, & R. H. Williams (Eds.), *The patient and the mental hospital.* Glencoe, IL: Free Press, 1957.

Noshpitz, J. D. Residential treatment of emotionally disturbed children. In D. X. Freedman & J. D. Dyrud (Eds.), *American handbook of psychiatry* Vol. V (2nd ed.). New York: Basic Books, 1975.

Paine, C. T. Resistance to change: Primary nursing versus therapeutic community. *Nursing Administration Quarterly,* 1981, *5,* 26–29.

Parsons, T. *The social system.* New York: Free Press, 1951.

Peplau, H. Interpersonal techniques: The crux of psychiatric nursing. *American Journal of Nursing,* 1962, *62,* 50–54.

Puskar, K. Structure for the hospitalized adolescent. *Journal of Psychiatric Nursing and Mental Health Services,* 1981, *19,* 13–16.

Rasinski, K., Rozensky, R., & Pasulka, P. Practical implications of a theory of the "therapeutic milieu" for psychiatric nursing practice. *Journal of Psychiatric Nursing and Mental Health Services,* 1980, *18,* 16–20.

Redl, F. The concept of a "therapeutic milieu." *American Journal of Orthopsychiatry,* 1959, *29,* 721–736. (a)

Redl, F. Strategy and techniques of the life-space interview. *American Journal of Orthopsychiatry,* 1959, *29,* 1–18. (b)

Rossi, J. J., & Filstead, W. J. (Eds.) *The therapeutic community.* New York: Behavioral Publications, 1973.

Rossman, P.G. A model for staff training in the psychiatric hospital treatment of adolescents. *The Journal of the American Academy of Child Psychiatry,* 1979, *18,* 559–570.

Rossman, P. G., & Knesper, D. J. The early phase of hospital treatment for disruptive adolescents. *Journal of the American Academy of Child Psychiatry,* 1976, *15,* 693–708.

Russakoff, L. M., & Oldham, J. M. The structure and technique of community meetings: The short-term unit. *Psychiatry,* 1982, *45,* 38–44.

Schwartz, M. S., & Shockley, E. L. *The nurse and the mental patient.* New York: Russell Sage, 1956.

Skinner, K. The therapeutic milieu: Making it work. *Journal of Psychiatric Nursing and Mental Health Services,* 1979, *17, 38–44.*

Stanton, A. H. Milieu therapy: A dialogue. *Mental Hospital,* 1963, *6,* 337–354.

Stanton, A. H., & Schwartz, M. S. *The mental hospital.* New York: Basic Books, 1954.

Strauss, A., Schatzman, L., Bucker, R., Ehrlick, D., & Sabshin, M. *Psychiatric ideologies and institutions.* New York: The Free Press of Glencoe, 1964.

Sullivan, H. S. *The interpersonal theory of psychiatry.* New York: W.W. Norton and Co., 1953.

Tudor, G. A sociopsychiatric nursing approach to intervention in a problem of mutual withdrawal on a mental hospital ward. *Psychiatry,* 1952, *15,* 193–217.

Whittaker, J. K. The ecology of child treatment: A developmental/educational approach to the therapeutic milieu. *Journal of Autism and Childhood Schizophrenia,* 1975, *5,* 223–237.

Wolf, M. A review of literature on milieu therapy. *Journal of Psychiatric Nursing and Mental Health Services,* 1977, *15,* 26–33.

BIBLIOGRAPHY

Berlin, I., Critchley, D., & Rossman, P. Current concepts in milieu treatment of seriously disturbed children and adolescents. In M. Shore & F. Mannino (Eds.), *Psychotherapy: Theory, research and practice* Vol. 21, Utica, NY: C. L. Hutson, 1984.

CHAPTER 15 PSYCHOPHARMACOTHERAPY

Linda S. Beeber

Pharmacotherapy is a frequent mode of treatment for patients seeking help in psychiatric settings. The psychiatric mental health clinical nurse specialist (PMHCNS) is often asked to contribute expert knowledge to the care of these patients. This chapter presents essential pharmacokinetic and medical treatment information to acquaint the clinical specialist with rational, acceptable standards of psychotropic drug use. Current uses of antipsychotic, antidepressant, mood-stabilizing, and antianxiety agents are presented with additional sections addressing the specialized needs of children, women, and the elderly. The emphasis throughout the chapter is on the use of the nursing process in caring for the person receiving medication. Through nursing interventions guided by the expertise of the clinical specialist, medication may be confined to an important yet adjunctive role in bringing about permanent psychosocial change in many patients.

Medicine's search to control and cure the symptoms of emotional disorders took a revolutionary turn in the 1950s with the introduction of chlorpromazine. By offering the chance to alter psychiatric symptoms rapidly without institutionalization and ongoing physical-restraint devices, chlorpromazine and its successors created optimism among both the sufferers of mental disorders and their helpers. Although medication offered the helpers opportunities to abandon time-consuming restraints and to work more closely with patients, paradoxically the ratio of professional nurses to mental patients did not increase (DHEW, 1974). Nurses' activities became linked with medication while the ongoing relationship with the patient was taken over by the nonprofessional. Peplau (1952) offered direction to professional nurses by introducing principles of therapeutic use of the nurse-patient relationship. The nurse could use the time and manageability provided by pharmacotherapy to offer corrective emotional experiences to the patient. When clinical specialists entered the picture, they brought expertise to the patient as well as commitment to improving patient care. Despite a discouraging slowness in professional nurses' return to ongoing relationships with mental patients, there have been promising attempts to combine the deliberative nursing process with the burgeoning body of technical information about psychotropic medication.

The astonishing growth of information concerning biochemical hypotheses about and treatments for emotional disorders demands that clinical specialists not only be current in knowledge of accepted drug therapies but also aggressive in articulating their use in individualized, health-cognizant client treatment plans. Accepted medical guidelines for the use of psychotropic medications often conflict with nursing diagnostic formulations that may include aesthetic and generative concerns not considered by the physician prescribing the medications. Clinical specialists must initiate and arbitrate these differences. Additionally, they must exercise their nursing expertise to ensure that psychotropic medication enhances rather than inhibits the client's functioning.

CLINICAL SPECIALIST ROLES IN PHARMACOTHERAPY

The clinical specialist delineates prevention and health-promotion principles for the patient receiving pharmacotherapy. Nursing occupies a pivotal role among psychiatric disciplines, a role that emerges clearly in the care of the patient treated with psychotropic medications. Using a shared humanities and science base, the nurse views the patient's medication regimen in a broad context and assesses the impact of chemical intervention on other variables besides the reduction of distressing symptoms. The nurse draws from experiences with individuals and families at many developmental stages in states of health and illness. The nurse systematically assesses and offers judgment about the interlocking variables that contribute to the patient's behavior and are affected by psychotropic medications. The nurse also evaluates the impact of medication on functional as well as dysfunctional aspects of the patient's behavior. Physiological capabilities such as sensoria, elimination, and exercise will be affected by the medication. The individual's abilities to dream, to love and be loved, to parent, and to pursue career goals will be affected.

Whether practicing as a single representative of nursing or in a nursing network, the nurse contributes specialized, accurate information drawn from many sources and identifies its relevance to the particular patient who is receiving a specific psychotropic medication. A physician will always be involved where medication is prescribed. The collaboration between medicine and nursing around medication issues requires skill, as the clinical area is circumscribed and the functional roles are often indistinct. Table 15.1 presents shared and independent nursing responsibilities during pharmacotherapy. In determining her specific nursing responsibilities, the clinical specialist needs to understand the peculiarities of both federal and state legislation relevant to nursing practice. Table 15.2 presents principles useful to the nurse caring for patients receiving pharmacotherapy. These principles guide

Table 15.1 Differentiation of Interdependent and Independent Medication Responsibilities of Nursing

Medico-Nursing (Shared) Responsibilities	*Nursing (Independent) Responsibilities*
Contributing expert *validated* observations of behavior patterns	Intervening to help the patient participate in the treatment process
Contributing information drawn from a comprehensive assessment of the patient that will influence or be influenced by psychotropic medication	Establishing specific, critical physiologic and behavioral baselines; evaluating the impact of medication on deviance from these baselines
Participating in the choice of medication group, route, dosage amount, and criteria for termination	Acting as health maintenance and health promotion advocate for/with the patient by preventing advance of adverse effects, intervening into treatment-related complications, intervening to improve health status and knowledge about health maintenance
Administering medication	Promoting interpersonal mastery toward the goal of enhancing positive medication effects
Introducing educative experiences about the effects of medication on the patient's system	Developing alternatives to medication for symptom reduction
	Evaluating impact of the patient taking medication on significant systems (family, career, community); intervening to disseminate mental health principles and to prevent the medication from becoming the sole focus for potential changes in the systems

Table 15.2 Principles of Nursing Intervention with Patients Receiving Psychotropic Medications

1. The nurse advocates on behalf of the patient toward the following pharmocotherapeutic goals:
   a. A single, correct medication for the *central* disorder suffered by the patient
   b. Dosage that is correct, safe, and changes according to the patient's needs
   c. A medication route that offers least potential for injury and most autonomous control by the patient
   d. Medication used in conjunction with intervention strategies toward permanent psychosocial improvement
   e. Medication discontinued at a specified point in time unless indefinite maintenance is chosen; indefinite maintenance requires fully informed consent by the patient
2. The nurse categorizes assessment and nursing diagnoses into:
   a. Physiologic and psychosocial response to the pharmacotherapeutic agent
   b. Psychosocial response to the symbolic meanings of pharmacotherapy (resistance, idealization, loss of control—see Tables 15.7, 15.14, 15.16)
   c. Wellness state: present—potential, related to pharmacotherapy
3. The nurse advocates for the patient's optimal health state by:
   a. Protecting healthy islands of personality functioning from interference by pharmacotherapy
   b. Utilizing interpersonal strategies to enhance and replace pharmacotherapy
   c. Introducing information about pharmacotherapy to the patient toward the goal of fully informed participation
   d. Preparing for and treating physiologic and psychosocial responses to pharmacotherapy
4. The nurse recognizes that countertransference issues will compromise professional judgments about medication and utilizes supervision to explore these issues
5. The nurse intervenes to keep the patient in charge of his own medication, avoiding, unless absolutely necessary, placing family members in charge of pharmacotherapy (This principle may lead to a decision to use an injectable, slow-release form of an antipsychotic rather than reinforcing the patient in the role of the "sick" member of the family system.)
6. The nurse views psychotropic medication as an adjunct to permanent change in the patient's relationships with other people; medication enhances interpersonal learning by reducing symptomatic behaviors that create interpersonal difficulties; nursing interventions center on creating new experiences in psychosocial learning

nursing interventions when medical guidelines conflict with the nurse's health-cognizant assessment of the patient.

Functional Roles of the Clinical Specialist: Expert Practitioner

Although a wealth of information about psychotropic drugs is presented in this and other texts, the nurse needs to continuously engage in updating his or her knowledge about pharmacologic treatment. An hour or two each month is usually sufficient time to review new research and to refresh knowledge of little-used medications. In clinical practice, using group leadership skills allows the nurse to intervene with several patients simultaneously as in medication groups.

Role Model

By performing an accepted, standard role of nursing (medication administration), the clinical specialist models advanced, comprehensive care of the patient. Clinical nurse specialists do much more than "give medications." They demonstrate the use of advanced concepts of nursing care for the patient on psychotropic medications. Often, due to the territorial overlap of physician, nurse, and patient, pharmacotherapy becomes an excellent theater in which clinical specialists model operational definitions of the nursing role.

Consultant and Teacher

The nurse not only suggests and formally teaches specific approaches to other nurses but also educates nurses in the process required for professionals to remain knowledgeable about current therapies being used with their patients. For example, the time spent studying drugs each month may evolve into a consultation-shared teaching group with nurse colleagues.

Researcher

As effectiveness and specificity of psychotropic medication develop, so too do groups of patients who are refractory to psychotropic medication. Examples of such groups include patients with medical conditions that contraindicate the use of such drugs, chronic schizophrenics who do not benefit from medication and are at risk for tardive dyskinesia, and patients who exercise their right to refuse medication but who continue to suffer severe symptoms. Nursing has excellent opportunities to research specific interventions with these groups since nursing interventions into social and behavioral spheres may constitute the major thrust of therapy for these patients. Some of these populations operate "outside" the health care system and could provide opportunities for research into the impact of nursing intervention with such groups without concomitant therapies.

PSYCHOTROPIC MEDICATIONS CURRENTLY IN USE: MEDICAL AND NURSING GUIDELINES

A number of medications have been found useful in treating the mentally ill. The first group to be discussed will be those used in treating psychotic individuals.

Antipsychotic Medications

Definitions and Terms

Psychosis is a term that describes the overt sympomatology in severe disorders that impair a person's ability to recognize reality, communicate, and maintain relationships with others (Wilson & Kneisl, 1979). The term psychosis gathers together a common aspect of many psychiatric syndromes, that is, the *persistent misevaluation of perceptions* (Klein, Gittelman, Quitkin, & Rifkin, 1980). *Organic* psychoses have a known neuropathologic toxin, degenerative process, disease entity, or trauma. *Functional* psychoses are presently understood as having no organic basis. Research is being done to find a biochemical abnormality, particularly in persons with schizophrenic disorders. Symptoms of functional psychosis are frequently associated with schizophrenic disorders (DSM-III, 1980, 215.1) and involve phenomena associated with disruption and disintegration of ego function. Such phenomena include regression with logic, behavioral and reality-testing disturbances, primitive defense structures, experiences of depersonalization, and omnipotent referential thought (Rosenbaum, 1970, pp. 108–111). Other functional psychoses include atypical and brief reactive psychoses (Task Force, 1980).

Medications used to treat the symptoms of psychosis are correctly called *antipsychotic medications.* To use any of the misnomers, "major tranquilizers," "neuroleptics," or "phenothiazines," distorts the primary purpose of these medications as agents that comprehensively reduce symptoms of psychosis. An antipsychotic agent will activate a withdrawn patient and reduce the delusions that prompt the suspicious patient to be fearful and agitated.

Figure 15.1 illustrates the current thinking on the pharmacologic action of antipsychotic medications.

Relevant Research Summary

1. Anatomical/physiological studies link dopamine depletion in Parkinson's disease with Parkinson's-like symptoms of the antipsychotics, suggesting that dopamine reduction is the pharmacodynamic focus.
2. Empirical studies show that amphetamines at normal doses exacerbate psychosis in schizophrenics. Amphetamines are known to increase dopamine activity, suggesting a correlation between dopamine excess/hyperactivity and psychosis. No evidence yet supports dopamine abnormalities in schizophrenics (Friedman & Kaplan, 1975; Snyder, 1976).

Clinical Guidelines for Use

1. Antipsychotics are superior to placebo in treating acute schizophrenia and preventing relapse (Hirsch, Gaind, Rohde, Stevens, & Wing, 1973; Rifkin, Quitkin, & Klein, 1977) and are superior to either psychotherapy or social manipulation (milieu therapy) alone (Davis, 1975; Klein et al., 1980; May, 1976). Of the five groups available, no one group of antipsychotics has proved superior (Klein et al., 1980). A useful approach is to become familiar with one preparation from each group and to choose a medication for its sedative qualities, potency, or patient tolerance to side effects.
2. High-potency preparations are more useful with elderly patients (Klein et al., 1980).
3. Only one antipsychotic should be used at a time (Klein et al., 1980).
4. Treatment should be evaluated by changes in consensually validated target symptoms.

Dosage

Dosage must always be determined by what is safe for the particular patient. Individual patients vary in tolerance to the antipsychotic agents. Rapid induction of antipsychotics (psychotolysis) and conservative induction of treatment are not mutually exclusive concepts when the patient is viewed comprehensively. A highly agitated, floridly symptomatic patient may respond quickly to psychotolysis and be capable of maintenance on a low dose. Ultimately, this patient will consume less medication over time than a patient inadequately dosed who requires a much longer time to respond, if a response occurs. Loaded single-dose, daily schedules maximize the long-acting nature of all antipsychotic agents, reduce side effects, and simplify the requirements for self-medication. Controversy exists over the

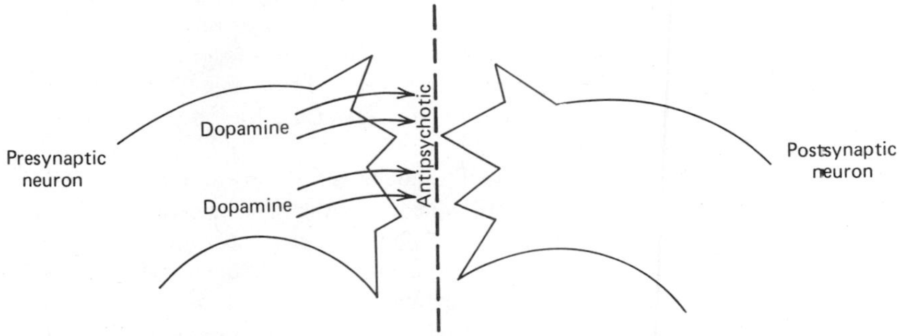

Figure 15.1 Theoretical pharmacologic action of antipsychotic medications. Dopamine hypothesis proposes that antipsychotics block the neurotransmitter dopamine at the postsynaptic neuron.

use of antiparkinsonian medications prophylactically as opposed to adding them when side effects appear (Klein et al., 1980; Shader, 1975). If adequate resources are available for the patient to be evaluated and to secure antiparkinsonian medication, it seems safer to avoid introducing a second medication before it is indicated.

The patient's long-term response to the drug is determined by changes in the less responsive target symptoms and by the appearance of side effects. Maintenance dosage should be set at the lowest dosage needed to prevent relapse. A 25% reduction of the acute treatment dose every one to three months may determine the maintenance dosage. Medication may often be discontinued within six months after a first psychotic episode and within one year after a second episode. When the patient's behavior indicates a pattern of relapses, indefinite management is usually considered (Kessler & Waletzky, 1981). Questions about dosage, the patient's resistance to continual medication, and the threat of tardive dyskinesia all require consideration at this time. Tables 15.3 and 15.4 present information about current antipsychotic medications and the medications used to treat the side effects commonly associated with these agents. The direct relationship between potency and side effects is illustrated by Table 15.3 as are the varying forms of available preparations. The antiparkinsonian drugs presented in Table 15.4 carry side effects that may exacerbate side effects of the antipsychotics and may also mimic psychotic symptoms. These preparations also vary in available forms. Tables 15.5 and 15.6 present side effects and adverse effects of the antipsychotics. Information is organized by assessment site to assist the nurse in continuous assessment of critical baseline data. Dystonias and orthostatic hypotension are side effects requiring anticipatory teaching and medication orders. The slower-onset side effects are noted through continuous assessment. Most side effects are effectively treated through dose reduction (Table 15.5).

Table 15.6 presents adverse effects. Note that tardive dyskinesia represents a permanent adverse effect that can be prevented by careful nursing assessment. The remaining adverse effects also are monitored by a continuous comprehensive assessment of the patient.

Nursing Interventions with the Patient Receiving Antipsychotic Agents

Antipsychotic medications have had the most powerful impact of all psychotropic drugs on nursing diagnoses and management of the acutely psychotic patient. Medical diagnostic categories are becoming increasingly discrete, an important advance given the development of more specific pharmaco- and psychotherapies. Nursing diagnostic categories are broad and concern patterns and clusters of behaviors. These categories reflect the current level of conceptual development in the profession. Consequently, clusters of behaviors associated with psychosis, as well as with healthy behaviors, become the basis for nursing diagnosis and intervention. Table 15.7 contains examples of frequent medication-associated behaviors in patients that are encountered by the nurse.

The patient's psychotic symptoms naturally induce anxiety in the nurse. Investigations of nurses' reactions to patients' symptoms will often reveal the transformation of a therapeutic "rationale" into a therapeutic "rationalization" for medication. Scrutinizing the decision to offer extra medication (or to pressure the patient to accept medication), to withhold medication, or to ignore the impact of medication reveals clues to unrecognized anxiety, anger, or overidentification in the nurse. Often, medication becomes a major issue in the nurse's interactions with the psychotic patient. When a patient regresses to infantile modes of thought, the nurse approaching with medication may become a nurturing figure, controller, poisoner, ally, authority, or alien being. The patient's perception of the nurse can shift

Table 15.3 Antipsychotic Medications: A Selected Listing by Chemical Groups with Characteristics Relevant to Nursing Care[a]

Chemical Group and Products	*Potency Compared to Chlorpromazine*	*Administration Forms*	*Side Effects*
Butyrophenones			
Haloperidol (Haldol) Droperidol (Insapine)	High[b] 1:50	Tablets, liquid, parenteral	High extrapyramidal side effects (EPS)
Phenothiazines			
Subgroup Aliphatic			
Chlorpromazine (Thorazine) Promazine (Sparine)	Low 1:1	Tablets, liquid, parenteral, suppositories Spansules (expensive; medication is slowly absorbed anyway)	High sedation High hypotension Low EPS
Triflupromazine (Vesprin)	Low 1:4 Potency makes this a slightly better choice where parenteral use of an aliphatic is desired.	Tablet, liquid, parenteral	
Subgroup Piperazine Trifluoperazine (Stelazine) Perphenazine (Trilafon)		Tablets, liquid, parenteral Perphenazine often in combination with amytryptaline; fixed-dose polypharmaceuticals are more expensive; doses of components cannot be altered	Low sedation Low hypotension High EPS
Fluphenazine (Prolixin, Permitil)	High 1:70	Tablet, liquid, parenteral Long-acting forms varying from 10–30 days duration; *use short form to rule out allergic response before using long-acting form*	Same
Acetophenazine (Tuidal) Thiopropazate (Dartal) Butaperazine (Repoise)	Moderate 1:8–10	Tablets only	Same
Carphenazine (Proketazine)	Low 1:4	Parenteral only	Same
Subgroup Piperadine			
Thioridazine (Mellaril)	Equal 1:1	Tablets, liquid	Lowest EPS of phenothiazines High hypotension High inhibition of ejaculation

Table 15.3 (*continued*)

Chemical Group and Products	*Potency compared to Chlorpromazine*	*Administration Forms*	*Side Effects*
Piperacetazine (Quide)	Moderate (1:10)	Tablets, parenteral	
Mesoridazine (Serentil)	Low (1:3)	Tablets, liquid, parenteral	
Thioxanthenes			
Thiothixine (Navane) Chlorprothixene (Taractan)	Equal 1:1	Tablets, Liquid, Parenteral	High sedation Low hypotension Low EPS
Oxoindoles			
Molindone (Moban, Endo)	Moderate 1:10	Tablets only	High sedation Low hypotention Low EPS; appears to prevent weight gain and promote weight loss in obese patients
Dibenzoxazepines			
Loxipine (Loxitane, Daxolin)	Moderate 1:10	Tablets only	

[a] New preparations and research are introduced so rapidly that the nurse is advised to consult the medication-specific literature and current medication publications for nurses for product specifications. Selections are included in the chapter bibliography. Characteristics such as sedation, side effect risk, and preparation options are helpful for delivery of nursing care.

[b] *High potency* means that a small amount of the medication will produce clinical effects similar to a much larger amount of chlorpromazine, the standard. A high-potency medication is quite useful if an intramuscular route is chosen, as it will produce less trauma. Psychotolysis is accomplished efficiently when high-potency medications are used. High-potency preparations cause less incidence of postural hypotension. Low-potency preparations are useful when the patient develops extrapyramidal side effects refractory to antiparkinsonian drugs (Klein, pp. 149–50). Ratios of Chlorpromazine to each product are given.

Table 15.4 Medications Used to Treat Acute Dystonic and Parkinsonian Side Effects of Antipsychotic Agents

Generic Name	*Administration Form*	*Side Effects and Adverse Effects*
Amantine (Symmetrel)	Tablet, liquid	
Antiparkinsonian agents		
Benztropine (Cogentin)	Tablet, parenteral	Antiparkinsonian agents are synthetic anticholinergic agents resembling atropine; side effects include: urinary hesitance, dry mouth, blurred vision; adverse effects include: bladder paralysis, paralytic ileus, aggravation of glaucoma, mental confusion, prostatic hypertrophy, toxic psychosis (difficult to distinguish from the functional psychosis being treated)
Biperiden (Akineton)	Tablet, parenteral	
Procyclidine (Kemadrin)	Tablet only	
Trihexyphenidyl (Artane, Piparol, Tremin)	Tablet, liquid	
Diphenhydramine (Benadryl)	Tablet, liquid, parenteral	

Table 15.5 Side Effects[a] of Antipsychotic Medications

Assessment Site	*Symptoms*	*Mechanism*	*Nursing Interventions*
1. Movement and coordination			
a. Dystonias	Rapid-onset contraction of skeletal muscles accompanied by pain; patient is frightened, often interprets side effect as a psychotic symptom; facial, jaw, neck muscles frequent sites; young male patients at high risk; occur early (1–2 weeks) in treatment or in conjunction with rapidly increased dosage	Interference with extrapyramidal tracts in central nervous system	a. PRN oral/injectible antiparkinson drugs should be prescribed when antipsychotic medications are begun b. Close scrutiny of *any* altered body sensation; use additional unobtrusive observation as patient may try to "hide" symptom c. Prepare patient to recognize onset and to plan an appropriate action (contact nurse, telephone clinic, etc.) d. Follow-up by dosage reduction and/or regular antiparkinson medications in divided doses e. Available medical treatments for acute dystonias include amobarbital (IM/IV), diphehydramine, calcium, caffeine, antiparkinsonian medication
b. Akinesia	General weakness, flaccidity of muscles; patient often "drops" tiredly into a chair or has difficulty opening doors, lifting objects. Often mistaken for fatigue, withdrawal, apathy	Interference with extrapyramidal tracts in central nervous system	a. Distinguish side effect from worsening psychosis, physical fatigue, physiologic deterioration b. Pursue dose reduction/antiparkinsonian agent c. Support, instruct patient about reversibility
c. Parkinson's-like syndrome	Rigidity, outward-rotating tremor of hands, shuffling gait, masklike face	Interference with extrapyramidal tracts in central nervous system	a. Pursue dose reduction/antiparkinson agent b. Support, instruct patient about reversibility

Table 15.5 (*continued*)

Assessment Site	*Symptoms*	*Mechanism*	*Nursing Intervention*
d. Akathesia	Jittery, hypermotoric sensation; patient cannot stand or sit still, describe "running while standing still" sensation; often rock while standing or sitting or pick up one, then another foot while sitting; mistaken for anxiety, autism		a. Differentiate symptoms of side effect from anxiety; anxiety: incremental, cause related; akathisia: stays the same, no causality, often aggravated by anxiety but persists after anxiety diminishes b. Pursue dose reduction/antiparkinson agent c. Support; reassure patient of reversibility
2. Skin and mucous membranes	Dry mouth	Interference with acetylcholine (anticholinergic)	a. Sugar-free lozenges, mouth rinses, low-caloric fluids b. Evaluate buccal cavity for fungus
Medication alert: Phenothiazines potentiate antihistamines	Photosensitivity		a. Use precaution when outside to limit exposure or use true sunscreen b. Monitor use of ultraviolet light sources for treatment c. Remember that dark-pigmented persons can sunburn
3. Cardiovascular system *Medication alert:* Phenothiazines 1. decrease effect of oral antigoagulants 2. in combination with high/overdose scopolamine or diuretics can cause hypotensive crisis 3. potentiate antihypertensives except quanethidine; oral hypoglycemics, reserpine	Hypotension/orthostatic hypotension	Interference with epinephrine (antiadrenergic)	a. Patient derived baseline—q. 12 hr measurement for three days; sitting and standing values b. Check BP 30 min postdose c. Pressure fall 5-mm significant d. Provide supervision when walking after sitting/sleeping; teach reliable patients to dangle feet; elastic stockings, isometric exercises before rising may help e. Consider dose reduction if continues

Table 15.5 (*continued*)

			f. Adrenalin *contraindicated* in acute hypotension episode; use neosynephrine or levophed
4. Gastrointestinal, genitourinary systems	Constipation	Anticholinergic	a. High fluid, roughage, regular eating routine, exercise b. Stool softener, suppositories c. Relaxation, diversion when toileting, warm po fluids
Medication alert: Antacids reduce uptake of antipsychotics	Impotence Ejaculatory inhibition		a. Foster relationship where patient can discuss personal issues b. Anticipatory guidence c. Pursue dose reduction or change to different medication *group*
	Menstrual irregularities		a. Assess/pursue diagnosis of pregnancy b. Encourage discussion
	Urinary hesitance	Anticholinergic	a. Baseline—intake/output b. Pursue medical evaluation of obstruction c. Withhold medication if symptomatic
5. Body shape/size	Breast enlargement, pseudolactation	Endocrine disruption	a. Explore patient's beliefs about cause, reactions b. Female—rule out pregnancy c. Support, advise of reversibility, encourage concealing dress
	Obesity/weight gain	Endocrine disruption; increased appetite due to effects on hypothalamus	a. Oral needs very important in psychosis—continue to meet but with low calorie foods b. Baseline—use patient's perception of correct weight to supplement norms

Table 15.5 (*continued*)

Assessment Site	*Symptoms*	*Mechanism*	*Nursing Interventions*
			c. Weight loss diet d. Change to Molindone may promote weight loss
6. Sensorium	Blurred vision	Anticholinergic	a. Baseline—examine retina and lens b. Magnifying lens/glasses help accommodate to print c. See adverse effects (See Table 15.6)
Medication and substance alert: Antipsychotics potentiate CNS depressants	Drowsiness		a. Load bedtime dose b. Switch to different group c. Caffeine in moderation
7. Laboratory studies altered by antipsychotic medications			

Test	*Alteration*
Alkaline phospatase *Bilirubin (serum, urine)* *Cerebral spinal fluid protein* *Cholesterol* *Fasting glucose* *Phorphyrins* *Pregnancy (frog)* *Steriods—170H* *Transaminase* *Urobilinogen*	*All false positive*
Estrogens (urine) *Iodine, protein bound* *Iodine, radioactive uptake* *Phenylketonuria*	*Inaccurate readings*
Uric acid (5HIAA) urine	*False positive and negative*

[a] *Side effect* is defined as a different pharmacodynamic result from the effect primarily sought (Martin, 1978).

Table 15.6 Adverse Effects[a] of Antipsychotic Medications

Assessment Site	*Symptoms*	*Mechanism*	*Nursing Intervention*
Rapid-onset adverse reactions			
1. Cardiovascular system	Cardiac arthymias; EKG abnormalities	Interference with epinephrine; idiopathic; exacerbation of preexisting cardiac disease	a. Preventative—EKG, history prior to starting pharmacotherapy b. Early recognition—compare cardiac indicators (apical/radical pulse) with patient-derived baselines c. Stop medication and seek medical evaluation d. Prepare for emergency cardiac intervention (periodic CPR update for psychiatric nurses is mandatory when pharmacotherapy is part of the treatment program)
2. Central nervous system	Seizures	Lowering of seizure threshold; may be due to preexisting seizure disorder or large doses of antipsychotic in a normal person	a. Preventative—history of seizure disorder; monitor dose increases; increase anticonvulsants in seizure disordered patients b. Prepare for emergency intervention into seizures
3. Movement and coordination	Oculo-gyric crisis—torticollis accompanied by spasm of extraocular muscles; head pulled to side, eyes drawn back in spasm		a. Preventative—recognize high risk groups; gradual increase of dosage b. Early recognition—use baseline for coordination; watch for secondary elaboration and explanation of developing symptoms, "I'm guilty—*I can't look you in the eye*" (due to extraocular spasm) c. Have prewritten order for po/IM antiparkinsonian or Benadryl and have medication handy

Table 15.6 (*continued*)

Assessment Site	*Symptoms*	*Mechanism*	*Nursing Intervention*
			d. Administer antiparkinson medication; support patient and reality test symptom and reversibility
Gradual-onset adverse reactions			
4. General physical health indicators and skin/mucous membrance a. Agranulocytosis: destruction of white blood cells	Elevated temperature, sore throat, malaise, bruising, nosebleeds	Blood dyscrasias—destruction of granulocytes, and monocytes leads to infections, hematologic symptoms (probably idiopathic)	a. Preventative—use caution with high risk populations (e.g., elderly females) b. Early recognition—viral symptoms should be evaluated, CBC done (not always reliable) c. In presence of symptom cluster, withhold medication and get medical evaluation
b. Cholestatic jaundice	Yellowing of skin, sclerae, acolic stool, discolored urine		a. Preventative—use caution with patients whose history includes liver damage b. Stop medication, get medical evaluation
c. Allergic reactions	Urticaria, dermatitis	Idiopathic hypersensitivity	a. Preventative—avoid contact with liquid forms; cleanse skin if patient drools or spits out medication b. Use po test dose of Fluphenazine before administering depot forms
5. Sensorium a. Retinitis pigmentation; opacities	Blurred vision, "spot" blindness	Idiopathic; deposition of medication in lens of eye	a. Preventative—encourage patient to report any vision disturbance b. Evaluate/seek evaluation of any vision disturbance

Table 15.6 (*continued*)

6. Movement and coordination			
a. Tardive dyskinesia frequently irreversible tics and generalized motor disorder; generally related to dose and duration of antipsychotic medication; worsened by antiparkinsonian medications and cessation of the antipsychotic b. Abnormal involuntary movement scale (AIMS) is a symptom-eliciting examination for early detection of tardive dyskinesia; copies can be obtained from the Pharmacologic/ Somatic Treatments Research Branch, Schizophrenic Disorders Section, National Institutes of Mental Health, Bethesda, MD 20857	Vermiform movements of tongue, fingers, toes rolling, motion of tongue behind teeth, protrusion of tongue (flycatching motion) grimacing, smacking, "rabbitlike" sniffing movements, choreiform movements of hands, pelvis, idiosyncratic repetitive movements of face, body, appendages	Damage to basal ganglia possibly due to prolonged dopamine depletion—leads to hypersensitivity of neurons to dopamine (rapid, continuous firing in presence of increased dopamine after medication is stopped)	a. Preventative—identify high risk populace (elderly, women, long-term users); consider whether medication is really necessary in light of symptoms or if some other method will work; if medication is the choice treatment, consider time-limited trial at lowest dose necessary b. Early detection—AIMS should be used to establish a premedicated baseline for movement; repeated exams should be done at intervals (weekly) and after drug holidays; concentrate on tongue, toes, fingers; make certain that tongue movements are not obscured by teeth or dentures; patients are often unaware of the movements, unlike dystonias; therefore, do not rely on the patient to report symptoms; plan periodic AIMS evaluations after the patient has discontinued the medication; if indefinite treatment is considered, patient should be apprised of the danger and make a fully informed consent for treatment; the nurse may need to advocate for patient in this situation; written consent is advisable

[a] *Adverse effect* is defined as a harmful pharmacologic result of a medication (Martin, 1978).

Table 15.7 Psychological Phenomena in Psychosis that Have an Impact on Medication Acceptance

Phenomenon	*Manifest Behavior Cluster*	*Nursing Intervention Options*
1. Regression	Confusion, logic disturbances, difficulty in determining self-other differentiation, omnipotence, timelessness, withdrawal, self-negation, reality processing faults	Clear and consistent interpretation of expectations to the patient; tell him what he needs to do Several forms of medication available to capitalize on those times when patient is able to exert autonomy; supports available when patient unable to assume responsibility (e.g., delivering medication to patient, long-acting depot preparation, reminding patient to take medications) Validation of patient's beliefs about medication will uncover teleological conclusions (e.g., "Angry is red; the tablet is red; therefore, if I take the pill I will be angry") Definition of boundaries (e.g. "Take *your* medication"); sensitivity to patient's fear of intrusion Protection from injection of harmful substances (e.g., patient associates positive trust of nurse with the medications she/he gives, therefore takes other pills indiscriminately in attempting to incorporate the nurse)
2. Massive anxiety requiring specific defensive structures		
a. Projection	Suspicion, fear of others, terror of others, hypervigilance, hypermasculinity, sensitivity to threats to competence, withdrawal	Provision of reality without challenging the defense "I am a nurse; I have no reason to hurt you with this medication; I am giving it to you because I want to help you." Provision of information in an open, planned manner can be reassuring Choose an antipsychotic that has little sedative S.E.; load bedtime dose to minimize sedation; sedating medication erodes the defense of hypervigilance and in-

Table 15.7 (*continued*)

Phenomenon	*Manifest Behavior Cluster*	*Nursing Intervention Options*
		creases anxiety; sedation may evoke feelings of sluggishness, passivity and threaten a hypermasculine, hypercompetent defense
b. Ambivalence	Erratic decision-making, inability to decide upon anything, decisions that vacilate between extremes	Consistency, persistence, frequent offers of medication will capitalize on the unstable nature of ambivalence Assured, confident insistence by a trusted nurse will encourage the patient to "side" with the feelings favoring alliance with treatment Ambivalence rarely causes emergencies; avoid using coercion unless the patient is endangered-endangering others as coercion will generally call forth more intensive ambivalence as anxiety increases
c. Altered perception	Hallucinations, delusions, illusions including bizarre kinesthetic and olfactory events and fixed delusions about disease, pregnancy and loss of body parts	See Table 15.5; patient must be protected from incorporating side/adverse effects into altered perception (In searching for meaning, the patient will offer elaborations to explain ocular changes, dystonias, etc.) Provision of clear, concise explanations without challenging the defense
d. Ritualism	Preoccupation with impulses particularly destructiveness	Allow ritual in medication procedure within limits Become absolutely consistent and predictable so that medication becomes a "ritual"

rapidly. Interventions need to be based on continuous assessment and flexible approaches that change as the patient changes. Table 15.8 presents significant variables that must be included in nursing assessment of patients receiving antipsychotic medications.

Planning Nursing Intervention

Pharmacotherapy is a shared, expert activity between medicine and nursing. Nurses are reluctant to share their information and educated opinion particularly in regard to diagnostic cues, noncoercive interventions that help the patient accept pharmacotherapy, and nonpathologic aspects of the patient that medication will enhance or disturb. However, such sharing is essential for the health and safety of the patient. The clinical specialist acts as a liaison during planning to ensure that information is accurately shared between disciplines.

A plan of care for the patient receiving antipsychotics needs to include the following points:

Table 15.8 Nursing Assessment When the Patient Receives Antipsychotic Medication

Dimensions in the Patient Prior to Receiving Medication	*Dimensions in the Patient When Medication Dosage Is Being Stabilized or Maintained*	*Dimensions in the Patient When Medication Is Being Discontinued*
1. Psychosocial response to the process of treatment with medication	1. Psychosocial response to the process of treatment with medication	1. Psychosocial response to the process of treatment with medication
a. Positive/negative experiences with medications in the past	a. Effect of corrective emotional experiences surrounding medication	a. Symbolic meaning to patient of stopping medication; potential to cooperate if medication is again necessary
b. Experiences of significant others with medication	b. Present attitudes of significant others toward patient's treatment with medication; perceptions of medication's impact on the patient	b. Significant others' response to patient stopping medication
c. Personal, cultural, religious values about medication	c. Impact of values on continuing cooperation	c. Impact of values on attitudes toward relapse and resumption of pharmacotherapy
d. Personal symbolic meaning of medication to patient (cure, ally, enemy, magic, etc.)	d. Perceptions of patient as to role of medication in therapeutic progress	d. Perceptions of patient regarding ability to remain symptom-free without medication
2. Psychosocial status: treatment-specific	2. Psychosocial status: treatment-specific	2. Psychosocial status: treatment-specific
a. Observed/validated/recorded target symptoms	a. Impact of medication on target symptoms; add new or more subtle target symptoms; status of target symptoms when dosage is reduced	a. Status of target symptoms during drug-free intervals
b. Stressors: behavioral patterns in response to stress; specific sources of stress (significant others, night, fatigue, anxiety in others, etc.)	b. Stressors: impact of medication on response to stress; impact of newly-learned interpersonal strategies on responses to stressful situations	b. Status of interpersonal coping behaviors during drug-free intervals; capacity for continuous use of interpersonal strategies when medication is stopped
c. Psychological phenomena and operative defenses that medication may enhance or disrupt (e.g., hypervigilence may be disrupted by sedating medication—anxiety will increase; hopelessness and loss of control may be interrupted by medication—anxiety will diminish; see Table 15.7)	c. Impact of medication on psychological phenomena	c. Patient's understanding of psychological phenomena and personal coping strategies

TABLE 15.8 (*continued*)

Dimensions in the Patient Prior to Receiving Medication	*Dimensions in the Patient When Medication Dosage Is Being Stabilized or Maintained*	*Dimensions in the Patient When Medication Is Being Discontinued*
3. Physiologic status	3. Physiologic status	3. Physiologic status
a. Critical baselines, insert patient-derived values (See Tables 15.9, 15.15 for baselines specific to medication group)	a. Impact of medication on critical variables; dosage levels, reduction of dosage—impact on variables	a. Impact of drug-free intervals on critical baselines (e.g., movement abnormalities with antipsychotic cessation)
b. Status of concurrent physiologic stressors (e.g., obesity, aging, pregnancy, disease, habits)	b. Interaction of medication and physiologic stressors; impact of interventions into physiologic stressors	b. Status of physiologic stressors
4. Comprehensive state of wellness	4. Comprehensive state of wellness	4. Comprehensive state of wellness
a. Developmental tasks being negotiated	a. Impact of medication on developmental task-seeking behavior (e.g., impotence and negotiation of intimacy and relationship role behavior)	a. Status of developmental task negotiation; impact of stopping medications
b. Islands of intact ego function that medication might enhance or disrupt (e.g. creativity, intellect, athletic/sexual prowess, alertness, delay of gratification)	b. Impact of medication on intact ego function	b. Status of ego functions
c. Self-care, self-restorative, self-actualizing activities (exercise, sexual activity, recreation, aesthetic-religious pursuits)	c. Impact of medication on self-restorative activities	c. Status of self-restorative activities

1. *Prior to medication*
   a. Scheduled, controlled observations to construct a behavioral "picture" and establish physiological baselines (see Table 15.9)
   b. Delineation of target symptom(s) and ascertainment of reliability among observers
   c. Delineation of *nonsymptomatic* target behavior to observe
   d. Reliable, planned routes of exchanging information
   e. Several different routes for administration and, as necessary, dosage options to allow for the maximum use of receptive moments in the patient's day; regular dosage will reduce the need for crisis management due to long action of antipsychotics
   f. Emergency antiparkinson medication orders,
   g. Written teaching plan delineating responsibilities of physician and nurse; content at this point to include essential information selected to match the patient's cognitive capacity; information must be compatible with the patient's operative defense stucture (e.g., the patient using denial will need only basic information whereas the bright, suspicious patient will require straightforward use of terms such as "antipsychotic");

Table 15.9 Suggested Patient-Derived Baselines for Evaluating Impact of Antipsychotic Medication

Baseline	*Remarks*
Laboratory studies (hemato/hepato panels EKG)	Use current established criteria
Temperature	Begin periodic assessment after two weeks on medication (agranulocytosis)
Blood pressure[a] (upright/reclining dirunal/nocturnal)	Decrease 5-mm upon standing up is significant indicator of orthostatic hypotension
Pulse[a] (rhythmn, rate)	Arthythmia, rate deviation should be evaluated using apical/radial measurement and notify doctor; EKG follow-up
Nonquantitative physiologic variables (bowel, sleep/waking cycle, eating habits, movement abnormalities, activity levels, skin, sexual practices, eyesight, menstrual cycle)	Use abnormal involuntary movement scale (AIMS) especially with high risk patients (see Table 15.6)
Weight	Combine normative developmental chart with patient's subjective appraisal
Seizure disorder[a], allergies; recent ingestion of medication, pregnancy	Document both investigation and results

[a] Critical measurements.

selected information with limits placed on demands for teaching will be necessary as a means of evading the patient's deep fear and distrust of medication

h. Interventions to establish alliance and facilitate acceptance of medications (see Table 15.7)

2. *During stabilization/maintenance*
   a. Evaluation of psychological and physiological responses to medication using patient-derived baselines—frequency will diminish as dosage is stabilized
   b. Schedule for observing the following tardive variables: hepatic, hematologic, ocular function; motor coordination (AIMS) see Table 15.6; subtle psychotic symptoms (associative looseness, suspicion, delusions) (Lion, 1978)
   c. Planned experiences in self-administration of medication and additional information about medication
   d. Health promotion interventions to reverse self-negation present in psychosis; restoration of abandoned hygiene, exercise, and nutrition
   e. Interpersonal interventions aimed toward helping the patient learn more effective social behavior and experience less interpersonal anxiety; *structured experiences* include group meetings, planned leisure activities, individual-group-family therapy, behavior therapy; *unstructured experiences* organized around a nursing diagnosis (Table 15.7) in which a spontaneous event is utilized by the nurse to explore and alter maladaptive behaviors in the diagnostic cluster
   f. Suppressive, self-controlled behaviors to reduce symptoms and anxiety (e.g., exercise, meditation, diversion, sublimatory activities [motor activity]
   g. Schedule for reducing dosage—preferably after interpersonal skills have been learned

3. *During conclusion*
   a. Criteria for cessation of pharmacotherapy
   b. Tentative schedule of trial drug-free intervals
   c. Schedule of AIMS evaluations subsequent to conclusion; patient is taught to recognize tardive dyskinesia (see Table 15.6)

d. Interpersonal/social support structure
e. Preparation for relapse; written plan should be constructed collaboratively with patient; such planning is presented with the hope that early intervention into relapse will prevent hospitalization

Medication Issues and Nursing Interventions

Tables 15.5, 15.6, and 15.7 have addressed specific nursing interventions regarding side and adverse effects and the patient's acceptance of medication. This section concentrates on several issues that commonly arise and require expert consultation by the clinical specialist.

ISSUE: PATIENT SAFETY AND NURSE EFFECTIVENESS. Establishing an alliance with a non-medicated, symptomatic patient hinges on the nurse's capacity to avoid identification with the patient's sense of fear and loss of control. Through relaying a sense of command, the nurse reduces the patient's anxiety. Though understandably anxious, the nurse needs to ensure patient safety through the following interventions:

1. Secure premedication baselines—use restraint and other safety precautions to allow access to the patient.
2. If intramuscular injections are necessary, use a high-potency choice in the gluteus maximus site well away from the sciatic nerve. Anxiety-provoking issues of exposure and sexual fantasies associated with the gluteus maximus site can be minimized by a professional manner on the part of the nurse. Adequate dosage early in treatment may result in lower total dosage of medication over a shorter duration.
3. The long-acting nature of antipsychotics offers the possibility of avoiding crisis management in favor of regular per os dosage. Careful observing will allow predictability of "symptom storms" and provide the chance to offer medication per os at nonstressful, receptive times. Regular injection of medication is superior to crisis dosage since the target symptoms are unlikely to wax according to blood level. Interpersonal means are more effective in a crisis than medication.
4. Quick intervention into side effects and complications concretizes the nurse's declaration of caring, an important paradigm in casting the nurse in the role of nurturing parent to the emotionally needy patient.

ISSUE: ANTIPSYCHOTIC MEDICATION AS ADJUNCT TO INTERPERSONAL CHANGE. Antipsychotics allow access to the highly symptomatic patient. Reduction of symptoms is not the end but the beginning for nursing intervention directed toward psychosocial change. Interventions helpful toward this end are discussed below.

1. Pharmacotherapy can be used as an interpersonal laboratory in which obstacles to collaboration are resolved. Rapport, decoding cryptic communication, and adapting to ambivalence require expertise by the nurse. Losing skirmishes when the patient needs control will not compromise therapeutic effects of these long-acting drugs and will allow the patient to experiment with taking control. Educative efforts will quickly allow the patient maximum control over medication.
2. Provision of interpersonal interventions lays the groundwork for psychosocial changes that the patient can make and that can reduce the need for medication. Consistency, structure, limits on impulsiveness, and the presence of persons less anxious than the patient are helpful interventions.

3. Encouraging investment in wellness-promoting behaviors is another route to interpersonal change that emerges in the context of pharmacotherapy. Intervention into side effects allows other issues of hygiene, nutrition, sexuality, and so on to be addressed by the nurse. Concrete changes in self-caring pave the way for low appraisals of self to be changed by the patient. Informed consumerism in regard to drug use is an example of self-caring that the nurse can teach; for example, fully informed consent to indefinite treatment with antipsychotics mandates expert teaching regarding tardive dyskinesia; conclusion of treatment with antipsychotics requires teaching about relapse and investment by the patient in seeking medication at the onset of relapse.

Mood-Stabilizing Medications

There are several groups of medications that are currently successfully used in the treatment of affective disorders.

Definitions and Terms

The term *mood* refers to a pervasive and sustained emotion that in the extreme, colors the person's perception of the world (Task Force, 1980). Extremes of mood ranging from intense, prolonged, exaggerated sadness to intense, prolonged, exaggerated happiness distort reality perception. The rigid, fixed nature of these extreme moods limits the adaptability of the extremely sad or happy person. These limitations create life difficulties ultimately causing the person to seek or be brought for help.

Extremes of mood are seen as linked by dynamic and clinical features and are described under one category, affective disorders, in the current psychiatric nomenclature (Task Force, 1980). Persons with disordered moods exhibit unilateral depression (unipolar disorder), alternate between depression and mania (bipolar disorder), or exhibit a mixture of the two states.

Depression is descriptive of a state of dejection and lowered activity. The term has become a psychiatric diagnostic category that includes qualities of lowered mood tone, difficulty in thought, and somatic changes (Haber, et al., 1982). Depression accompanied by suicidal thoughts and actions is a threat to life. Investigations indicate that the depressive syndromes are a heterogeneous group of disorders that share depressive mood as a core feature (Klein et al., 1980,). Research also suggests that distinguishing unipolar depressions with endogenomorphic symptoms is useful for the purposes of pharmacotherapy, since patients with these symptoms respond to antidepressant medication (Klein et al., 1980). This approach eliminates confusing variables such as presence/absence of a precipitating event, severity/longevity of symptoms, and recidivism. Endogenomorphic depressions are characterized by an autonomous (not related to a life incident), pervasively impaired capacity to experience pleasure or to respond appropriately to anticipated pleasure. Deinvestment in the environment and its events occurs. Usual symptoms accompanying endogenomorphic depression include obsessional thinking, guilt, helplessness, low self-esteem, somatic disturbances, pervasive sadness with crying, weight disturbance (usually loss), sleep disorders (usually insomnia), and diurnal fluctuations that are usually more severe in the morning and decrease as the day goes on. Tri/tetracyclic antidepressants are the medications of choice in such disorders. Antipsychotics may also be used when agitation or psychotic features are present (Klein et al., 1980).

Mania or a symptom cluster of pressured speech, euphoria, flight of ideas, hyperactivity, belligerence, grandiosity, spending sprees, and insomnia (Shader, 1975) alternating with a state of depression distinguishes bipolar disorders. Euphoria, an exaggerated happy mood, is a core feature (Task Force, 1980). The "happiness" associated with the manic state lacks the elusive quality of "well-being" or satisfaction. The euphoric person seems to be perched precariously on the edge of hopelessness. Depressive themes of disrupted self-worth and isolation from interpersonal relationships are expressed as grandiosity and intrusiveness. Extreme forms of mania (manic delerium) can be life-threatening. Most patients with bipolar features require hospitalization (Klein et al., 1980).

Lithium carbonate is a potent "normalizer" of euphoric mood and manic symptoms. Lithium acts to reduce labile mood but does not extinguish anxiety. Prophylactic treatment using lithium prevents recurrent manic and depressive episodes. Figure 15.2 illustrates the theorized pharmacologic action of mood stabilizing medications.

Relevant Research Summary

1. Studies of sleep and wakefulness correlate levels of serotonin (5HT) and norepinephrine (NE) with shifts in these functions. Depletion of 5HT induces insomnia (Friedman & Kaplan, 1975,), whereas hypothalmic norepinephrine seems to mediate euphoria and depression and influence muscle tone in anxiety (Friedman & Kaplan, 1975).

2. Empirical studies involve an exploration of a link between 5HT and NE and the clinical symptoms of disrupted sleep, motor and cognitive retardation, anxiety, and mood disruption present in depression.

Clinical Guidelines for Use

TRICYCLIC ANTIDEPRESSANTS. Tricyclic antidepressants are subject to idiosyncratic metabolism by individuals and require individualized dosage (Shader, 1975). Klein et al. (1980) recommend imipramine 50 mg/day as a beginning dose. This dosage is increased by 50 mg every four days until major improvement is noted. Shader (1975) recommends a 25 mg test dose followed by an orthostatic hypotension evaluation with subsequent 25 mg increments every two days in divided doses. As these medications are slow-acting, a single dose regimen similar to the antipsychotics may be used if side effects are not a problem.

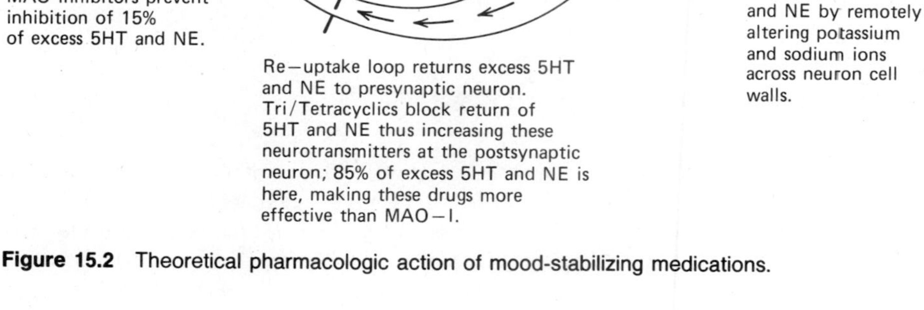

Figure 15.2 Theoretical pharmacologic action of mood-stabilizing medications.

Orthostatic hypotension and urinary retention may require a slower increase in dose (Klein et al., 1980). A trial of four to six weeks at an adequate dosage is necessary before a different antidepressant is tried. Many treatment failures are the result of inadequate dosage. Evaluation of target symptoms is useful in measuring medication effectiveness. Target symptoms include vegetative signs—sleep disturbance, anorexia, constipation—and the loss of pleasure previously described in the endogenomorphic picture.

Maintenance of the patient on antidepressants is recommended for about six months at approximately 50% of the acute treatment dosage. The medication is discontinued gradually while watching for reemergence of symptoms. After a six-month maintenance period, a decision is necessary regarding using the medication prophylactically (Klein et al., 1980).

MAO-INHIBITORS. Monamine oxidase inhibitors are generally not the first choice for treatment of depression due to their lesser efficacy and greater lethality. All other medications are withdrawn one week prior to beginning treatment with monamine oxidase inhibitors. Dietary restrictions should also begin before introducing these medications. Medication is started at a low level. Since these drugs can cause euphoria, a large noontime dose can assist in sleeping. One needs to teach the patient to anticipate orthostatic hypotension.

LITHIUM CARBONATE. Mania can be treated with Lithium or initially with an antipsychotic medication adding Lithium after the acute symptoms subside and the patient becomes more receptive. An aliphatic phenothiazine antipsychotic may assist the patient to sleep. High-potency, low-sedating antipsychotics (e.g., butyrophenone) may be used if sleep is not a problem. A high dosage may be necessary. Klein et al. (1980) state that manic patients require the largest dose of phenothiazines of all psychiatric patients.

Cooperative patients may be placed on Lithium only, but a lag of six to ten days will occur before therapeutic effects take place. Generally, therapeutic effects include a "flattening" of mood variations. The patient will be able to experience appropriate happiness without euphoria (Klein et al., 1980). Renal patency, absence of cardiac disease, and tolerance of normal dietary sodium intake are essential when using these medications. Monitoring blood levels is also essential, since individuals vary in renal excretion of Lithium.

Maintenance dosage is generally 0.6–1.2 mEq/liter. Regular plasma Lithium levels are obtained and clinical signs observed. Plasma Lithium should never exceed 2.0 mEq/liter. Using Lithium is preferable to antipsychotics in manic patients because of its lower-risk, long-term effects (Klein et al., 1980). It is crucial that patients be warned of the possibility of toxicity if a fluid/electrolyte imbalance occurs. Table 15.10 provides a picture of selected antidepressant and antimania medications by chemical group, side effects, and therapeutic action.

Nursing Intervention with the Patient Receiving Mood Stabilizing Agents

Unlike the patient with psychotic symptoms, patients with symptoms of depression and euphoria generally do not arouse uncanny or fearful responses in others until their symptoms become life-disrupting. Consequently, the undemanding, depressed individual and the productive, though erratic, euphoric person may not seek or be referred for treatment until

Table 15.10 Antidepressant and Antimania Medications: A Selected Listing by Chemical Groups and Characteristics Relevant to Nursing Care

Chemical Group and Products	*Side Effect Comparison*	*Action Comparison*
Antidepressants		
Tricyclics		
Imipramine (Tofranil, Presamine, Sk-Pramine, Janimine, Imavate)	Sedation, hypotension, dry mouth, blurred vision, constipation	Imipramine responders may have low levels of urinary MHPG
Trimipramine (Surmontil)	Same	All block serotonin reuptake
Amitriptyline (Elavil, Endep, Amitid, Amitril)	High sedation, hypotension	Amitriptyline responders may have normal to high levels of urinary MHPG
Doxepin (Sinequan, Adapin)	Highest sedation of tricyclics	
Desipramine	Less dry mouth, blurred vision, constipation	Block norepinephrine reuptake "Therapeutic window" required (i.e., not reaching or exceeding a specific dosage produces no desired pharmacodynamic effect)
Nortripytline (Aventyl, Pamelor)		
Protriptyline (Vivactyl)		
Amoxapine (Asendin)	Less dry mouth, blurred vision, dizziness, constipation	Blocks both serotonin and norepinephrine; reuptake may have quicker onset (4–7 days) than other tricyclics
Tetracyclics		
Maprotiline (Ludiomil)	Less dry mouth, blurred vision, hypotension, constipation, fewer cardiac side effects	Blocks norepinephrine reuptake
Triazolopyridine		
Trazodone (Desyrel)	Sedating Virtually no anticholinergic side effects, low cardiotoxicity, low postural hypotension	Blocks serotonin reuptake
Monamine Oxidose Inhibitors		
Phenelzine (Nardil) Tranylcypromine (Parnate)	Blurred vision, dry mouth, constipation, urinary hesitance, excessive activity and jitterness	Blocks intracellular degradation of norepinephrine at receptor site, increases dopamine and serotonin

	Blood Level—Starting	*Blood Level—Maintenance*	*Blood Level—Toxic*
Antimania agents			
Lithium carbonate (Eskalith, Lithane, Lithonate, Lithobid spansule)	1.5 mEq/liter 1500–2500 mg/day	0.5–1.0 mEq/liter 600–1800 mg/day	over 2.0 mEq/liter

Each daily 300 mg $LiCO_3$ increase raises blood concentration by 0.25 mEg/liter

Table 15.11 Side Effects of Antidepressant Medication

Assessment Site	*Symptom*	*Medication Group*	*Mechanism*	*Nursing Intervention*
1. Cardiovascular system *Interaction alert:* Tricyclics block antihypertensive effect of quanethidine (Ismelin)	Orthostatic hypotension (5.0-mm drop upon standing)	TCA[a] MAO	Anticholinergic	Preventive—BP baseline and orthostatic regimen; teach patient to dangle legs after lying down and to stand slowly; elastic stockings; supervision at night; handrails
	Tachycardia, palpitations	TCA MAO	Anticholinergic	Monitor BP baseline; provide information and support to patient
2. Skin and mucous membranes	Dry mouth	TCA MAO	Anticholinergic	Mouth rinses, sugarless lozenges
	Unpleasant taste	TCA		Educate patient—may incorporate taste into delusions of poisoning and punishment
	Sweating	TCA		Comfort measures, education
3. Gastrointestinal system	Constipation	TCA MAO	Anticholinergic	Aggravates existing constipation from depression; begin high fluid, high bulk diet prior to administration of antidepressants Monitor baseline to prevent impaction
	Nausea, anorexia, mild diarrhea	Lithium		*Transient* at beginning of therapy; if persistent, evaluate for toxicity
4. Central nervous system	Drowsiness, fatigue	TCA Lithium		Frequent, short rests; protect from injury—driving, operating machinery; educate patient; generally transient TCA—persistence may indicate change in group Lithium—observe for toxicity

Table 15.11 (*continued*)

5. Genitourinary system	Bladder atony	TCA MAO	Autonomic interference	Monitor intake and output Urine acidifier (cranberry juice) for patients with history of UTI
	Polyuria	Lithium		Transient at onset of therapy; persistent, evaluate for toxicity
	Delayed ejaculation, impotence, inhibited orgasm	MAO	Autonomic interference	Patient education important as this side effect aggravates self-doubt and perceived inferiority
6. Sensory organs	Blurred vision	TCA	Autonomic interference May be aggravation of congestive glaucoma	Assessment variables: blurred vision accompanied by pain around eyes or rainbows around lights may indicate acute congestive glaucoma
7. Body size and coordination	Weight gain	TCA	Reversal of depressive symptomatology	Reduction diet and patient education
	Fine tremor	Lithium TCA		Educate patient; no measures usually necessary

[a] Withdrawal symptoms associated with sudden cessation of TCAs include nausea, headache, vomiting, chills, abdominal cramps, insomnia, anxiety, irritability.

his/her symptoms have escalated to self-endangering or suicidal actions. The person who is sufficiently mood-distressed to require medication is often quite tolerant of his symptoms. This tolerance extends to the patient's significant others. For example, the nurse perceives that antipsychotic medication combats symptoms that torment the patient. However, antidepressant medications, in particular, seem to produce results that are not dramatic, slow in coming, and that the patient may greet with ambivalence. Lithium does not extinguish the anxiety present in mania but it will "normalize" mood swings. Knowing these aspects of the drugs can prevent the nurse from undervaluing the impact of medication for the depressed and euphoric patient who may also be undervaluing the medication as an outgrowth of disrupted self-worth.

It is essential that the nurse understand behavior clusters that appear in the depressed and euphoric patient and that affect his or her medication acceptance. Familiarity with the medications used to stabilize mood will help prevent nontherapeutic responses by the nurse. "Contagion" of mood is a powerful factor in working with these patients and the nurse who remains hopeful and balanced can be therapeutic with the patient. Though a powerful ally, medication will not replace the need for the nurse to be introspective and watchful of her own countertransference responses to these patients. Table 15.11 illustrates areas of assessment, symptomatic behavior, and nursing interventions according to antidepressant medication group. Table 15.12 highlights the sites of major adverse effects of antidepressant medications and appropriate nursing interventions.

Psychosocial Assessment

Target symptoms characteristic of depression include vegetative signs (anorexia, insomnia, motor retardation, and constipation). Target symptoms used for psychosis (Table 15.7) may be used for the manic patient who will receive antipsychotics before receiving Lithium.

Table 15.12 Adverse Effects of Antidepressants

Assessment Site	*Symptom*	*Medication Group*	*Nursing Interventions*
1. Cardiovascular system	Aggravation of preexisting cardiac disease especially conduction defects	TCA	Evidence points to low or no cardiotoxicity in young to middle-aged persons without preexisting cardiac disease; may even be antiarrhythmic in ventricular arrythmias Monitor cardiac baseline Use apical/radial values Prepare for emergency cardiac support
2. Gastrointestinal system	Paralytic ileus	TCA	Data indicate rare adverse effect; conjunctive use of atropine with TCA significant Seek medical evaluation if symptoms develop
3. Central nervous system	Agitation, psychosis	TCA	Withhold medication (can occur with rapid increase of dosage) Seek medical evaluation

Other target symptoms in mania include hyperactivity, euphoria, insomnia, and grandiosity. *Suicidal urges are present in depression and mania and must be evaluated and noted in the nursing assessment.* Particularly useful to document are known behaviors prodromal to suicidal acts (withdrawal, verbal threats, and euphoria). Medication is a frequent means to suicide in the depressed or manic patient.

Subsequent to beginning treatment with antidepressants, the nurse may note signs of improvement before the patient verbalizes feeling better. Since suicide is quite possible when the patient seems to be improving, the nurse needs to assess suicidal cues during the stabilization-maintenance period of antidepressant use in particular. Overcompliance and requests for extra medication may mean a suicide attempt is in the making. Table 15.13 illustrates nursing emergencies with patients on mood-altering medications and appropriate emergency interventions.

A plan of care for the patient on antidepressants or Lithium should include the following points:

1. *Prior to medication*
   a. Controlled observations focused on diurnal variations in symptoms, prodromal suicidal behaviors, and physiologic baselines
   b. Delineation of target symptoms
   c. Delineation of nonsymptomatic target behavior
   d. Reliable, planned routes of exchanging information
   e. Nonmedication means to alleviate severe vegetative or euphoria-related conditions (e.g., constipation, anorexia, electrolyte imbalance, hypo- or hypermotor behavior
   f. Dietary restrictions begun (MAO-I)
   g. Written teaching plan devised
   h. Interventions to alleviate blocks to acceptance of medication (see Table 15.14)
2. *During stabilization/maintenance*
   a. Evaluation of psychosocial/physiologic responses to medication; suicide assessment is particularly important; central nervous system signs of toxicity are essential to monitor in the lithiumized patient (see Table 15.15)
   b. Schedule for observing tardive variables: variables associated with antipsychotic medications if used (see Table 15.5), mood and sleep normalization, prodromal signs of latent psychosis with antidepressant use
   c. Planned experiences in self-administration of medication; assessment of self-destructive potential with medication; additional information such as Medic-Alert band for MAO-I, hypertension, and lithium toxicity
   d. Health promotion interventions to reverse consequences of disrupted self-worth; exercise and movement programs are especially helpful in depression
   e. Interpersonal interventions (Table 15.14 contains nursing diagnoses helpful in planning care.)
3. *During conclusion*
   a. Schedule and criteria for concluding pharmacotherapy (antidepressants)
   b. Collaborative decision to continue lithium indefinitely with written informed consent by patient
   c. Schedule of AIMS evaluations when antipsychotic agent discontinued
   d. Interpersonal/social support structure
   e. Preparation for relapse including written plan for patient to follow

Table 15.13 Nursing Emergencies with Mood-Altering Medications

Emergency	*Symptoms for Assessment*	*Intervention*
Overdose Tri/tetracyclic antidepressants Lethal dose: 10–30 times daily dose	Agitation, restlessness, rapid speech, dry mouth, urinary retention, mydriasis, absent bowel sounds, hypotension, hyperreflexia, convulsions Cardiac symptoms: widening of QRS complex to 100 msec or more (Biggs, 1977), sinus tachycardia, T-wave changes, ventricular tachycardia	Emergency intervention 1. Notify emergency services for transfer to intensive care unit of a hospital 2. Induce vomiting, gastric lavage 3. Monitor pulse, blood pressure, prepare for cardiac emergency Medical measures may include: 1. Physostigmine salicylate 1–3 mg IV; Neostigmine or Pyridostigmine for atropine effects (controversy over usefulness of these agents) 2. Cardiac medications and evaluations by cardiac specialist 3. Rebound of symptoms common in 72 hr after overdose
Hypertensive crisis MAO-inhibitor Interaction with dietary tyramine (a pressoramine normally inactivated by monamine oxidase in the gut) and certain medications	Throbbing occipital/temporal headache radiating frontally and generalizing Elevated BP, sweating, nausea, vomiting, restlessness, stiff neck	Nursing intervention 1. This symptom complex is generally remitting and requires notification of physician followed by support and symptomatic relief
	Sudden severe hypertension (use patient baseline to diagnose hypertension) Palpitation, sweating, chest pain, headache	1. This symptom complex represents more severe syndrome requiring emergency medical intervention; if followed by intercerebral hemorrhage, death may result 2. Medical treatment may include phentolamine (Regitine) IV, Chlorpromazine (Thorazine) IM Prevention 1. Assessment of capacity to manage complex dietary/medication restrictions 2. Educational preparation 3. Dietary restrictions—cheese (aged), beer, wine, pickled foods (herring, saurkraut), live yeast, yeast extracts, fermented dairy products (yogurt), soy sauce, fava beans, chicken livers, smoked salmon, raisins, snails, coffee, chocolate

Table 15.13 (*continued*)

Emergency	*Symptoms for Assessment*	*Intervention*
		Interaction alert: 1. Barbiturates, alcohol 2. Sympathomimetics (ephedrine, tricyclic antidepressants) 3. Amphetamines, cocaine, diuretics (partial listing) 4. Educate patient to inform physicians of MAO inhibitor therapy when being treated with *any* medication and to avoid nonprescription medications 5. Two to three weeks must elapse after discontinuing MAO-inhibitor before restrictions can be lifted 6. Medic-Alert bracelet should be worn by patient
Lithium toxicity	Central nervous system symptoms are highly responsive to toxic levels of Lithium: somnolence, ataxia, slurring of speech, confusion, slowed thinking, metallic taste Other toxic symptoms: persistent gastrointestinal disturbance (nausea, vomiting, diarrhea) persistent thirst and urination, hypotension, pulse irregularities, EKG abnormalities, coarse tremors of the hands hyperreflexia, athetoid movements, seizures, coma	Prevention 1. Use baseline functions to constantly assess CNS indicators 2. Educate patient to seek medical attention during any condition disruptive of fluid/electrolyte balance 3. Educate significant others to assess CNS function (confusion will keep patient from doing this autonomously) 4. Withhold Lithium if signs of toxicity present; administer fluids and NaCl 5. Seek emergency medical evaluation 6. Medic-Alert bracelet

Planning Nursing Intervention

PREMEDICATION PHASE. The depressed and euphoric patient requires a comprehensive plan that includes health restoration and prevention of further illness. Depressed patients require immediate planning to remedy vegetative symptoms by nonmedication means since the pharmacotherapeutic effect of tricyclics and MAO-inhibitors will be delayed. Fluid and electrolyte imbalances due to neglect need to be corrected especially in the euphoric patient who needs Lithium. Interpersonal strategies to alter observed behavior clusters need to be planned. Dietary restrictions and education need to be planned for the patient who might receive MAO-inhibitors.

STABILIZATION-MAINTENANCE PHASE. Planning is necessary to include baseline monitoring of target symptoms in the depressed patient in order to objectively judge efficacy and prevent suicide. A structure for monitoring sensitive central nervous system indicators of toxicity should be developed for the patient receiving Lithium.

Table 15.14 Psychological Phenomena in Depression and Mania that Have an Impact on Medication Acceptance

Phenomenon	*Manifest Behavior Cluster*	*Nursing Intervention Options*
Disrupted self-worth	Ruminative expressions of worthlessness and guilt unchanged by provision of reality; grandiose expressions unchanged by provision of reality Both behaviors lead to refusal of medication due to feelings of worthlessness or unperceived need for medication	Maintenance of "compromise" stance by nurse by identifying with neither extreme view held by the patient; offering carefully chosen perceptions different than the patient's own view (timing is important here) Encouraging medication; again, consistency utilizes the receptive "windows" present in ambivalence
	Self-neglect; will not take medication as a self-caring expression; will resist being "helped"	Avoid using terms such as "helpful," "help you get better" or self-caring terms; choose neutral expression, "Here is the medication."
Preoccupation with self in regard to anxiety, hostility, internal perception of emptiness	Projection and displacement of hostility on to nurse; expressions range from withholding, apathy, passivity, devaluation of nurse of the depressed patient to direct hostility, threats, sarcasm, mockery, and hypercontrol of the euphoric patient; if medication-giving becomes a predictable time to interact with the nurse, these feelings will be acted out around medication; devaluing or idealizing medication can express anger and dependency	Avoid personalizing the medication as an extension of the self; do not refer to medication as an expression of caring—"neutralizing" the medication-giving will remove medication from the issue of control Provide predictable times not connected with medication to interact with patient
	Distractibility, confusion, misperception, forgetting	Provide functions for patient as long as necessary (e.g., do not insist on autonomy in regard to medication as long as anxiety is high)
	Suicidal preoccupations; medication is a frequent method of suicidal action	Observe for lifting of depression that may be evidenced by *increased* anxiety (no longer bound into depressive delusions or hallucinations), *increased* somatisizing (return of sensation), increased hostility (less internalization of hostility) Observe for suspicious actions (sudden compliance in a resistive patient may mean hoarding medication for an overdose)

Table 15.15 Suggested Patient-Derived Baselines for Evaluating Impact of Mood-Stabilizing Medications

Baseline	*Remarks*
Laboratory studies	Use current established criteria
EKG (rhythm/conduction defects)	
Hepatic panel (MAO)	
Renal studies (Lithium)	
Blood pressure	
Orthostatic hypotension regimen	For tri/tetracyclics
Hypertensive picture	For MAO-inhibitors
Pulse	Arhythmia, rate deviation should be evaluated using apical/radial measures and notify physician; EKG follow-up
Fluid/kidney function	
Intake-output	For tri/tetracyclics, MAO-I and Lithium
Urine specific gravity	For Lithium
Nonquantitative physiologic variables	
Bowels, sleep/waking activity levels, skin, eyesight, urination (muscular)	For tri/tetracyclic A.D.
Dietary habits (tryptophan, tyramine ingestion)	For MAO-inhibitors
Movement abnormalities	If antipsychotic/antidepressant combination is used, use AIMS exam
Weight	Reversal of trend (loss/gain) during depression will indicate efficacy of TCAs
Gastrointestinal function, thirst, hand tremor, central nervous system functioning (alertness, speech clarity, thought clarity)	Specific for Lithium carbonate
Suicidal cues using patient-derived prodromal cues as suicidal "target symptoms" (e.g., withdrawal, elation, alcohol abuse, etc.)	Specific for TCAs and MAO-inhibitors
Seizure disorder, allergies	Document both investigation and results
Recent ingestion of medication	
Pregnancy	

CONCLUSION PHASE. An AIMS evaluation should be planned if the patient has been treated with an antipsychotic agent.

Nursing Interventions

Nursing interventions appear in Tables 15.11 through 15.15. Additional interventions are presented here. In the premedication phase, depressed patients require interpersonal interventions with symptoms of disrupted self-worth and self-preoccupation prior to treatment with antidepressants.

Medication Issues and Nursing Interventions

Tables 15.11–15.15 address specific nursing interventions into side and adverse effects, emergencies, and the patient's acceptance of mood-altering medications. Other issues requiring expert consultation by the clinical nurse specialist are discussed below.

ISSUE: COUNTERTRANSFERENCE TOWARD THE PATIENT WITH DISRUPTED SELF-WORTH. In severe depression, patients may refuse medication because of an intense belief in their unworthiness or delusions of requiring punishment, hence "poisoning" by medication. Conversely, medication can be seized upon as "the answer" as an outgrowth of both the patient's intense dependency on and ambivalence (love-hatred) toward significant others. For example, a patient who has a significant relationship with a nurse may praise the nurse for being "caring enough to give me medication." This expression may be a hostile devaluation of the nurse and an expression of the patient's passive idealistic expectation of cure through medication. Interpersonal interventions made by the nurse prior to pharmacotherapy will establish that antidepressants alter symptoms not the life patterns that cause and perpetuate depression. The positive, relatively stable presence of the nurse who offers specific approaches to help the patient alter fixed behavior clusters will help reduce the patient's extreme refusal and idealization of medication prior to its use. Euphoric patients may often refuse medication due to grandiose notions that defend against feelings of diminished self-worth. Patience, support of the patient's defenses, and setting limits on a few critical behaviors need to precede the use of medication, if possible. These actions tell the patient that the nurse sets limits around safety issues. They also reinforce the autonomy needed by the patient to defend against catastrophic helplessness and hopelessness.

ISSUE: SELF-CARING IN DEPRESSED AND EUPHORIC PATIENTS. Suicide and adverse reactions to Lithium and MAO-inhibitors are important nursing considerations with mood-altered patients. Careful education and concrete planning for emergencies are necessary. As the patient assumes responsibility for self-medication, the danger of overdose or dietary manipulation increases for the patient taking antidepressants and MAO-inhibitors. Patients on Lithium may miss the hyperenergia of mania and stop their medications. The most critical need for the nurse working with patients in this phase is to establish a viable alliance with them so that they feel comfortable in communicating suicidal or demoralizing episodes. Nurses who may identify with the omnipresent hopelessness in these patients will find such episodes anxiety-provoking. The nurse needs to be alert that his or her anxiety does not prevent identification or critical prodromes in these patients. Behaviors expressing abandonment themes are important. Missed appointments, missed medications, and any trends toward severing ties with significant others are all cues of hopelessness. The nurse's anxiety over the patient's hopelessness may surface in many forms. Relief that this difficult patient has not arrived for medication class or has not called the clinic to discuss a seemingly endless array of medication side effects may be expressions of anxiety. Feelings of relief in the nurse toward a potentially suicidal patient are a clue to trigger immediate introspection and a comprehensive examination of recent events in the clinical picture of the patient. Only then can the nurse be sure that the patient's behavior is not an indication of diminished self-worth and a possible indication of suicidal intent.

Nursing Assessment

For patients in the premedication phase, see Table 15.8. Physiological observations should include the nursing baselines in Table 15.15.

Anxiolytic Medications

Anxiolytic medications are used to treat the symptoms of extreme anxiety. The rationale, treatment protocol, and the clinical specialist's role in the use of these medications will be discussed in the following section.

Definitions and Terms

Anxiety is a subjectively painful warning of impending danger (Wilson & Kneisl, 1979). Anticipatory in nature, the complex physiological responses may arise in predictably threatening situations such as separation from significant people or confrontation with strangers, or in unanticipated situations, anticipation of pain, humiliation, or loss of self-esteem, and internal conflicts between opposing motivations (Klein et al., 1980; Wilson & Kneisl, 1979). Since anxiety is a preparation for "survival" actions, preparatory responses form the symptoms as differentiated from the distortion of reality in psychosis and the alteration of mood in affective disorders. Table 15.16 organizes phenomena seen in moderate to high anxiety states and the nursing interventions with these phenomena. Anxiolytic medications are used to treat symptoms of anxiety. Klein et al. (1980) encourage conservatism in using anxiolytic agents as patients are often reassured about their capacity to master the feelings by not being treated with medication. Even panic states remit fairly rapidly and, except for patients in extraordinary agony or free-floating anxiety (i.e., no specific stress or psychological state), panic anxiety can be approached conservatively. Dissociative reactions, histrionic personality disorders, phobic disorders, obsessive-compulsive disorders, psychophysiologic disorders or factors, and personality disorders have not been shown to be responsive to treatment with anxiolytic agents (Klein et al., 1980).

Table 15.16 Phenomena Associated with Moderate to Panic Levels of Anxiety and Nursing Intervention Options in Addition to/in Lieu of Medication

Phenomenon	*Symptoms*	*Nursing Intervention Options*
Preparedness for personally-defined or source-obscured threat to survival	Obvious signs of muscle tension; twitching, hypermotoric movements	Physical activity (stretching, rhythmic and aerobic exercise) Bathing, hydrotherapy Deconditioning exercises, autosuggestion Biofeedback training
	Autonomic nervous system activity; bowel, urination frequency; perspiration, tachycardia, tachypnea	Monitor baselines for pulse, respiration Allow and protect relief behaviors (urinating frequently) Observe for environmental events which increase anxiety and create a "stressor" baseline
	Vigilant, hyperalertness, scanning, insomnia	Succinct, relevant preparation for any interpersonal or environmental change or known stressor Adequate light, visual field Physical measures for sleep enhancement
Disrupted problem-solving ability; diminished capacity for learning more effective interpersonal patterns	Distractibility, distorted focus of attention (a single detail), inattention, selective retention of parts of content	Plan new interpersonal learning experiences to occur at predictable low anxiety point; reduce stimuli Short, succinct content with frequent repetitions Check retention of content at remote point from new experience Supportive emotional environment with flexible structure apparent and "felt" limits on disrupted behavior

Proposed Pharmacologic Action of Antianxiety Medications

The site and pharmacologic action of the antianxiety medications is not known. Meprobamate and the benzodiazepines act through the inhibitory neurotransmitter gamma-aminobutyric acid (GABA), which produces muscle relaxant and anticonvulsant effects. Whether GABA is involved in the antianxiety effect is unknown. Proposed sites of action for the antianxiety drugs are the limbic system (affect alteration), the reticular-activating system (sensory reduction), the median forebrain bundle (altering reward and punishment systems), and the hypothalamus (remote effects of anxiety) (Hollister 1982).

Relevant Research Summary

1. The DSM-III has designated a core event (namely, spontaneous panic attacks) as differentiating a group of anxious patients who may have a pathophysiological aberration. Experimental intravenous infusion of lactate induces panic attacks in this group of patients but not in normal controls. The finding has been replicated consistently, but the meaning is not understood. Additionally, anxiety without known precipitants has been chemically reproduced in susceptible experimental subjects suggesting increased beta-adrenergic receptor activity as a basis for panic disorders (Klein, 1982). Klein (1982) suggests that the core panic episode initiates a sequence of secondary anticipatory anxiety and tertiary Phobic avoidance.
2. Empirical trials have demonstrated that imipramine and monoamine oxidase inhibitors block panic attacks. Benzodiazepines reduce anticipatory anxiety but do not help panic attacks (Klein, 1982). Beta-adrenergic blockers have a weak antianxiety effect, especially on the physical aspects of anxiety (Klein, 1982).
3. Comparison of behavioral methods of treatment and pharmacotherapy have generally shown pharmacotherapy combined with exposure (progressive confrontation experiences with the feared situation) to be the most effective form of the treatment combinations systematically studied (Liebowitz and Klein, 1982).

Clinical Guidelines for Use

Anxiety may be seen as a familiar landmark in navigating through the multiple demands of modern life. Anxiety is as syntonic with modern life as the fear of our ancestors produced by the many threats to their existence. Anxiety is not tolerated well in American culture. Media presentations depict relaxed, ideal males and females who seem immune to everyday terrors of meeting new people in strange situations, establishing an identity in a period of tremendous role redefinition (especially for women), and succeeding in careers where self-fulfillment and creativity are "basic" requirements.

The tremendous popularity of the anxiolytic medications speaks to the need for a rational approach to their use. No one enjoys experiencing or watching another person experience painful anxiety. Yet, this useful warning of threats to well-being is often treated symptomatically without a concurrent search for either a cause or a permanent solution. An argument can be made that the subjective discomfort of anxiety is a potential source of motivation for necessary change. The inherent danger in anxiolytic medication is the eradication of a warning behavior and the redefinition of an essentially useful process (anxiety) into a pathological, drug-sensitive entity. Anxiety at high levels, however, is counter-productive as it constricts one's capabilities for learning more effective approaches to interpersonal situations. Table 15.17 gives a listing of anxiolytic medications by chemical group and characteristics relevant to nursing care.

Table 15.17 Anxiolytic Medications:[a] A Selected Listing by Chemical Group with Characteristics Relevant to Nursing Care

Chemical Group and Products	*Administration Form*	*Side Effects of Anxiolytic Medications*
Glycerol derivatives	All tablet form except SK-Bamate, which has liquid form	Sedation Muscle weakness Withdrawal syndrome (rare occurrance of convulsions) Abuse Excitement in elderly patients
Meprobamate (Equanil, Miltown, SK-Bamate)		
Tybamate (Solacen, Tybatran)		
Benzodiazepines		
Chlordiazepoxide (Librium, SK-Lygen, A-poxide)	Tablets	
Diazepam (Valium)	Tablets, parenteral	
Oxazepam (Serax)	Tablets only	*Interaction alert:* Alcohol and CNS Depressants are potentiated
Chlorazepate (Tranxene)	Tablets only	
Flurazepam (Dalmane)		
Temazepam (Restoril)		
Halazepam (Paxipam) Alprazolam (Xanax)	Tablets only	
Diphenylmethane derivatives		
Hyrdoxyzine (Atarax, Vistaril)	Tablets, liquid, parenteral	

[a] Additional groups of medications being used in panic and phobic disorders include imipramine, Monoamine oxidase inhibitors, and beta-adrenergic blockers (Klein, 1982, pp. 85–88).

Five guidelines are useful in the administration of antianxiety medications:

1. High and moderate degrees of anxiety respond appropriately to anxiolytic medication; low to moderate levels of anxiety can be mobilizing and need not be medicated. Figure 15.3 depicts behaviors and learning potential along the anxiety gradient.
2. Prescription of anxiolytic medication should be done by a psychiatrist.
3. Anxiolytic medication should be given in conjunction with recognized treatment for interpersonal difficulties.
4. Anxiolytic medication should be given on a *time-limited basis* as iatrogenic and psychological dependence are inevitable. A date for terminating the medication should always be part of the treatment plan and alternatives to pharmacotherapy identified.
5. Anxiolytic medications may be used for sleep induction but, again, *only on a time-limited basis.*

Anxiolytic medications have also been useful in treating acute alcohol withdrawal. Anxiolytic use with alcohol withdrawal should include:

1. The treatment of *withdrawal symptoms* (GI disturbance, muscle cramps, insomnia, irritability, memory/concentration loss), sympathetic nervous system instability (elevated pulse, hypertension, diaphoresis, fever) occurring between six and 78 hours after cessation of drinking.
2. Sympathetic nervous system symptoms, dehydration, or hallucinosis are criteria for hospitalization (Shader, 1975,).
3. Oral benzodiazepines are preferred for use in conjunction with vitamin, fluid and electrolyte replacement.
4. *Antipsychotics are contraindicated* (seizure-causing).

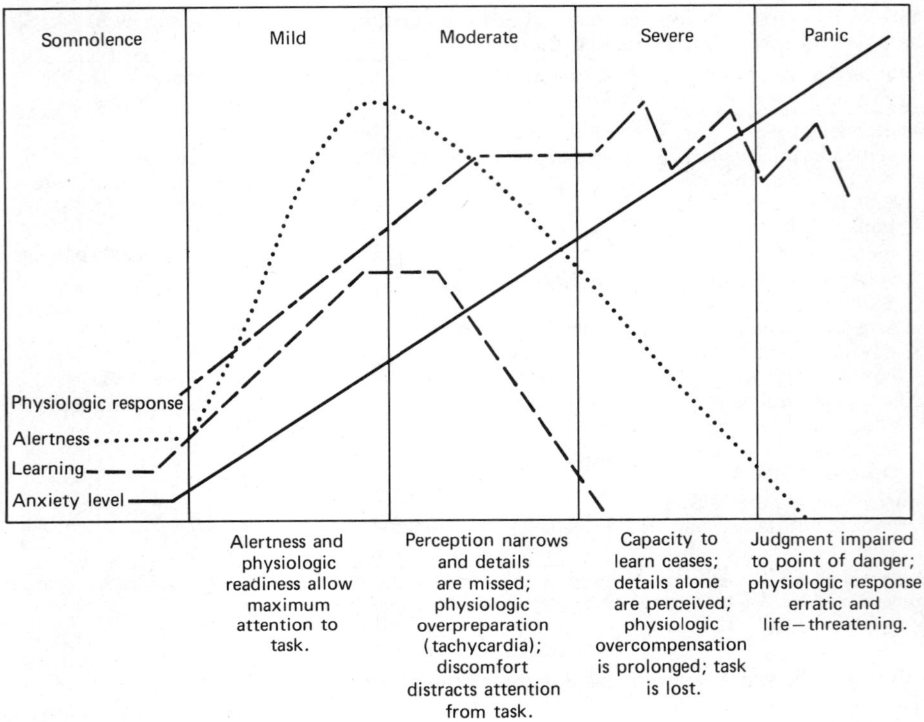

Figure 15.3 Behavior and learning potential along the anxiety gradient.

5. Maintenance of REM sleep seems essential in reversing withdrawal symptoms; hence anxiolytics are preferable to barbiturates that suppress REM sleep (Shader, 1975).
6. Surveillance of liver function is essential during withdrawal.

Dosage

Antianxiety preparations are long-acting and may be given in a single loaded dosage at bedtime to capitalize on hypnotic side effects. An empirical approach to determining dosage is recommended. Five- to seven-day treatment trials are suggested except in chronic "trait" anxiety where longer trials (with concomitant psychological dependence) are used (Hollister, 1982).

Nursing Interventions with the Patient Receiving Anxiolytic Medications

Planning Nursing Intervention

Clinical nurse specialists have the opportunity to explore interpersonal issues with a patient and ultimately to reduce the need for anxiolytic medications. The nonspecificity and abuse potential of these medications are very strong. The nurse acts in a preventive manner when interventions other than medication are offered. Clearly, a medication is less time- and energy-consuming than an individualized intervention. However, every time a nurse offers to sit with an anxious preoperative patient or to pace with or give supportive words to a hypermotoric patient a chance at prevention has been seized.

The concept of learning new behaviors in interpersonal situations is useful in working with the anxious patient if the effect of the anxiety gradient on learning is understood (Figure 15.3). From this standpoint, anxiolytic agents can be useful if they are followed by planning and providing experiences in interpersonal learning while anxiety is low. A nursing care plan needs to include using the therapeutic relationship to explore interpersonal or other nonmedication means to reduce anxiety. Practicing these techniques when symptoms are controlled by medication will allow an associative link between the action taken and a feeling of calm. After repetitive "practice," the patient may repeat the action without medication in a moderately stressful situation. When the patient has achieved some confidence through mastery, an experimental "trial by fire" may be attempted with assurance that support and retrials are available. The objective of nursing intervention is to substitute interpersonal solutions for medication and to terminate medication as rapidly as possible.

SPECIAL CONSIDERATIONS IN THE USE OF PSYCHOTROPIC MEDICATIONS

Despite advances in diagnosing mental disorders in adults and children, correct interpretation of psychological and behavioral information is often a matter of clinical judgment. The absence of "hard data" through research encourages subjectivity. Disturbed mentation and behavior is profoundly disturbing to others. Pressure by people other than the patient can frustrate clinicians and encourage them to prescribe psychotropic medication. Psychotropic medication then shifts from being an adjunct of treatment to become, instead, an agent of social control.

Unfortunately, nurses too may exert pressure toward using psychotropic medication with disturbing patients. The clinical specialist can alter this process by assisting others to learn effective interpersonal techniques and to view medication as an adjunct to other forms of treatment. This section discusses selected populations who frequently receive psychotropic medications and the nursing role in regard to their special needs. Additional resources appear in the bibliography to be used as guides to understanding racial, age, gender, cultural, and socioeconomic differences that complicate the evaluation of psychological distress and create populations prone to receiving psychotropic medications in our society.

Women and Psychotropic Medications

In reviewing data derived from investigation of patterns of psychotropic medication use in Canada and the United States, Cooperstock (1981) makes these conclusions about gender differences:

1. Women receive more medication of all kinds than men; the greatest difference between the two groups, however, is in psychotropic drugs where the prevalence of *women using prescribed anxiolytic medications on a steady basis is double that of men.*
2. Women receive 70% of their prescriptions from general practitioners and are more likely to receive anxiolytic medication for nonspecific symptoms than are men (who are more likely to receive physical therapies and laboratory tests).
3. In studies done in long-term facilities for the elderly, women were more frequently diagnosed as "anxious" by staff than were men. When the diagnosis of anxiousness was held constant between the two genders, *more women received psychotropic medication.*

4. Women who work outside the home or attend interest groups and clubs or engage in sports use fewer psychotropic drugs than women who are not involved outside the home (general health level must be considered a confounding variable, however).
5. Gross differences between genders in regard to psychotropic medication exist in poorly defined entities such as neurotic and psychosomatic disorders. As severity of symptoms increases, gender, socioeconomic, and cultural variance for psychotropic drug use decreases.
6. Peak use of psychotropic medication by women occurs in middle age.

Cooperstock (1981) postulates that greater psychotropic drug use among women occurs because:

1. Women do not clearly define their symptoms and thereby incur psychotropic prescriptions as a response from frustrated physicians.
2. Women are four times more likely to report symptoms of anxiety to others than are men, and women make greater use of social and treatment networks than do men.
3. Women self-label symptoms as "psychiatric" and accept the role of patient more willingly than do men.

As a women's profession, nursing shares both problems and change potential wherever women are treated with psychotropic medication. The capacity to remain objective with troubled women is difficult, and a female patient's interpersonal difficulties may often correspond to threatening and unsolved situations in the nurse's own life. Conversely, the predelection of women to seek out networks in times of stress may be channeled by nurses into supportive and educative groups that explore the proper use of medications and alternatives to their use. The nurse can assist women in clarifying symptomatology and in seeking physician specialists, particularly psychiatrists, for help. This involves helping the women to work through the perceived stigma of a psychiatric problem. Clinical specialists need to ascertain that the theoretical constructs used in planning care for women represent valid hypotheses in feminine psychology. Nursing research into alternatives to medication such as utilizing women's networks is desperately needed. Research would be especially useful in regard to the "minor" symptoms that are quite amenable to change through interpersonal means.

Pregnant and Lactating Women

The notion of the placental "barrier" has changed and the placenta is now viewed as a selective filter across which most potential teratogens pass. First trimester exposure to teratogens may produce obvious deformity, whereas exposure during subsequent trimesters may result in physiological, biochemical, or microscopic deformities and behavioral disturbances in the newborn (American Academy of Pediatrics, 1982). Establishment of teratogenic potential for psychotropic medications has been hampered by the paucity of research methodology in evaluating the subtle malformations from exposure to teratogens during late pregnancy. Consequently, only one psychotropic medication, *Lithium,* is clearly contraindicated for use in pregnancy. Animal studies, however, point to possible teratogenic potentials of other psychotropic medications.

Lactation is a complex process in which the predicted pharmacokinesis of psychotropic medication is altered. Information is presently limited to reports of acute toxic reactions in nursing infants. Table 15.18 summarizes human and animal research to date concerning the impact of psychotropic medication on fetal and infant development. The American Academy of Pediatrics (1982) offers the following recommendations for use in pregnant and lactating women:

1. No psychotropic medication should be given to a pregnant or lactating woman unless absolutely necessary.
2. If medication is chosen, the most effective drug with the least side effects should be used.
3. Whenever possible, a psychotropic medication should be withdrawn prior to conception.
4. *Lithium is contraindicated during pregnancy,* but there is no evidence to contraindicate the use of other psychotropic medications when deemed necessary.
5. A woman receiving psychotropic medications may breastfeed if evidence regarding the particular medication indicates no danger for the infant. The infant should be assessed continuously.

The importance of the nurse offering interpersonal interventions and strategies to the psychiatric patient is no more dramatic in importance than in the care of the pregnant or lactating woman. Until research defines the role of psychotropics in fetal and infant development, conservatism is the obvious preventive approach. Nurses who possess crisis intervention skills can diagnose and facilitate reintegration at a higher level when pregnancy or birth has created a transitional life crisis for the woman and her family. There is no demonstrated reason to prohibit breastfeeding by the mother treated with psychotropic agents and the nurse may need to intervene to support the mother's wish to nurse her infant. Anxieties of helpers and family members may result in efforts to separate the mother and infant or to overmedicate the mother. The nurse needs to facilitate bonding between mother and infant by providing direction, education, and interpersonal presence and intervention to assure safety without overmedication.

Implications for the use of the clinical specialist's skills in liaison nursing are clear. Providing factual information and effective interventions to maternal-child and community health nurses will allow greater opportunities for a positive birth and bonding experience. Often, the successful negotiation of this critical event catalyzes more complex integration of the mother's personality and increases her self-esteem. Medication may cease to be necessary following successful negotiation of the mothering role.

Children and Psychotropic Medications

Children are not miniature adults. They exhibit a variable response to psychotropic medications. Predictable variances in response to psychotropic drugs (paradoxical effects) by children have become the desired therapeutic effect of certain drugs. Stimulants, normally adrenergic in adults, produce sedation in children and are used in hyperactive states. Urinary hesitance, a side effect of tricyclic antidepressants, is utilized to control enuresis. Unfortunately, little substantive research on pharmacokinesis of psychotropic medication in children presently exists and few placebo-controlled studies on efficacy have been completed. Consequently, empiricism continues to dominate decision-making in regard to psychotropic medications with children.

When one considers the developmental and social vulnerability of the child, clinical guidelines are essential in reducing subjectivity when the child's symptoms are disturbing to a

Table 15.18 Impact of Psychotropic Medications on Fetal and Infant Development

Group	*Animal Studies*	*Human Studies*	*Conclusions*
Antipsychotics	Fetal exposure resulted in structural malformation, impaired learning, reduction of spontaneity, increased susceptibility to seizures, alteration in neurotransmitter levels, and alteration of dopamine receptor sites; Perphenazine concentrates in milk of ewes whereas haloperidol does not exceed serum levels; behavioral/neurochemical aberrations persistent after exposure ended	Contradictory evidence; incidence of congenital malformations contradicted by evidence showing no increased risk; Chlorpromazine appears in milk when maternal serum levels exceed 16 mg/ml but no consistent relationship exists between plasma level and breast milk concentration	
Mood-stabilizing medications Tricyclics Lithium	Morphologic and behavioral aberrations after imipramine exposure in utero	Imipramine but not amytriptyline found in breast milk after acute ingestion (may differ when regularly ingested); fetal and neonate abnormalities: cardiovascular (Epstein's anomaly), congenital goiter, hypothermia, cyanosis, bradycardia, shallow respirations, diminished suck, hypotonia, EEG changes, diabetes insipidus Lactation: Lithium milk concentration = ½ maternal serum. Infant serum Lithium is equal to Lithium milk concentration. 0.6 mEq/liter level in infants produces lethargy, cyanosis, hypotonia, poor suck	Contraindicated in pregnancy
Anxiolytics	Abnormal arousal and motor behavior after prenatal exposure to diazepam; One incidence of weight loss	Conflicting reports of oral-facial deformities following diazepam exposure; increased incidence of cesarean section, fetal heart rate aberrations, depressed Apgar, hypotonia, poor suck; conflicting studies indicating as high as 4.5 times severe abnormalities in fetuses exposed to chlordiazepoxide; other studies do not confirm such a high rate; metabolites of diazepam have been found in breast milk but no information yet about rate or effects of concentration; one incident reported of infant weight loss, EEG changes, lethargy	

family or school system. Considerable pressure may be placed on a helping system to control the child's behavior when, in fact, the child is not subjectively bothered by his own symptoms. Whereas tremendous controls are placed on physicians' conduct in researching psychotropic drugs in children, very few controls are placed on prescribing these drugs for children. Empiricism, the need for social control and ease of prescription become factors that increase the likelihood that the child with disturbed behavior or psychological functioning will receive psychotropic medications. Klein et al. (1980) suggest the clinical guidelines presented in Table 15.19. Table 15.20 presents the stimulants that are used *only* in children to treat attention-deficit disorders.

Although far from overwhelming, evidence indicates the possibility that psychotropic medication interferes with learning, nutrition, sleep, and physical growth in children. These findings demand that the nurse emphasize the use of nonmedication treatments for children and work for their success. The comfort of nurses in life-style settings enhances the access of the child to professional help while playing, learning, eating, and living at home with the family. The clinical specialist is able to adapt complex treatment methodologies to a variety of settings as well as interpret the regimen to other professionals. The nurse draws upon his/her developmental preparation to advocate for the child at critical developmental periods. The clinical nurse specialist is a consultant to generalist nurses in schools and community and hospital settings to provide specialized, developmentally appropriate mental health interventions that can offer permanent change.

The child is intrinsically capable of greater change than the adult because of developmental flexibility. Consequently, medication standards used for adults (e.g., maintenance antipsychotics) must never be used for the child. The nurse must advocate for continuous assessment and change in the treatment program to mirror the child's continual cognitive and emotional growth. Resistance to reevaluating an *effective* medication will be strong, but must occur since the child may be showing improvement through learning and maturation, not medication. The clinical nurse specialist can use expanded skills in group and family intervention to alter attitudes and to educate parents of symptomatic and nonsymptomatic children in regard to effective parenting patterns.

Psychotropic Medication and the Elderly

As the population of aging persons increases, the exposure of these persons to psychotropic medication becomes more prevalent. Natural disruptions of integrity such as losses of significant relationships, declining health, restricted mobility, and reduced economic power increase pressures on the elderly. Persons who have successfully coped in previous stages of life may develop symptoms of emotional distress. Symptoms of psychosis and depression are commonly treated with antipsychotics and antidepressants. Anxiolytic agents are used to reduce moderate to severe states of anxiety (Shader, 1975). Psychotropic medication for the elderly needs always to be considered an adjunct to environmental, supportive, and familial therapies. The symptoms need to be evaluated and weighed against the frequent medication complications that can occur in this age group. Relatives and caretakers often find the symptoms more distressing than does the elderly patient.

Significant alterations in physiological function of elderly persons affects psychotropic drugs in the following manner (Shader, 1975):

1. Duration of action is extended and potency is increased.
2. Drug peaks, time of onset, and half-life are altered; generally, predictable times of onset are delayed and the half-life is extended.

Table 15.19 Medication-Responsive Disorders in Children

Disorder	*Type of Psychotropic Medication Used*	*Comments*
Moderate to severe attention disorders with hyperactivity (mild forms may be managed through environmental manipulations—structured classrooms, parent support, education, treatment)	Dextroamphetamine Methylphenidate (refer to Table 15.20)	1. Dosage and schedule are highly variable between individuals 2. Child should be removed from the drug *during each school year* for several weeks to evaluate need 3. Parents should not be allowed to alter dosage 4. Withdrawal should occur over a one to two week period; follow-up should occur 5. Medication must be coordinated closely with efforts at school and home, preferably in an interdisciplinary setting
Pervasive developmental disorders	Antipsychotics (refer to Table 15.8) Side effects that appear in children: drowsiness, increased appetite, enuresis (Thioridazine), photosensitivity (Chlorpromazine), dry mouth, blurred-vision (rare), nasal congestion (rare), acute dystonias, transient dyskinesia upon *withdrawal;* high potency drugs more likely	1. Antipsychotics are the *only* group demonstrated to be effective 2. *Exert symptomatic control* where marked agitation, hyperactivity, poor sleep, mood lability are present 3. *Do not exert an antipsychotic effect* (alteration of the core psychotic disorder) as in adults—specificity for agitated symptoms make these drugs of little value with withdrawn, mute children 4. *Never used as the only treatment modality*
Separation anxiety (school phobia)	Imipramine (no data justifies use of benzodiazepines in children for anxiety)	1. Only demonstrated in a single investigation 2. Symptomatic decrease but not necessarily increased school attendance 3. Recommended maximum treatment duration is eight weeks with an additional eight-week trial if symptoms have remitted 4. Used as an adjunct to supportive-directive treatment programs
Enuresis	Tricyclic antidepressants (no difference among compounds) Side effects that appear in children: dry mouth, drowsiness (rare), sweating (rare), constipation (rare), mild	1. Effect is generally noted within one week 2. Short-term use advocated; *conditioning techniques preferable to medication* due to long-term benefit and reduced danger

Table 15.19 (*continued*)

Disorder	*Type of Psychotropic Medication Used*	*Comments*
	tremor, blood pressure alterations, EKG changes with absence of clinical signs, gastrointestinal distress when drug suddenly withdrawn	3. Treatment effect ends when drug discontinued with high relapse rate; role as an adjunct to long-term interventions preferable 4. Withdrawal of drug should be gradual. 5. *Maximum dose recommended is 5 mg/kg* due to cardiac toxicity

SOURCE: Adapted from Klein, D., et al. *Diagnosis and drug treatment of psychiatric disorders: Adults and children,* 2nd ed. Baltimore: Williams and Wilkins, 1980.

3. Concommitant medical problems frequently potentiate therapeutic and side effects (e.g., hypotension exacerbates existing confusion). Generally, *one-third to one-half the adult dose is given to the elderly adult.*

Nurses find crisis theory most useful in addressing and intervening with the elderly person. All along the human maturation pathway, critical periods challenge the resources of the person. At any stage, symptoms of distress may appear as a result of temporary loss of

Table 15.20 Medications Used in Treating Childhood Attention-Deficit Disorders

Generic Compound and Product	*Comments*
Amphetamine (Benzedrine)	
Dextroamphetamine (Dexedrine)	General dosage range is 10–25 mg/day; not recommended for children under three years old
Methylphenidate (Ritalin)	General dosage range is 30–60 mg/day; not recommended for children under six years old
Magnesium pemoline (Cylert)	General dosage range is 25–125 mg/day

Side Effects of Stimulants

Assessment Site	*Symptoms*	*Nursing Intervention*
Gastrointestinal system	Anorexia	Establish baseline eating pattern before medication is begun Watch for dose-related variation with compensation (child may make up for low daily intake by increasing food at night) Appetite enhancements; allow food preferences, separate eating from disciplinary activities

Table 15.20 (*continued*)

Generic Compound and Product		*Comments*
	Gastrointestinal disturbances	Give medication after meals Slow increment in dosage at onset of treatment
Central nervous system	Insomnia, delay of onset of sleep	Baseline sleep record with *onset* recorded Load morning dose Earlier bedtime or later awakening time
Cardiovascular system	Tachycardia	Pulse baseline Seek medical evaluation if prolonged
	Mood changes—lability, sadness, lethargy	Recommend dosage reduction Educate parents and child to this possibility
	Adverse Effects of Stimulants	
Assessment Site	*Symptoms*	*Nursing Intervention*
Growth rate	Reduction in growth rate, more vulnerability in taller children, appears minor and may reverse over time with compensatory growth May be related to anorexia or interference with growth hormone production during sleep (by-product of insomnia)	Monitor growth rate
Liver function	Elevated SGPT/SGOT may indicate liver damage Values accurate only with magnesium pemoline	Baseline monitoring of lab tests Withhold medication if values abnormal
Central nervous system	Hallucinations	Withhold medication Seek further psychiatric evaluation for pervasive developmental disorder

coping ability. The nurse's capacity to diagnose and to assist in a favorable crisis resolution may make medication unnecessary or, at least, ensure that the use of medication is brief. The elderly experience multiple losses that make them a crisis-prone population whose needs are best served by intervention that avoids the use of psychotropic medication. Although major personality change is generally not possible for an elderly person, behavioral and physically comforting interventions are quite helpful. Mobilizing a viable network of supportive persons often prevents the use of medication and promises more effective postcrisis adaptation. Recognizing cultural defensiveness concerning death and loss issues in the elderly will guide the nurse in determining that the patient receives psychotropic medications only when necessary and, then, in conjunction with other therapies and on a time-limited basis.

SUMMARY

Synthesis of new psychotropic compounds will continue and increasingly focus upon symptom- and disorder-specific medications. The call for research in special populations will undoubtedly lead to as many new pharmacotherapies as nonsomatic therapies. Proliferation of groups of patients for whom medication cannot be used will also occur. It is within these populations that nursing may validate through research the effectiveness of interpersonal and behavioral methods for control and cure of emotional disorders.

Symptom-specific medication raises the spectre of social control of feeling states, which, despite its fictional sound, has already been argued in the use of medication with women, prisoners, and school children (Hallek, 1971). Recent litigation by mental patients regarding the right to refuse medication has created dilemmas for mental health professionals. Unanswered questions lie between the extremes of patients' rights to refuse medication and helpers' mandates to treat the mentally disordered. Helpers', particularly nurses', rights to safety in working with potentially aggressive and abusive patients are threatened by these unanswered dilemmas. The clinical nurse specialist as a multidimensional nursing leader can influence the development of knowledgeable interpersonal interventions within the context of psychopharmacotherapy. Through these contributions, the clinical nurse specialist can enhance the future care of the mentally ill.

REFERENCES

American Academy of Pediatrics Committee on Drugs. Psychotropic drugs in pregnancy and lactation. *Pediatrics,* 1982, *69,* 241–244.

Biggs, J. T., Reisenberg, R. A., and Zeigler, V. E. Overdosing the tricyclic patient. *American Journal of Psychiatry,* 1977, *134,* 461–462.

Cooperstock, R. Women and psychotropic drugs. In E. Howell & M. Bayes (Eds.), *Women and mental health.* New York: Basic Books, 1981.

Davis, J. Overview: Maintenance therapy in psychiatry 1: Schizophrenia. *American Journal of Psychiatry,* 1975, *132,* 1237–1245.

Department of Health, Education and Welfare Division of Nursing. *Source book on nursing personnel* (HRA 75–43). Bethesda, MD: DHEW, 1974.

Friedman, A., & Kaplan, B. *Comprehensive textbook of psychiatry* (2nd ed.). Baltimore: Williams & Wilkins, 1975.

Haber, J., Leach, A., Schudy, S., & Sideleau, B. *Comprehensive psychiatric nursing* (2nd ed.). New York: McGraw-Hill, 1982.

Hallek, S. *The politics of therapy.* New York: Science House, 1971.

Hirsch, S. R., Gaind, R., Rohde, P. D., Stevens, B. C., & Wing, J. K. Outpatient maintenance of chronic schizophrenic patients with long-acting fluphenazine: Double-blind placebo trial. *British Medical Journal,* 1973, *1,* 633–637.

Hollister, L. Drugs for treating anxiety. In W. Modell (Ed.), *Drugs of choice 1982–1983,* St. Louis: C. V. Mosby, 1982.

Kessler, K., & Waletzky, J. P. Clinical use of antipsychotics. *American Journal of Psychiatry,* 1981, *138,* 202–209.

Klein, D. F. Medication in the treatment of panic attacks and phobic states. *Psychopharmacology Bulletin,* 1982, *18,* 85–90.

Klein, D. F., Gittelman, R., Quitkin, F., & Rifkin, A. *Diagnosis and drug treatment of psychiatric disorders: Adults and children* (2nd ed.). Baltimore: Williams & Wilkins, 1980.

Liebowitz, M. R., and Klein, D. F. Unresolved issues in the treatment of agoraphobia with panic attacks. *Psychopharmacology Bulletin,* 1982, *18,* 109–114.

Lion, J. *The art of medicating psychiatric patients.* Baltimore: Williams & Wilkins, 1978.

Martin, E. *Hazards of medication* (2nd ed.). Philadelphia: J. B. Lippincott, 1978.

May, P. Pharmacotherapy in relation to alternative treatment methods. In B. Sedvall (Ed.), *Antipsychotic drugs: Pharmacodynamics and pharmacokinetics.* New York: Pergamon, 1976.

Peplau, H. *Interpersonal relations in nursing.* New York: Putnam, 1952.

Rifkin, A., Quitkin, F., & Klein, D. F. Fluphenazine deconate, oral fluphenazine and placebo in treatment of remitted schizophrenics, II. Rating scale data. *Archives of General Psychiatry,* 1977, *34,* 1215–1219.

Rosenbaum, P. *The meaning of madness.* New York: Science House, 1970.

Shader, R. *Manual of psychiatric therapeutics.* Boston: Little Brown, 1975.

Snyder, S. The dopamine hypothesis of schizophrenia: Focus on the dopamine receptor. *American Journal of Psychiatry,* 1976, *133,* 197–202.

Task Force on Nomenclature and Statistics. *Diagnostic and statistical manual of mental disorders* (*DSM III*) (3rd ed.). Washington, DC: American Psychiatric Association, 1980.

Wilson, H. S., & Kneisl, C. R. *Psychiatric nursing.* Menlo Park, CA: Addison-Wesley, 1979.

BIBLIOGRAPHY

Appelbaum, P. Can mental patients say no to drugs? *New York Times Magazine* (March 21, 1982) pp. 46–59.

Appleton, W. Fourth psychoactive drug usage guide. *Journal of Clinical Psychiatry,* 1982, *42,* 12–27.

Campbell, M. Psychopharmacology. In S. Harrison (Ed.), *Basic handbook of child psychiatry* Vol. III. New York: Basic Books, 1979.

Eisenberg, G. Ethical aspects of the right to refuse medication. *Psychiatric Quarterly,* 1981, *53,* 93–99.

Parry, H. J., Balter, M. B., Mellinger, G. D., Cisin, I. H., & Manheimer, D. I. National patterns of psychotherapeutic drug use. *Archives of General Psychiatry,* 1973, *28,* 769–783.

Rodman, M. *Pharmacology and drug therapy in nursing.* Philadelphia: J. R. Lippincott, 1979.

Salzman, C. A primer on geriatric psychopharmacology. *American Journal of Psychiatry,* 1982, *139,* 67–74.

Simpson, L. (Ed.). *Drug treatment of mental disorders.* New York: Raven Press, 1979.

Willie, C., Kramer, B, & Brown, B. (Eds.). *Racism and mental health.* Pittsburg: University of Pittsburg Press, 1973.

PART FOUR SPECIAL ISSUES FOR SELECT POPULATIONS

While psychiatric mental health nursing requires knowledge and skill in specific therapeutic modalities, successful application requires an understanding of the special issues specific to various populations of clients. Part Four is focused on Standards I, IV, V, and X of the American Nurses' Association's (ANA) *Standards of Psychiatric and Mental Health Nursing Practice* (ANA, 1982) and issues common among clients from minority cultural groups, clients in general hospital settings, women, the chronically mentally ill, and alcoholics are addressed. While clients from these populations all have unique, individual needs, they also share problems with others of their group that stem from their place in the structure of society. Successful therapy demands that these issues be considered together with presenting psychopathology.

The different definitions of mental health and illness held by Western psychotherapists and lay people from minority cultural groups are discussed in Chapter 16. The importance of understanding and incorporating the client's world view by discussing psychotherapeutic work with clients of Japanese and Chinese descent are illustrated.

In Chapter 17, the consultation and liaison roles in nonpsychiatric, general hospital settings are presented. A distinction is made between these two interrelated roles, and the processes are illustrated with clinical examples.

In Chapter 18 the impact of stereotyping and prejudice on women as both providers and clients in mental health settings is discussed. Among the issues explored are differences in the definitions of mental health and illness for men and women; the significance of increasing rates of mental illness for women; differences in therapist attitude toward male and female clients; and the effects of prejudice on the education and practice of the psychiatric mental health nurse specialist.

The multidimensional problems of the chronically mentally ill are explored in Chapter 19. Central to the suggestions for intervention with these clients is a sensitivity to the issues of powerlessness and helplessness. Numerous intervention strategies are recommended that realistically accept the client's limitations but that facilitate an optimal level of client control through the cultivation of "positive dependence."

In Chapter 20, the multidimensional problem of alcoholism is discussed. Physiological, genetic, and family systems perspectives of alcoholism are presented. It is stated in Chapter 20 that each system is a necessary framework for care at different stages of treatment. However, Bowen's family systems therapy is an essential approach if fundamental change is to occur in the way the alcoholic client functions in his or her intimate social milieu.

In Part Four insights are offered into the special problems of client groups most commonly encountered in the practice of psychiatric mental health nurse specialists.

CHAPTER

16 BRIDGING CULTURAL DIFFERENCES

Roxy Schlesinger

The purpose of this chapter is to explore an area within the field of mental health that is commonly neglected by clinicians, namely, the impact of culture on mental health and mental illness and relevant treatment issues. Two particular cultural groups, Asian-Americans of Chinese and Japanese ethnicity, will be discussed to provide the reader with concrete examples illustrating the major concepts presented throughout the chapter. The conclusion addresses the expanding field of "transcultural nursing," including some specific implications for the psychiatric mental health clinical nurse specialist.

NATURE OF CULTURE IN SOCIETY

A survey of the anthropological literature reveals that an accurate, universally accepted definition of culture is simply nonexistent. Two anthropologists, Kroeber and Kluckhohn (1952), conducted a thorough investigation of the social science literature and found 164 meanings of culture. Loosely defined, however, culture is a way of living made up of ideas, beliefs, symbols, and values. As such, it defines an individual's world view.

All human beings are exposed to a constellation of cultural views throughout their lifetime, and their perceptions, values, and behaviors are greatly affected by such exposure. Psychiatric mental health nurses must not lose sight of the fact that this factor invariably holds true for both nurse and patient. It has been repeatedly demonstrated if the culture of the therapist varies significantly from that of the patient, certain problems will arise in the course of treatment (Leighton, 1981). Culture has a profound effect on two vital psychological functions: cognition and affect. Furthermore, different cultures and subcultures condone different ways of experiencing, expressing, and sharing emotions. Cultural, social, psychological, and biological dimensions of human existence are interconnected and interrelated with each other in such a way that they cannot be easily separated.

Since the work of Benedict on cultural relativity, the molding force of culture has received the attention of anthropologists, sociologists, psychologists, and psychiatrists (Odejide, 1979). Those who subscribe to the postulates set forth by proponents of cultural determinism maintain that a *basic personality type* exists for any given society. However, in their classic article, Kluckhohn and Mowrer (1944) cautioned that "recognition of culture as one of the determinants of personality is a great gain, but there are some indications that this theoretical advance is tending in some professional circles, to obscure the significance of the other determinants" (p. 1).

The determinants of personality are multiple, and the formation of the character structure of individuals involves a complex interplay of biological, psychological, social, and environmental factors. In addition, all human behavior reflects both universal elements and those elements that vary from culture to culture. Such behavioral variations represent differences in value orientations between cultures.

CULTURAL INFLUENCES ON ROLE EXPECTATIONS

The Role of Patient

Ruth Benedict (1938) contended that patients are culturally conditioned into the patient role. Parsons' (1951) model of the *sick role* enlarges on this idea by clearly illustrating the social aspects of the sick role. He differentiates between illness, which is the disease process, and the sick role, which is an institutionalized role socially learned. Within this model, sickness is a form of deviant behavior that affords societal members with a socially sanctioned and institutionalized way to avoid the stresses of daily living. After assumption of the sick role has been legitimized (in Western society by a physician accepting a person as a patient), the patient has two primary rights and two primary responsibilities. The patient has the rights to be exempt from his or her normal social role responsibilities and to be cared for until he or she recovers. In return, the patient has the responsibilities to acknowledge the sick role as undesirable and to seek technically competent help and cooperate with this help in getting well.

In societies that make a distinction between diseases of the mind and diseases of the body (as in Western society), the Parsonian model must be modified somewhat with respect to mental illness. Segall (1976) states that individuals who undergo psychiatric care for emotional illnesses are, like their physically ill counterparts, committed to recovery. However, while physically ill patients are usually not stigmatized by their diseases, those with mental illnesses often encounter stigmatization and rejection. Furthermore, many therapists believe that excusing mentally ill patients from all social responsibility is not only unnecessary but counterproductive. Indeed, in the Western world "whereas the behavior of the physically ill patient is expected to be marked by passivity, submission, and dependency, that of the mentally ill patient is expected to be marked by action, independence, and self-direction in relation to the therapist" (Foster & Anderson, 1978, p. 155).

The Role of Healer

Universals in Curing Roles

Common characteristics in healer roles include specialization, selection and training, sense of a professional image, expectation of payment, and belief in healers' powers. Furthermore, healers tend to be regarded with ambivalence by the public (Foster & Anderson, 1978).

Modern Western medicine is highly *specialized.* In addition, Western society accommodates further specialization by providing for "nonestablishment" treatment alternatives such as spiritualism, faith healing, and ethnic folk medicines. While the degree of specialization found within traditional societies is less, the various curing roles are distinguished from one another.

Selection and training in Western society are generally conscious decisions and lengthy training is required. A personal decision to become a curer is sometimes involved in traditional societies. For instance, herbalists and midwives often learn necessary curing skills from close relatives. One who wishes to become a "witch doctor" may study for years with an older witch doctor who is already established as a curer. Remuneration for this apprenticeship is expected in the form of lavish gifts.

The supernatural is present to some extent in both Western and non-Western societies. For example, in Catholic countries, Christ and the saints are thought to be endowed with curing powers or to transfer these special powers to human beings. In traditional societies, certain persons may be forced by spiritual beings to become curers, often against their will. The *shaman* exemplifies the type of curer who is elected by a spirit.

As mentioned above, in those non-Western societies where the art of healing is rather sophisticated, students must pay for their apprenticeship period. In Western society, as well, students are expected to pay for their education and training. Certification, required in both Western and non-Western societies, is accomplished by different methods. Legal certification in the West involves passing a standardized examination. In non-Western societies, healers are "initiated" by established shamans through culturally prescribed ceremonial rituals following completion of their training.

In all societies, curers identify themselves as professionals and express their *professional image* by costume and behavior. In the Western world, a different image is portrayed by healers of the body and by those who treat mental disorders that is clearly manifested by their divergent styles of dressing. Among non-Western peoples the shaman possesses certain ritual objects that distinguish him from both laymen and other types of curers (midwives and herbalists). Contrary to popular belief, healers in all societies expect *payment* for services rendered. Moreover, healers in some societies demand to see the fee for service before accepting the patient for treatment; a practice analogous to admission procedures in many U.S. hospitals. Another common myth is that the traditional curer's approach to the patient is always friendly and supportive. In actuality, the range of personality styles and attitudes toward the patient found among non-Western healers is at least as great as that found in the Western world. According to Foster and Anderson (1978), "non-Western curers can on occasion be just as formidable as the most aloof American doctor" (p. 112).

In all societies, most healers *believe in their curative powers.* Although Westerners often doubt the integrity of shamans, most of these traditional healers are truly attempting to help their patients and have complete confidence in their ability to do so (Foster & Anderson, 1978).

Finally, in all societies, the public sector harbors *ambivalent feelings* toward their own healers. The reason for this paradox seems to be related to control issues and the exercise of power. It is to our healers to whom we must turn and depend on in times of great need. We expect them to use their curative powers to restore us to a state of wellness. Yet it is also natural for people to fear and mistrust those who exercise power over them.

Healers' Attention to Nonmedical Demands

The social context is important in determining whether or not societal demands of a nonmedical nature will be dealt with in the psychotherapeutic situation. Seguin (1974) speaks of the powerful influence of the native healer and how he employs it "to modify the net of human relationships of his patients" (p. 299). The relationship is not merely between therapist and patient and privacy is not respected, as is the case in most forms of Western psychotherapy. In many non-Western societies, sessions are conducted in full view of the public. Healing sessions often take place in groups with the accompaniment of music, song, and the ingestion of beverages prepared from native plants. According to Seguin (1974), this aspect of the psychotherapeutic encounter facilitates the rearrangement of family and community life. The solutions to problems are considered to reside primarily within the patient's relationship with significant others. Western psychiatry traditionally focuses on the individual patient and how he might actively "work out" his problems.

Foster and Anderson (1978) point out that public curing rituals reflect much more than cultural tradition. The social dimensions of the patient's illness are being attended to. For instance, the patient may have fallen out of balance with nature and society; social therapy for the entire group assures all spectators that the interpersonal stresses that have caused the illness are being properly dealt with. In addition, some societies attribute illness to the anger of deities, ghosts, spirits, and witches. When illness is explained in such personalistic terms, public demonstration of the healer's powers helps allay the peoples' fears. Onlookers can clearly see that human beings are able to protect themselves against supernatural forces.

The Therapeutic Interview

The therapeutic interview takes place in all societies, yet the manner in which it is conducted varies across cultures. Variations in therapeutic style reflect differences in views related to disease etiology, as well as cultural and ideologic differences. Nevertheless, Jerome Frank (1972) has identified a few commonalities underlying psychotherapy that transcend cultural boundaries. These commonalities have been succinctly paraphrased by Wittkower and Warnes (1974) as follows:

1. An intense, emotionally charged confiding relationship with a helping person.
2. A rationale or myth that includes an explanation of the cause of the person's distress and that is compatible with the cultural world view shared by the patient and therapist. Also, supplying a conceptual scheme for what seems to the patient to be a group of nonsensical symptoms provides powerful reassurance to him. Essentially, then, the functions of the rationale and ritual, rather than their specific content and form, are what really count.
3. Provision of new information concerning the nature and sources of the patient's problems and alternative ways of dealing with them.
4. Strengthening the patient's expectations of help through the personal qualities of the therapist, enhanced by his status in society and the setting in which he works.
5. Provision of success experiences that further heighten the patient's hopes and also enhance his or her sense of mastery, interpersonal competence, or capability.
6. Facilitation of emotional arousal, a prerequisite of attitudinal and behavioral changes (pp. 566–567).

Unfulfilled Role Expectations

Wittkower and Warnes (1974) state that "problems arise if treatment procedures created, developed, and practiced in one cultural area are transposed to another" (p. 569). Psychopathology can be understood only when the therapist is thoroughly familiar with the patient's culture and world view. Such an understanding is a prerequisite for the deliverance of psychiatric treatment that is meaningful to the patient.

In those areas of the world where mental illness is attributed to supernatural forces, patients are unlikely to derive any benefit from treatment by a Western-trained mental health professional. Quite understandably, help is sought from persons believed to be able to control supernatural powers (that is, shamans, priests, medicine men, and witch doctors). "In fact, in these countries, even if psychologically disturbed patients submit themselves to medical help for symptom removal, they may afterwards turn to the traditional healer for effective removal of the assumed cause" (Whittkower & Warnes, 1974, p. 567). Additionally, in many developing countries, the need for group approval is much stronger than in the West; hence, psychiatric treatment is generally conducted in a group setting instead of on an individual basis.

Language barriers present another obstacle to the deliverance of psychiatric care cross culturally. Wilson, Ries, and Bokan (1980) point out the distortions and misinterpretations that can result from the use of translators. In still other instances, a therapist may experience feelings of guilt for using a treatment modality in conflict with accepted cultural norms. Finally, even within the Western world, difficulties may arise in the course of psychotherapy owing to differences in race, religion, socioeconomic status, and ethnicity between patient and therapist.

Because of the factors mentioned above, patient expectations in relation to the therapist's role and function may not be met when cultural differences prevail. Suspicion and mistrust of the therapist result, and treatment failure is inevitable. Hence, it is imperative that Western therapists obtain knowledge of and sensitivity to other cultures.

CONCEPTS OF NORMAL AND ABNORMAL

Universal Definitions

Concepts such as illness and wellness have been defined as universally generalizable. However, even when so defined, they are acknowledged to be influenced by cultural factors. Illness is a state in which the human organism's response to stressors is ineffective (Paxton, 1976). However, the prevalence of various illnesses (both physical and emotional) are affected by a multiplicity of cultural factors. Some of the cultural factors that may influence disease rates are race, ethnicity, geographic location, and socioeconomic status. Poverty as a factor in disease causation has important implications for mental health care providers. It has been argued that the *survival life-style* of people in poverty perpetuates emotional difficulties. Paxton (1976) defines a survival life-style as "a way of life which dictates action directed toward meeting the most basic needs for the maintenance of life" (p. 129). All energy expended by the individual is directed toward maintaining life rather than fulfilling it. Such a life-style, which reduces the individual's ability to adapt to the stresses of daily living, is clearly not conducive to the promotion of mental health. Indeed, prolonged and continual threat to the integrity of the individual may lead to emotional disintegration.

Wellness also has been defined so as to be universal in scope. According to Paxton (1976) "Wellness is facilitated by the dynamic interaction of energy systems for the maintenance of a balanced state" (p. 132). A variety of culturally related factors interact to promote wellness behaviors in man. Need fulfillment is prerequisite to wellness. Since need fulfillment is affected by biological constitution, ability to cope with stress, and physical and emotional environmental conditions, these factors likewise influence wellness.

Culturally Derived Definitions

Some authors have argued that labels such as normal and abnormal and wellness and illness are not simply objective states affected by cultural conditions, but are themselves culturally defined. Labeling (or societal reaction) theory provides a convenient framework from which the culturally derived definitions can be examined. Labeling theory was originally developed within the field of sociology and dealt with social definitions of deviance (Becker, 1963) and mental illness (Scheff, 1966). According to this theoretical orientation, the predominant characteristics of the behavior patterns constituting mental illness in Western societies are as follows:

1. These behaviors represent deviations from what is believed to be normal in particular sociocultural groups.
2. The norms against which the deviations are identified are different in different groups.

3. Like other forms of deviation, they elicit societal reactions that convey disapproval and stigmatization.
4. A label of mental illness applied to a person whose behavior is deviant tends to become fixed.
5. The person labeled as mentally ill is thereby encouraged to learn and accept a role identity that perpetuates the stigmatizing behavior pattern.
6. Individuals who are powerless in a social group are more vulnerable to this process than others.
7. Because social agencies in modern industrial society contribute to the labeling process, they have the effect of creating problems for those they treat rather than easing problems (Murphy, 1976, p. 1019).

Clearly, this school of thought places heavy emphasis on learning and the social formulation of normative standards. It is consistent with the idea of cultural relativity, or the view that "normal" behavior in one culture may be considered highly abnormal in another.

Today, many anthropologists contend that past investigators overemphasized the importance of the molding force of culture. However, the debate over the relative importance of universal and cultural definitions of mental illness continues. Based on her own cross-cultural research, Murphy (1976) asserts that "in widely different cultural and environmental situations sanity appears to be distinguishable from insanity by cues that are very similar to those used in the Western world" (p. 249). El-Sendiony (1977) likewise agrees that "mental diseases are basically the same all over the surface of our planet, although the symptoms are more or less molded by cultural factors" (p. 229). Avoiding the issue of the universality of mental diseases, Foster and Anderson (1978) state that the labeling of abnormal behavior is universal to both Western and non-Western societies. What varies cross culturally seems to be (1) the contexts in which mental illness is accorded attention, (2) the seriousness with which it is viewed, and (3) the treatment rendered to those afflicted with emotional disorders (pp. 81–82).

Psychiatric Definitions

Psychiatric definitions of mental illness assume a universal generalizability of the syndromes described. A major problem encountered in conducting cross-cultural studies of psychiatric disorders is the temptation to fit data into these preconceived categories. Psychiatric diagnostic categories already exist in the minds of Western researchers and have meaning within the context of Western culture. It is questionable whether these categories transfer to other cultures.

The problem is compounded by the difficulty in differentiating between *primary* and *secondary* symptoms. "Primary symptoms appear early in the course of the illness and are manifestations of basic dysfunction. Secondary symptoms, which occur later as illness progresses, represent the patient's reaction to illness, resulting from attempts to deal with 'inappropriate' behavior. The characteristics of secondary symptoms depend largely on the patient's social and cultural background" (Schlesinger, 1981, p. 26). Foster and Anderson (1978) state that "Western-trained psychiatrists lacking familiarity with the world of the patient may find it difficult to distinguish priority of symptoms" (p. 94). The practical problems posed by this dilemma are self-evident.

Perhaps much of the ambiguity in documenting and defining normality and distrubance cross culturally could be eliminated if a conceptual distinction were made between the two terms psychiatric abnormality and sociocultural deviance. A *psychiatric abnormality,* on the one hand, constitutes an unmistakable personal disturbance and is abnormal behavior that is universally recognizable in that its symptom criteria are culture free. *Sociocultural deviance,* on the other hand, is a form of social maladaption in which normality or abnormality of a particular behavior is situationally determined and relative to the norms of a given community (Draguns, 1977; Tseng & Hsu, 1978). The extent to which our psychiatric diagnostic categories fit this theoretical definition of psychiatric abnormality is still open to debate and research.

Cross-Cultural Classification of Mental Illness

In the early 1960s, the psychiatric profession began to recognize the public health aspects of its discipline. Many governments adopted generally accepted classification systems in order to more easily identify mental health needs and facilitate planning efforts. At that time, the World Health Organization (WHO) embarked on a program of standardization of psychiatric diagnosis classification and statistics, attempting to help countries reach a consensus on classification. This project required a major international collaborative effort involving over 40 countries. An internationally acceptable glossary evolved as a result of this program, based on descriptions of abnormal behavior rather than on theories of causation. The new classification system represents a compromise, at best, and continual evaluation of its usefulness will be necessary. For instance, further research is needed to understand better and to define certain culture-specific disorders. Such research calls for a concerted effort in the field of cross-cultural psychiatry, which is a high priority of the newly revised mental health program of WHO (Sartorius, 1978).

Cross-cultural investigations of mental disorders are currently being conducted in hopes of finding critical clues to the cause, pathological course, and response to treatment of mental disorders. Unfortunately, the results of these studies are often conflicting and/or difficult to interpret. Sartorius (1978) has identified three principal factors that may account for most of these problems:

1. Lack of clear definitions of culture and its components.
2. Disagreements on the scope and boundaries of the concept of mental disorders.
3. Methodological deficiencies.

The ambiguity in the definition of culture has already been addressed elsewhere in this chapter. Interestingly, some anthropologists contend that similarities between cultures outweigh the differences, which are so heavily emphasized. More specifically, these anthropologists believe in "a basic unity of man across cultures, which is reflected in common personality types, common basic strategies of dealing with stress, and common basic forms of psychological disturbance" (Sartorius, 1978, p. 81). In fact, it is plausible that variations within a given culture may be as great as the differences between cultures. Cox (1977) likewise cautions clinicians about the common "tendency to exaggerate the relevance of cultural factors and so overlook the universal validity of much clinical methodology and descriptive psychopathology" (p. 216). Moreover, many psychotherapeutic techniques have been shown to be effective in treating the same problems all over the world (Tseng & McDermott, 1975).

In the search for clear definitions of psychiatric concepts that will be applicable in diverse settings, WHO sponsored the International Pilot Study of Schizophrenia (WHO, 1973).

This is the largest investigation undertaken to deal with this problem. It has involved mental health workers from nine countries across the globe and resulted in the largest number of patients (1,200) assessed in a standardized way in different cultures. Data obtained indicate that a syndrome of schizophrenia indeed exists in all cultures studied. Furthermore, the study validated the feasibility of international collaborative endeavors in which psychiatrists from widely divergent cultures use identical assessment tools and together make their diagnoses. Follow-up of the patients (Sartorius, Jablensky, & Shapiro, 1977) revealed that, in general, patients in developing countries have a better prognosis than those in the developed nations, lending support to the importance of sociocultural factors in the outcome of mental illness.

Another WHO-sponsored investigation (Sartorius, 1974) has developed standardized methods for the cross-cultural assessment of depression. This study involved initial evaluation and follow-up of 600 patients in five countries. Results indicated marked similarities in basic depressive pathology in patients from different cultural groups (that is, primary symptoms), although there were significant differences in interviewing styles and in symptoms manifested by patients in different populations (that is, secondary symptoms). From a societal reaction viewpoint, one might speculate that the differing presentations of depressive illness in the patient groups resulted at least in part from cultural variations in the interviewing techniques employed. In any event, it seems that a comprehensive investigation of interviewing strategies, and their applicability in settings other than that in which they originated, is indicated.

Methodological problems in cross-cultural studies of mental disorders are numerous. Traditionally, these studies have been characterized by lack of premorbid and longitudinal follow-up information, ethnocentrism, and excessive concern with culturogenesis. Still other difficulties include inadequate assessment of cultural variables, failure to consider anthropological findings regarding normative behavior in the same settings, employment of conventional epidemiological methods, and poor definitions. Not suprisingly, the validity of results obtained from such studies is questionable (Manaschreck & Petri, 1978). Advances in research designs and methodology are needed (1) to develop further and to refine cross-cultural classifications of mental illness and (2) to develop and conduct meaningful studies of culture and its impact on mental health.

TREATMENT, GOALS, AND TECHNIQUES

Psychotherapy

Psychotherapy refers to "a therapeutic process of psychological interaction which takes place between the therapist and patient, the latter who in his suffering consults the former with the aim of seeking relief from his problems" (Tseng & Hsu, 1978, p. 297). In intercultural psychotherapy, the differences between therapist and patient introduce an interaction of cultural variables. This makes the process infinitely more complex than ordinary psychotherapy (Schlesinger, 1981). These ramifications will be explored more fully in a subsequent section dealing specifically with the applicability of Western psychiatry to Asian-Americans of Chinese and Japanese ethnicity.

Pharmacotherapy

Medications are no different than other aspects of treatment in that they have meaning in relation to the social context in which they are prescribed (Amarasingham, 1980). When physicians prescribe medication, they are attempting to treat a diagnosed illness and/or alleviate the patient's symptoms. Yet the prescribed medication invariably assumes additional meaning in relation to the patient's social world, which sometimes leads to noncompliance.

As already discussed, all members of a given culture give credance to an *explanatory model* of illness which defines the nature of illness, its appropriate treatment, as well as the types of relationships within which treatment can occur. It follows that all patients arrive at the treatment setting with a preconceived system for understanding and classifying medication. "A patient who has a coherent explanatory model of his own will be motivated to reject any competing model that is presented to him" (Amarasingham, 1980, p. 355). The patient derives cognitive satisfaction from the model's logical consistency, as well as emotional gratification from its linkage with other cultural symbolic domains. Furthermore, it often incorporates treatments that are both convenient and socially satisfying for the patient. Finally, it may also include symbolic meanings that permit the expression of conflicts in relation to the illness through manipulation of certain objects and substances.

Before prescribing medication, it is necessary to explore the patient's explanatory model to ascertain his theories and assumptions about medication. If some aspect of taking a prescribed drug is inharmonious with his world view, the clinician might attempt to explain the medication in terms that are congruent with the patient's belief system. This approach is not always possible, and patients sometimes choose not to comply with drug treatment regimes, thereby preserving internal cognitive consistency. Clearly, a complex interplay of social and cultural determinants exists in the realm of drug therapies and related compliance issues (Amarasingham, 1980).

APPLICATION TO ASIAN-AMERICANS

In this era which acknowledges and encourages cultural pluralism, psychiatric mental health nurses must be aware of the manner in which human behavior is affected by both present and past cultural influences. They need to understand to what extent conceptions of mental illness are culturally biased and when diagnostic and therapeutic approaches need to be modified to take into account the world view of a particular cultural group. The case of Asian-Americans will be used as an example.

Asian-Americans comprise a significant proportion of the U.S. population, yet it would be a mistake to assume that even this subgroup is a homogeneous cultural group. The group includes both foreign and American-born Asians from East Asia (China, Indonesia, Japan, Korea, and the Philippines) and South Asia (Bangladesh, India, Pakistan, and Sri Lanka). Such a heterogeneous group represents multiple religions, cultures, languages, and histories. The following discussion will focus on Asian-Americans of the East Asian group (those of Chinese and Japanese ethnicity) and explore the applicability of Western psychiatry to these two cultural groups.

Asian Perspectives

Chinese folk medicine philosophies strongly influence most other Asian health traditions. Therefore, the folk medicine beliefs and practices of the various Asian groups are very similar to those of the Chinese. In addition, Chinese medicine, constituting an entire medical system, is the most prevalent in public usage. A fundamental difference between the Chinese system of medicine and that of many Western cultures is that, traditionally, the former emphasizes prevention, whereas the latter focuses on crisis intervention. In order of importance as preventive measures, Chinese medicine includes all of the following techniques:

philosophy, meditation, nutrition, martial arts, herbology, acumassage, acupressure, moxibustion (the burning of moxa, an herb with a scent similar to marijuana), acupuncture, and spiritual healing (Chow, 1976). Since the medical systems of other Asian groups have much in common with that of the Chinese, one might logically conclude that preventive medicine is an integral component of Asian health care systems in general.

Chinese-Americans

Western and Chinese Medical Systems

A dual system of medical care exists in Chinese-American communities consisting of Western medicine and Chinese medicine. Since this dual system of medical care is available, a Chinese-American psychiatric patient may select either system or (as is often the case) choose to use both forms of care simultaneously.

Chinese medicine consists of a wide variety of traditional healing practices passed on from one generation of folk practitioners to the next. The value system of Chinese medicine reflects what is important to this population, such as mutual dependence, exertion of rational control over emotion and impulse, and living in harmony with others and with nature. These same values influence how mental illness is defined, manifested, interpreted, and responded to by Chinese-American patients (Gaw, 1982).

Help-Seeking Behavior

Various investigators have found that Chinese patients are kept within the family for prolonged periods of time during the initial phases of their illnesses. In fact, many are isolated within the home and interpersonal contacts are severely restricted. The family is generally extremely tolerant of even floridly psychotic behavior, unless the patient becomes violent and/or highly disruptive. At this point, professional consultation is usually sought. Unfortunately, in most cases the patient's condition has deteriorated to such an extent that admission to a psychiatric facility is mandatory. Interestingly, once the patient's psychiatric disorder has been publicly acknowledged, there is decreasing acceptance of the patient by the family. The family's high tolerance level in the early stages of the patient's illness may be attributed to a sense of family loyalty and a feeling of obligation to take care of the unfortunate member. Yet one must not overlook other possible contributory factors that would tend to discourage consultation with mental health care providers, particularly the strong stigma attached to mental illness by the Chinese (Lin, Tardiff, Donetz, & Coresky, 1978) and the lack of bilingual mental health workers sensitive to the cultural needs of Chinese patients in mental health facilities (Gaw, 1982).

Psychiatric Evaluation and Treatment

The psychiatric evaluation and treatment of Chinese-Americans should be sensitive to these patients' cultural characteristics and needs. Western evaluation of patients most commonly involves a focus on the individual patient and is aimed primarily at individual therapy. Even in group therapy situations, the patient enters the group without consideration of his familial relationships. This approach is incongruent with the life-style and values of Chinese patients, where the primary unit is the family rather than the individual. Gaw (1982) emphasizes the importance of engaging the family in the interview and treatment process. He states that "family involvement in the management of the patient's problems is natural to Chinese Americans" (p. 25). Moreover, the active involvement of families in caring for their sick members and their high tolerance of abnormal behavior can be highly advantageous from a therapeutic standpoint by promoting the institution of family therapy.

Yet any therapist who undertakes family therapy must remember that the familial structure is patriarchal and relationships within the family unit are vertical. Consequently, an open challenge to authority could never be tolerated in a Chinese society (Schlesinger, 1981; Hsu & Tseng, 1974). Finally, perhaps psychiatric facilities could form mental health teams to make home visits to provide early intervention and treatment of a sick family member, thereby preventing greater morbidity owing to long delays in seeking help (Gaw, 1982). Such a preventive approach is apt to be accepted by a sizable number of Chinese-Americans in light of (1) the heavy emphasis traditional Chinese medicine places on prevention and (2) the strong stigma associated with psychiatric hospitalization.

The therapist must be sensitive to the healing system to which the patient subscribes. The traditional Chinese family is a continuous network, tracing back to countless (known and unknown) ancestors and looking forward to future unknown descendants. A feeling of linkage, belonging, and involvement prevails, one which transcends the life of any particular individual. Those Chinese-Americans who subscribe to traditional cultural values believe that one's behavior does not simply affect one's self. Among the ancient Chinese, "there was a belief that a good life that one was experiencing might be due to the virtues of an ancestor. Similarly, the troubles of this life might be helping an ancestor who was suffering in the Chinese equivalent of purgatory" (Reid, 1979, p. 679).

On the other hand, Chinese-Americans who have become more or less acculturated to American ways will subscribe to Western cultural values. A major area of difference between the Eastern and Western worlds involves their respective religious orientations. In their eagerness to acculturate, many Chinese-Americans have denied their past religious beliefs and practices (such as Taoist or Buddhist) and adopted Christian ethics. However, Krieger and Zussman (1981) contend that it is highly unlikely that individuals can completely disregard their past. These researchers suggest that "instead of fighting these beliefs, the patient can be encouraged to integrate them with his new life" (p. 249).

From a psychotherapeutic standpoint, cultural and religious beliefs have important clinical implications. Owing to embarrassment, Chinese-Americans may not reveal their belief in traditional practices until a good therapist-patient rapport has been established and the patient feels that the therapist is respectful of his or her cultural background. "An understanding of the patient's belief system can assist the psychiatrist to appreciate the reaction of the patient to certain bodily phenomena and to explain therapeutic procedures in such a way that the patient will understand" (Gaw, 1982, p. 23).

The most effective approach to the patient depends on his level of sophistication in relation to understanding mental health concepts and the role of mental health professionals. Thus, the therapeutic situation must be individualized for every Chinese-American patient, taking into account such factors as the patient's degree of acculturation, educational background, and familiarity with the Western medical care system. Because of the stigma attached to mental illness, the less acculturated Chinese-Americans frequently present for treatment with somatic complaints. If a patient is not amenable to "talking therapy," it is advisable to start from "where the patient is." The content of the interview can slowly shift from a superficial somatic level to a deeper psychological level after a therapeutic alliance has been formed. In addition, Chinese-American patients may resent an initial interview that probes into "embarrassing" family, social, and personal issues. If the patient does not speak English, the use of a translator (one familiar with the patient's dialect, not merely one who speaks Chinese) is helpful in overcoming the language barrier and allaying the patient's anxiety (Gaw, 1982). Finally, the authoritarian relationships characterizing traditional Asian families extend to the therapeutic relationship as well. The therapist is viewed as the patriarch and respected as the authority figure. Indeed, the Western ideal of the therapist as a neutral, nonjudgemental, and somewhat passive individual is contrary to the patient's expectation of the therapist's active and instructive role as helper (Schlesinger, 1981).

As previously mentioned, some Chinese-Americans use Western and traditional Chinese medical systems simultaneously. Consequently, these patients may take both Western drugs and Chinese medicines. If concern arises about an adverse drug interaction, the patient can be advised that mixing Western drugs and Chinese herbs is unsafe because of possible undesirable side effects. Should the patient insist on ingesting both types of medication, it is best to discourage him from taking them at the same time. It is difficult to predict what drug actions may take place with these combinations (Gaw, 1982). Finally, when prescribing psychotropic drugs, a lower therapeutic dosage of antidepressants and tranquilizers is recommended for Chinese patients, as well as for other patients of Asian origin (Yamamoto, Fung Lo, & Reece, 1979).

Japanese-Americans

Help-Seeking Behavior

Japanese-Americans also tend to underutilize mental health services. A cross-cultural study of clinic utilization recently conducted in Hawaii substantiated the assertion that psychiatric help-seeking behavior is greatly affected by ethnicity. Kinzie and Tseng (1978) reported that Caucasians were significantly overrepresented in proportion to the population while other groups, particularly Japanese, were substantially underrepresented. Furthermore, Caucasians were apt to be self-referred, presenting with subjective complaints of anxiety and depression. Japanese patients, on the other hand, were more likely to be brought into the clinic after a crisis or severe mental illness and exhibited more socially disruptive behaviors. Kinzie and Tseng (1978) believe that the tendency of Japanese-Americans to avoid psychiatric facilities, using them only for crises and severe emotional distress, indicates that problems of a more minor nature are handled effectively within the family unit or via other social networks. Yamamoto (1982) also relates that, throughout the United States, Asian-Americans underutilize mental health services. He largely attributes this to the high stigma attached to mental illness.

Diversity Within a Cultural Group

The Japanese-American group is a heterogeneous one and, therefore, is not easily stereotyped. The *issei,* or first-generation Japanese who originally came to the United States, are now part of America's elderly population. These individuals continue to hold on to old and cherished Japanese traditions, such as filial piety. For the Japanese, filial piety means loyalty to an extended family in contrast to the extended clan loyalty of the Chinese (Benedict, 1946). A substantial proportion of the *nisei,* or second-generation Japanese-Americans, has been able to advance appreciably gauged by their impressive educational and occupational achievements. The third generation, the *sansei,* present different types of problems than their ancestors. They are more Americanized and consequently encounter the same emotional difficulties as do most young Americans. Typically the *yonsei,* or fourth generation, have essentially acculturated. They frequently select spouses with ethnic backgrounds different from their own and identify with the majority culture in general. Clearly, "planning programs for individuals and for communities among the Japanese requires a thoughtful consideration of the different needs depending on generation, social class, geographic data, diagnostic situation, and so on" (Yamamoto, 1982, p. 39).

Implications for Mental Health Care

In light of the varied socialization patterns found among Japanese-Americans, the clinician's approach will differ depending on whether the patient's value orientation is predominantly

Japanese or American. If the patient's life-style and world view are mainly Japanese, he or she must be evaluated and treated as an "interdependent" family member. Heavy emphasis should be placed on social interactions, interdependency, hierarchical relationships, and empathy. A keen awareness on the therapist's part of the significance of close family ties is essential. Japanese families often work together, eat together, and may bathe and sleep together. Furthermore, this "togetherness" extends throughout the individual's lifetime. The traditional Japanese hospital permits a family "representative" to remain at the hospital, sleep in the same room, and cook meals. Continuation of the family's daily routines is an important consideration in rendering patient care (Yamamoto, 1977).

Many of the principles and recommendations cited in the previous section dealing with the psychiatric evaluation and treatment of Chinese-Americans are also applicable to Japanese-American patients. While those points will not be reiterated, they are all based on an appreciation of and keen sensitivity to the patient's cultural characteristics and needs.

Japanese Introspective Therapies

Different treatment methods for anxiety disorders and personality disturbances have been developed in Japan. Two forms of therapy, Morita and Naikan, which include introspection and specific instructions by the therapist, have been described in the literature. A great deal about Japanese culture is divulged through exploration of these two treatment modalities (Schlesinger, 1981).

Morita therapy was developed by Dr. S. Morita approximately 60 years ago. This form of therapy is relatively group centered, ritualistic, and behavioristic (Reynolds & Kiefer, 1977). It involves placing patients in isolation for one to two weeks and gradually increasing their activity level. In Japan, life is not built on feelings but on productive activity; an individual's self-worth is dependent on achievement. The aim of Morita therapy is to involve patients in the needs of the moment so that they forget about their intrapsychic problems. Patients are told by the therapist that although they cannot control their thoughts, they are nonetheless responsible for their behavior. The therapist instructs his or her patients to develop an awareness of what is happening from one moment to the next. The purpose of this introspection is to focus on external reality rather than on disturbing inner feelings and problems, thereby preventing excessive rumination and potential exacerbation of symptoms. The ultimate goal of therapy is to improve overall functioning, not merely symptomatic relief. Near the end of hospitalization, patients participate in group discussions and, upon discharge, are given the opportunity to join the "Morita Group" as outpatients.

In *Naikan therapy* (which originated with prison inmates), patients are told to sit alone in a small, enclosed, boothlike area. They are instructed by the therapist to think about the past in blocks of three-year periods, beginning from birth and continuing to the present. The entire day is occupied with introspection. Each patient's thoughts must center on past relationships with significant others and, more specifically, on what was received from each person, what was given to that person in return, and what problems that person encountered as a result of the patient's behavior. It is imperative that the appropriate memories are recalled together with the proper feelings of obligation attached to these memories. Therapy is usually terminated after approximately one week of intense introspection.

Both of the above therapies have foundations in Japanese culture. According to Yamamoto (1977), there are important characteristics common to both forms of therapy: 1) introspection, 2) directions to guide thinking, 3) expectations of behavior to suit Japanese values, and 4) the objective of creating a person who fits into the Japanese way of life, including filial piety, achievement orientation, and a strong sense of obligation and responsibility. Also, while the origins differ, both are based on Japanese Buddhist beliefs and past Chinese Confucian influences.

Therapy for Asian-Americans

This discussion has identified several crucial issues that must be taken into account when rendering psychiatric care to Asian-Americans of Chinese and Japanese ethnicity. The discussion of Morita and Naikan therapies illustrates how cultural values influence the therapeutic process and its goals. The American ideal of independence and self-sufficiency is clearly at variance with the popular Asian notion of interdependence within the family unit. Certainly, if adequate mental health services are to be provided for Asian-Americans, culturally relevant diagnostic and treatment methods must be devised and implemented (Yamamoto, 1978).

IMPLICATIONS FOR PSYCHIATRIC MENTAL HEALTH NURSING

The branch of nursing that incorporates an understanding of culture in the nursing care of clients is called *transcultural nursing.* Brink (1976) defines it as "the fusion of nursing and anthropology in both theory and practice" (p. 1).

Psychiatric mental health nurses are becoming more and more involved with treating ethnic minority groups. Moreover, there exist in America many other ethnic groups that do not occupy minority status but for whom cultural differences between patient and therapist are nonetheless of paramount importance in the healing process. "The advent of community mental health and the increased awareness of minority group issues have brought a special focus on the practical relevance of culture in serving the physical and mental health needs of these populations" (Foulks, 1982, p. 239). For these reasons, it is imperative that the psychiatric mental health nurse specialist incorporate the insights and perspective of transcultural nursing into his or her clinical practice.

Human beings are social and cultural beings, and their needs are satisfied primarily through interpersonal interactions. In psychotherapeutic situations, misperceptions and misunderstandings based on cultural differences often lead to poor treatment outcome. Nurses must modify their traditional view of "cooperative" and "uncooperative" patients and instead adopt a holistic perspective that takes into account the cultural, social, and psychological dimensions of human behavior. "Most important, we need to consider *how* cultural differences in behavior between the staff and the patient influences the quality of care to patients, families, and social groups" (Leininger, 1978, p. 134).

Psychiatric mental health nurse specialists possess a high degree of proficiency in therapeutic and interpersonal skills. In their "expanded nurse role," these professional nurses are expected to assume responsibility for the advancement of nursing theory and therapy. Specific functions of the clinical specialist include therapy, teaching, research, consultation, supervision, management, and coordination of patient care. Kohnke (1978) cites Gordon as according special significance to the *change agent* function of the clinical specialist's role. As change agents, clinical specialists occupy a unique position that undoubtedly facilitates successful accomplishment of these various functions. In relation to cultural issues pertinent to mental health, clinical specialists must make use of their knowledge and skills in three major areas: education, research, and clinical care.

Educational and research activities are closely related to one another. As educators, clinical specialists can influence and modify both attitudes and behaviors of other professional nurses and students of nursing. Teaching efforts should be directed toward increasing awareness of the European roots of American psychiatric theory and practice, thereby helping to eradicate the narrow ethnocentrism that generally prevails in our Western society. Mandatory courses on cultural diversity should be included as part of the basic curricula of schools of nursing. As researchers, clinical specialists can study the mental health beliefs and practices of ethnic groups. Information obtained from systematic research investigations should be disseminated to interested nurses via lectures, symposia, and publication in textbooks, journals, and newsletters.

As clinicians, clinical specialists must function as role models for their peers. Acting in this capacity, they are in an ideal position to initiate and implement change. Whenever planning and delivering direct patient care, psychiatric mental health nurse specialists should appropriately address the cultural dimension of the patient's overall health status. Finally, when called on to assume the consultant role, clinical specialists are provided an opportunity to encourage their professional colleagues to incorporate the critical domain of culture into planning and carrying out more personalized patient care.

SUMMARY

This chapter has explored the impact of culture on the definition and expression of mental health and mental illness and explored resulting treatment issues. Two Asian-American groups, Chinese-Americans and Japanese-Americans, were discussed in depth to illustrate the necessity of considering cultural patterns and beliefs when offering psychiatric nursing care. Finally, implications for the role of the psychiatric mental health nurse specialist were addressed.

REFERENCES

Amarasingham, L. R. Social and cultural perspectives on medication refusal. *American Journal of Psychiatry,* 1980, *137*(3), 353–358.

Becker, H. *Outsiders.* New York: The Free Press of Glencoe, 1963.

Benedict, R. Continuities and discontinuities in cultural conditioning. *Psychiatry,* 1938, *1,* 161–167.

Benedict, R. *The chrysanthemum and the sword.* Cambridge, MA: Riverside, 1946.

Brink, P. J. (Ed.). *Transcultural nursing: A book of readings.* Englewood Cliffs, NJ: Prentice Hall, Inc., 1976.

Chow, E. Cultural health traditions: Asian perspectives. In M. F. Branch & P. P. Paxton (Eds.), *Providing safe nursing care for ethnic people of color.* New York: Appleton-Century-Crofts. 1976.

Cox, J. L. Aspects of transcultural psychiatry. *British Journal of Psychiatry,* 1977, *130,* 211–221.

Draguns, J. G. Problems of defining and comparing abnormal behaviors across cultures. *Annals of the New York Academy of Sciences,* 1977, *18,* 664–675.

El-Sendiony, M. F. The problem of cultural specificity of mental illness—A survey of comparative psychiatry. *International Journal of Social Psychiatry,* 1977, *23(3),* 223–230.

Foster, G. M., & Anderson, B. G. *Medical anthropology.* New York: John Wiley & Sons, Inc., 1978.

Foulks, E. F. Discussion: Relevant generic issues. In A. Gaw (Ed.), *Cross-cultural psychiatry* Littleton, MA: John Wright PSG Inc., 1982.

Frank, J. D. Common features of psychotherapy. *Australian and New Zealand Journal of Psychiatry,* 1972, *6,* 34–40.

Gaw, A. Chinese Americans. In A. Gaw (Ed.), *Cross-cultural psychiatry.* Littleton, MA: John Wright PSG Inc., 1982.

Hsu, J., & Tseng, W. S. Family relations in classic Chinese opera. *International Journal of Social Psychiatry,* 1974, *20(3–4),* 159–172.

Kinzie, J. D., & Tseng, W. S. Cultural aspects of psychiatric clinical utilization—A cross-cultural study in Hawaii. *International Journal of Social Psychiatry,* 1978, *24(3),* 177–188.

Kluckhohn, C., & Mowrer, O. H. Culture and personality: A conceptual scheme. *The American Anthropologist,* 1944, *46,* 1–29.

Kohnke, M. F. *The case for consultation in nursing: Designs for professional practice.* New York: John Wiley & Sons, Inc., 1978.

Krieger, M. J., & Zussman, M. The importance of cultural factors in a brief reactive psychosis. *Journal of Clinical Psychiatry,* 1981, *42(6),* 248–249.

Kroeber, A. L., & Kluckhohn, C. *A review of culture: A critical review of concepts and definitions* (monograph). Papers of the Peabody Museum of American Archeology and Ethnology, Vol. 47, No.1, Cambridge, MA: Harvard University, 1952.

Leighton, A. H. Culture and psychiatry. *Canadian Journal of Psychiatry,* 1981, *26(8),* 522–529.

Leininger, M. *Transcultural nursing: Concepts, theories, and practices.* New York: John Wiley & Sons, Inc., 1978.

Lin, T. Y., Tardiff, K., Donetz, G., & Goresky, W. Ethnicity and patterns of help-seeking. *Culture Medicine and Psychiatry,* 1978, *2(1),* 3–13.

Manaschreck, T. C., & Petri, M. The atypical psychoses. *Culture, Medicine and Psychiatry,* 1978, *2(3),* 233–268.

Murphy, J. M. Psychiatric labeling in cross-cultural perspective. *Science,* 1976, *191,* 1019–1028.

Odejide, A. O. Cross-cultural psychiatry: A myth or reality. *Comparative Psychiatry,* 1979, *20(2),* 103–109.

Parsons, T. *The social system.* Glencoe, IL: The Free Press, 1951.

Paxton, P. P. Epidemiology in health and disease. In M. F. Branch & P. P. Paxton (Eds.), *Providing safe nursing care for ethnic people of color.* New York: Appleton-Century-Crofts, 1976.

Reid, T. F. Psychosocial structure in China. *Arizona Medicine,* 1979, *36(9),* 679–681.

Reynolds, D. K., & Kiefer, C. W. Cultural adaptability as an attribute of therapies: The case of Morita psychotherapy. *Culture, Medicine and Psychiatry,* 1977, *1(4),* 395–412.

Sartorius, N. Description and classification of depressive disorders. *Pharmakopsychiatrie, Neuro-Pharmokologie* 1974, *7,* 76–79.

Sartorius, N. Diagnosis and classification: Cross cultural and international perspectives. *Mental Health and Society,* 1978, *5(1–2),* 79–85.

Sartorius, N., Jablensky, A., & Shapiro, R. Two year follow up of patients included in the WHO international study of schizophrenia. *Psychological Medicine,* 1977, *7,* 529–541.

Scheff, T. J. *Being mentally ill.* Chicago: Aldine, 1966.

Schlesinger, R. Cross-cultural psychiatry: The applicability of Western Anglo psychiatry to Asian-Americans of Chinese and Japanese ethnicity. *Journal of Psychosocial Nursing and Mental Health Services,* 1981, *19(9),* 26–30.

Segall, A. The sick role concept: Understanding illness behavior. *Journal of Health and Social Behavior,* 1976, *17(2),* 162–168.

Seguin, C. A. What folklore psychotherapy can teach us. *Psychotherapy and Psychosomatics,* 1974, *24(4–6),* 293–302.

Tseng, W. S., & McDermott, J. F. Psychotherapy: Historical roots, universal elements, and cultural variations. *American Journal of Psychiatry,* 1975, *132(4),* 378–384.

Tseng, W. S., & Hsu, J. Suggestions for intercultural psychotherapy. In M. H. Logan & E. E. Hunt (Eds.), *Health and the human condition: Perspectives on medical anthropology.* North Scituate, MA: Duxbury Press, 1978.

Wilson, L. G., Ries, R., & Bokan, J. Transcultural psychiatry on an American psychiatric ward. *Hospital and Community Psychiatry,* 1980, *31(11),* 759–762.

Wittkower, E. D., & Warnes, H. Cultural aspects of psychotherapy. *American Journal of Psychotherapy,* 1974, *28(4),* 566–573.

World Health Organization. *Report of the international pilot study of schizophrenia.* Geneva: WHO, 1973.

Yamamoto, J. An Asian view of the future of cultural psychiatry. In E. F. Foulks, R. M. Wintrob, & Westermeyer (Eds.), *Current perspectives in cultural psychiatry.* New York: Spectrum Publications, Inc., 1977.

Yamamoto, J. Therapy for Asian Americans. *Journal of the National Medical Association,* 1978, *70(4),* 267–270.

Yamamoto, J. Japanese Americans. In A. Gaw (Ed.), *Cross-cultural psychiatry.* Littleton, MA: John Wright PSG Inc., 1982.

Yamamoto, J., Fung, D., Lo, S., & Reece, S. Psychopharmacology for Asian Americans and Pacific Islanders. *Psychopharmacology Bulletin,* 1979, *15(4),* 29–31.

BIBLIOGRAPHY

Beiser, M., Benfari, R. C., Collomb, H., & Ravel, J. L. Measuring psychoneurotic behavior in cross-cultural surveys. *Journal of Nervous and Mental Disease,* 1976, *163(1),* 10–23.

CHAPTER 17 PSYCHIATRIC CONSULTATION AND LIAISON

Mary Kay Simmons

During the past 20 years, psychiatric consultation and liaison have evolved as significant roles for the master's-prepared psychiatric mental health clinical nurse specialist.

This chapter will define the concept of psychiatric consultation and liaison and discuss the development of the role. Next, the types of consultation, lines of authority, and preparation for the role will be presented. Both the consultation and liaison processes will be discussed and clinical illustrations provided. Finally, steps in evaluating the effectiveness of the process used will be discussed.

DEVELOPMENT OF CONSULTATION-LIAISON PSYCHIATRY

Consultation-liaison psychiatry began with the development of psychiatric units in general hospitals and was first described in 1902 at Albany Hospital. The establishment of a psychiatric unit in the hospital made psychiatrists more available and visible within the general hospital setting. Collaboration and consultation then began between psychiatry and the medical-surgical divisions. The concept of liaison psychiatry was formally introduced in 1929 by a psychiatric consultant at Cornell Medical School, George W. Henry, who envisioned a hospital-based psychiatrist available for consultation to other physicians (Henry, 1929).

Concurrent work in liaison psychiatry was being done by the Commission on Medical Education, organized by the Association of American Medical Colleges in 1925. The commission's final report was published as the Lowell Report in 1932 and emphasized the importance of integrating psychiatric teaching into the curricula of general medicine, pediatrics, and neurology (Lipowski, 1974).

Developments in psychosomatic medicine in the 1920s supported and expanded the role of the psychiatric consultant by recognizing that mind and body are one interfacing complex. In 1924, funds from the Rockefeller Foundation established five psychiatric liaison departments within general hospitals. This funding implemented the recommendations of the Lowell Report and provided for the interplay between psychiatry and medicine.

World War II played an important role in strengthening the position of consultation-liaison psychiatry. It was imperative that psychiatry and medicine work closely together to treat war-connected illnesses in an effective and efficient manner.

In the 1950s and 1960s, increased specialization and advanced technologies resulted in a greater emphasis on the disease process. Intensive care units were expanding and patients were living longer. Both these changes created new psychological stresses to which consultation-liaison psychiatry responded. New, effective psychopharmacology developed and medications became a new tool for the psychiatrist and helped strengthen the working relationship between psychiatry and medicine. The psychiatrist could now use medications to help control patients experiencing psychiatric problems on a medical ward.

ROOTS OF PSYCHIATRIC NURSING CONSULTATION

Psychiatric consultation-liaison nursing developed in tandem with psychiatry's consultation development. With more psychiatric units established within general hospitals, the psychiatric nurse became more visible and available to consult with medical-surgical nurses regarding the psychiatric problems of their patients. Johnson (1963) from Duke University Medical Center was the first to describe a nursing consultation service. From this evolved the role of the psychiatric consultation-liaison nurse, a person who did not assume direct responsibility for patients on a medical-surgical unit but worked with the staff on those units to help them better understand the emotional concerns of their patients.

In "The evolution of psychiatric liaison nursing," Nelson and Schelke (1976) envision today's psychiatric-liaison consultant nurse in a multifaceted role: (1) consultation directed at solving an immediate patient care problem and improving the observation, assessment, and intervention skills of the staff nurses, (2) teaching via conferences with the patient care team and by serving as a role model, and (3) providing direct, specialized psychological care to patients and their families.

By the early 1970s, the University of Maryland and Yale University had recognized the need for specific training and provided a "track" for liaison nursing in their graduate nursing programs. The deinstitutionalization of the mentally ill brought more of the psychiatric population to the general hospital and created a need for more psychiatric consultation within the general hospital. In response, many hospitals created psychiatric consultation teams of which the nurse became an integral member, bridging psychiatric and medical-surgical nursing care (Lewis & Levy, 1982).

PSYCHIATRIC CONSULTATION AND LIAISON

Though psychiatric consultation and liaison are interwoven processes, for clarity they will be discussed separately.

Consultation

The term *psychiatric consultation* instead of *mental health consultation* will be used in this chapter. Gerald Caplan, generally seen as the father of mental health consultation, describes consultation as a professional interaction between a specialist (the consultant) and the consultee, with the goal of solving a problem in which responsibility for the client remains with the consultee (Caplan, 1964). Additionally, Caplan clearly points out that the consultant is not only trying to assist the consultee regarding a specific problem but is also educating the consultee, thereby reducing areas of possible future misunderstanding.

Varying definitions of psychiatric consultation (DeLougherty, Gebbie, & Newman 1971; Lewis & Levy, 1982; Lipowski, 1975) have similar components: there are at least two people, one of whom is less knowledgeable and in need of assistance with a problem (the consultee). The problem may relate to different levels: to a specific patient, to a program, or to a system of employment. In every case, however, the goal of consultation is always to provide information that will assist the consultee in more effective problem solving.

In this process, the consultee experiences support and empathy from the consultant rather than judgment and evaluation. While direct responsibility for decision making and patient care remain with the consultee, the consultant's role is to assist in definition of the problem, collection of data, formulation of a care plan, and allowing staff to express conflicts and to ventilate feelings (Davis & Nelson, 1980).

Lipowski (1981) described consultation as being "the cornerstone of the liaison psychiatrist's clinical service, without which he would lose his *raison d'etre*" (p. 807). There is debate in the literature concerning the relative value of consultation and its related function, liaison. These two functions, consultation and liaison, are interdependent and require successful experiences in both areas for one and/or the other to be successful.

Liaison

Z. J. Lipowski is to liaison what Gerald Caplan is to consultation. Lipowski defines *liaison* as regular contact with clinical staff by a mental health worker to enhance the psychosocial aspects of patient care and prevent disruptions in care through active participation in clinical rounds and communication. Additionally, staff members are educated regarding the psychological and social issues that add to the stresses imposed on patients and caregivers (Lipowski, 1979).

Robinson, a forerunner in liaison nursing, defines liaison as sorting out all of the influences contributing to the communication gap between patient and care-givers, with mutual understanding of the ultimate goal. Through the successful resolution of a critical situation, increased awareness and expanded, shared experience will result in correct perceptions of motives and actions (Robinson, 1974).

It is clear that liaison is an extension of the consultation process by meeting the client's psychological needs (Lehmann, 1983), providing preventive management (Hackett & Cassem, 1978) and facilitating relationships (Lewis & Levy, 1982).

Differences Between Consultation and Liaison

Consultation and liaison are separate and distinct, but interdependent, activities. Psychiatric consultation occurs when a psychiatric expert evaluates the psychosocial aspects and behavior of a patient or program and gives an opinion regarding diagnosis, management, and prevention of mental disorders to a nonpsychiatric colleague. This procedure generally occurs over a limited time and does not require ongoing contact once the consultation is complete.

Liaison occurs in the context of an ongoing relationship between psychiatric experts and nonpsychiatric colleagues in which mediation, interpretation, and communication are the main functions. Liaison mediates and interprets patient or system behaviors to nonpsychiatric colleagues by communicating individual and group psychodynamics and *building a context* within which care-specific consultations are useful.

Other Definitions

Consultation is sometimes confused with other areas of performance/interaction: supervision, collaboration, and therapy. Briefly, a supervisor is a senior person usually in the same profession as the supervisee who is definitely responsible for both the work of the supervisee and quality assurance within the agency. Aspects of clinical supervision are discussed in Chapter 23. A collaborator shares responsibility for the patient in the context of a relationship between more experienced and less experienced colleagues within a specialty.

Finally, consultation and therapy differ in crucial ways: The focus of consultation is on the consultee's work functioning, whereas the focus of therapy is on the client's adaptation to living. The private life of the consultee is not explored; the private life of a patient in psychotherapy must be explored.

Types of Consultation

For the most part, Caplan (1964) is the primary source for defining types of consultation. He divides consultation into two major divisions: Division A focuses the consultant on a case problem approach and Division B focuses on administrative problems dealing with programs or policies of the institution. He further subdivides each division into two consultation types.

A-1: Client-Centered Case Consultation

The consultee employs a consultant to evaluate the client's problems and advise the consultee how to deal more effectively with the problem. The primary goal is to provide the consultee with alternatives for working with the client, while education of the consultee is a secondary goal.

A-2: Consultee-Centered Consultation

Here, education of the consultee is the primary purpose, using current client problems as a focus.

B-1: Program-Centered Administrative Consultation

The consultee asks for assistance in program planning and evaluation, using the consultant's skills in administration, social systems, and mental health, and education is secondary.

B-2: Consultee-Centered Administrative Consultation

Again, the primary goal is education of the consultee regarding program development and organization.

Lewis and Levy (1982) similary purpose direct and indirect consultation as follows:*

Direct (Client-Centered)	*Indirect (Consultee-Centered)*
The patient and/or family are interviewed. Psychological treatment is provided by the liaison nurse as indicated.	A consultee-centered/case-centered meeting is held. The patient and/or family are not interviewed.
Specific nursing intervention is planned and may be indicated.	Specific nursing intervention is planned and initiated.
A consultee-centered/case-centered meeting is held with further intervention planned.	Further consultee-centered/case-centered meetings are held as needed.
The consultation is documented in the patient's record by the liaison nurse.	The consultation is documented in the patient's record by the patient's nurse.
Follow-up, reassessment, and evaluation are ongoing.	Follow-up reassessment, and evaluation are ongoing.

Forms of Liaison Activities

The most popular activity described by Lipowski (1975) is a series of regularly scheduled discussions with the consultant regarding staff reactions to difficult patients and the strains imposed by such patients as well as regarding the patients themselves.

* From Lewis, A., & Levy, J. *Psychiatric liaison nursing.* Reston, VA: Reston Publishing, 1982, p. 87. Reprinted with permission of Reston Publishing Co., a division of Prentice-Hall.

A regularly scheduled conference is the usual form for liaison activity. The liaison person and the group requesting liaison agree upon a meeting time, duration, and problem focus. Teaching, mediation, and relationship-building between the group and liaison person are the primary functions of these conferences.

THE NURSE AS PSYCHIATRIC CONSULTANT

In 1977, Pranulis stated to the American Psychosomatic Society that "Nursing does not carry the stigma of pathology as does the psychiatrist, the connotation of testing as does the psychologist or of poverty or do-gooder as does the social worker" (Garant, 1977, p. 75). Nurses are trained to view people in a holistic manner and concern themselves with patients' physical and psychosocial well-being. Since the family and environment are very important in treating and caring for a patient, the nurse's traditional training and role provide an excellent base for training in psychiatric consultation and liaison.

Preparation for the Role

There is consensus in the nursing literature that the clinical nurse specialist is best suited for a consultation-liaison position (Berarducci, Blandford, & Garant, 1979; Bilodeau & O'Connor, 1978; Blake, 1977; Burch & Meredith, 1974; Davis & Nelson, 1980; Garant, 1977; Goldstein, 1979; Johnson, 1963; Kuntz, Stehle, & Marshall, 1980; Lewis & Levy, 1982; Przepiorka & Bender, 1977; Robinson, 1974). The clinical nurse specialist holds a master's degree, is a practitioner with expertise in a special area, and functions as a role model, consultant, educator, change agent, and researcher. Graduate training increases knowledge in psychopathology, psychodynamics, research, and clinical experience with individuals, families, and groups (Garant, 1977).

The nurse also needs to have had experience in general nursing as a staff nurse or as a supervisor in medical-surgical, maternal and child health, or in public health, as well as in psychiatric nursing. An understanding of organizational systems and general hospital systems as well as the organizational structure, operational policies, and practices and goals of the institution involved are critical knowledge areas for the psychiatric nurse consultant.

Theoretical Framework and Skills

Consultation-liaison nursing is a multifaceted role that includes assessment, problem identification, treatment planning and evaluation, and expected outcome. The nurse consultant transmits information clearly and concisely to the client, family, and colleagues and assists the consultee to enhance his or her skills in patient observation, assessment and intervention.

The theoretical framework from which a consultation-liaison nurse works is synthesized from many sources. Theories of learning, personality, systems, consultation-liaison, crisis, problem solving, staff management, organization and development, stress and stress reduction, and knowledge of psychopharmacology and cultural and ethical norms are all part of the psychiatric clinical nurse specialist's knowledge base.

The goals of psychiatric consultation-liaison nursing are described by Lewis and Levy (1982):

1. To demonstrate and to teach mental health concepts and their application in clinical nursing practice

2. To effect appropriate psychiatric and nursing intervention
3. To support nurses in continuing to provide quality nursing care
4. To promote and to develop the professional and personal self-esteem of the nurse
5. To encourage, among the members of the nursing staff, tolerance of situations in which immediate and/or effective intervention or resolution is unattainable*

Skills, a theoretical base, and clear goals are not sufficient in themselves to effect change. The staff and the consultee need to respect the consultant and desire to implement suggestions she or he makes. It is the responsibility of the consultant to nurture and cultivate a collaborative relationship with the consultee so that trust, respect, and equality between the two professionals exist and contribute to the consultative process.

Organizational Placement of the Consultation-Liaison Nurse

There appear to be three possible administrative placements for the consultation-liaison nurse. Most frequently, the consultation-liaison nurse is placed within a nursing service, following the belief that one's own discipline offers the most support. Within departments of nursing, the consultation-liaison nurse could report to one of the following: the director of staff education, the coordinator of psychiatric nursing services, the psychiatric nursing supervisor, the director of nursing for staff and project development/research, the assistant director of nursing, or the director of nursing.

The consultation-liaison nurse may also be placed within a department of psychiatry, generally as part of a multidisciplinary team. The director of the consultation-liaison service is usually a psychiatrist and the immediate supervisor of the consultation-liaison nurse, with the department chairperson having ultimate responsibility. This structure necessitates the consultation-liaison nurse having a good working relationship with the director of nursing who supports the position even though not having direct line authority for it.

Third, the psychiatric consultation-liaison nurse may be a private consultant hired on a contractual basis for a specified period of time to deal with specific requests within the hospital or organization.

Numerous psychiatric consultation-liaison nurses function independently either hired by the department of nursing or on a contractual basis also through the department of nursing. When working independently, it is important for the nurse to establish a collaborative relationship with a psychiatrist for psychiatric back-up, which would include reviewing the psychiatric cases having a complex medical component, a need for medication, or assistance in determining a diagnosis.

Clinical supervision is best sought from an experienced consultation-liaison nurse whenever possible. When this is not possible, supervision from an experienced psychiatrist or psychologist is acceptable and encouraged.

In all organizational structures, it is imperative that the consultation-liaison nurse be in a line position and not in an administrative position in which she or he would have authority over the consultee. The consultant must be administratively free and professionally available to the consultee in order to define the problem at hand and assist in the resolution of it.

* From Lewis, A., & Levy, J. *Psychiatric liaison nursing,* 1982, p. 17. Reprinted with permission of Reston Publishing Co., a Prentice-Hall Co., 11480 Sunset Hills Road, Reston, VA 22090.

THE CONSULTATIVE PROCESS

Consultative Readiness

Cherniss (1978) postulates that consultees differ in their readiness for consultation and that readiness can, in part, be conceptualized in terms of the existing relationship between the consultant and the consultee. Her Consultation Readiness Scale (CRS) defines six levels of consultation readiness:

Level 1. No relationship. At this level, there has been no prior consultant-consultee contact or there is a hostile, indifferent, or apathetic consultee but, in either case, the consultant's primary task is the development of an amicable relationship.

Level 2. Social relationship only. At this level, there is amicable, informal social contact between the consultant and the consultee. However, the consultee does not readily engage in discussion of work-related issues. A mutual discussion of work-related issues becomes the primary task.

Level 3. Limited work relationship. One type of consultee at this level is clearly distressed and wants help but seems defensive and not open to modifying behavior. The second type readily engages in discussion of problems when approached by the consultant but does not effectively participate in the development and implementation of solutions. The task is to identify the factors preventing the consultee from accepting and implementing possible solutions. One can then develop consultation strategies to remove the problem and allow more productive consultation.

Level 4. Adequate work relationship. At this level, the consultee is open to consultant-initiated contact concerning problems and cooperates in the development and implementation of solutions to problems. The consultant's task becomes assisting the consultee to identify problems suitable for consultation so that contacts will be initiated around relevant problems.

Level 5. Informal work relationship. Consultees at this level initiate contact with the consultant whenever a potential problem is identified and effectively participate in the development and implementation of solutions. The consultant's task is to encourage the consultee to develop better relationships with potential consultees at lower readiness levels.

Level 6. Reciprocal work relationship. Consultees at this level may not only seek consultation when it is needed but also become active advocates with other potential consultees and are willing to help the consultant expand consultation services. True reciprocity exists at this highest level (Cherniss, 1978).

At all levels, the process of consultation will be largely the same. Termini and Ciechoski (1981) describe a seven-step process summarized in Table 17.1.

It is important for the consultant to determine the urgency of the need for consultation. Listening to the content of the conversation and the tone and affect of the consultee will provide this information. Once the urgency is determined, the consultee is informed how soon the consultant will be able to respond. Four hours is the usual response time, with the maximum being 24 hours. The longer the consultant takes to respond, the less likely the consultee is to be interested in the recommendations or to request services in the future.

Data Collection

Data collection begins when the consultant receives the request and tries to determine the question to be addressed, the clarity of the consultee's question, and whether or not there

Table 17.1 Steps in the Consultation Process

I. Request for consultation
  A. Face-to-face contact or telephone contact
  B. Consultant impression of initial contact
II. Data collection
  A. Consultant impression from request
  B. Consultant-consultee meeting
  C. Patient (family) interview
  D. Information from medical record
  E. Consultant knowledge of theoretical concepts
III. Assessment
  A. Consultant interpretation and synthesis of data from all sources
  B. Consultant application of theoretical concepts
C. Consultant diagnosis of needs of patient (family)
  D. Consultant diagnosis of needs of consultee
IV. Plan of action
  A. Consultant recommendations to patient (family)
  B. Consultant recommendations to consultee
  C. Consultant documentation of assessment, diagnosis, and recommendations
  D. Consultee recording of nursing care plan
  E. Consultant-consultee identification and redefinition of roles
V. Implementation of plan

Client-Centered Relationship	*Consultee-Centered Relationship*	*Consultant-Patient (Family) Relationship*
A. Establishment of contract and mutual goal agreement	A. Establishment of contract and mutual goal agreement	A. Establishment of contract and mutual goal agreement
B. Application of nursing process methodology	B. Application of nursing process methodology	B. Application of nursing process methodology
C. Reference point is patient and his illness	C. Reference point is theme interference resolution	C. Reference point is patient (family) and illness
D. Interactional flow of communication is on patient problem	D. Interactional flow of communication is on consultee problem	D. Interactional flow of communication is on patient (family) psychiatric/psychosocial problem
E. Consultant-consultee collaboration with nursing and other staff on patient care	E. Consultant-consultee collaboration with nursing and other staff on patient care	E. Consultant collaboration with nursing and other staff on patient care
F. Modification of nursing dependent upon acquisition of new knowledge and skills by consultee	F. Modification of nursing care dependent upon resolution of theme interference	F. Modification of patient care for nursing and other staff dependent upon psychiatric therapeutic relationship
IV. Evaluation		
A. Consultant-consultee evaluation of nursing care	A. Consultant-consultee evaluation of consultee	A. Consultant patient (family) evaluation of psychotherapy
B. Consultant-consultee evaluation of consultant care	B. Consultant-consultee evaluation of consultation	B. Consultant evaluation of therapeutic role of psychotherapy
C. Consultant-consultee staff evaluation of patient care, consultation process, and collaboration process	C. Consultant-consultee staff evaluation of patient care and collaboration process	C. Consultant-staff evaluation of patient care and collaboration process
		D. Consultant's generalizations of problems and issues for own growth, for evaluation, and for research

Table 17.1 (*continued*)

Client-Centered Relationship	*Consultee-Centered Relationship*	*Consultant-Patient (Family) Relationship*
VII. Termination		
A. Termination of immediate consultation request	A. Termination of consultant-consultee relation ship	A. Termination of patient (family) relationship
B. Availability for future consultation	B. Availability for future consultation	B. Referral for further treatment to community agencies

SOURCE: M. Termini & M. Ciechoski, The consultation process, *Issues in Mental Health Nursing*, 1981, *3*, 77–88. Used with permission.

is confusion, anger, or frustration regarding the question. A meeting between the consultant and consultee needs to take place as quickly as possible in order to begin collecting data and exchanging information.

The medical record, chart, or file is the next useful area in which to acquire pertinent information. It provides information about the patient's current medical and surgical illness and treatments, previous medical and psychiatric history, social history, age, race, religion, address, occupation, marital status, and next of kin.

Next, an interview with the patient and/or the patient's family is necessary, but only after the consultee has prepared the patient for the interview. This critical step is impaired if the consultee is uncomfortable introducing a psychiatric team member, if he or she fears the patient will be angry or afraid of a psychiatric interview, or if the consultee does not understand the interview process. If such is the case, it becomes a perfect opportunity for the consultant to educate the consultee about the nature of a psychiatric intake interview and to assist him or her in clarifying fantasies or questions while demonstrating the "why" and "how to" of preparing the patient for an interview.

The consultant is explicitly identified as a psychiatric consultant and explains openly and honestly who requested the interview and the reasons for the request. The consultant seeks to learn the patient's feelings and conceptualization concerning hospitalization, various diagnostic procedures, and other issues, as well as the reason for psychiatric consultation. A psychiatric evaluation includes a mental status exam to evaluate the appropriateness of the patient's general appearance, relatedness to the interview, speech functioning, thought process, homicidal/suicidal ideation, use of defense mechanisms, motor functioning, anxiety level, judgement, and insight. The consultant then assesses the patient's family and support systems, observing the interaction of the patient with the family. Patients often ask questions or express feelings that they do not feel comfortable asking of their nurses and medical staff.

Finally, the consultant outlines points to be raised with the consultee, ensuring insofar as possible that the patient will follow through by continuing to identify his or her needs and with recommendations as how best to meet them. This process allows the patient to ask questions and to participate in developing treatment plans.

Assessment

A combined and flexible theoretical framework comes into play as the consultant utilizes an integration of relevant theoretical frameworks to develop a formulation: a coherent explanation of the problems that indicated the need for the initial consultation.

Termini and Ciechoski (1981) describe two distinct dimensions of the nurse-patient relationship that are involved in the consultant's assessment: (1) what *knowledge* or *skills* does the consultee need to provide adequate patient care and (2) what *attitudes, values,* or *behavior* by the consultee interfere with the delivery of nursing care? If present, such attitudes, values, and behavior create *theme interference:* "These interfering themes, that is, personal biases, preconceptions, mind sets, or value judgements about the patient or other caretakers, may be detriments to the development of a helping and collaborative relationship" (Termini & Ciechoski, 1981, p. 81).

The consultant must be very careful in relaying information back to the consultee and should evaluate the nature and history of the existing relationship with the consultee since, as described above, the consultant-consultee relationship has its own developmental sequence. If the relationship is ongoing, open, and supportive, the consultant may explicitly describe the theme interference with the consultee within a theoretical context applicable to the situation. However, if this is the first experience with the consultee and the consultant is uncertain of the level of the relationship at present, then one would not share the theme interference identified. Information sharing is generally structured around diagnosis and recommendations to assist the consultee in management. The treatment plan is discussed by both consultant and consultee with the patient and/or family.

Plan of Action

The plan of action consists of the recommendations provided by the consultant in terms of specific nursing interventions. For example, one might recommend that a primary nurse be assigned to explain all procedures and treatments before they occur in order to lessen a patient's anxiety or to place a large clock and calendar next to the bedside of a recent stroke patient to improve orientation.

The consultant writes a report for the chart to include the data collected, assessment, diagnosis, formulation, and recommendations. The consultant works with the nursing staff to ensure that documentation of the recommendations occurs in the nursing care plan. In this way, the information obtained can be systematically and uniformly transmitted to all nursing personnel who will come in contact with the patient.

Implementation of Plan

When making recommendations, the consultant keeps in mind the type of consultation involved (see Table 17.1). At times, the patient, or family, needs psychiatric or other care beyond or outside the consultee's skill. Given adequate indication, and in a manner explicit to all, the entire consultant-consultee-patient structure may shift radically with the consultant taking a *direct* role in the care of the patient (Termini & Ciechoski, 1981).

If the consultant has identified theme interference as the key issue, the consultation becomes consultee-centered, and both consultant and consultee agree on the desired goal and the time available to achieve it. The consultee provides the necessary information about the consultee-patient relationship, and the consultant provides the theoretical framework necessary to identify and explain the theme interference in useful terms. A successful result requires the consultee to adopt new attitudes and to learn new knowledge and skills necessary to resolve the problem.

When the consultation is a patient-centered one, the consultant's role, though direct, always seeks a better understanding of the patient and the illness through an exchange of information with the consultee regarding the patient's behavior and needs. The consultant provides a psychosocial framework to assist the consultee to better understand the patient's behavior and to identify appropriate nursing interventions to help control or modify that behavior when necessary. After this process, the consultee will modify the nursing care plan to reflect the knowledge and skills learned during the consultation.

In all consultation relationships, the nursing process is utilized. In both patient- and consultee-centered relationships, the consultee documents the care plan and the consultant documents psychiatric therapautic practice in the consultant-patient relationship. Group conferences are held to discuss the patient's care and allow incorporation of recommendations into the patient's care plan (Termini & Ciechoski, 1981).

Evaluation

Ongoing evaluation regarding the effectiveness of the consultative process is essential and will differ according to the type of consultation done and the existing relationship between the consultant and the consultee. Information concerning the structure, process, and role performance of the consultation are obtained in order to improve one's consultant skills, create a database for research, and strengthen the collaborative relationship with the consultee.

Termination

Termination follows the evaluation process when the goals of consultation have been achieved. If further psychiatric care will be needed, the consultant identifies appropriate resources and facilitates the patient's transfer to an appropriate agency while ensuring continuity of care. If the consultant is working primarily with the consultee, a review of the evaluation may raise new problems, in which case the consultant may reinitiate the consultation process. If no problems are identified, the process is concluded and assurance is given of future availability.

Clinical Application of the Consultative Process

A clinical nurse specialist in oncology requested a consultation concerning a 34-year-old, divorced mother of two, recently diagnosed as having carcinoma of the ovaries. The psychiatric nurse consultant met with the oncology specialist to discuss the case and to plan preparation of the patient for the consultation. The consultant reviewed the chart for an overview of the clinical picture and obtained the nursing staff's impressions of the patient's condition and attitude. After this preparation, both the consultant and the purpose of the interview were introduced to the patient. The consultant established whether or not the patient knew a psychiatric consultation had been requested and explored the patient's feelings about and understanding of such an interview.

Mrs. P. explained that she had two children, ages 9 and 11, who were being taken care of by neighbors and family. Her ex-husband lived in another town but was quite active with the children on weekends. The patient and ex-husband had a supportive relationship and were able to talk freely. Ovarian carcinoma had been recently diagnosed, and the patient had been referred to this hospital for treatment. Her ex-husband, parents, doctors, and friends knew of her diagnosis; her children did not. Mrs. P.'s physical condition had deteriorated rapidly, leaving her partially paralyzed and in considerable pain. She had asked to talk with a psychiatric staff member to help her cope with her debilitation and to help her prepare herself and her children for her death. The interview with the patient included a mental status exam, developmental history, and psychosocial history. No family members were available to interview.

Clinically, the patient was a well functioning woman with no preexisting psychiatric diagnosis or personality disorder. She was anxious and angry about the devastated condition of her body and poor prognosis. Her physiological crisis was destroying her usual psychological balance. Mental status exam and interview revealed no abnormalities indicative of brain metastases, but this possibility was monitored carefully in view of her diagnosis.

The consultant's nursing diagnosis was that the patient's life-threatening disease had impaired her ability to function, removed her from her natural environment and support system, and overwhelmed her usual coping style. The consultant saw the patient on a regular basis, offering therapy directed toward helping the patient set her life in order before her death. The consultant was also available to the nursing staff, who were overwhelmed and uncertain about how to deal with the patient as she deteriorated. The consultant established that she was available if the patient wished a family meeting with her two sons and possibly her ex-husband. These recommendations were shared with the patient, nursing staff, and consultee, all of whom agreed to the meeting.

The consultant was instrumental in facilitating communication between the patient and health care team, and between the patient and her family, especially her children. As the patient progressed from fear and anger to acceptance, she was able to say goodbye and plan for her children's future (Kubler-Ross, 1972). The patient eventually was transferred to her community hospital and died within two weeks.

Following the patient's transfer, the consultant met with the oncology specialist and health care team to evaluate the effectiveness of the consultation by asking the following questions: Were there any unfinished issues that interfered with the health care team's level of functioning? Were questions answered appropriately? Were there any other unresolved issues? Once these questions were answered, the psychiatric consultant could terminate the process, leaving the door open for future contact and consultation.

THE LIAISON PROCESS

Defining the Process

Liaison is the development of a working relationship between a consultant, a psychiatrist or psychiatric mental health nurse or other mental health professional, and the staff of a ward or unit or clinic. Goals of liaison work include creating optimal conditions to help prevent, detect, and manage psychiatric disorders; mediating in patient-staff conflicts; and teaching (Lipowski, 1981). In the early days of psychiatric consultation and liaison nursing, liaison was considered to be of principal importance, with consultation being secondary. As more time was spent on nonpsychiatric units assisting the nursing staff in problem solving and sensitizing them to the psychosocial needs of their patients, it became evident that direct patient contact was valuable. Thus, the liaison process gradually developed a more legitimate role.

Frances Lehmann (1983) believes that the liaison process can be compared to the traditional nursing process. Both are interpersonal, orderly, mutual problem-solving activities working to effect change, and both require active participation. Lehmann's description involves four steps common to nursing and liaison: assessment, planning, implementation, and evaluation (see Figure 17.1). Liaison adds orientation and termination phases to these four.

Orientation Phase

The liaison nurse becomes familiar with the clinical area, makes personal contact with the staff, contacts the system's decision maker, and learns the organizational structure, communication network, and nature and scope of services provided.

Both sides need to explicitly define the tasks and functions of the liaison nurse, particularly if the people involved are unfamiliar with or have misconceptions about the role of a liaison nurse. Such clarity will preclude two possible problems: unrealistic staff expectations and distortion of the purpose of liaison work.

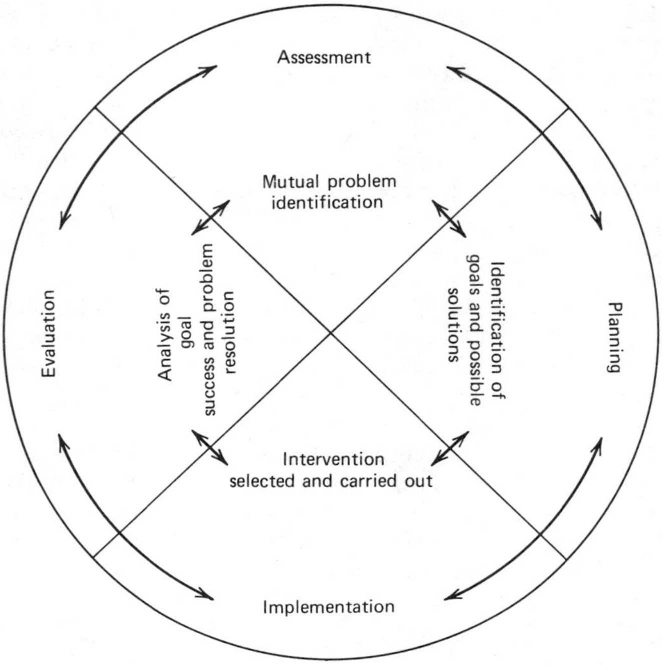

Figure 17.1 Stages of the liaison process (From F. G. Lehmann, Liaison nursing: A model for nursing practice. In G. W. Stuart & S. J. Sundeen (Eds.), *Principles and practice of psychiatric nursing,* (2nd ed.), St. Louis: C. V. Mosby, 1983, p. 693.)

A smooth and successful liaison relationship requires both formal and informal communication networks using common terminology; the liaison nurse avoids unnecessary psychiatric terms. Questions that guide the user to a new view of the problem are more advantageous than advice.

Discussions need to be, for the most part, confidential, and this is conveyed to the staff. The liaison nurse needs to communicate openly without taking sides. To accomplish this, making the relationship safe is essential. A professional focus is maintained and information available to the liaison nurse is only used for problem solving and never to harm any person or the agency. If a staff member begins to share personal troubles, the liaison nurse needs to intervene, tactfully encouraging the individual to seek more appropriate help. To preserve the nature of the relationship, a liaison nurse does not recommend therapy for a staff member (even if it appears to be indicated) during the liaison process.

Two levels exist in the liaison process that help in the ongoing clarification of expectations: the informal liaison process, in which there is continual negotiation by both parties about the development and modification of the ground rules of the relationship, and the formal liaison process, an explicit written agreement delineating the specific services to be rendered and the parameters of the complementary activity. Basic points that are important in this contract include: (1) a brief description of the problem situation, (2) expected goals, (3) estimated time to be used on the project, (4) means of compensation for the time, and (5) the key department and personnel involved, including the contact person (Lehmann, 1983).

A liaison contract is not a legal document, but simply an agreement between professionals to clarify expectations and help avoid misrepresentation or ambiguity.

The work phase begins once the orientation and contract have been completed and negotiated. This phase encompasses four stages (demonstrated in Figure 17.1)—assessment, planning, implementation, and evaluation (Lehman, 1983).

Assessment

Here the liaison nurse and the user identify goals and ensure ongoing planning, interpretation, and evaluation. The conceptual framework useful for mutual problem solving in consultation (Hollister & Miller, 1977) is useful here as well. A diagnostic inventory is necessary. Does the consultee lack (1) knowledge (absence of necessary information), (2) skill (recognition of the problem but not how to deal with it), (3) objectivity (interference by the consultee's feelings or reactions), or (4) confidence?

If the problem relates to a lack of knowledge or skill, problem-solving strategies can frequently generate mutually developed, new approaches to the problem. When lack of objectivity is the problem, Caplan's strategies for "theme interference" are useful. With a lack of confidence, the consultant's sensitive emotional support will frequently strengthen the consultee and increase her or his confidence (Hollister & Miller, 1977). Hollister and Miller further describe the following nine strategies:

Stress analysis and modification. Both the staff and the liaison nurse list the stresses, such as demands, conflicts, pressures, and expectations, that appear to be causing the problem. Unchangeable stresses are eliminated from the list. The remaining stresses are mutually evaluated to determine if they can be decreased, deferred or, eliminated. If so, a plan is constructed to modify them.

Trait-cause analysis. This strategy focuses on the behavior trait or attitude that appears to be causing the problem. The staff and liaison nurse list the possible causes for this behavior, looking at areas that previously may not have been considered. This approach exemplifies the saying, "Don't treat the symptoms, treat the cause." A typical example would be that, when a patient repeatedly uses a call light, one needs to consider why this is occurring. Perhaps the reason is that the patient is overanxious or feeling isolated and abandoned. The nurse can then allot more time to the patient, thus focusing on the cause and not the symptom.

Listing emotional needs. The user identifies the emotions that could be behind the problem behavior. The liaison nurse then assists in identifying the patient's possible unmet emotional needs. Together, the liaison nurse and the user mutually design a plan to meet these unfulfilled needs.

Reduction of energies. An attempt is made to rechannel unwanted behavior into acceptable behavior. The user and liaison nurse mutually explore alternative behaviors for the patient/client that would be more emotionally satisfying and less destructive.

Temporary use of a defense. The user and liaison nurse evaluate the patient's use of defense mechanisms. A person with a series of stresses may overutilize certain defense mechanisms to get through the crisis. When this situation is identified, the user needs to encourage the use of these familiar defenses as well as offer support until the crisis passes or the patient chooses a better solution. To illustrate, when a patient first realizes he is quadraplegic after a traumatic injury, denial is appropriate until the shock wears off and more realistic thinking occurs. The user does not challenge this denial and is available for support.

Behavior modification contracts. This strategy involves identifying undesirable behaviors as well as desirable behaviors, with a goal of limiting the undesirable behaviors and encouraging more appropriate behaviors. A plan is developed to help the staff work out a contract with the patient that clearly identifies undesirable behaviors and when they generally occur. Both the staff and patient need to agree upon a positive program that reflects emotional rewards such as extra privileges, praise, and recognition to reinforce desirable behaviors. For example, every time an encopretic child on a pediatric ward uses the toilet appropriately, he is given points that add up to rewards appropriate to his developmental age. The child also receives praise and encouragement for giving up the undesirable behavior and successfully using the desired behavior.

Adverse stimulus. This is a tricky strategy and needs to be carefully planned. To begin with, the user and liaison nurse need to decide reasonable consequences for undesirable behaviors. The plan is discussed with the patient/client. A contract is agreed upon and discussed openly with appropriate staff. Consistent and immediate consequences need to be reinforced whenever an undesirable behavior occurs in order for this strategy to work.

Mobilizing peer pressure. This strategy identifies the group within the staff that is exhibiting undesirable behavior. The plan utilizes group processes to develop new behaviors designed to mobilize peer control and to lessen the attention directed toward the undesirable behavior. This is an effective approach when there is more than one person exhibiting the unwanted behavior.

Education for the desired behavior. This strategy assumes that the patient, staff, or client is ignorant of appropriate behaviors for certain situations. An educational program is developed that explicitly describes and illustrates the desired sets of behaviors for specific situations. This strategy is a useful preventive method that can stifle undesired behavior before it becomes a problem.

Planning

Planning follows assessment in the work phase, as the liaison nurse reframes the original problem so the user can now look at it objectively. Mutually understood concepts are essential in developing a plan that is practical and feasible for the setting, the talents and skills available, and the rights and well-being of all those who will be affected by the change.

Implementation

The user alone decides which interventions to try given the setting involved, the skills available, and the situation at hand. Generally, several different interventions are necessary before the best ones are found. This stage ends when an intervention has been functional long enough to evaluate its outcome.

Evaluation

Evaluation determines how well the intervention met the stated goals and if it can be done without the liaison nurse. Since one is measuring the results and not how the results were obtained, the staff members need to understand that their skills are not being evaluated. Evaluation is complete once it is determined how successfully the problem has been resolved and whether any additional problems have occurred (Lehmann, 1983).

Termination Phase

The main tasks of this phase are report writing and terminating the relationship. Both will be influenced by the liaison nurse's personality, the setting in which the liaison activity takes place, and the contract.

A written report, addressed to the organization, not to individual staff members, outlining the experience is essential. Lehmann (1983) suggests including: (1) the purpose and dates of and activities during the process, (2) a statement of the identified problem, (3) an assessment of the situation, (4) alternative plans for problem resolution, (5) specific interventions, and (6) suggestions on how to evaluate the interventions.

Clinical Application of the Liaison Process

A head nurse called a psychiatric liaison nurse with whom she had worked previously to discuss a problem. The head nurse and her staff had recently been assigned to a larger ward in the hospital, where the head nurse was to become head nurse for the now-combined staffs and services. Identified problems included: intolerance for new ideas, lack of cohesiveness, hostility, competition, unwillingness to share staff between the two services, resentment from the old staff about being invaded by a new head nurse and her staff, and resentment from the new staff about moving to a larger combined service floor and sharing their head nurse. These problems had begun to affect the quality of patient care.

The two agreed that weekly meetings on each shift for a month would be a suitable way to begin, and the head nurse prepared her staff with a timetable for meetings and by discussing the purpose of the meetings. She agreed to come to the first meeting on each shift to share her concerns and to list the problems she had noted since the merger of the two services.

At the first meeting, the head nurse presented her concerns. She and the liaison nurse emphasized that the purpose of the meetings was to enhance patient care, that finding fault or placing blame were unimportant, and that the working conditions of the staff had to be improved in order to improve patient care.

The liaison nurse understood the difference between a psychotherapy group and staff support group. Staff support groups do not identify staff as patients; their sole function is to improve patient care by providing support for staff and they focus on specific identifiable issues. Group discussion is strictly confined to these issues and absence of staff due to emergencies is not interpreted as resistance. In this situation, rotating membership cut attendance of the meetings and this may have occurred because of variable staff working schedules or work patterns that disrupted regular attendance. Confidentiality was probably breached, as important issues had to be discussed outside the group with medical and nursing hierarchies to effectively resolve problems and promote change (Eisendrath, 1981).

The first meeting set the tone; ground rules were established and trust strengthened as staff became acquainted with each other and the liaison nurse and specific problems related to patient care were discussed.

The second meeting went into the interplay between patient care problems and staff behavior and the liaison nurse introduced an explanation for the identified problems. She told the staff that she believed they were experiencing a loss of identity and were going through the grief process.

Information regarding the grief process and systems theory was introduced at the third group meeting (while keeping the focus on patient care). The liaison nurse illustrated the relationship between grief and staff behaviors and brought up hypothetical examples. Exploring this concept allowed the staff members to verbalize their thoughts and feelings and move on to resolution. The liaison nurse then introduced conflict-resolution theory to help solve problems and implement new interactions.

By the fourth meeting, the staff nurses were more cohesive as a working group and the quality of patient care had improved. The head nurse, liaison nurse, and staff reviewed the purpose and goals of the meetings and what problems had been solved. They also used the time to identify any unresolved problems or new problems that needed attention and to suggest additional actions.

After the last group meeting, the liaison nurse and head nurse reviewed the work accomplished and discussed the goals achieved and any possible unfinished business. The head nurse was pleased with the new level of functioning and believed it was important for the staff to work together as a group for a time before any further liaison support groups would be effective. The liaison nurse agreed. She assured the head nurse that a written report would follow within a short period of time to summarize and highlight the progress of the work group.

SCOPE AND ISSUES OF CONSULTATION-LIAISON NURSING PRACTICE

Psychiatric consultation-liaison nursing has expanded beyond the hospital. However, the majority of psychiatric consultation-liaison nursing positions still exist in general hospitals. DeLougherty et al (1971) divided clinical consultation and liaison work into medical and nonmedical settings. Medical settings include hospitals, clinics, and community-based agencies, all offering care and service of some type to the "sick" individual. Here, consultees have some responsibility for the health of their clients and the consultants assist in solving a problem in some way related to the clients' mental health. Nonmedical settings include schools, welfare agencies, and judicial systems. Consultees in this situation do not assume responsibility for clients' well-being and the consultant must not attempt to alter this relationship.

Peer Support and Review

Consultation-liaison work is exciting and stimulating, requiring an active and inquisitive mind. Often, the position is unique within the clinical setting, which leads to frustrations arising from isolation, widely varied staff expectations, difficulties in setting priorities, lack of feedback, resistance, lack of authority, lack of time, and lack of peer identification.

An appropriate support system is essential to help the consultation-liaison nurse deal with the problems described. Consultation-liaison nurses who work independently need to seek out peers with whom to share experiences, identify similar aspects of their work, and gain support through problem-solving strategy sessions. Peer support may often be found outside one's own agency.

Lewis and Levy (1982) found that the peer group (1) provides a safe and supportive environment to discuss all of the ramifications of being a psychiatric liaison nurse; (2) provides confidentiality while discussing clinical issues, achieving better understanding, receiving feedback, and identifying strategies for problem resolution; (3) identifies research areas and role expansion; and (4) promotes professional identity, development, and collegiality. Administrators may also be supportive through role legitimization, encouragement, and guidance.

Consultation-liaison nurses working as part of a multidisciplinary team can use the team for support whenever this is appropriate. Working rounds, team meetings, and collaborative working relationships all contribute to lessening the inevitable frustrations of consultation-liaison. Seeking out nursing peer support groups for support and feedback to assist in maintaining one's identity as a nurse and a psychiatric clinician is also helpful.

Research

Traditionally, nursing has not taken a very active role in the research field. Yet, the consultation-liaison nurse works in a fertile area for research including identifying patterns of utilization of consultation or patients' coping styles within the hospital setting. As nurses become more skilled and confident in initiating research, consultation-liaison nurses will begin to pursue studies in the field.

Accurate and detailed record-keeping is vital, both for research purposes and documentation of effectiveness. An intuitive feeling of satisfaction is not sufficient to justify the continued existence of the role of the psychiatric consultation-liaison nurse, especially in times of budgetary crisis (Nelson & Schelke, 1976). Only documentation of the numbers and types of consultations and liaison activities, teaching requests, and professional activities will provide the necessary data to support the existence of the role.

Evaluation of Consultation-Liaison Nursing

Psychiatric consultation-liaison nurses realize the importance of continual professional growth and evaluation of clinical practice. Lewis and Levy (1982) identify three aspects of evaluation—the formal process, the informal process, and the identification and role of the evaluator(s).

Formal evaluation looks at the specific tasks and responsibilities of the consultation-liaison nurse. Areas covered might include: (1) direct and indirect consultation, (2) communication skills, (3) interpersonal skills, (4) teaching skills, (5) liaison activities, (6) leadership and/or professionalism, and (7) academic advancements (Lewis & Levy, 1982). The formal evaluation also includes feedback received from consultees regarding their understanding of the information provided by the consultant, their understanding of why a consultation was necessary, and their expectations and reaction to the consultation-liaison process.

Informal evaluation consists of the subjective thoughts, feelings, and perceptions of the consultation-liaison nurse regarding his or her profession. Consultation and liaison requests are often complex and personalized by the consultee. In order to evaluate success or failure, one looks at both the technical and personal skills of the consultant, including the quality of the consultation alliance, the transference issues between consultant and consultee, and the ability of the consultant to take into consideration those aspects that influence his or her success or failure. For example: (1) Were the consultant's recommendations and intervention suggestions implemented? (2) Did these recommendations relieve or ameliorate the problem? (3) Were the goals of the consultation obtained? (4) Was the consultee-consultant alliance strengthened by the consultation process? Other methods of obtaining informal evaluation information would be through peer audit, peer review, and information obtained from a clinical supervisor.

The third part of the evaluation process identifies appropriate and qualified people who can evaluate the clinical work of a consultation-liaison nurse. Often an unqualified person (someone not trained or experienced in consultation-liaison) is appointed to evaluate the clinical performance of the consultation-liaison nurse. If this step occurs, it is the responsibility of the consultation-liaison nurse to request and, if necessary, design an appropriate evaluation structure.

However stressful, comprehensive evaluation is a basis for personal and professional growth and ideally is accomplished with input from a skilled supervisor and peers and feedback from consultees (Lewis & Levy, 1982).

SUMMARY

Psychiatric nursing has evolved from custodial care to interactive nursing practice. Specialization in nursing has been a crucial part of this evolution. Over the past 20 years, consultation-liaison nursing has evolved as a specialty in tandem with the corresponding specialty in psychiatry.

Consultation as described by Gerald Caplan is a professional interaction between a specialist (the consultant) and the consultee, with the goal of solving a problem. In the process, responsibility for the client remains with the consultee. Consultation also offers education to the consultee.

Liaison also is a relationship between a specific individual and a specific staff over a defined period of time. Lipowski defined psychiatric liaison as regular contact by a mental health worker with the clinical staff to enhance the psychosocial aspects of patient care. Liaison concerns mediation, interpretation, and communication issues related to a patient's or system's behavior. Staff education is also a goal.

Consultation and liaison are two distinct, though interdependent, mutually supportive activities. There is a consensus that the psychiatric mental health clinical nurse specialist prepared at the master's level is best suited for this specialized work. These nurses have special expertise in this area and can be role models, consultants, educators, change agents, and researchers.

REFERENCES

Berarducci, M., Blandford, K., & Garant, C. The psychiatric liaison nurse in the general hospital. *General Hospital Psychiatry,* 1979, *1,* 66–72.

Bilodeau, C., & O'Connor, S. Role of nurse clinician in liaison psychiatry. In T. Hackett & N. Cassem (Eds.), *Massachusetts General Hospital handbook of general hospital psychiatry.* St. Louis: C. V. Mosby, 1978.

Blake, P. The clinical specialist as nurse consultant. *Journal of Nursing Administration,* 1977, *7*(10), 33–36.

Burch, J., & Meredith, J. Nurses as the core of a psychiatric team. *American Journal of Nursing,* 1974, *74*(11), 2037–38.

Caplan, G. *The theory and practice of mental health consultation.* New York: Basic Books, 1964.

Cherniss, C. The consultation readiness scale: An attempt to improve consultation practice. *American Journal of Community Psychology,* 1978, *6*(1), 15–21.

Davis, D., & Nelson, J. Referrals to psychiatric liaison nurses. *General Hospital Psychiatry,* 1980, *2,* 41–45.

DeLougherty, G. W., Gebbie, K. M., & Newman, B. M. *Consultation and community organization in community mental health nursing.* Baltimore: Williams & Wilkins, 1971.

Eisendrath, S. Psychiatric liaison support groups for general hospital staff. *Psychosomatics,* 1981, *22*(8), 685–694.

Garant, C. The psychiatric liaison nurse: An interpretation of the role. *Supervisor Nurse,* 1977, *8*(4), 75–78.

Goldstein, S. The psychiatric clinical specialist in the general hospital. *Journal of Nursing Administration,* 1979, *9*(3), 34–37.

Hackett, T., & Cassem, N. (Eds.). *Massachusetts General Hospital handbook of general psychiatry.* St. Louis: C. V. Mosby, 1978.

Henry, G. W. Some modern aspects of psychiatry in general hospital practice. *American Journal of Psychiatry,* 1929, *8,* 481–499.

Hollister, W., & Miller, F. T. Problem-solving strategies in consultation. *American Journal of Orthopsychiatry,* 1977, *47*(3), 445–450.

Johnson, B. S. Psychiatric nurse consultant in a general hospital. *Nursing Outlook,* 1963, *11*(10), 728–729.

Kubler-Ross, E. *On death and dying.* New York: Macmillan, 1972.

Kuntz, S., Stehle, J., & Marshall, R. The psychiatric clinical specialist: The progression of a specialty. *Perspectives in Psychiatric Care,* 1980, *18*(2), 90–98.

Lehmann, F. G. Liaison nursing: A model for nursing practice. In G. Stuart & S. Sundeen (Eds.), *Principles and practice of psychiatric nursing.* St. Louis: C. V. Mosby, 1983.

Lewis, A., & Levy, J. *Psychiatric liaison nursing.* Reston, VA: Reston Publishing Co., 1982.

Lipowski, Z. J. Consultation-liaison psychiatry: An overview. *American Journal of Psychiatry,* 1974, *131*(6), 623–630.

Lipowski, Z. J. Psychiatric liaison past, present and future. In R. O. Pasanau (Ed.), *Consultation-liaison psychiatry.* New York: Grune & Stratton, 1975.

Lipowski, Z. J. Consultation-liaison psychiatry past failure and new opportunities. *General Hospital Psychiatry,* 1979, *1*(1), 3–10.

Lipowski, Z. J. New prospects for liaison psychiatry. *Psychosomatics,* 1981, *22*(9), 806–809.

Nelson, J., & Schelke, D. A. The evolution of psychiatric liaison nursing. *Perspectives in Psychiatric Care,* 1976, *14*(2), 61–65.

Przepiorka, K., & Bender, L. Psychiatric nursing consultation in a university medical center. *Hospital Community Psychiatry,* 1977, *28*(10), 755–758.

Robinson, L. *Liaison nursing: Psychological approach to patient care.* Philadelphia: F. A. Davis Co., 1974.

Termini, M., & Ciechoski, M. The consultation process. *Issues in Mental Health Nursing,* 1981, *3,* 77–88.

BIBLIOGRAPHY

Hazlet, C., & Rappaport, L. Mental health consultation. In L. Bellak (Ed.), *Handbook of community psychiatry.* New York: Grune & Stratton, 1964.

CHAPTER

18 STEREOTYPES AND PREJUDICE: WOMEN AS CLIENTS AND PROVIDERS

Anne J. Davis

The status of women since antiquity has been profoundly influenced by prevailing philosophical, social, and economic factors. This chapter highlights how certain of these factors have negatively affected women socially, educationally, and professionally. Specific issues discussed will be the effects of sexual stereotypes and prejudices on women as providers and clients in mental health, different definitions of mental health and illness for men and women, significance of increasing rates of mental illness for women, differences in therapist attitudes toward male and female clients, and the effects of prejudice on the education and practice of the psychiatric nurse clinical specialist.

HISTORICAL OVERVIEW

Being defined as a problem or as different in negative ways is nothing new for women. Aristotle (384–322 BC) viewed the male by nature as superior and the female as inferior. This theme runs throughout Western philosophical thought and has had a major impact on our taken-for-granted world. Even today many men and women believe that women are inherently inferior. Aristotle and other thinkers defined a woman as a mutilated or incomplete man, a thesis that has enjoyed a long and persistent history culminating in Freud's theory of woman in the nineteenth century (Agonito, 1977).

Most nineteenth century novels caricature or idealize women. Only after 1860, with the writings of individuals like George Eliot (Mary Ann Evans), was progress made towards more complexity and an abandonment of the Victorian simplified stereotype (Basch, 1974; Hardwick, 1974). Remnants of these early stereotypes die hard. For example, as recently as 1955, Barzun, an educator well known to the general public, wrote that although it took hard work, the minds of women students could be forced out of their conventionality and made to cope with abstractions. One could speculate that this statement received little response at the time because it fit the stereotype for women.

The Second Sex (de Beauvior, 1953), published in English translation in the early 1950s, did not reach a wide audience in this country at that time. A decade later, the *Feminine Mystique* (Friedan, 1963) raised questions and led to a beginning examination of definitions, myths, and problems of women. It became a landmark document for what was to be the new or revived women's movement. This social movement has had many goals including the examination of the stereotype of women in our society.

Lest we think that the social context for changes in women's roles is very recent, we need only to look briefly at historical data to disabuse ourselves of that notion. And, while we look, we need to remember that change in social role is not necessarily always change in one direction leading to a better situation for the people involved. Change is dynamic and complex and often results in a mixed situation that also includes unintentional consequences.

Conflicting View of Women

For example, from the seventeenth century onwards, the evolution towards a capitalist mode of production deeply affected women's societal role. The industrial revolution and capitalist concentration disrupted the family production unit within which women had played an important part (Trevelyan, 1976). The decline in home industry and increasing specialization meant, among other things, that female labor became devalued (Clark, 1919). This situation increased markedly during the first decade of the nineteenth century with the full effects of the Industrial Revolution that had begun in England and then took hold in the United States. Women faced the dilemma of working for starvation wages in dying sectors of the economy or depending financially on a family to which they could not easily make a financial contribution. This latter solution became increasingly approved by a society that prescribed for a woman in the home an ornamental, metaphysical, and morally inspiring role (Houghton, 1957). In a paternalistic society, women were venerated as the embodiments and guardians of domestic bliss, yet at the same time they were considered frail creatures all too likely to yield to sexual temptation. So, to keep those of the middle and upper classes pure, society deemed it fitting that they be surrounded by many children while their husbands went about their worldly business, which included trips to the brothel (Calder, 1976; Marcus, 1977).

Unmarried women found themselves first in a social and then an economic impasse. The word *spinster* changed from designating the trade of the spinning girl, a legal and economic reality, to mean an unmarried woman. This latter meaning held a value judgment. The pejorative connotation of the term, used first in 1719, showed that a specific professional problem that resulted from economic and social upheavals led to a lack of respect for the unmarried woman on the cultural level (Bodichon, 1857). Having lost her role as an economic producer and deprived of the all-encompassing roles of wife and mother, she became something of a social outcast. Paradoxically, the law favored this single woman, the spinster, over married women. Eighteenth and nineteenth century law, grounded in patriarchal Roman law, vested legal existence only in the head of the family (Watt, 1965). The spinster's legal position was from every point of view identical to that of men but her public and political rights were the same as the married woman's, that is, all women had the status of a minor in these social arenas. No women could be members of professions nor could they be admitted to universities.

Women in the Work Force

For women of the lower class or women who had never married and had to work, economic exploitation became a common experience. The 1851 census indicated that three-quarters of unmarried women worked or lived on their own earnings (Milne, 1867). In 1865, one-third of all women over 21 years of age in England were independent workers (Martineau, 1865). These and other similar writings regarding women and work led to the recognition that the view of woman's place as being only in the home was dogma and not fact. This in turn led to discussion focused on woman's education that had as its chief aim at that time to make women ornaments and the soul of the family. Such an education was obviously resting on a falsification of the facts.

In the United States, though industrialization meant that many of the goods and services that women traditionally produced in their homes were increasingly provided by the market economy, it must not be overlooked that industrialization also brought ever-increasing numbers of women into the paid labor force. In 1890, women constituted 17% of all workers in the labor force and this number represented 18% of the total female population. These numbers continued to increase as the nineteenth turned into the twentieth century. Recent figures indicate the number of women in the labor force along with statistics showing pay disadvantage, job opportunities, and where women work (Table 18.1). Although the recession and unemployment of the 1980s has had an impact on women's employment, women continue to enter the labor force in increasing numbers.

In addition to these economic changes in the nineteenth century, other changes occurred in women's lives. By the late 1860s, while Mill (1869) argued for the right of women to vote and an end to the legal subordination of married women to their husbands, the movement for sex equality had already gathered considerable momentum both in England and in the United States. Fifty years later, American women won the right to vote. They had made one step toward being defined as people and as adults, but many aspects of the stereotype remained.

These brief historical remarks indicate that changes occurred in women's roles with regard to their economic, legal, and social status especially during the latter nineteenth and early twentieth centuries. One could assume that these changes would lead to a less stereotyped

Table 18.1 Some Basic Facts about Working Women

Women in the labor force	1962, 38.0%; 1972, 43.9%; 1982, 52.9%. (In the last 20 years, 24.5 million women have joined the labor force, compared with 13 million men.)		
Pay disadvantage	1962	Men,	$ 5,474
		Women,	$ 3,062
		Women's pay as share of men's, 56%	
	1972	Men,	$10,202
		Women,	$ 5,903
		Women's pay as share of men's, 58%	
	1982	Men,	$20,260
		Women,	$12,001
		Women's pay as share of men's, 59%	
Job opportunities	Proportion of management jobs held by women 1971, 10.9%; 1976, 14.9%; 1980, 19.2%		
Where most women work	Women as proportion of all persons employed as:		
	Secretaries, typists		98.3%
	Receptionists		97.3%
	Bank tellers		93.5%
	Telephone operators		92.9%
	Nurses, dietitians, therapists		92.6%
	Bookkeepers		91.1%
	Cashiers		86.2%
	Librarians, archivists, curators		82.8%
	Health technicians		72.3%
	Salesclerks		71.2%
	Teachers (noncollege)		70.6%

SOURCE: Growing impact of women in the U.S. labor force. *San Francisco Chronicle*, August 16, 1982, p. 5.

response to women, and in some respects this is the case, but such an assumption needs close examination. Although some strides have been made, in many instances women are still defined as second class or unimportant.

ISSUES INVOLVED IN ROLE CHANGE FOR WOMEN

This discussion focuses on two aspects of women's changing roles: family role and work role outside of the home. With very few exceptions, women enact one or the other or both of these roles in our society.

In all human aggregations, one finds differentiated behavior, the specialization of individuals in specific domains of behavior, and particular complements of specializations called division of labor. To examine these concepts, the everyday tasks that have to be performed in every family in order to keep things going become one useful set of variables for study.

Traditionally, husbands did "men's work," which was strenuous and dangerous, and wives did "women's work," which was centered in the home. There has been much discussion in recent years about the American family's alleged abandonment of this traditional division of labor. As more women have taken jobs outside the home, there has been some pressure on husbands to lighten the double workload that falls on their working wives. Basically, shared work becomes the ideal if not the reality rather than the old division of labor.

To a considerable extent, the idea of shared work seems incompatible with the most efficient division of labor. Much of the progress in modern economy rests on the increasing specialization of its division of labor, although such an arrangement does have its problems, such as worker alienation.

Work Roles Within the Family

Blood and Wolfe (1960) conducted a study in which they examined the division of labor in American families by asking questions as to how the responsibility for eight household tasks was allocated. They found that the predominant picture reveals specialized tasks performance along traditional sex lines. The reason was not so much that contemporary Americans are conservative in principle, since they have altered their pattern of decision making to fit the times. Rather, the same bio-social reasons that shaped the traditional family still supply the differential resources men and women bring to marriage. Where resources differ, the modern family adjusts its division of labor accordingly. Blood and Wolfe concluded that the criterion that governs the contemporary division of labor in the family is not custom but equity, and an equitable division of labor depends on the resources of time, energy, and skill that each family member can contribute to the common task.

The married woman of today functions increasingly in two worlds as her husband has done for some time. She does this in a society that provides images and ideals of how marriage should be lived and how each is to play out his or her role within marriage. The prevailing idea of marriage in our society has been a romantic one combining the values of love and freedom. The freedom referred to has for the most part been the freedom to choose a partner. More recently, this idea of freedom has extended in attitude or expectation, if not always in fact, to include the idea that those who have freely chosen each other will permit each other to seek a greater or lesser degree of success and identity in work. Therefore, there is an inherent, if rarely acknowledged, contradiction between the traditional idea of marriage and the emancipation or possibility for role change of women. Role change for women implies major choices, possible stresses, and risks largely unknown in Western societies until recently. For example, the dimensions of many present-day marriages include high standards of sharing, understanding, and accomplishment, together with the expectation that middle-class women will function regularly in those spheres formerly thought of as masculine while continuing aspects of those functions traditionally regarded as feminine. This is no small order and will have effects on everyone, not just married women. Such role functions may be a profile of Super Woman in that this standard for woman's performance may become a stereotype foisted on American women with as much rigidity as those role functions from the past. It is characteristic of American optimism, somewhat tarnished recently but still a part of the national picture, that we expect ambitious targets to be attained and experience the guilt of personal failure when they are not.

Marriage has been called a social contract. In the past, it was a contract in which property rights were settled and a religious sacrament established eternal bonds in addition to a personal contract. Now it is mostly a personal contract in which both persons work to make the relationship a meaningful one wherein the rights of each to realize his or her hopes and desires are upheld. Dangers exist in such a demanding contract. Failure in this case may not be seen as failure of a moral code, or of a social class, or even of a system but of the individuals involved. Thus, the woman question is not merely a struggle for women alone but for everyone. Perhaps it always was but was not so openly acknowledged to be so.

Working Women and Working Mothers

To have a fuller understanding of working women, it is useful to begin with a basic profile of American women in general based on 1982 data (Table 18.2). According to one Census Bureau Report, married women are entering the labor force in higher numbers and at younger ages, leading to increased family income. In addition, this trend will continue as women's work experience grows (Gallup, 1982). During the past decade, women accounted for 60% of the growth in the labor force, with married women responsible for a large share of the increase. By March, 1980, 51% of all married women were in the labor force compared with 24% in 1950. A large share of the growth came among women with children under six years of age, with 45% of these women working or seeking jobs in 1980, up from 30% in 1950. Participation of this age group allows women more time and experience on the job, which may widen career opportunities and advancements and could result in higher income levels for women. But other factors tend to push family income down. One such factor is the structure of the family. For example, during the 1970s, there was a 53% increase in the number of households maintained by women with no husband present. By 1980, they totaled 8.5 million or 15% of all family households. These households tend to have significantly lower incomes than those with a male earner. Women head 50% of all poor families in the United States. With the continuing growth of separation, divorce, and children born out of wedlock, increases in families maintained by women will likely have a dampening effect on the overall growth rate of household and family incomes. In addition, divorce and postponement of marriage will also likely lower average household earnings by creating more single-income households of people living alone. The study from the U.S. Census Bureau listed 1980 median household income as $21,390, up from 1979 but actually representing a net decline in real income because of inflation.

Freudian Stereotypes of Women

We can look to Freud for input on the subject of women and their social roles. His pioneering work in psychoanalytic theory had its largest impact in general during the 1940s and 1950s.

Table 18.2 Basic Profile of American Women in 1982

Number	Women constitute more than half of the population, 119.9 million females comprising 51.3% of the total population. In 1992 there will be 130.3 million women but their proportion of the total population will remain the same. At present 88.4 million women are 18 years of age or older.
Age	The average age of women is 31.9 years and of men 29.3 years. Females as a group are getting older, and by 1992 women will, on the average, be 34.5 years old, and by the year 2000 they will be 36.8 years of age.
Race	Of every seven American women, six are white. Of all American women, 101.6 million or 85% are white. Blacks constitute 14.6 million women or 12%, and 2.9 million women are of other races.
Life span	Women live longer than men. The average woman lives a little more than 78 years, which is nearly eight years longer than the average man. This gap in life expectancy is widening, since figures show that 20 years ago the difference between men and women was a little more than seven years.
Education	Women are now more likely to attend college than in the past. Among persons aged 18–24, 35% of women are enrolled in college compared to 34% of men. About 30.4% of lawyers are now women and 24.4 percent of doctors.
Marriage	More women are now putting marriage off. Just over half of the women aged 20–24 have never been married, compared with 35.8% in 1970 and 28.4% in 1960. However, 83% of women ultimately do marry.
Families	There has been a sharp rise in the number of families headed by women. More than one in seven, or 9.1 million, families are now headed by women. The number has risen since 1970, largely because of climbing divorce rates.
Children	Women in general want fewer children. Of childless married women aged 18–24, 23% expect to have one child or none and 72% expect to bear two or three children. Only 5% expect four or more. These plans, if fulfilled, mean little population growth.
Political power	Women have an edge in numbers at the polls. Women of voting age are 52.2% of all Americans aged 18 and over. With women living longer than men, the proportion is growing.

SOURCE: G. Gallup, Poll on women and job bids, *San Francisco Chronicle,* August 16, 1982, p. 5.

The famous phrase "Anatomy is destiny" gained importance in the American conscious at the time of World War II and immediately afterwards. Women were viewed as a deviation from the norm of masculinity and were best described as masochistic, narcissistic, and passive. Essentially, to be fulfilled sexually and maternally was woman's most important goal. It was understood that, though women's "penis envy" could create problems for them in properly adjusting to their feminine role, no truly normal feminine women would aspire to masculine work and life-styles. Together with the right to vote and admission to the hallowed halls of institutions of higher learning society also gave women the belief that sexuality is all determining. The sexual aspect in personality was not considered a component but all encompassing. If women did work outside the home, they should certainly try to find suitable feminine vocations and not be overly concerned with their work. This attitude, of course, took little of the realities of women's lives into account, especially lower-class women. Most if not all middle- and upper-class women were made to feel that something was wrong with them emotionally if they did not find total fulfillment in the traditional female roles.

The post–World War II era, a time of larger families and togetherness, was when the boys came marching home and back into the labor force to do many jobs that women had done in their absence. During the 1960s, women and social scientists began to question the Freudian orthodoxy that fit nicely with folk wisdom to support the female stereotype.

The basic question was: If other cultures start from the same biological base and elaborate very different structures for the woman's role, why must women's differences and subordination be innately determined? This question takes into account cultural and social differences and the effects these factors have on sex-role socialization and performance. Men could no longer be viewed as innately aggressive, abstract thinkers and doers while women were innately nurturers and passive receivers. The stereotype for both women and men received more serious criticism than ever before.

One aim of role choices and changes should be the valuing of all roles in our society. Not all work is highly regarded or self-fulfilling for many women or men. Many people have dull, uninteresting jobs although in our society to have any job is better than having no job. The roles of homemaker and parent are fulfilling for many women and, in some instances, where traditional roles have reversed, they are also fulfilling for men. Change not only means that women have more opportunities and can work outside of the home, but change also can mean that society has a change of attitude towards traditional women's work, which includes wives, mothers, nurses, teachers, and so on. Sometimes the flavor of "true women's liberation" is laced with the notion that women should pursue a career and preferably not in a traditionally defined women's occupation. Is it possible that one rigid stereotype is being pushed and exchanged for another?

Women have been told by society's experts that working outside of the home and motherhood are antagonistic sorts of activity. Indeed, working has been viewed as a rejection of children and the maternal role: Either you are a good worker or a good mother. One empirical study addressing this point noted that if a woman shows a certain amount of interest and involvement in her work, whatever it is, the prognosis is better for her interest in and enjoyment of motherhood (Sears, Macoby, & Levin, 1957). The authors suggest that enjoyment of outside work and motherhood may well be reflections of an underlying style of dealing with whatever life situations the individual woman finds herself in. A psychiatrist whose practice is mostly women patients has said that this dichotomy would seem not to be between motherhood and career, but between women who do well in both and women who do well in neither (Rheingold, 1967).

Although this section has not been a complete presentation of the research on the topic and has tended to gloss over possible class and other differences, the point should be made nevertheless that more research needs to be done in the area of working women.

EQUALITY IN THE MARKETPLACE

It will not surprise anyone with the most cursory acquaintance with legal realities to read that the law has often accorded very different treatment to women and men solely because of sex. Voting rights, jury service, right to a separate domicile, causes of action for loss of consortium, capacity to enter into binding agreements and to sue and be sued, change of citizenship upon marriage to an alien, change of name upon marriage, and age of attaining majority are some of the more glaring areas in which the law has at times treated people differently due to their sex. Sex-discriminatory rules of law are by no means relics of the past. Sex-biased legal inequality continues as a fact of life (Kanowitz, 1969). In addition, although laws change to remedy some of the inequality, attitudes continue to affect women in negative ways and serve to cause stressful situations in some cases.

To develop this point more specifically, women in this country continue to receive the short end of the salary stick. Although Congress passed the Equal Pay Act in 1963 (equal pay for equal work), women still are paid far less than their male counterparts. According to recent Labor Department statistics, women working full time received an average of

$224 per week in 1981 compared to $347 per week for men, a difference of 35.5%. For every $100 a man earned, women earned just $64.70. Some economists have long held that women earn less because of their relative inexperience, which prevents them from holding high-paying positions. In 1981, Labor Department figures show, however, that women received considerably less than men in the same occupations. For example, men averaged $366 per week in sales work, women only $190, a difference of 48%. Where male salaried lawyers average $574 per week, females average $407. Men cooks average $202 per week; women cooks average $148. Men service workers such as janitors, cleaners, and so on, received $238 per week but women only $170 per week. According to another study conducted in 1980, women constitute the poorest people in the United States. Ninety percent of those receiving minimum Social Security benefits are women; 69% of food stamps are issued to households headed by women; 61% of all Medicare enrollees are women; 80% of households receiving money from the Aid to Families with Dependent Children program are headed by women. Three out of every four Americans living in poverty (by federal government definition) are women (Shearer, 1982). Some of these figures reflect the difference in male/female longevity but they all illustrate the economic and social standing that women have in this society. One can predict that as recent federal governmental cutbacks occur, affecting women more than any other group since they are more dependent on federal agencies, we will see more social and familial disorganization and more evidence of psychological stress.

Although women now constitute more than 40% of the labor force, as mentioned previously, the public perceives little progress towards equalizing employment opportunities for them. In fact, comparison of a 1982 Gallup survey with one taken in 1975 reveals that fewer women now (41%) than seven years ago (49%) perceive that equal job opportunities exist for the sexes. A concomitant number (an increase from 46% to 54%) believe that women are discriminated against in employment. In both this and the earlier poll, 46% of men thought women had equal job opportunities and 50% did not. Women with formal jobs outside of the home did not believe that women had equal opportunities in the marketplace, and women without formal jobs took the opposite stance (Gallup, 1982).

In another area, unequal treatment flows from persistent but, in many cases, false ideas about women. As mentioned earlier, 51% of all married women in the United States work outside the home. This is over 25 million women. Like men, they pay Social Security taxes on an individual basis. But the government awards benefits on a family basis. Thus, both married women who work and the much smaller group of men and women who never marry receive smaller benefits related to taxes than the married "head of household" with a dependent spouse. Another inequality of the present rules is that the married couples where both husband and wife work receive on the average smaller benefits related to taxes paid than if the family income had been the same but the wife had never worked. The benefits of two-worker retired families average about 17% less than those of a one-worker family with the same income covered by Social Security (Ricardo-Campbell, 1982).

Once a woman decides to work outside the home, she finds only a limited number of jobs available. When a society experiences economic "hard times" such as the recession of 1982, this limitation takes on special meanings. In some instances, women do better at finding a job than do men in some occupational groupings but since women are already concentrated in certain industries and occupations these can absorb only so many additional women. As of March, 1974, 76% of all employed women worked in the service sector (Hayghe, 1974). Within the service sector, women tend to be concentrated in specific industries that have traditionally employed them. For example, in 1973, women made up 46% of retail trade employees, more than 80% of hospital employees, and 61% of elementary and secondary school teachers, but only 42% of college and university faculty members (Waldman & McEaddy, 1974). One indication of the limited job opportunities open to women is that half of all working women work in just 21 of the 250 occupations listed by the Bureau of the Census. One-quarter of all employed women work in only five jobs: secretary-stenographer, household worker, bookkeeper, elementary school teacher, and waitress (Hedges, 1979).

A somewhat different but important issue, that of turnover, reflects employer beliefs that women workers are less likely than men to stay on the job and, therefore, they are justified in discriminating against them. Even if it was true that women on the average were more likely to quit their jobs than men, this would not justify treating individual women as if they all conformed to the average (Blau, 1978). We have no data to answer the question of turnover in a definite way. When we examine averages, men tend to stay on the job longer than women, but this can be misleading. Other factors such as age and marital status are not always taken into account. The public's view of the turnover problem developed at a time when the typical woman worker was young, single, and apt to leave work permanently when she married. This situation is no longer the case. What needs examination is whether women receive the same incentives to stay on the job as do men. Employer practices that restrict women to low-paying, dead-end jobs and deny them access to training programs encourage turnover. Sometimes the lack of maternity leave forces younger women to leave their jobs permanently. Thus, something of a vicious circle becomes established with regard to turnover and the attitudes toward it.

All of the above remarks lead us to the conclusion that women suffer from a stereotype in our society that affects their work opportunities and social and economic status in negative ways.

SPECIAL POPULATIONS

Many girls and women experience conflict between traditional notions of femininity and occupational or intellectual achievement (Laws, 1976). Women's potential for occupational achievement is underdeveloped, underutilized, and underrated in our society even today. This conflict, a complex but potent factor, affects sex-role socialization as well as achievement and career orientation on the job for those women who do work outside of the home. Conflicting values and the resulting ambivalent attitude toward the job that some women experience has great implications, especially for those occupations traditionally defined as women's work, such as nursing.

Minority Women

Previous comments in this chapter have demonstrated discrimination against women in the work place, but some women experience a double dose of discrimination. Many minority women, for example, suffer from their status as both women and minority group members. The term "minority women" means women of races other than white and white women of Spanish decent. This group composes more than 18% of the female population in our country and more than five million of them work outside the home. Data show us that minority women are not uniformly disadvantaged. For example, Asian-American women are very close to white women in occupational status and salary earnings. Mexican-American women are entering the labor force in increasing numbers but the low educational level for many, especially in the Southwest, and the high proportion of families with preschool children mean that those who do obtain jobs outside the home will experience disadvantages.

The labor force status of black women greatly changed from 1960 to 1970 in that more of them sought white-collar clerical and female-dominated professional occupations. This shift improved their status more than their income. The Native American woman confronts the most difficult situation because she finds herself caught between staying on the reservation, where she has little opportunity or power, or leaving it and rupturing traditional kinship ties (Almuguist & Wehrle-Einhorn, 1978). The usual pecking order with regard to economic status from highest to lowest is: white male, black male, white female, and black female. This last category includes some other minority women as well as black women.

As of the mid-1970s, minority women constituted 16% of all women in the U.S. labor force. Numerous studies have been conducted focusing on women employees, but this term has generally meant white women. Studies of black workers have focused on black men almost exclusively, and research on other minority women is scarce. Not only are women who work at home and are an important factor in the overall economy essentially invisible, but in much of our data minority women also tend to be invisible. This fact in itself can cause us to raise questions about society's attitude toward women in general and toward minority women in particular.

Older Women

The median age of women workers is now 42 years, or about the same age as men workers. Marriage no longer takes many women out of the work world and mothers of school-age children are more likely to be working than not. The work experience of mature women differs from that of men and younger women in several important ways. The kind of jobs they do, the rewards they seek from work, and the manner in which work becomes woven into the patterns of their lives point to a certain set of constraints that affect the work decisions of women in midlife (Rosenthal, 1978). Older women must compete with young women for traditional female jobs in a work world where many employers (men) prefer young women. Blue-collar jobs at low skill levels employ the largest proportion of older women workers. In addition, women with jobs tend to work an average of 10 hours per week longer than men or housewives (longer if they are employed full time) due to the double duty of work at home and work outside the home (Time Use Studies, 1973). The traditionally defined role structure of the nuclear family also can serve to limit a woman's choice of job possibilities. This line of reasoning goes as follows: Older women have fewer job opportunities because their skills are obsolete. They withdrew from the labor force to attend family needs and after some years have returned. There are two assumptions here that may not be true for many older women workers. First, it assumes that women had job skills initially and, second, that jobs open to them require some skill. The first assumption has a middle-class bias and the second one overlooks the type of jobs available to older women.

In summary, these special categories of women, minority status by race and/or age, are much more complex than indicated here. More data are needed and the task then becomes one of examining these data in light of mental health issues for all women including minority and older women.

MENTAL HEALTH ISSUES FOR WOMEN

Over the past 20 years, the number of people receiving psychiatric help has more than doubled. Of this number, women have been overrepresented in proportion to their numbers in the population (Chesler, 1971, 1972). No one knows why this situation exists. One factor, the male/female stereotypes, allows women to seek help and thereby enter the mental health system whereas men are more likely to enter the criminal justice system. Another factor may be that people accept psychological treatment more readily and have greater knowledge of available facilities where they can obtain help. In addition, people live more stressful lives and this may be especially true for women, particularly those working in the labor force in larger numbers for the first time.

Sex Differences in Symptomatic Behaviors

Statistics on women in psychiatric treatment reveal some striking patterns. Women with certain life-styles and in certain age ranges experience certain types of disorders more than other types (Bernard, 1971). These patterns may provide some clues as to which factors contribute to psychological disorder in women.

Married women seek psychological help more than married men, while single women by this measure seem better adjusted than single men. Married women, the most heavily represented group in psychiatric treatment, use both hospitalization and private psychotherapy more than any other group.

The age at which women experience a particularly high risk for psychological disorders gives us an additional clue as to what experiences might be stressful. Although people of all ages seek psychiatric treatment, especially large numbers of women in their late thirties and forties do so. Women appear more likely to seek help for some disorders than for others. According to a late 1950s study, the feelings and behaviors prevalent among women in treatment most often fall into a category labeled "turning against the self" (Phillips & Rabinovitch, 1958). Women more often experience feelings of inadequacy and inferiority, excessive guilt, and depression. Suicide attempts are between six and ten times more common for women than for men. By comparison, the disorders prevalent among men typify "turning against others" such as antisocial behavior, low control over violent impulses, and breaking social conventions by abusing drugs and alcohol. We do not know what causes this difference between men and women and, lacking biological evidence, we look at the social and situational context of men's and women's lives to understand them.

On the one hand, the medical model in psychiatry attempts to explain all psychological stress and disorders as consequences of faulty genes, physiology, or biochemistry. Such explanations leave little room for variations in one's life roles and expectations and do not take into account the social context. However, biological factors cannot be dismissed since much recent research supports this explanation. The psychodynamic model, on the other hand, emphasizes responses to stress that one learned in early childhood and minimizes the role played by the very real conflicts in the person's adult life.

Real factors experienced by adults such as economic hardship, racial or sexual stereotyping, and discrimination may also be psychologically stressful. The types of stress that people encounter are to some extent influenced by their sex, age, race, and socioeconomic status. Another explanation of the sex-stereotyped pattern of psychological disorders suggests that differences in the stressful situations faced by each sex lead to the disparity in men's and women's responses. This means that an individual's sex role significantly determines the subjective meaning and importance of a stressful occurrence. Women, as members of a low-status group, often have less power than men in interpersonal relationships, in political life, and in occupational roles. Low status and low power can result in lowered self-esteem, feelings of worthlessness, feelings of powerlessness and submissiveness, and suppression of anger.

Yet another explanation holds that the difference between people who cope successfully with stressful situations and those who develop psychological disorders can be found in their capacity for dealing with stress. People who use ineffective or limited coping mechanisms may be more likely to develop psychological disorders than others. One common limitation of possible behavior comes from sex-role stereotypes. Perhaps people whose behavior conforms to rigid sex-role expectations will be less capable of coping with a broad range of stressful situations. People who hold extremely masculine or feminine self-perceptions perform poorly in situations requiring more flexibility in behavior (Bem, 1975). No direct evidence, however, supports the idea that people whose behavior in stressful situations conforms rigidly to sex stereotypes are at higher risk for mental disorder.

Stress, Sex Roles, and Coping

The person's sex role strongly affects the subjective significance of stressful events. Sex-typed interpretations of life events tend to occur in areas of experience where the culture maintains rigid prescriptions for appropriate sex-role behavior. In the United States, for example, generally speaking, marriage has different meanings for men and women, so marital discord may affect both but may affect women more. This difference reflects role investments and self-esteem.

Four common components of women's experiences have received attention in the literature: marital roles, aging, socioeconomic status, and female physiology. Of course, not all women experience these factors as stressful. The great majority of women cope successfully with these experiences and avoid actual disorder.

A survey of psychiatric treatment facilities' clientele shows that the incidence of psychological disorders is higher among married women than married men and lower among single women than single men (Cannon & Redick, 1973). This survey and other such findings do not provide grounds to condemn all marriages or marriage per se. But they do help one to examine aspects of this situation. In marriages, women often lose more legal and social autonomy. Additionally, working women generally play fewer major roles in the workplace, and the housewife role is ascribed to a woman when she marries as opposed to being achieved by her. Occupational roles for both men and women are achieved roles. Society expects people in ascribed roles such as housewife to perform competently, and, therefore, they receive few rewards though failures are dealt with harshly. The reverse is true for achieved roles. Yet another strain on married women emerges from reductions in the requirements and status associated with the traditional mother and housewife roles.

These differences in values and attitudes can lead to different reactions in numerous stressful events. Direct evidence concerning women's class backgrounds and role strains leading to psychological disorder is scarce. However, we do know that role strains can differ according to class status (Lopata, 1971). Again, another common component of women's experiences, their physical characteristics, can produce stressful situations. As a culture, we value feminine youth and physical beauty.

Historically, women have had lower social status and fewer legal rights than men. This inequity has led to a number of negative consequences such as loss of self-esteem, feelings of powerlessness, economic hardship, and less control over external events (Dohrenwend, 1973). But do any of these consequences make women more likely to experience stress? Some evidence points to a correlation, but caution must be exercised due to flaws in design, sampling problems, and lack of data. Obviously, more research is needed on this topic.

Many women experience these stresses and cope. What determines whether stresses will lead to psychological disorder or successful coping? The psychological disorders prevalent among women are passivity, low self-esteem, guilt, helplessness, and feelings of inadequacy.

Therefore, one can conceptualize women with psychological disorders as those who exhibit exaggerations of the feminine stereotype (Bem, 1975; Frieze, 1978). However, much research fails to demonstrate that women's personalities differ from men's (Maccoby, 1966). Specifically, sex differences in dependence, passivity-activity, nurturance, and self-esteem failed to emerge clearly with samples of normal children and adults. One possible conclusion points to sex-role extremes as associated with psychological disorder and not reflective of the general population.

With regard to women's response to psychological stress, there is much that is not known. However, in the meantime, we must use language and concepts to order the raw data of experience. We can easily fall back on stereotypes that are negative in this culture for women. It is easy for mental health professionals to stereotype women and to proceed with psychotherapy or other treatment according to this stereotype. For example, twice as many women as men have used minor tranquilizers, 50% more women than men have used barbiturates, and three times as many women are reported using amphetamines for medical purposes. Drug company advertisements have supported certain images and stereotypes. In these ads, men are sick and women are neurotic. This is complicated because several interacting variables come together. Women are more apt to seek help from others, but also physicians are more apt to view women as neurotic and to prescribe corresponding drugs for them.

THEORIES OF FEMININE PERSONALITY

The early twentieth century witnessed a profound change in psychology, which revolutionized our view of human behavior. This change, of course, was Freud's pioneering work in psychoanalysis. Today, in the United States, much of the field of personality development has been derived from the psychoanalytic tradition. Many people both in the general population and in mental health professions question the validity of numerous Freudian concepts; however, a brief examination of selected ones shows their influence and impact on female sex-role stereotyping.

Many of Freud's speculations about women remain basic to psychoanalytic theory today despite the lack of corroborating research data. Freud described both sexes as "little men." Maleness was the norm and femaleness was a deviation from that norm. Because girls lack a penis, both boys and girls view them as inferior. This traumatic discovery causes the girl to hold the mother responsible for her loss, and, because the mother lacks the highly valued penis, Freud believed that the mother and all females become greatly devalued in the eyes of both girls and boys. The girl regards men with profound envy and joins all males in disdaining women. The girl's penis envy motivates her to renounce her love for her mother and turn to her father, while at the same time she renounces her clitoris and shifts her erotic focus to the vagina, the mature female sex organ according to Freud (who viewed the clitoris as masculine).

The girl acquires her superego and her feminine identity from her mother but, because of these basic developmental differences, Freud believed that women cannot develop as strong a superego as men since the motive for its formation is lacking. Women remain forever morally and ethically undeveloped compared to men.

Additionally, Freud believed that the libido functions less effectively in women than in men. The libido, essentially active or masculine, becomes more constrained in the woman. This means that the normal process of female development demands more sexual repression than does male development.

Freud did recognize the limited, tentative nature of his formulations about women and, in 1933, said during a speech, "If you want to know more about femininity you must interrogate your own experiences or turn to the poets, or else wait until science can give you more coherent information" (in Strause, 1974). Science has presented more coherent information since Freud's words of 1933. But many clinical practitioners continue to adhere to the original notions, which fit into a cultural, social stereotype of women with a masculine bias and a basic belief in the biological inferiority of women. This is not a formulation that lends itself easily to testing, since it is more a matter of value and subjective belief. This assigning of values to biology has caused widespread criticism of Freud's theory of women, although it did fit with Victorian values. Even if clinicians do not believe these concepts in their entirety, they can, nevertheless, retain the attitudes toward women that accompany them.

Freud takes the male as the norm for his theories and sees the female as an inadequate male. Numerous problems arise with this approach. A woman is not a man, and males and females exist with certain inherent and socially conditioned differences. Assigning one sex a higher value than the other has had profound negative consequences for both sexes but especially for women.

Karen Horney (1967) emphasized the importance of social and cultural values as the context for biophysical phenomena. She proposed the then-radical notion that women might have a psychology of their own, not derived from analogies to men. Horney shared Freud's belief that penis envy was a regular feature of a girl's development but she differed from Freud in a number of important ways. She viewed penis envy as, among other things, the girl's recognition of the superior social status awarded to males. Although emphasizing the anxiety in female development, as well as that in male development, Horney specifically rejected psychoanalytic concepts about female masochism. She demonstrated that cultural factors such as lack of effective outlets for sexual expression for women, the belief in the inferiority of women, the economic dependence of women on men, and the restriction of women to emotionally centered spheres of life could adequately account for the female tendency toward masochism.

Clara Thompson (1964) believed that neurotic traits were more a product of culture than of one's sex. She realized that biological factors could not be ignored; however, she thought that psychological difficulties resulted from a sociohistorical situation that could not adequately provide for the fulfillment of biological needs. Like Horney, Thompson argued that many of the behaviors of women that a Freudian analyst probably would interpret as penis envy actually resulted from envy of male status. In a patriarchal and competitive culture, women could be expected to experience envy apart from biological sex differences. Thompson questioned Freud's assertion of the biological base for such "feminine traits" as narcissism, weak superego, and psychic rigidity and, for all of these, she offered convincing social explanations. She believed that one of modern woman's most serious conflicts concerns childbearing. She wrote that women were socialized to believe that adequate sexual fulfillment, including childbearing, was not compatible with self-development and creative self-expression. This attitude was at least partly a result of lack of social supports for creative activity for the woman with children. Thompson also challenged Freud's concept of the equivalence of a penis with a baby and stated that childbearing is a sufficiently biological function to have value for its own sake. She said, "Surely, only a man could have thought of it in terms of compensation or consolation" (1964, p. 232).

Jung's use of masculine and feminine archetypes gives a biological as well as a spiritual basis to the traditional male and female stereotypes. His theories could assist in providing a scientific rationale for the traditional roles of women and men. However, his emphasis on the integration of the male and female aspects of one's personality can also be viewed as one means of achieving androgyny.

Erik Erikson accepts most basic principles of Freudian personality theory, but he emphasizes the social and cultural factors in continual interaction with the biological factors, which he says are basic to all sex differences, including differences in personality. He believes that a woman's potential for motherhood creates the central focus of her identity and that her other personality characteristics derive in large part from her childbearing and child-rearing potential. He regards her participation in nonmothering roles as secondary to her primary function. Erikson emphasizes the positive aspects of femininity as part of his tendency to stress health rather than pathology. He disagreed with Freud that normal functioning could be understood completely from the study of pathology and believed that many of Freud's ideas do not apply to normal women and girls. He developed the concept of womb envy and thinks it more important than penis envy. Generally, Erikson is helpful due to his efforts to reinterpret the psychoanalytic view of femininity in a more positive and primary light, his recognition of the importance in feminine personality of a woman's maternal functions, and especially his understanding of male psychology with regard to women. However, he still sees women's natural maternal function as the determinant of her personality and underestimates the weight of social factors in determining a woman's personality. His turn away from Freud's negative view of women to a romantic, idealized, maternal view of women tends to be equally male-identified. Although these theories have given us a profoundly different view of the human species, they also have maintained basic stereotypes of women as well as men. Therefore, it might be useful to examine selected research on sex differences in personality.

SEX DIFFERENCES IN PERSONALITY

Many people hold the stereotype in our society that women are passive, dependent, quiet, gentle, unintelligent, and generally inferior to the average man. We think of the average adult man as active, aggressive, independent, neither quiet nor gentle, intelligent, and superior to women. How valid are these stereotypes? In many instances, the data remain incomplete or inconsistent; however, it might be the case that the actual differences between the sexes are not as great as many believe. Many studies have either failed to find the expected differences or have found them to be relatively small.

The studies of aggression have yielded a large number of consistent findings. More than 48 studies reviewed by Oetzel (1966) found that males exhibit more aggressive behavior than females. What does this sex difference mean? Aggression is usually conceptualized in terms of overt, physical behavior; however, a good definition must include an underlying motive. Several indications point to the possibility that females may not differ much from males in aggressive drive or motivation. In nonphysical measures of aggression, the differences become clear and, in some of these instances, females express more aggressive behavior than males. Strong evidence does support the hypothesis that males behave more aggressively than females at all ages. However, other research suggests that these sex differences in overt aggression may be partly due to the masculine sex-typing of aggressive responses. This situation means that females recognize that the culture has defined aggressive behavior as unfeminine and, therefore, they will experience anxiety when responding aggressively and will limit aggression to private or permissive situations or express it in an indirect way. This belief would be especially true for overt physical aggression, the type of aggression maximized by sex-role differences.

The usual definition of dependency—reliance on others for help, approval, and attention—involves a number of different but related behaviors. Psychologists usually focus on two dependency-related behaviors, suggestibility and conformity. Although many believe that females are more passive and dependent and more easily influenced than are males, empirical verification of these stereotypes remains much less clear than the support for the aggressive stereotype. Recently, the legitimacy of the assumption that females tend to be more dependent at any age has been questioned. Current research fails to show consistent sex effects in dependency-related behaviors (Maccoby & Jacklin, 1974).

Recent studies have also created doubt on the generality of this sex difference. Women's supposedly greater interest in other people does not seem to result in their having more ability to judge emotions (Tagiuri & Petrullo, 1958) or develop more sensitivity to social cues (Maccoby & Jacklin, 1974). Some indication of sex differences in empathy has been found. Studies measuring a social orientation in task situations have usually found no sex differences (Ruble, 1975; Ruble & Nakamura, 1972). Several findings contradict the stereotype that females are more cooperative than males (Cook & Stingle, 1974). Basically, the extent of sex differences in social orientation remains inconclusive at present.

Mass media and popular fiction fill our minds with the stereotype that women are more emotional than men. The emotional woman becomes flustered in a minor crisis. She is sensitive, fearful, and anxious, and she cries easily. However, we need to realize that sex bias exists in what behaviors become thought of as emotional. Emotionality usually refers to fearfulness, anxiety, moodiness, and neuroticism as opposed to acting-out behaviors and maladjustments that fit the male stereotype. Research on emotionality tends to support the stereotype that females are more emotional than males, at least after early childhood. However, investigators examining anxiety and fearfulness have mostly used paper-and-pencil measures and these present numerous problems. Therefore, some studies have attempted to avoid these problems by using physiological measures of emotionality. They assume that increases in physiological indicators such as heartbeat, pulse, or respiration indicate an increase in emotional arousal. In contrast to overt behavioral or self-reported studies, which usually report females to be more emotionally responsive, physiological measures yield inconsistent results.

Such factors as physical attributes, intellectual capacity, personality traits, and perceptions of how others view one affect one's self-concept. Differences in self-concept on psychological measures refer to level of positive or negative self-evaluation. Males are stereotyped as being more self-confident than females, but empirical verification of this stereotype has been weak except in achievement-related areas. Few studies have directly compared the levels of positive self-concept of males and females on standardized scales. Studies, using one of the standard personality scales, either have not examined sex differences or have not found any (Coopersmith, 1967; Primavera, Simon, & Primavera, 1974). Of 39 comparisons of various measures of self-esteem, females scored high on 9, males on 6, and no differences were found on the remaining 24. The sexes do not seem to differ on generalized measures of self-esteem. For studies of achievement-related competence or expectations for success, however, it has been fairly well established that females perceive themselves as less competent than men. Females have relatively negative evaluations of their own abilities, performance, and likelihood of future success as compared to males.

The study of stereotypic traits and values provides a more indirect approach to self-concept. There have been numerous indications that society more highly values men and masculine attributes than it does women and feminine attributes. Because masculine activities are generally preferred over feminine activities, many more women than men recall a desire to be men. Consistent with this general trend, occupational prestige decreases when increased proportions of women enter a given profession. Stereotypic feminine attributes are devalued relative to male attributes; nevertheless, females do not show a consistently less positive self-concept than males except in areas related to achievement.

Finally, what kinds of generalizations can we draw concerning sex differences in personality? Little data support the notion that many strong and consistent personality differences exist between males and females. It appears, however, that when studies in a specific area are taken as a whole, the resultant differences lie in the direction of the predominant stereotype. Of all the traits listed, the strongest difference can be found in physical aggression. But it must be noted that this reporting of research findings has in no way dealt with methodological, sampling, research bias, and other problems that can have major effects on findings.

THE THERAPIST AND SEX-ROLE STEREOTYPES

The replacement of maladaptive behavior, thought, and feeling patterns with more positive and more socially acceptable ones that also promote growth for the individual remains the goal of mental health services. The choice of specific goals of therapeutic change for individual patients is strongly influenced by the therapist; therefore, the question of therapist sex bias becomes an important one.

Several studies of therapists demonstrate that, for the most part, their images of women conform to traditional stereotypes and can best be described as somewhat negative (Broverman, Clarkson, Rosenkrantz, & Vogel, 1972; Fabrikant, Landau, & Rollenhagen, 1973; Nowacki & Poe, 1973). The first Broverman study (1970) gave female and male clinicians a list of adjectives and asked them to indicate which adjectives characterized a healthy male, a healthy female, and a healthy adult without reference to sex. These clinicians' answers highly differentiated sex roles. They described the male as more logical, more independent, and less emotional than the female. Those adjectives that they used to describe a healthy male also characterized a healthy adult without reference to sex, but those used to describe a healthy female did not match with the healthy adult. This result means that women are placed in a double bind: If they act like women they are not being healthy adults, and if they act like healthy adults they are acting like men. Therapists viewed women in a negative way and, importantly, the characteristics they used to describe them they often use to describe mentally ill individuals. Kjervik and Palta (1978) replicated the Boverman study with 125 master's prepared nurses. They found that these nurses considered healthy adults more like men than women. This implies that they thought of adults as males and of females as a separate class.

How do these negative sex-role stereotypes operate in actual therapist-client relationships? Here the evidence is very sparse indeed. Psychotherapy is a difficult subject for study; it is highly unstructured and private and occurs over an indeterminate period of time. Additionally, the therapist's goals and values remain most often implicit rather than explicit and are conveyed to the client only in subtle ways such as nonverbal cues. Psychological testing, easier to explore for research purposes, has been examined.

Psychological tests, often given prior to therapy and used to formulate diagnosis and to assess the client's strengths and weaknesses, show evidence of sex bias in the administration, scoring, or interpretation, as has been documented by Harris (1974). This evidence that psychological testers may shift their evaluation of the client's personality or behavior according to the client's sex could point to possible sex bias in the therapeutic interactions as well.

Zeldow's (1978) empirical review of sex differences in psychiatric evaluation and treatment becomes important here. He reviewed 25 studies, nearly all of them published since 1970. Though such studies offer ample evidence of the responsiveness of behavioral scientists and mental health professionals to charges of sexist clinical practices, Zeldow says that they do not provide sufficient grounds for more than tenuous conclusions. The proper research question is not whether sex-related biases in clinical practice exist; instead, we must ask what aspects of psychiatric treatment, practiced by whom, tend to be influenced by the sex of the patient and under what circumstances. By itself, the sex of a patient or client rarely acts as a factor in determining diagnosis, prognosis, degree of psychopathology, or treatment goals. A large and possibly diminishing minority of clinicians hold separate standards of mental health for men and women. We do not know in what ways such sex-role stereotyping affects the help that women receive from mental health professionals. However, we do not need more research to state that it is inappropriate for a therapist to assume that a female client's problems will be solved or ameliorated by entry into, or more complete commitment to, traditional roles such as marriage, homemaking, and child-rearing.

Research results indicate with frequency that the patient's sex must be considered in combination with other variables in order for sex-related treatment and assessment differences to emerge. Four general areas of sex bias and sex-role stereotyping in psychotherapeutic practice have been delineated: fostering of traditional sex roles, bias in expectations and devaluation of women, sexist use of psychoanalytic concepts, and responding to women as sex objects.

The most strident claims of sex discrimination in this field cannot be supported by current research evidence. On the other hand, research has, to date, concerned itself insufficiently with the connection between its paper-and-pencil measures of clinician intentions and actual clinical behavior. Many of the published studies that show evidence of sex-related biases need replication. Further research must attempt to approximate more closely actual clinical conditions and to avoid a shot-gun approach to research by selecting variables for study with an eye to their theoretical and previously demonstrated relevance.

EFFECTS OF STEREOTYPES ON PSYCHIATRIC MENTAL HEALTH CLINICAL NURSE SPECIALISTS

Just as society deprives women of their proportional share of the social, economic, and political values, so similar gender inequalities can be found in the health field. One factor of this inequality is that, although women account for about 60% of the contacts with physicians, medicine remains a male-dominated system. Interestingly enough, at the turn of the century, physicians constituted about 80% of all health care givers while at the present time they constitute about 12%. Health care provided by numerous different people in a complex division-of-labor system depends on women employees to a large extent. It has been argued that the health industry is not simply a service industry but a powerful instrument of social control, replacing organized religion as a prime source of sexist ideology and a major enforcer of sex roles (Ehrenreich & English, 1973).

Stereotypes of Women as Providers of Care

Cleland (1971) has made it very clear that the problems of women in the society account for many of the problems encountered by nurses as an occupational group. Women have functioned in health care positions that can best be described as supportive. This tends to be the case with most, if not all, traditionally defined female occupations. The status of a female occupation in a male-dominated culture becomes problematic due to stereotypes. These stereotypes serve to maintain the status quo socially and economically.

This factor means that, for economic and sociopolitical reasons, those in power can use the stereotypes of both men (rational, adventuresome, strong, dependable, etc.) and women (emotional, passive, weak, undependable, etc.) to continue the distribution of opportunities as presently organized and to maintain societal structures that impact on these opportunities. This situation, in turn, has an impact on such questions as who can function by performing what tasks, who can be paid what amount and by whom, and who can be involved in what kinds of decisions?

Generally speaking, over the years, in this country, nurses have been employed by patients while student nurses did the ongoing work in hospitals for those who could not afford private nurses. After World War II, a shift occurred in employment patterns and most nurses now work for some type of agency such as a hospital, health clinic, or doctor's office. Such groups have been referred to as semiprofessionals in the literature. This concept implies that semiprofessions in comparison to professional groups are more bureaucratic and subject to numerous rules governing not just the central work tasks but extraneous details of conduct on the job (Katz, 1969). Such sociopolitical and economic realities have importance for nursing as a whole and affect all nurses including those who define themselves as practitioners. Underlying this definition of semiprofessional, one finds at work, to a large extent, the stereotypical images of women.

It has only been in this century that we in this country have begun to address the ethical issue of equality. Inequality has been the norm for many centuries and has been reflected in the haves and have-nots of our society such as men and women, whites and blacks, and so on. These deeply rooted prejudices have become a part of our taken-for-granted world. That is to say, *of course,* everyone knows that men are more intelligent than women, that men are more dependable than women since they do not get so emotional about situations. Or, so goes the often unexamined belief underpinning all sorts of decisions having to do with what is right and proper for members of our society. Nursing has historically been subjugated to medicine in large part not because what nurses do is unimportant but for socioeconomic reasons that are laced with traditional stereotypes. This historical reality makes it difficult, but not impossible, for nursing to create and implement new roles such as nurse practitioners and clinical nurse specialists even though data support the need for such roles in our society. Such difficulty can become monumental in an era of scarcity coupled with a glut of physicians in the work force. Stereotypes will be used consciously and unconsciously to maintain the status quo. Such stereotypical definitions are extremely functional to those in decision-making positions who determine the sociopolitical and economic arrangements in the work world of health care.

Social, Political, and Economic Effects

The first necessity for those in clinical nurse specialist roles as well as for other nurses is to think of their work world in these economic and sociopolitical terms as well as the usual clinical terms. One cannot fully understand the forces that affect one's work world without these concepts. And, importantly, one cannot change the larger structural world surrounding one's work without such an understanding. Only as we view situations from various perspectives can we understand, plan, and change. Being a good practitioner is not enough. In order to provide health care, we must examine the larger issues and concepts in order to get the whole picture. In this process, we need to remember that economic, social, and political concepts serve as our most practical tools because they give us ways of organizing the raw data of experience and of viewing the world in which we live and work.

Potential for Discrimination Within the Speciality

As clinical nurse specialists examine their own world from the perspective of these socioeconomic factors, they should also extend their insights into the nature of their work. Both research and our experience of the everyday world indicate that women, including those who function as clinical nurse specialists, often harbor negative feelings and attitudes towards women. They, like others socialized in this culture, can and do stereotype women into such categories as "just a housewife," "an aggressive career woman," "a dumb blond." Importantly, we must realize that our knowledge is often biased in that data are gathered from a sample of men and models are constructed based on these data; when women do not fit the model, they are labeled as deviant or "less than." The model itself does not receive another examination to determine how well it measures what it is supposed to measure (Gilligan, 1982).

Women constitute not only the majority of those who seek help from the mental health service delivery system but women also constitute many, if not most, of those who provide these health services. If one accepts these two statements as facts, then they force one to examine one's own attitudes and behaviors regarding women in general, for stereotyping does not begin with patients and clients. We are sexist when we say such things as "I prefer a man boss to a woman boss," "I don't like to spend my time only with women because I find men so much more interesting," "I would never go to all of this trouble to make this cake if women only were going to be there," etc.

Much of this sexist attitude is out of our awareness but comes to the surface in our language and specifically in those behaviors that reflect these stereotypes. When we call women by their first name without some relationship to permit that behavior and the other's permission to do so or when we join the men at their lunch table so that we do not have to interact with the "girls," we may be viewing the situation from the perspective of stereotypes. This is not to say that all women are wonderfully engaging socially or professionally but then neither are all men.

Clinical nurse specialists have many opportunities to break through these narrow stereotypes of women as they work with women clients. One of the most important factors to emerge from the women's movement together with awareness of social and economic oppression is the notion of friendship between and among women that can serve as a support system. When we expand the concept of relationships to go beyond the usual female-male couple and the family unit, we have a larger reality within which to function, to perceive, and to evaluate situations. Surely the days when both female nurses and male physicians told women that they would be better when they got married and had children have become relics from our recent past. Some women may want and need to marry and have children; other women may want and need not to marry and still have children; others may want and need neither to marry nor have children; still others may want and need to marry and not have children. The social movement referred to as the women's movement has attempted to establish choices for women, and only as clinical nurse specialists understand and act on this ideal, which is in part a reality, can women who come to them for help begin to experience what it means to be a woman in the fullest sense. Any use of stereotypes is problematic; therefore, we as health professionals must develop mechanisms to become more aware of those we hold for both women and men. The first such mechanism is self-awareness and awareness of others with regard to sex and sex-role stereotypes.

It has been common historically for men and women to blame women for any number of things, including mental illness. The literature refers to this as blaming the victim. Examples of blaming can be found in the following. Rape victims historically have felt guilt because, among other things, the social establishment told them that "they got what they had asked for." Police, courts, health professionals, and others still blame rape victims, but this has begun to change to some extent. One reason for this change can be found in women who will not put up with such sexist biases on the part of others. And this behavior has grown out of knowledge about the facts involved in rape. Another factor influencing this change has been a heightened awareness on the part of the establishment.

Some believe that a part of the debate regarding abortion can be traced to our unconscious beliefs and attitudes about women being blamed because they caused the fall of man. We have been told since before the golden days of Greece that women are morally inferior and therefore blameworthy.

All of these sex stereotypes and the blaming of the victim become and remain problematic because they are most often out of our awareness. They also still seem for many to be normal ways of thinking and behaving. Any clinical nurse specialist who has not examined these stereotypes in therapeutic relationships with women might possibly be of limited therapeutic value to these clients. As mentioned earlier in this chapter, the Broverman studies (1970, 1972) showed that mental health professionals do not differ in their negative stereotypes of women from the population in general. This fact should not surprise us since we received our socialization in a sexist environment in which we did not examine and question the assumptions underlying these attitudes and behaviors towards women.

This chapter has given no specific clinical example as such because the assumption has been made that these sex and sex-role stereotypes permeate most if not all situations, both social and therapeutic. When one makes that assumption, it puts one on guard against oneself. All clinical nurse specialists need constantly to examine and probe their own attitudes, beliefs, and behaviors to avoid sexist thinking and behavior. This is no easy task, for the reasons already stated; such attitudes, beliefs and behaviors have become part of our taken-for-granted world, always the most difficult aspect of reality to perceive and examine. Such an examination has the potential of also demonstrating the disparity between one's ideal self and one's real self. The possibility exists for many of us that we will never be able to break out of our sex stereotypes completely, but that does not relieve us of the professional and ethical obligation to try. One needs to be very honest with oneself but that, after all, is central to being therapeutic with any client or patient.

SUMMARY

This chapter began with a brief glimpse of the historical aspects of stereotypes of women. It then moved to examine some of the issues involved in role changes for women with a major focus on married women and married mothers. These comments received further elaboration within the context of the notion of equality in the marketplace. A brief discussion focused on special populations, here limited to minority women and older women, and the double-barreled situation in which they live and work.

The chapter then turned to an examination of mental health issues for women, with particular attention to the concepts of stress, sex roles, and coping. Theories of feminine personality that provide us with theoretical frameworks for clinical practice were shown to have major sex biases and stereotypes in them. And, to extend this line of reasoning, a section of the chapter was given over to a discussion of sex differences in personality studies. Do men and women differ psychologically, and if so, in what ways? That serves as the basic question for the personality studies reported here.

Then the chapter presented a brief look at the therapist's sex-role stereotyping with special emphasis on what effects such stereotyping has had on the clinical nurse specialist as a woman herself and as a professional working with women clients.

Two points have been made several times in this chapter. Stereotyping women and, by indirection, men can have grave consequences both for individuals and for society. Such attitudes, beliefs, and behaviors have become so ingrained in us that we often cannot see them, and therefore we victimize ourselves as women, as well as victimizing other women, our clients and patients.

REFERENCES

Agonito, R. (Ed.), *History of ideas on women.* New York: Putnam Publishing Group, 1977.

Almuquist, E. M., & Wehrle-Einhorn, J. L. The double disadvantaged: Minority women in the labor force. In A. H. Stromberg & S. Harkess (Eds.), *Women working: Theories and facts in perspective.* Palo Alto, CA: Mayfield, 1978.

Basch, F. *Relative creatures.* New York: Shocken Books, 1974.

Bem, S. L. Sex role adaptability. *Journal of Personality and Social Psychology,* 1975, *31,* 634–643.

Bernard, J. The paradox of the happy marriage. In V. Gornick & B. K. Moran (Eds.), *Women in sexist society.* New York: Basic Books, 1971.

Blau, F. D. The data on women workers, past, present, and future. In A. H. Stromberg & S. Harkess (Eds.), *Women working: Theories and facts in perspective.* Palo Alto, CA: Mayfield, 1978.

Blood, R. O., & Wolfe, D. M. *Husbands and wives: The dynamics of married living.* New York: Free Press, 1960.

Bodichon, B. *Women and work.* London: Sherwood, Gilbert & Piper, 1857.

Broverman, D., Clarkson, P., Rosenkrantz, P., & Vogel, S. Sex role stereotypes and clinical judgments of mental health. *Journal of Consulting and Clinical Psychology,* 1970, *34,* 1–7.

Broverman, D., Clarkson, P., Rosenkrantz, P., & Vogel, S. Sex role stereotypes: A current appraisal. *Journal of Social Issues,* 1972, *28,* 59–78.

Calder, J. *Women and marriage in Victorian fiction.* New York: Oxford University Press, 1976.

Cannon, M. S., & Redick, R. W. *Differential utilization of psychiatric facilities by men and women* (U.S. 1970, Department of HEW, NIMH). Washington, DC: U.S. Government Printing Office, 1973.

Chesler, P. Women as psychiatric and psychotherapeutic patients. *Journal of Marriage and Family,* 1971, *33,* 746–759.

Chesler, P. *Women and madness.* Garden City, NY: Doubleday, 1972.

Clark, A. *Working life of women in the seventeenth century.* London: Livingstone, 1919.

Cleland, V. Sex discrimination: Nursing's most pervasive problem. *American Journal of Nursing,* 1971, *71*(8), 1542–1547.

Cook, H., & Stingle, S. Co-operative behavior in children. *Psychological Bulletin,* 1974, *81,* 918–933.

Coopersmith, S. *The antecedents of self-esteem.* San Francisco: Freeman, 1967.

de Beauvoir, S. *The second sex.* New York: Knopf, 1953.

Dohrenwend, B. S. Social status and stressful life events. *Journal of Personality and Social Psychology,* 1973, *28,* 225–235.

Ehrenreich, B., & English, D. *Complaints and disorders: The sexual politics of sickness.* Old Westbury, NY: The Feminist Press, 1973.

Fabrikant, B., Landau, D., & Rollenhagen, J. Perceived female sex role attributes and psychotherapists' sex role expectations for female patients. *New Jersey Psychologist,* Winter 1973, pp. 13–16.

Freud, S. Some psychical consequences of the anatomical distinction between the sexes. In J. Strouse (Ed.), *Women and analysis.* New York: Grossman, 1974.

Friedan, B. *The feminine mystique.* New York: Norton, 1963.

Frieze, I. H. Attributions of success and failure in internal and external barriers to achievement in women. In J. Sherman & F. Denmark (Eds.), *Psychology of women: Future directions of research.* New York: Psychological Dimensions, 1978.

Gallup, G. Poll on women and job bias. *San Francisco Chronicle,* August 16, 1982, p. 5.

Gilligan, C. *In a different voice: Psychological theory and women's development.* Cambridge: Harvard University Press, 1982.

Growing impact of women in U.S. labor force. *San Francisco Chronicle,* August 16, 1982, p. 5.

Hardwick, E. *Seduction and betrayal.* New York: Random House, 1974.

Harris, S. *The influence of patient and therapist sex in psychotherapy.* Unpublished manuscript, Rutgers, The State University of New Jersey, 1974.

Hayghe, H. *Marital and family characteristics of the labor force* (Report No. 173. U.S. Department of Labor, Bureau of Labor Statistics). Washington, DC: Government Printing Office, March 1974.

Hedges, J. N. Women workers and manpower demands in the 1970s. *Monthly Labor Review,* June 1979, p. 19.

Horney, K. *Feminine psychology.* New York: Norton, 1967.

Houghton, W. E. *The Victorian frame of mind.* New Haven: Yale University Press, 1957.

Kanowitz, L. *Women and the law.* Albuquerque: University of New Mexico Press, 1969.

Katz, F. E. Nurses. In A. Etzioni, *The semi-professions and their organization.* New York: Free Press, 1969.

Kjervick, D. K., & Palta, M. Sex role stereotyping of assessment of mental health. *Nursing Research,* 1978, *27,* 166–171.

Laws, J. L. Work aspirations of women: False leads and new starts. *Signs,* 1976, *1*(3), 33–50.

Lopata, H. Z. *Occupation: Housewife.* New York: Oxford University Press, 1971.

Maccoby, E. E. Sex differences in intellectual functioning. In E. E. Maccoby (Ed.), *The development of sex differences.* Palo Alto, CA: Stanford University Press, 1966.

Maccoby, E. E., & Jacklin, C. N. *The psychology of sex differences.* Palo Alto, CA: Stanford University Press, 1974.

Marcus, S. *The other Victorians.* New York: Bantam Books, 1977.

Martineau, H. Nurses wanted. *The Cornhill Magazine,* 1865, *11,* 409–433.

Mill, J. S. *The subjection of women.* Bungay, England: Richard Clay Ltd., 1869.

Milne, J. D. *Industrial and social position of women in the middle and lower ranks.* London: Livingstone, 1867.

Nowacki, C. M., & Poe, C. A. The concept of mental health as related to sex of person perceived. *Journal of Consulting and Clinical Psychology,* 1973, *40,* 160.

Oetzel, R. M. Annotated bibliography. In E. E. Maccoby (Ed.), *The development of sex differences.* Palo Alto, CA: Stanford University Press, 1966.

Phillips, L., & Rabinovitch, M. S. Social role and patterns of symptomatic behaviors. *Journal of Abnormal and Social Psychology,* 1958, *57,* 181–186.

Primavera, L. H., Simon, W. E., & Primavera, A. M. Relationship between self-esteem and academic achievement. *Psychology in the Schools,* 1974, *11,* 213–216.

Rheingold, J. C. *The fear of being a woman.* New York: Grune & Stratton, 1967.

Ricardo-Campbell, R. Social security: The working woman's burden. *Washington Post,* September 20, 1982.

Rosenthal, E. R. Working in mid-life. In A. H. Stromberg & S. Harkess (Eds.), *Women working: Theories and facts in perspective.* Palo Alto, CA: Mayfield, 1978.

Ruble, D. N. Visual orientation and self-perceptions of children in an external cue-relevant or cue-irrelevant task situation. *Child Development,* 1975, *46,* 669–676.

Ruble, D. N., & Nakamura, C. Y. Task orientation versus social orientation in young children and their attention to relevant social cues. *Child Development,* 1972, *43,* 471–480.

Sears, R. R., Maccoby, E. E., & Levin, H. *Patterns of childbearing.* Evanston, IL: Row, Peterson, 1957.

Shearer, L. It's tough to be a woman. *Washington Post,* April 18, 1982, p. 7.

Strause, J. (Ed.). *Women and analysis.* New York: Grossman, 1974.

Tagiuri, R., & Petrullo, L. (Eds.), *Person perception and interpersonal behavior.* Palo Alto, CA: Stanford University Press, 1958.

Thompson, C. M. *Interpersonal psychoanalysis: The selected papers of Clara M. Thompson.* New York: Basic Books, 1964.

Time use studies reveal plight of working women: Everyday life in 12 countries has common design. *ISR Newsletter,* Autumn, 1973, pp. 6–7.

Trevelyan, G. M. *A shortened history of England.* New York: Penguin Books, 1976.

Waldman, E., & McEaddy, B. Where women work. *Monthly Labor Review,* May 1974, p. 6.

Watt, I. *The rise of the novel.* Berkeley: University of California Press, 1965.

Zeldow, P. B. Sex differences in psychiatric evaluation and treatment. *Archives of General Psychiatry,* 1978, *35,* 89–93.

BIBLIOGRAPHY

Tangri, S. S. Determinants of occupational role innovation among college women. *Journal of Social Issues,* 1972, *28,* 177–199.

U.S. Department of Labor. *Manpower Report of the President, April 1975.* Washington, D.C.: U.S. Government Printing Office, 1975.

Walker, K., & Granger, O. Time and its dollar value in household work. *Family Economics Review,* Fall 1973, pp. 8–13.

CHAPTER 19

THE CHALLENGE OF CHRONICITY

Susan M. Godschalx

Chronic mental illness imposes tremendous losses on people, including the loss of a sense of being normal. It inhibits one's ability to form satisfying, intimate relationships, limits one's financial productivity, and restricts available life-styles. The unpredictability of the course of chronic mental illness prevents clients from planning long-term goals, and physical problems occur secondary to medication. Further complicating the situation, these losses are usually first realized during young adulthood, when loss is extremely difficult to manage (Silver & Wortman, 1980). Helping clients with chronic mental illness discover personal meaning in life that transcends the limitations of their illness is, indeed, the challenge of chronicity.

This chapter describes chronicity, intervention strategies which minimize client problems, and the therapeutic relationship with chronic clients. Research questions are identified. However, the focus of this chapter is on providing a conceptual framework and suggesting intervention strategies that will enable the psychiatric mental health nurse to increase the client's quality of life.

CHRONICITY: A MULTIDIMENSIONAL CONDITION

Chronicity is defined as a client condition characterized by a lack of significant improvement in level of functioning over several years. It can be viewed on a continuum; some clients eventually and gradually change more than others. The extent to which chronicity is viewed as problematic will depend on the therapist's expectations and whether the chronicity is due to changeable or unchangeable factors.

Mental health professionals are trained primarily in the "talking therapies" which require certain emotional and cognitive resources often impaired in chronic mental illness. When a therapist expects to cure the client with chronic mental illness, chronicity is seen as a severe problem. If the therapist tackles it at all, she or he frequently ends up feeling frustrated, angry, and helpless. As a result, working with "chronics" has been considered less prestigous than working with healthier clients who benefit from "real therapy." This notion is unfortunate and stems not from the nature of the client, but from misunderstanding chronic illness and setting inappropriate goals.

Chronicity can be caused by any or all of the following three factors: psychopathology, institutionalization, and how the client psychologically manages the awareness of loss. Some aspects (for example, possible genetic predispostions) may be less changeable than others (for example, grieving vs. denying loss). Understanding the factors that contribute to persistent lack of change, or chronicity, will help the psychiatric mental health nurse appreciate why it occurs and identify areas for potential client growth.

Psychopathology

There are approximately two million chronically, severely mentally ill people in the United States (Goldman, Gattozzi, & Taube, 1981; U.S. Government Printing Office, 1978).

"Chronic mental illness," which technically says nothing about severity, has come to refer to a group of severe, persistent mental and/or emotional disorders that significantly affect one's ability to function. People with chronic mental illness usually fall into the diagnostic categories of schizophrenia and major affective and borderline personality disorders. No one knows for sure what group of conditions must exist for these illnesses to occur; and we do not know how to cure them. Researchers have reported findings that suggest there is a physiological base or predisposition to chronic mental illness. Discovering what factors may trigger or prevent the onset of this predisposition remains a challenging area of research.

While research is inconclusive in the area of explaining chronic mental illness, numerous studies have described the client experiencing it. We know that these individuals are extremely vulnerable to stress. Stressors of any kind can overwhelm the ego and stimulate acute psychotic symptoms and drastic mood and/or behavioral changes. These symptoms are usually controllable with appropriate dosages of antipsychotic medication (or lithium carbonate for bipolar disorders). In addition to periods of acute symptomatology, the client experiences incapacitating residual symptoms: lack of motivation, inability to problem solve around daily life situations, poor judgement, poor impulse control, an inability to form satisfying, intimate relationships, and chronic social anxiety (Gersten, 1981; Test & Stein, 1978; Waters, 1981). Unfortunately, these are not alleviated by psychotropic drugs. Emotionally painful acute symptoms compounded by these residual deficits make chronic mental illness a truly disabling disorder.

Institutionalization

Another factor that contributes to chronicity is institutionalization. Institutionalization is not just hospitalization, but a process of systematically assuming responsibility for the client and thereby decreasing his or her self-determination and ability for self-care. The effects of this process were dramatically seen in discharged state hospital patients in the 1960s and 1970s and were described by Goffman (1961). Many of these people were unable to care for themselves in society because they had been taken care of for so many years. This process can occur whenever responsibility for self-determination and self-care are systematically taken away in mental health centers, nursing homes, or within families (Goldman et al., 1981).

The effects of institutionalization are crippling. Clients begin to believe that they are truly incapable of making decisions or caring for themselves, resulting in helplessness, lack of motivation, and decreased self-esteem. Institutionalization can cause chronicity, or persistent lack of change, even in persons without chronic mental illness. For clients with residual deficits, institutionalization complicates the assessment process and increases the tendency toward chronicity.

Psychological Style of Managing Loss

The third factor affecting chronicity is how the client psychologically manages the awareness of loss. As previously stated, clients experiencing chronic mental illness suffer many losses and they cope with the awareness of these losses using one of several psychological processes. The clinically observable outcome of these psychological processes is a defensive style. A defense style is one's method of protecting the self from threat of ego disorganization and reduced functioning (Adams & Lindemann, 1974). Ego strength, or the ability to maintain one's sense of self, determines the client's choice of psychological defense. A model for understanding these defense styles is proposed in Figure 19.1. Four clinically distinct outcomes result from the way clients psychologically manage loss. These defensive style outcomes are adaptation, depression, avoidance, and aphanisis.

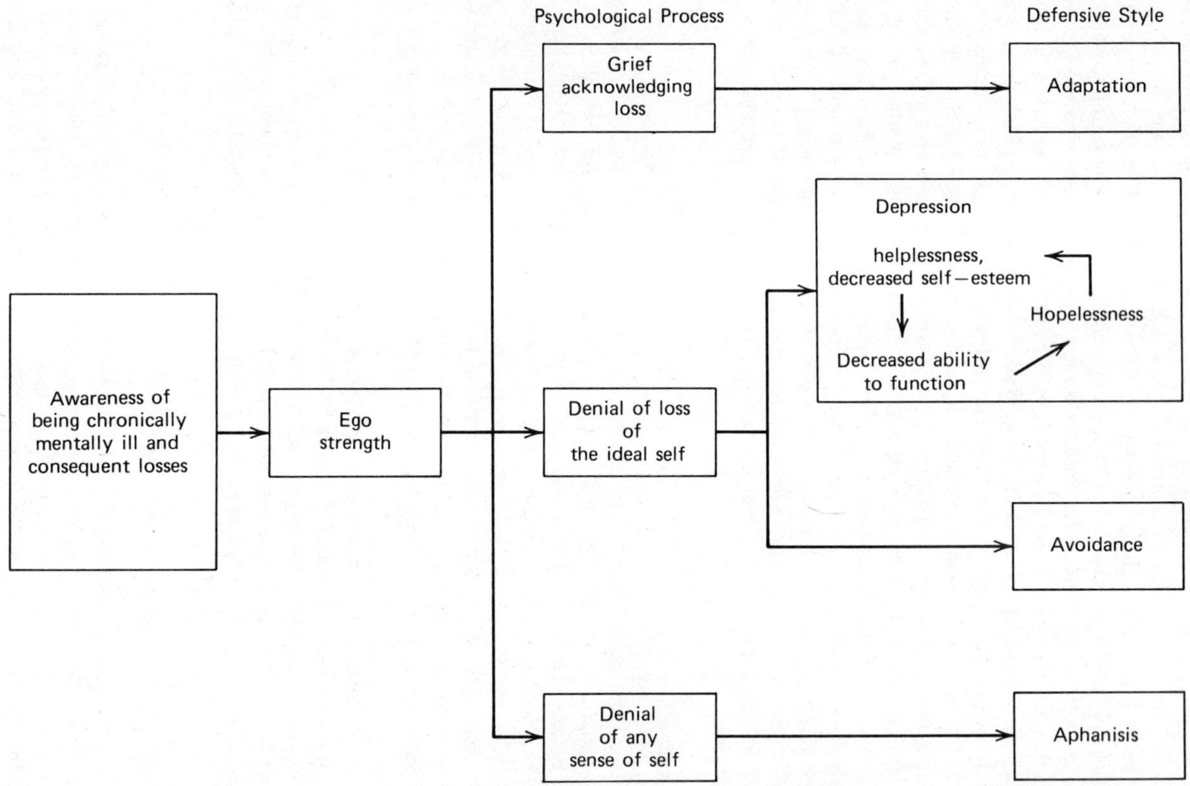

Figure 19.1 Psychological styles of managing the awareness of loss.

Recently, the term postpsychotic depression (PPD) has become popular in the literature. Unfortunately, various authors define PPD very differently. For clarity, the term postpsychotic depression is avoided here. Rather, phenomena are described according to their dynamic and clinical characteristics.

Grief and Adaptation

The first, and healthiest, way for the client to deal with the awareness of loss is through grief and adaptation. Dynamically, the grieving client acknowledges that loss has indeed occurred. Through the process of acknowledging the unattainability of the ideal self, the client is able to reinvest in a new ideal self and eventually reformulate goals, values, and a perception of him- or herself that integrates the illness into a sense of self (McGlashan, 1982; Miller, 1983; Roth, 1970; Russell, 1981; Smith, 1971). The outcome of grief, unless the client shifts into denial and depression (McGlashan, 1982; Meyersburg, Ablon, & Kotin, 1974) is adaptation. Adaptation is defined as "coming to terms existentially with the reality of chronic illness as a state of being, discarding both false hope and destructive hopelessness. . . . It demands the reorganization and acceptance of the self so that there is a meaning and purpose to living that transcends the limitations imposed by the illness" (Feldman, 1974, p. 290).

Clinically, the grieving client may appear "depressed." Tearfulness, lack of motivation, and suicidal ideations are common. Grieving clients, however, express much more curiosity about their illness than depressed clients. While grieving clients verbally describe experiences of loss, usually with intense affect, depressed clients do not. Grieving clients feel they cannot cope with life, refuse to set goals for themselves, and may be labeled "problem patients." As the grieving process continues, the psychological release of "what might have been" gives energy for reinvesting in life. Questioning, trying on new roles, developing a supportive peer group, and viewing oneself as "different" rather than sick are clinical characteristics of the adapting client (Feldman, 1974). As clients experience new limitations and losses resulting from their illness, grieving and adapting recur.

Depression

In contrast to the psychological choice of grief and adaptation, other clients deny that loss has occurred and experience depression. Clients with chronic mental illness are particularly vulnerable to denial and depression for several reasons. First, the intangibleness and unpredictability of symptom exacerbation predisposes the client to denial. Second, the weak ego boundaries clients experience make facing loss extremely difficult. Finally, most clients experience a very severe illness. Viney and Westbrook (1981) reported that illness severity has a great impact on anxiety level and use of depression. Roth (1970) has suggested that when loss is very great, the psychological risk of grieving is much more difficult. For these reasons, clients with severe, poorly controlled illnesses are prone to using the defensive style of denial and depression.

Depression is defined as a "fundamental psychobiological response to the experience of helplessness in the face of persistent discrepancies between actual states . . . and an ideal state of satiation and power" (McGlashan, 1982, p. 125). In depression, the inevitability of loss is denied. The ideal self is clung to yet experienced as unattainable (Smith, 1971). For example, clients with chronic mental illness often deny the severity and chronicity of their illness (for example, "I may have had problems once when I was in the hospital, but I'm okay now and don't need my medication") yet decompensate when medication is refused. This unwillingness to acknowledge the loss of normality (denial), combined with the inability to regain normality, stimulates helplessness and decreased ability to function.

The client complains of confusion, lack of energy, weight loss (or gain), and insomnia. Suicidal ideations can develop as clients observe their decreased functioning and experience hopelessness, compounding their helplessness and decreased self-esteem. Depression can become a stable, chronic defense used by clients to avoid awareness of the losses inherent in their illness (Kotin, 1976; Meyersberg et al., 1974). Because of these dynamics, the true signal of a client overcoming depression is not euphoria, but grief (Roth, 1970; Smith, 1971).

Avoidance

The third clinically distinct defensive style clients use to manage the awareness of loss is avoidance or "sealing over" (McGlashan, Levy, & Carpenter, 1975; Visotsky, Hamburg, Goss, & Lebovits, 1961). The avoiding client uses denial yet, for reasons unknown, does not experience helplessness or decreased self-esteem. McGlashen and Carpenter (1981) discovered no difference in level of functioning between schizophrenic clients who had grieved and those using avoidance. Apparently, avoidance may be a nondebilitating defensive style for some clients.

Clinically, clients using avoidance appear involved with their day's activities. They focus away from their mental illness, ignoring that compartment of themselves, and focus on daily activities and relationships. They frequently minimize symptoms, have little or no curiosity about their illness, and prefer to "let past be past." Only when they are unable to ignore their illness (for example, when psychotic symptoms significantly increase) do these clients experience anxiety, helplessness, and decreased self-esteem. After taking psychotropic medication to eliminate the psychotic symptoms, they again successfully ignore their illness.

Aphanisis

The fourth defensive style identified is aphanisis. Aphanisis means "obliteration of drive," or ceasing to struggle (McGlashan, 1982). Dynamically, the client not only denies the loss of an ideal self, but also regressively denies any sense of self. This defensive style has been compared to the infant's apathy following an unsuccessful protest. Despairing, the infant gives up expecting that his or her needs will be met and withdraws by increasing a physiological stimulus barrier. The client in aphanisis uses two psychological strategies aimed at withdrawal and isolation to maintain an existence with minimal awareness of any inner conflict. The first involves blocking out all internal stimuli (thoughts, emotions, sensations) and external stimuli (conversation or events). Therapists working with chronically mentally ill people see clients sitting alone for hours, not being entertained by hallucinations, yet not bored. Perhaps this may be a clinical example of obliterating stimuli.

When the client is unable to eliminate all stimuli, McGlashan (1982) proposes a second strategy, scotomatizing. Scotomatizing refers to the process of focusing all of one's energies on one particular stimulus to the exclusion of everything else. Again, the client isolates from the environment and even from personal thoughts and feelings but this time by solely concentrating on one stimulus.

The tremendous energy used in these defenses leaves the client complaining of a lack of energy and motivation. Other clinical symptoms include anhedonia, social isolation, and complaints of "being stuck" or empty. The client is very withdrawn and lives a wooden-like existence, yet in spite of this inner deadness, rarely demonstrates suicidal intent (McGlashan, 1982; Raskin, 1970).

Aphanisis is more stable than any of the other defensive styles. It has not been described in general rehabilitation literature, however. Are there factors peculiar to chronic mental illness that predispose clients to use this regressive, debilitating defense? Further research is needed to describe thoroughly and explore this defensive structure and its impact on client functioning.

PROBLEM AREAS FOR THE CHRONIC CLIENT

Chronic mental illness imposes special problems on all clients. Frequently experienced problems are dependence/independence conflicts, decreased self-esteem, helplessness, and inadequate living resources. The following discussion describes why these problems occur for clients with chronic mental illness, identifies treatment goals, and suggests treatment strategies for each problem (see Table 19.1). Minimizing these problem areas increases the client's experienced quality of life, which is the goal of all therapeutic intervention.

Dependence/Independence Conflict

Dependence/independence conflicts pose problems for many clients. For the chronically mentally ill client, this conflict is intensified for several reasons. First, the weak ego boundaries and ambivalence of the schizophrenic complicate the normally difficult process of separation/individuation. Second, demands and limitations of chronic illness necessitate that clients rely extensively on others to live their healthiest. This "positive dependence" is a comparatively healthy life-style given that the alternative is an exacerbation of one's illness (Craig & Hyatt, 1978; Feldman, 1974; Krauss, 1980; Greenberg, Weltz, Spitz, & Bizzozero, 1975; McGlashan et al., 1975; Slavinsky & Krauss, 1980). Positive dependence focuses on a greater-than-usual involvement with a supportive group of people. This can be distinguished clinically from an unhealthy dependence that is characterized by the client refusing to accept any responsibility (Feldman, 1974).

Achieving a "positive dependence" requires the psychological task of acknowledging loss and the behavioral task of discovering one's optimal level of independence through a trial-and-error process. Depressed clients may experience significant dependence/independence conflict because they deny the loss of the ideal self, including their capability to lead an independent life. When the client experiences an inability to be "normally" independent, helplessness increases and the depressive cycle deepens.

Because many clients with chronic mental illness experience ambivalence, deny the limitations of their illness, and yet require "greater-than-usual" support, dependence/independence conflicts are a major problem. The goal of therapeutic intervention for this problem is that the client experience positive dependence with minimal conflict. The suggested treatment strategy for the dependence/independence conflict is *to support positive dependence.*

The therapeutic relationship is the client's primary resource for minimizing dependence/independence conflicts. Within the relationship, the client can explore experiences of helpless-

Table 19.1 Problems and Goals for the Client Experiencing a Chronic Mental Illness

Problem	*Goal*
Dependence/independence conflict	Client experiences positive dependency and conflict is minimized
Decreased self-esteem	Client experiences positive self-esteem
Helplessness	Client experiences a perception of control
Inadequate health and living resources	Client has ongoing financial, housing, medical, and occupational resources

ness and, hopefully, with the therapist's acceptance and empathy, strengthen the ego and begin to acknowledge loss. During the behavioral task of discovering an optimal independence, the client may need directives when symptoms become life threatening, particularly if the client has not acknowledged the limitations of his or her illness. The following case study illustrates these strategies and process.

Jane is a 36-year-old woman with chronic undifferentiated schizophrenia who denies the losses associated with her illness and frequently experiences severe depressive episodes. Recently, Jane decided to move out of her parents' home to be on her own; she had been dependent on them for six years. During her individual therapy time, she shared that living alone would signify that she was "well." Shortly after moving into an apartment, Jane experienced hallucinations that led to suicidal ideation. When she reached the point of no longer engaging with the therapist because the voices were telling her that if she talked with the therapist, they would kill her, the focus of the relationship switched from a supportive problem-solving mode to a supportive directive one. Asking her to remember past experiences in which she trusted the therapist and recovered decreased her paranoia. Meeting with her several times a day, when needed, communicated care and enabled her to continue trusting the relationship. By firmly stating that the therapist believed she would recover from this present episode gave her some hope that motivated her to continue to work with the therapist. Once she could agree to work with the therapist in keeping herself alive, she was supported in choosing alternatives that ensured her safety rather than continuing directives. With this firm support, Jane decided not to stay alone in her apartment but to stay in the crisis center for a few days, to take her medication, and even to give the therapist her car keys for the 24 hours she was most suicidal. Her acute symptoms subsided and Jane again assumed responsibility for her own well-being.

Frustration with her inability to be "normal" stimulated helplessness but also a curiosity about her experience. During Jane's individual time, the increased psychotic symptoms were relabeled as a consequence of her illness instead of personal failure. This allowed her to stop blaming herself. The therapist and client discussed what being "well" meant, encouraging her to question the validity of cure as the goal of therapy. But Jane remained unable to accept the loss of her ideal "no illness" self.

About this time, Jane had to terminate seeing a private psychiatrist she had seen for many years. This termination proved to be particularly painful but therapeutic for Jane. She had been hoping that her ideal "no illness" self was not really lost and would be regained in therapy with this person. Helping Jane identify this assumption, encouraging her to think about the realistic possibilities of this person having a "cure" that no one else knew about, and intensively supporting her over several months enabled Jane to acknowledge that she had a serious illness and that life could still be meaningful.

Without the internal pressures to deny her illness, Jane has been able to decide that she feels the best when she is living with someone with whom she can discuss her threatening hallucinations. Jane moved into an apartment with two friends and is now functioning well. In reflecting on her process of acknowledging loss and discovering positive dependence, Jane shared the following: "I used to like thinking that nothing was wrong with me; then when I'd see how I'd burned my stomach or something, I'd think of suicide. Maybe recognizing that I have a serious problem is the first step to my being able to get better. I sure am glad I don't have to burn myself or think about ways to kill myself in my apartment anymore." Jane has minimized her dependence/independence conflict by psychologically acknowledging loss and behaviorally exploring her current optimal level of "positive dependence."

Decreased Self-Esteem

Decreased self-esteem is such a major problem that many authors cite increasing self-esteem as crucial to quality of life (Adams & Lindemann, 1974; Dimond & Jones, 1983; McGlashan et al., 1975; Silver & Wortman, 1980). The stigma of being mentally ill can be more detrimental to self-esteem than the illness itself (Dimond & Jones, 1983). To be locked up is demoralizing and humiliating. Being hospitalized in a state mental institution is viewed as equivalent to (or worse than) being a convict. This intense prejudice against mentally ill people significantly compounds injury to the client's self-esteem. The goal of treatment for the problem of decreased self-esteem is that the client experience positive self-esteem. Strategies to accomplish this goal include clarifying values, identifying strengths, relabeling the client's condition, strengthening social support, and acknowledging sexuality.

Clarifying Values

The myth of normality contends that one must be normal in order to lead a happy, satisfying life (DeLoach & Greer, 1981). Challenging this myth encourages clients to acknowledge the discrepancy between the actual and ideal self and redefine values and aspirations that bring the actual and idealized selves into a closer fit. This process can be done by identifying people society calls successful but who are not happy, and using values clarification exercises. A man, feeling dejected after 21 years of chronic schizophrenia, commented after listing what he valued, "Why, not one of these has anything to do with being mentally ill or not!" This strategy helps clients question mental illness as an obstacle to happiness.

Identifying Strengths

Clients with mental illness often assume that because they have a mental illness, all other aspects of themselves are defective as well (Strauss, 1975). This destructive tendency can be countered by the therapist identifying and encouraging the client to use areas of strength.

A 19-year-old woman had been a pianist before a psychotic episode the year before. Since then she rarely played the piano. Realizing this strength, staff took time to ask and listen to her play. Soon other clients also were asking her to play for them. Their applause and compliments helped her feel proud of her ability, increasing her self-esteem.

Intelligence is another strength often overlooked. Assessing for this resource and encouraging clients to use their intelligence (by returning to school or discussing their concerns using a more advanced vocabulary) increases self-esteem, perception of control and, potentially, their living resources as well.

Relabeling the Client's Condition

Many clients perceive themselves as being "sick." This cognitive label is both inaccurate and nontherapeutic. First, in many ways the chronically disabled client lives a very different life than does someone who is "sick." The client is active in treatment, compliance remains necessary even when symptoms disappear, and the goal of therapy is increasing the quality of life, not cure (Dimond & Jones, 1983). Second, the perception of oneself as sick is nontherapeutic. Being "sick" is traditionally a passive role, encouraging the process of institutionalization. Additionally, seeing oneself as "sick" encourages an expectation of cure, predisposing the client to denial and depression.

To avoid these problems and encourage positive self-esteem, the therapist can suggest that the client is "at risk" for symptom exacerbation rather than sick. Being "at risk" implies an ongoing condition over which the client has some degree of control, encouraging self-determination and self-care. Self-worth increases as assumptions about oneself as a capable adult are congruent with behavior.

Strengthening Social Support

Clients with chronic mental illness have difficulty establishing and maintaining social relationships. Yet social support is frequently correlated with quality of life. Kemp and Vash (1971) cite it as a critical resource for people with severe, disabling illness. Strengthening the client's social support from family and peers increases client self-esteem.

The therapist strengthens the client's social support from the family by establishing and maintaining communication with the family. It is extremely important to communicate respect and concern for the stresses the client imposes on the family. Unless the therapist is warm and accepting, the family will assume that the therapist blames them for the client's problems and will react with hostility or aloofness. Paranoid clients may fear therapist-family contact. Processing this concern by asking what the client fears might happen, reassuring the client against unreasonable fears, and discussing specifically what will happen decreases paranoia.

Second, the therapist can strengthen family social support by facilitating client-family communication. Families may withdraw from the client emotionally, physically, and/or financially owing to the client's excessive illness-related demands, the client's own hopelessness, and/or the client's bizarre behavior (Strauss, 1979). Family sessions to resolve conflict or discuss goals and expectations can prevent this withdrawal (Adams & Lindemann, 1974; Dimond & Jones, 1983). For example, the family may need help in identifying ways to meet the client's positive dependence needs without exhausting themselves. The therapist may educate the family about the "at risk" role to decrease the family's tendency to isolate the "sick" member (Strauss, 1975). Alternatively, the family may request help in confronting a client assuming a completely dependent role and abdicating all responsibilities within the family system.

A group approach to educating families about their relative's mental illness has recently become popular. Most programs focus on a fairly small group (10–16 family members) and present a structured sequence of information at a leisurely pace, offering time for questions and exercises. Involving family members in this type of program may be yet another way to increase family support for the client.

Loneliness, and fear of loneliness, is a major concern of many clients due to social isolation. A peer social support group is another resource the therapist can help the client draw upon to minimize the self-esteem threat of social isolation. A peer social support group is a small group of people who experience similar problems and concerns as a result of illness. The groups are usually informal and are a very supportive resource to clients for several reasons. First, a client in the process of reformulating goals, values, and a perception of self that integrates his or her illness can see others who have gone through this same process and have successfully created a new life-style (McGlashan et al., 1975). Likewise, the client using denial may be encouraged to acknowledge loss seeing friends who have adapted.

Second, the client can experience being needed as help is given to other clients with problems. Being needed is necessary for positive self-esteem and is significantly different from being welcome (MacKinnon, 1977; Visotsky et al., 1961). Clients need to be needed. A peer social support group provides this role as peers rely on one another. Officially recognizing clients' support of each other by giving special privileges and responsibilities to members of the support group may increase group prestige and self-esteem.

Third, clients frequently have time with nothing to do, particularly clients whose illness prevents employment. A social support group can provide these clients with a role of socializing, and perhaps volunteering, that gives them something they "do" all day. Being expected somewhere provides a sense of being needed and increases self-esteem.

Fourth, the support group is one environment in which the client can share experiences of past craziness, helplessness, and fears for the future. It is not acceptable to discuss mental illness in "normal" types of groups; it is in this one. A peer social support group is also more tolerant of drastic changes in level of functioning. Whereas the client would be outcast from other groups, a group of people also experiencing mental illness will be more likely to tolerate strange behavior.

Finally, a third method to strengthen the client's social support involves pets: clients have found that owning and caring for a pet can increase self-esteem. An animal's dependence on the client gives a sense of being needed. Additionally, pets provide an outlet for touch. Many clients do not experience intimate relationships and have withdrawn from their family of origin. Whom can they touch? An animal wanting to be petted and scratched may be meeting this very human need. Lovejoy (1983) has shared how having a pet helped keep her paranoia from interfering with her life. Normally she was unable to distinguish between a safe and dangerous environment, which was preventing her from living in an apartment. However, she could rely on her dog to bark if someone was approaching. When the dog was quiet she knew she was safe. For several problems the client may confront, such as a lack of being needed, lack of touching relationships, or for symptom management, the psychiatric mental health nurse may suggest a pet.

Sexuality

There is an unwritten rule in our society that says: Only normal, young, and beautiful people enjoy sexuality. Consequently, many clients avoid discussing concerns about their sexuality and experience tremendous guilt over sexual feelings. Directly asking about concerns the client has regarding sexuality, providing information about contraception, or suggesting alternatives to harmful practices (such as using glass as a vibrator) can prevent unwanted stressors and health problems and increase self-esteem as the client realizes the therapist accepts him or her as a person.

Helplessness

Helplessness is the perception and expectation that situational outcomes are uncontrollable (Abramson, Garber, & Seligman, 1980). Clients with chronic mental illness often experience helplessness because of the unpredictability of symptom exacerbation. Clients who deny the loss of their ideal self are especially vulnerable. As they cling to their ideal self, a sense of inefficacy develops when reality confronts them. Their expectation of being ineffective in controlling situations results clinically in depression (McGlashan, 1982).

Attribution theory contends that when people feel helpless, they ask why. What a person attributes, or credits, his or her helplessness to influences whether or not helplessness will be generalized to all situations. There are three attributional dimensions to helplessness: internal–external, stable–unstable, and global–specific.

The internal–external continuum focuses on self–other. Internally oriented people will most likely attribute helplessness to factors within themselves (for example, a lack of inner emotional strength). In the same situation, an "external" client may cite the faulty judgement of others to explain current helplessness. Contrary to popular assumption, internal attributions are not necessarily more healthy than external attributions. People who use internal attributions tend to experience a greater loss of self-esteem when faced with perceived failure (Abramson et al., 1980; Lewis, 1982).

The second attributional dimension, stable–unstable, determines the chronicity of attribution. Because internal attributions tend to focus on personal characteristics, or "I," they also tend to be more stable than external attributions. Viewing hospitalization as a result of biochemical illness is likely to be a more stable attribution than attributing it to a response to temporary stress.

The global–specific continuum determines the extent to which attributes are generalized to situations. Does the attributed cause influence all of one's functioning or just a specific area? For a detailed explanation of attribution theory and helplessness, the reader is referred to *Human Helplessness* (Garber & Seligman, 1980).

The antidote for helplessness is a perception of control. Averill (1973) postulated that there are three types of control: behavioral, cognitive, and decisional. Behavioral control refers to the availability of a response that may directly influence or modify the objective characteristics of a threatening event. Decreasing uncertainty is the crux of behavior control. Cognitive control refers to ways that events can be interpreted that reduce the stress of the awareness of illness. Decisional control refers to the opportunity to choose among various courses of action. Each of these modes of control are extremely useful tools for decreasing helplessness and encouraging a perception of control. Useful intervention strategies include providing information, teaching specific skills, goal setting, problem solving, tailoring to locus of control, and distinguishing between spirituality and mental illness.

Providing Information

Knowledge about one's illness can increase self-esteem and decrease helplessness (Hoffman, 1981; McGlashan & Carpenter, 1976; Miller, 1983; Pilsecker, 1981). However, like all interventions, providing information must be based on assessment of the client. Clients attributing helplessness to a temporary response to stress or successfully using avoidance may not want, or benefit from, information. An individual client's desire for information also fluctuates over time (Lowery & DuCette, 1976; Visotsky et al., 1961).

Given these assessment concerns, the therapist can provide information to increase a sense of cognitive control. The nurse should give accurate information that acknowledges the limits of our understanding. While remaining hopeful about growth, the therapist should not encourage false hope. Comparing chronic mental illness to another less stigmatized illness with a similar course, such as diabetes, is an effective way to educate clients. Neither diabetes nor mental illness is life threatening when under control; both significantly affect the ability to function when not controlled. The treatment of both illnesses involves medication for a long period of time, even when symptoms disappear. The concreteness of diabetes and its treatment helps clients better understand their own intangible mental illness. Additionally, no one would blame a person for having diabetes or think him or her less a person. This comparison decreases the stigma of mental illness which may help clients acknowledge their illness and begin to work actively with the therapist toward better symptom management. Thus, the client receives a sense of behavioral control.

Another aspect of providing information is to teach some of the professional jargon specific to the client and his or her care. This also increases the perception of control (Mailick, 1979). Knowing that b.i.d. means "twice daily" allows the client to read prescriptions. Knowing what "schizoaffective disorder" means enables the client to converse intelligently with professionals as adult to adult rather than as the traditional sick patient to doctor.

Teaching Specific Skills

Teaching clients specific skills to increase their ability to manage increases self-esteem and perception of control, as well as minimizes the interference of symptoms in their life. Short-term planning and warning symptom identification are two of these skills. Dimond (1980) interviewed 36 hemodialysis patients to examine the relationship between short-term planning and adaptation. Short-term planning referred to organizing one's daily schedule to meet the demands of illness. The four dependent measures of adaptation were morale, changes in social functioning, number of medical complications, and stability of physical status. One of the strongest relationships was found between short-term planning and stability in physical status. Dimond hypothesized that short-term planning increased clients' control over their lives. By making plans that increased predictability, they actually decreased stress and resulting physical complications. Perhaps clients with mental illness can use short-term planning as well to increase predictability in their daily lives and influence the course of their illness. It is accepted that stress exacerbates symptoms of mental illness. Might short-term planning decrease symptoms? Clinical research applying this theory to a chronically mentally ill population is needed to validate this hypothesis.

Learning one's own warning symptoms is another skill that increases ability to manage symptoms and behavioral control (Feldman, 1974; Strauss, 1975). A warning symptom is an identified symptom that cues the client to eminent symptom exacerbation. The client with a bipolar disorder may identify one or two symptoms (such as sleeping less than five hours per night or changing clothes more than twice a day) that then alert the client so that preventative action can be taken. The nurse, by observing fluctuation in client functioning, can suggest individualized warning symptoms. One client experiencing paranoid schizophrenia would decide to move from his apartment every time his paranoia was beginning to increase. Recognizing that concrete warning symptom enabled him to feel more in control of his paranoia.

A corrollary strategy involves teaching clients to distinguish between normal and abnormal changes. For example, a woman with a severe bipolar disorder went into crisis when she noticed any mood fluctuation, fearing another onslaught of depression or mania. Teaching her to recognize the difference, by identifying the warning symptoms of abnormal changes, significantly decreased her anxiety and increased her perception of control.

Goal Setting

Short-term planning has been discussed, but goal setting in general can be an effective tool for increasing the perception of decisional control (Kemp & Vash, 1971; Seeman & McGree, 1982). Goals should be highly visible and probably attainable. When a long-term goal is set, intermediate goals also should be set to encourage the client (Visotsky et al., 1961). The criteria by which to measure progress should be concrete, for example, how many days a week one will attend day treatment (Dimond & Jones, 1983; Miller, 1983). However, when decompensation occurs, which is inherent in the illness, clients may interpret their decreased ability to function according to the criteria as failure, causing hopelessness. Comparing oneself to a referent group of people with similar problems may give clients an alternative criteria for progress and a more accurate picture of adaptation as they see others fighting symptoms and continuing on.

When clients set goals without taking into consideration their degree of psychopathology, institutionalization, and style of managing loss, they usually fail to attain the goal and experience hopelessness. Depressed clients may insist on unrealistic goals, denying the limitations of their illness. While these experiences will stimulate hopelessness and helplessness, they also can be used to encourage the client's curiosity and potentially open the way toward acknowledging loss. Clients who resist setting any goals for themselves may need help distinguishing changeable from unchangeable aspects of their life. Finally, clients with poorly controlled illnesses may benefit from setting goals that pertain to their life in general, avoiding illness-related goals. The increased quality of life associated with the perception of control is, fortunately, more a function of control over one's life than over one's illness (Lewis, 1982).

Problem Solving

Integral to planning and goal setting is problem solving, which also gives the client experiences in cognitive and decisional control. Problem solving is a process of the therapist and client working together to define the problem, consider alternative strategies, determine the best solution, and evaluate the results after the client has used that strategy. It is an active, creative process that mobilizes the client to deal with day-to-day problems.

Clients who frequently experience ambivalence, weak ego boundaries, paranoia, poor judgement, and few resource alternatives find problem solving daily life situations difficult. Developing a budget or declining an invitation are extremely stressful and encourage a sense of helplessness. Supporting the client in this process can decrease client anxiety and helplessness. This process proceeds best within an ongoing trusting relationship.

A woman with a 15-year history of chronic schizophrenia and multiple hospitalizations called a therapist because her daughter had been assaulted by her ex-husband. After she shared her anger and confusion, they problem solved around a course of action. This decreased her anxiety and overwhelming sense of helplessness. It also encouraged her to continue to take care of herself. Before she hung up the phone, she commented, "You know, my daughter is doing alright, but she doesn't have a mental illness. I do, and I need your extra support right now, is that OK?" This woman has accepted that illness does impose limits in her life and so can take steps to ensure her well-being. A great majority of individual and group therapy time with people experiencing chronic mental illness is spent problem solving. Through this experience of cognitive and decisional control the client can experience a higher quality of life.

Tailoring to Locus of Control

The psychiatric mental health nurse can maximize the perception of control by assessing locus of control and tailoring interventions to the client's style. Locus of control refers to a fairly stable preference for interpreting outcomes as being the result of external situations and people, or the result of one's own actions. Whereas locus of control and attributional dimensions both describe beliefs about the relationship between one's response and situational outcomes, locus of control is considered to be a more generalized, stable view of life while the attributional dimensions apply specifically to responses to helplessness.

Knowing the client's locus of control and attributions for helplessness, the nurse can tailor therapy to potentiate quality of life. Clients with an external locus of control benefit most from group experiences, receiving advice from other clients and other external sources of support. On the other hand, internally oriented clients might perceive greater control by examining multiple options for treatment and actively participating in decision making (Dimond & Jones, 1983). After their study of locus of control in diabetics, Lowery & DuCette (1976) suggested that clients with an internal locus of control may actually experience greater helplessness if information they are given about their illness does not lead to their being able to control their illness. These data have significant implications for internal-oriented clients with chronic mental illness, since very little information that can be shared will necessarily increase control over their illness. Emphasizing what will impact on their illness (for example, medication) and recognizing the limits of a therapist's knowledge may prevent setting the client up to expect greater control than therapy offers.

At this point the literature is inconclusive, and even contradictory, about the value of one type of locus of control or attribution over the other. If attributions can be altered, would encouraging external attributions to situations of helplessness preserve self-esteem for the chronic mentally ill? Clients do seem relieved when failure is attributed to their illness rather than to personal failure. Would encouraging specific, rather than global, attributions encourage clients to use their other strengths? Further study is necessary to examine the nature of locus of control, attribution change, and these relationships. Until the literature more clearly identifies otherwise, the nurse should assume that neither locus of control or attributional style is "better." Rather, the nurse therapist, through assessing this dimension and modifying the treatment plan, can enhance the perception of control for clients using each style.

Clarifying Spirituality and Mental Illness

Finally, some clients gain the perception of control in their lives by knowing that God cares for them and is in control. Unfortunately, society's separation of the secular from the spiritual has discouraged therapists from helping clients to use this powerful resource. Yet a basic assumption of most nursing models is that an individual is not a divided, but a whole, integrated being (Carson, 1980; Slimmer, 1980). The nurse can maximize this resource of faith in God by acknowledging the client's spirituality and distinguishing between mental and spiritual realms. Because spirituality is part of being human, when clients become psychotic, delusions or hallucinations often contain spiritual content in much the same way that human sexuality stimulates sexual delusions or hallucinations. Clients frequently confuse spirituality, their relationship to God, with the psychotic spiritual content of their hallucinations. For example, a client shared that her voices were telling her she was demon possessed, and since she was demon possessed God could no longer care for her. Orienting her to the clear distinction between her relationship with God and her mental illness decreased her anxiety and protected her perception of control in knowing that God cares for her and is in control. Identifying warning symptoms that distinguish spirituality from delusional material also may help clients experience cognitive control. Both of these strategies are based on the nurse's acknowledging spirituality and being receptive to the spiritual concerns of the client.

Inadequate Living Resources

The residual deficits resulting from chronic mental illness can be extremely incapacitating. As a result, most clients have inadequate basic living resources. Most live below the poverty level. Some can manage very low stress employment; others cannot. For those unable to work, decreased funding at the federal, state, and local levels make even the basic living resources difficult to obtain. Difficulty with interpersonal relationships, paranoia, ambivalence, and poor health habits cause clients difficulty in obtaining and maintaining resources. The goal of intervention for this problem is that clients have ongoing financial, housing, medical, and occupational resources. Strategies the nurse can use include drawing on social resources and assessing health status.

Social Resources

To ensure effectively that the client has adequate living resources, the nurse therapist must learn what resources exist and how to use them. For example, it is important to know the criteria for Social Security Disability to identify and help eligible clients receive financial assistance. Knowing what documents will be required of the client applying for welfare can save the client frustration and stress and help the client to receive money and food faster. This basic knowledge is necessary before the nurse can help coordinate system resources.

Actively coordinating and interfacing directly with other agencies on behalf of the client is an integral role in therapy with many chronically ill clients (Levy, 1979; Slavinsky & Krauss, 1980). The degree to which the therapist assumes the role of systems advocate depends on assessment of the individual client.

Even chronically mentally ill clients vary greatly in their ability to function. Some clients may need a protective payee to ensure adequate food and housing; others may own their own home. Determining how actively to intervene may be difficult, but it is therapeutically important. Assuming too much responsibility decreases client self-esteem and the perception of control; assuming too little leaves the client without needed resources, causing symptom exacerbation and possibly rehospitalization.

It has been said that if one can make it through the paperwork of financial assistance systems, one does not need the money. To some degree, this is true. Clients who are unable to maintain any employment will most likely need the therapist's assistance to obtain help. This process may mean sitting down with the client and filling out application forms, giving addresses of agencies, and bus money for transportation, or even going to the agency with the client. The presence of the therapist is particularly helpful for paranoid clients who would not be able to interact with many strangers by themselves.

Coordinating with occupational resources is frequently needed to provide employment experiences at varying levels of functioning. A job of some type, be that regular employment, workshop or other "sheltered" employment, volunteering, or selling cigarettes to other clients within a peer social support group, provides an important sense of being needed.

Assessing for Health Problems

Chronically ill clients frequently have poor health care habits that predispose them to physical illnesses. Obesity, thyroid dysfunction, infections, and vitamin deficiencies are common health problems. All of these physical problems impact on the client's psychological sense of well-being. Psychiatric mental health nurses must familiarize themselves with physical complications that may result from long-term medication use and continually assess for these problems.

Complaints about physical symptoms should be evaluated carefully. Even clients with delusions around physical symptoms can, and do, become ill. Their "crying wolf" makes these clients a serious risk for major medical complications.

It is easy to forget that clients with chronic mental illness can experience other mental illnesses as well. There is the need to assess for these. Schizophrenia does not prevent personality disorders, for example. Surely some clients with chronic schizophrenia also experience depression unrelated to the awareness of losses involved with this illness.

Health care resources are probably even more difficult for the client to obtain than financial resources. Keeping a file of low cost health clinics keeps track of the resources that do exist. Although there is no easy solution, nurses have a responsibility to observe for health problems and identify appropriate health care resources. By learning about systems, actively coordinating them, and assessing for potential health problems, the nurse therapist can attempt to ensure that the client has ongoing basic living resources. During these frugal economic times, this is indeed a challenge.

THE THERAPEUTIC RELATIONSHIP

The therapeutic relationship has been referred to in the preceeding discussion. However, because it is the nurse's primary tool and the client's greatest resource, it merits specific discussion. This section describes the relationship with chronically ill clients, identifies strategies using the therapeutic relationship to impact on problems, and addresses particular needs of clients using each defense style.

Developing Trust

Acceptance and empathy are crucial elements in the development of trust. Trust makes the therapeutic relationship a powerful tool in promoting optimal client well-being. Acceptance operationally means avoiding unrealistic expectations for client progress. Expecting progress predisposes the therapist to feel frustrated and disappointed when periods of decompensation, inherent in chronic mental illness, occur. The client quickly senses therapist disappointment, interprets his or her own behavior as failure, and the therapist's disappointment as rejection (Seeman & McGree, 1982). Instead, the therapist should actively encourage progress toward goals, but expect none. Encouraging progress allows the therapist to exult with the client during good times yet be supportive during times of increased symptomatology. The therapist and client become a team, working together to minimize the intrusion of symptoms in the client's life and increasing the quality of life.

Empathy refers to a process in which the therapist communicates care for the client by listening to and understanding experiences from the client's perspective. This understanding, combined with professional knowledge, is shared with the client and becomes potentially useful to the client in understanding his or her experience. For example, the therapist conveys empathy by acknowledging that psychotic experiences seem real, rather than discounting the client's experience. Empathy and acceptance encourage trust, which makes the relationship a therapeutic tool.

Patience

Growth occurs over long periods of time. For example, grieving takes time. The nurse must be patient and allow the client time to struggle with the awareness and implications of loss, reformulate goals, and eventually achieve a new sense of self. Patience is crucial in working with chronically ill adults (Garant, 1980; Kotin, 1976; McGlashan & Carpenter, 1976). This quality is facilitated by focusing on present functioning or broadening one's time frame to growth that has occurred over years. For example, a client with chronic schizophrenia frequently became impatient with herself, which increased her stress level and stimulated hallucinations. Looking back several years to a time when she was hospitalized almost every three months helped her appreciate, and accept, her own progress. Placing importance on present functioning and long-term gains also gives the therapist material about which to be enthusiastic and decreases the emphasis on the unknown future course of the illness (Mailick, 1979).

Reaching Out

Clients not only desire someone to listen honestly to their feelings and concerns, but also to ask about their experiences. Recently, an 18-year-old client was asked, "How does it feel knowing that you've been crazy?" She responded with astonishment, then with tears, and said, "I say to myself, Why me?" She went on to express great relief that someone had encouraged her to talk about her frightening experiences in a state hospital. Because of the stigma of mental illness, the nurse must directly ask about the client's perception of themselves and their "being crazy." They want to talk about it. The therapist need only ask.

In settings that involve long, informal contacts between clients and nurse, it is easy to forget that regular therapy appointments are still essential to develop and maintain trust. The nurse should set aside time that is uniquely the client's, regardless of the presence or lack of acute symptoms. Also, therapist and client should consistently meet in a private office, not in a public area. This approach communicates the nurse therapist's trustworthiness and care for the client and avoids getting into a pattern of rewarding decompensation with attention.

Avoiding Withdrawal

Chronically mentally ill clients are often not the most charming of people. Their hygiene may be poor and their public behavior embarrassing. Because of this, and an unrealistic expectation for change on the part of the therapist, avoiding psychological withdrawal from the client is a major task within the therapeutic relationship. Mutual withdrawal (Tudor, 1952) begins when the therapist interprets the client's persistent lack of change as failure and consequently makes fewer and fewer attempts to empathize with the client. Ironically, the client from whom one feels the greatest tendency to withdraw needs therapist involvement the most.

Recognition of psychological withdrawal is the cornerstone to preventing its harmful influence (Bachrach, 1979; Shea & Hurley, 1964; Slavinsky & Krauss, 1980). Signs of withdrawal include (1) labeling the client, for example, as hopeless, which legitimatizes the therapist's psychological pulling away; (2) avoiding individual time or charting that both require thinking about the client and treatment; (3) humoring the client rather than taking needs and concerns seriously; and (4) dealing with the client by spontaneously inventing rules and policies rather than processing issues. Case conferences and clinical supervision can help the nurse become aware of signs of withdrawal.

Gaining Self-Awareness

Finally, the therapist's attitudes and beliefs impact on the client. This includes beliefs about chronic mental illness. Friedmann, Procci, and Fenn (1980) studied the effect of therapist's prognosis on client functioning. In four case studies, they described significant changes in functioning when the therapist communicated positive, encouraging expectations. Others, too, warn that a therapist's disappointment and encouragement are communicated to the client (Dimond & Jones, 1983; Lovejoy, 1982; Seeman & McGree, 1982). Experiential, value clarification exercises can increase the nurse therapist's awareness of personal values that may infiltrate the therapeutic relationship.

There has been a change in professional jargon over the past years. In contrast to focusing on growth, today therapists talk about "preventing decompensation" and "maintaining the client in the community." Perhaps this is an unfortunate byproduct of genetic studies and the widespread use of medication. Learning more about the physical aspects of these illnesses has altered our hope for growth in clients, possibly too much so. Exactly how this change from encouraging growth to encouraging maintenance has affected clients would be an interesting area of study.

The therapeutic relationship is an important resource for the client with chronic mental illness. Far from being ineffective or too costly, the therapeutic relationship is an essential tool for helping severely ill clients deal with the problems they face and increasing their quality of life. Nursing is only beginning to explore the dynamics involved in living with chronic mental illness. Studies remain on the descriptive level and focus on correlating demographic variables rather than exploring the experience of chronic mental illness. Consequently, much of the material in this chapter, particularly intervention strategies, has been derived from literature discussing other chronic illnesses. Clearly, the value of these strategies for the chronically mentally ill needs to be validated by research. However, in its absence, clinical examples were provided to increase the validity of the approaches recommended.

SUMMARY

In this chapter an attempt was made to provide the psychiatric mental health nurse with a framework from which to effectively work with clients experiencing chronic mental illness. The major problems of these clients were discussed and intervention strategies aimed at increasing the client's quality of life were suggested.

REFERENCES

Abramson, L. Y., Garber, J., & Seligman, M. E. P. Learned helplessness in humans: An attributional analysis. In J. Garber & M. E. P. Seligman (Eds.), *Human helplessness: Theory and application.* New York: Academic Press, 1980.

Adams, J. E., & Lindemann, E. Coping with long-term disability. In G. Coelho, D. A. Hamburg, & J. E. Adams (Eds.), *Coping and adaptation.* New York: Basic Books, 1974.

Averill, J. R. Personal control over aversive stimuli and its relationship to stress. *Psychological Bulletin,* 1973, *80,* 286–303.

Bachrach, L. L. Planning mental health services for chronic patients. *Hospital and Community Psychiatry,* 1979, *30,* 387–393.

Carson, V. Meeting the spiritual needs of hospitalized psychiatric patients. *Perspectives in Psychiatric Care,* 1980, *18,* 17–20.

Craig, A. E., & Hyatt, B. A. Chronicity in mental illness: A theory on the role of change. *Perspectives in Psychiatric Care,* 1978, *16,* 139–154.

DeLoach, C., & Greer, B. G. *Adjustment to severe physical disability: A metamorphosis.* New York: McGraw-Hill, 1981.

Dimond, M. Patient strategies for managing maintenance hemodialysis. *Western Journal of Nursing Research,* 1980, *2,* 555–568.

Dimond, M., & Jones, S. L. *Chronic illness across the life span.* Norwalk, CT: Appleton-Century-Crofts, 1983.

Feldman, D. Chronic disabling illness: A holistic view. *Journal of Chronic Disease,* 1974, *27,* 287–291.

Friedmann, C. T. H., Procci, W. R., & Fenn, A. The role of expectation in treatment for psychotic patients. *American Journal of Psychotherapy,* 1980, *34,* 188–196.

Garant, C. Stalls in the therapeutic process. *American Journal of Nursing,* 1980, *80,* 2166–2169.

Garber, J., & Seligman, M. E. P. (Eds.). *Human helplessness: Theory and application.* New York: Academic Press, 1980.

Gersten, E. Mental health issues of the severely disabled psychiatric client. In M. Davis (Ed.), *From dependence to independence.* Boulder, CO: WICHE, 1981.

Goffman, E. *Asylums.* Garden City, NY: Anchor Book, 1961.

Goldman, H. H., Gattozzi, A. A., & Taube, C. A. Defining and counting the chronically mentally ill. *Hospital and Community Psychiatry,* 1981, *32,* 21–27.

Greenberg, I. M., Weltz, S., Spitz, C., & Bizzozero, D. J. Factors of adjustment in chronic hemodialysis patients. *Psychosomatics,* 1975, *16,* 178–184.

Hoffman, B. F. To tell or not to tell. *Schizophrenia Bulletin,* 1981, *7,* 369–371.

Kemp, B. J., & Vash, C. L. Productivity after injury in a sample of spinal cord injured persons: A pilot study. *Journal of Chronic Disease,* 1971, *24,* 259–275.

Kotin, J. Discussion. *American Journal of Psychiatry,* 1976, *133,* 19.

Krauss, J. B. The chronic psychiatric patient in the community: A model of care. *Nursing Outlook,* 1980, *28,* 308–314.

Levy, N. B. The chronically ill patient. *Psychiatric Quarterly,* 1979, *51,* 189–197.

Lewis, F. M. Experienced personal control and quality of life in late-stage cancer patients. *Nursing Research,* 1982, *31,* 113–119.

Lovejoy, M. Expectations and the recovery process. *Schizophrenia Bulletin.* 1982, *8,* 605–609.

Lovejoy, M. Treatment and community support from the client perspective. Paper presented at *Learning and Sharing: Community Support Systems for the Chronically Mentally Ill,* Salt Lake City, March 1983.

Lowery, B. J., & DuCette, J. P. Disease-related learning and disease control in diabetics as a function of locus of control. *Nursing Research,* 1976, *25,* 358–362.

MacKinnon, B. L. Postpsychotic depression and the need for personal significance. *American Journal of Psychiatry,* 1977, *134,* 427–429.

Mailick, M. The impact of severe illness on the individual and family: An overview. *Social Work in Health Care,* 1979, *5,* 117–128.

McGlashan, T. H. Aphanisis: The syndrome of pseudo-depression in chronic schizophrenia. *Schizophrenia Bulletin,* 1982, *8,* 118–134.

McGlashan, T. H., & Carpenter, W. T. Postpsychotic depression in schizophrenia. *Archives of General Psychiatry,* 1976, *33,* 231–239.

McGlashan, T. H., & Carpenter, W. T. Does attitude toward psychosis relate to outcome? *American Journal of Psychiatry,* 1981, *138,* 797–801.

McGlashan, T. H., Levy, S. T., & Carpenter, W. T. Integration and sealing over. *Archives of General Psychiatry,* 1975, *32,* 1269–1272.

Meyersburg, H. A., Ablon, S. L., & Kotin, J. A reverberating psychic mechanism in the depressive processes. *Psychiatry,* 1974, *37,* 372–386.

Miller, J. F. *Coping with chronic illness: Overcoming powerlessness.* Philadelphia: F. A. Davis, 1983.

Pilsecker, C. On educating schizophrenics about schizophrenia. *Schizophrenia Bulletin,* 1981, *7,* 379–382.

Raskin, D. E. Masked depression in chronic schizophrenia. *Psychiatric Quarterly,* 1970, *44,* 575–582.

Roth, S. The seemingly ubiquitous depression following acute schizophrenia episodes. *American Journal of Psychiatry,* 1970, *127,* 91–98.

Russell, R. A. Concepts of adjustment to disability: An overview. *Rehabilitation Literature,* 1981, *42,* 330–338.

Seeman, M. V., & McGree, H. Treating depression in schizophrenic patients. *American Journal of Psychotherapy,* 1982, *36,* 14–22.

Shea, F., & Hurley, E. Hopelessness and helplessness. *Perspectives in Psychiatric Care,* 1964, *2,* 32–38.

Silver, R. L., & Wortman, C. B. Coping with undesirable life events. In J. Garber & M. E. P. Seligman (Eds.), *Human helplessness: Theory and application.* New York: Academic Press, 1980.

Slavinsky, A. T., & Krauss, J. B. Mutual withdrawal or Gwen Tudor revisited. *Perspectives in Psychiatric Care,* 1980, *18,* 194–203.

Slimmer, L. W. Helping students to resolve conflicts between their religious beliefs and psychiatric-mental health treatment approaches. *Journal of Psychiatric Nursing and Mental Health Services,* 1980, *18,* 37–39.

Smith, J. H. Identificatory styles in depression and grief. *International Journal of Psychoanalysis,* 1971, *52,* 259–266.

Strauss, A. L. *Chronic illness and the quality of life.* St. Louis: C. V. Mosby, 1975.

Strauss, A. L. Chronic illness. In A. L. Strauss (Ed.), *Where medicine fails.* New Brunswick, NJ: Transaction, 1979.

Test, M. A., & Stein, L. E. Community treatment of the chronic patient: Research overview. *Schizophrenia Bulletin,* 1978, *4,* 319–347.

Tudor, G. A sociopsychiatric nursing approach to intervention in a problem of mutual withdrawal on a mental hospital ward. *Psychiatry,* 1952, *15,* 193–217.

U.S. Government Printing Office. *Task panel reports: The president's commission on mental health* (Vol. 2). Washington, DC: U.S. Government Printing Office, 1978.

Viney, L., & Westbrook, M. T. Psychological reactions to chronic illness-related disability as a function of its severity and type. *Journal of Psychosomatic Research,* 1981, *25,* 513–523.

Visotsky, H. M., Hamburg, D. A., Goss, M. E., & Lebovits, B. Z. Coping behavior under extreme stress. *Archives of General Psychiatry,* 1961, *5,* 423–448.

Waters, J. H. Needs of the chronically mentally ill adult: Implications for mental health services. In M. Davis (Ed.), *From dependence to independence.* Boulder, CO: WICHE, 1981.

BIBLIOGRAPHY

Brissett, D. Toward a clarification of self-esteem. *Psychiatry,* 1972, *35,* 255–263.

CHAPTER 20

THE ALCOHOLIC CLIENT AND FAMILY

Mary Ann Walsh Eells

There is an emergent and rapidly developing literature about alcoholism, and although tomorrow's discoveries may change our views it is possible to discern a certain focus and direction in the many theories being proposed, investigated, and used today. Because it is unrealistic to review all the theoretical perspectives relevant to alcoholism, this chapter is written in the spirit of Occam's razor, that the explanations of alcoholism should first be sought in terms of what is known and whether it is efficacious in practice. Included in this chapter are some of the current issues and newer concepts from advances in research and theory organized within the conceptual models of the disease concept of alcoholism, the developmental psychodynamic model, the neurophysiological model, the genetic familial transmission model, and the Bowen family systems model. Some of these advances promise to organize and integrate differently what we now know about alcoholic clients and their families. The apparent strengths and limitations of the perspectives are discussed as are their implications for the psychiatric mental health nurse specialist.

Although alcoholic clients and their families are the focus, many of the principles apply also to those who abuse other substances. A beginning knowledge on the part of the reader is assumed or can be gained from well developed resources such as the book edited by Estes and Heinemann (1982).

The various theories being advanced today are actually conceptual models in that they are comprised of more or less interrelated components. The models provide different perspectives, although in many ways they are also complementary and sometimes overlapping. In order to compare them to a given standard, Prigogine's general systems theory model of systems undergoing change will be utilized.

One of the tenets of general systems theory is that systems have only a few major purposes that are fundamental. One of these purposes is simply to remain viable. In order to do so, there must be a uniqueness in a system's patterns. Without uniqueness, it would melt into its environment and cease to exist as a separate entity. The second major purpose is that a system must reliably maintain its unique patterns. The third major purpose is that the system must reproduce these patterns over time so that the patterns are maintained in an uninterrupted fashion. Whether these patterns are functional or dysfunctional does not matter; the fact is that any pattern at all that is unique, reliable, and reproduced over time is life-giving to its system, even if the pattern is alcoholism or another addiction.

PRIGOGINE'S MODEL OF SYSTEM CHANGE

Prigogine, Nicolis, and Babloyantz (1972; also Prigogine, 1980) have proposed a model that shows the basic process a system undergoes as it changes. First, the system regularly produces innate and acquired coherent sets of behavior that are unique to the system. If the system never learned anything new, eventually these well known sets of behavior would wear down, in that they would no longer fit new situations encountered and would no longer work. Feedback received from the environment would show that these old behaviors are not working, but the system would doggedly reproduce them since at least they are unique and reliable and can be reproduced consistently. A certain gratitude should exist for having such sets of behaviors; otherwise, a system would be required to learn everything anew each day. Also, they need only a low order of input of resources to work. If this set of behaviors is no longer working, entropy or disorder begins to pile up in the system's environment. To the extent that the system keeps using the behaviors anyway, the system's energy becomes depleted. Nevertheless, such nonworking sets of behavior are relentlessly reproduced and exhibited out in the environment.

The alcoholic client and his or her family can be compared to a system that is tightly interconnected with various components and processes that maintain addiction. The alcoholic's boundary with the external environment permits very few exchanges. It is usually impervious to negative feedback which, if accepted, would be corrective in changing the behaviors. This fact is especially true when the alcoholic has been drinking. Until satiated, his boundary permits one important type of exchange, the intake of alcohol. Although the actions taken are not working for him, the alcoholic keeps reproducing the same behaviors and becomes depleted of energy. We now know that his or her innate behaviors no doubt include a genetic inheritance that sustains addiction in strong force. When these patterns are plotted on a graph, their cyclic and homeostatic nature becomes readily apparent.

Prigogine describes a second set of behaviors, which are new behaviors being learned. They require a higher order of input consisting of better information and resources being exchanged across a boundary that selectively accepts them. As the new behaviors are being formed, dissonance internal to the system is set up since the new behaviors are often different from, and even in opposition to, the old behaviors. The new behaviors are also displayed out in the environment and the system receives feedback that corrects errors. This helps to shape the new behaviors. Though all this activity and disequilibrium is unsettling to the system, it is necessary, and, when enough has happened, a plateau or lull occurs. Suddenly, however, the system reintegrates and learns the new behavior. At that time, the system rocks to a new rhythm, integrating the new and old behaviors, and a high level of energy is experienced. A new and more optimal level of functioning is reached and entropy or disorder is decreased significantly. In order to reach this state, however, note that the system has had to undergo a risky period of disequilibrium. This is the process of change that must occur in order for the alcoholic client to sober up. Yet, it is the very process that is mightily resisted by the forceful patterns of addiction prevailing at each level of the system. Even in the external environment of the addiction system, fixed patterns prevail that sustain addiction. The family of the alcoholic is an example.

From experiences with these alcoholic systems and environments so resistive to change the following conceptual models have emerged for the understanding and treatment of alcoholism. Each model makes a unique contribution at a different level in alcoholic systems. The professional role required by each is somewhat different.

THE DISEASE CONCEPT OF ALCOHOLISM

Jellinek (1960) was the first to conceptualize alcoholism as a disease, fully describe its different syndromes, and subsequently popularize the disease concept. Its wide acceptance plays an important role in freeing the alcoholic from stigma and blame for his illness. At least the physical aspects of the disease concept were fully accepted by the members of Alcoholics Anonymous, who even today tell new members that they suffer from an allergy to alcohol. However, they have not accepted as enthusiastically the psychological aspects of the disease concept, and most members claim that continued abstinence alone will solve these problems.

Though most professionals accepted Jellinek's disease concept in principle, the nature of the disease of alcoholism continued to be hotly debated. The major issues include: (1) Is alcoholism a single disease or is it several diseases? (2) Are biological, psychological, and social variables equally contributory or can just one of these suffice for the development of alcoholism? (3) Is alcoholism hereditary, genetic, or acquired? (4) Does alcoholism progressively worsen over time or are plateaus reached? (5) Are the continuous and episodic types of drinking patterns only different forms of the same disease or are they different diseases? (6) What is the best type of treatment?

A unitary model of alcoholism as a disease eventually emerged. Pattison, Sobell, and Sobell (1977) described the underlying assumptions of this model as the view that alcoholism is a progressive, permanent, and irreversible condition unique to alcoholics, who experience irresistible physical or psychological compulsions to drink alcohol and who have lost control over initiating or stopping drinking. However, Pattison et al. (1977) also marshalled research findings to dispute the unitary disease concept. Instead, they supported the concept of a "multivariate alcoholism syndrome." Their view acknowledged the associated environmental influences and was representative of the thinking of many professionals in the field. Some of the propositions of the multivariate model include: (1) several syndromes of alcoholism exist, (2) anyone could develop alcohol dependence given the opportunity of a sufficiently long and intensive period of alcohol ingestion, (3) alcoholism could stablize at any level of severity, (4) alcoholism is reversible, (5) abstinence bears no relationship to rehabilitation, (6) there is no unique metabolic processing of alcohol, and (7) patterns of alcohol intake may be modified and controlled so that drinking is no longer a problem.

Out of this type of thinking emerged many experiments and studies. Some experiments attempted to prove that alcoholics could control their drinking (they could not). Some studies hypothesized that social environments could precipitate alcoholism (some individuals succumbed, others did not). Other studies hypothesized that the psychological aspects of the disease, presumably learned, could be unlearned (unfortunately, no proof has been forthcoming that there are lasting effects of such unlearning).

Types of Alcoholism

Over the years, many research studies have supported the consistent clinical impression that different types of alcoholism exist, at the very least two types. One is characterized by continuous, usually daily drinking, and the other by periodic binge drinking.

Goodwin (1979) has described two other types of alcoholism, familial and nonfamilial, which may be important in determining patterns of hereditary transmission. Prevention, intervention, and rehabilitation measures would vary for the two different groups. He characterizes the *familial* type by (1) a family history of alcoholism, (2) early onset, (3) severe symptoms that require treatment at an early age, and (4) the absence of other psychopathology. The *nonfamilial* type is characterized by (1) no family history of alcoholism, (2) later onset in life, (3) symptoms that are milder, and (4) the presence of other psychopathology. Goodwin's categories are congruent with the types of alcoholism often described as primary and secondary. Eells (1984) has suggested the probable need for revision of Goodwin's criteria for special population groups, particularly women. Because of the potentially damaging stigma of alcoholism for women, those who come from families with the inheritable type of alcoholism may vigorously postpone heavy drinking early in life, only to succumb later to addiction. According to Ashley (1977), women alcoholics as a group experience a rapidly developing and severe pathophysiology, which categorizes them with Goodwin's familial type.

Wartburg (1980) has theorized that the various types or expressions of alcoholism among different populations are related to a genetic polymorphism of human liver deoxyhydrogenase. This syndrome may produce as many as nine different genetic forms of alcoholism that range from an extremely aversive reaction following alcohol ingestion to a very rapid metabolism of alcohol and increased tolerance for high blood levels of alcohol. This theory fits with clinical observations of families with alcoholism, which almost always include both teetotalers and alcoholics. As the technical problems in the measurement of acetaldehyde are resolved, more definitive studies should be forthcoming. Eventually, different genetic types probably will be incorporated in the available criteria and guides for assessment. For the time being, the practical need for making some determination of the alcoholic's status is resolved primarily through the use of the Diagnostic and Statistical Manual for Mental Disorders (DSM-III; American Psychiatric Association, 1980).

Using the DSM-III

It is relatively simple to assess the client for alcoholism using DSM-III if its limitations are recognized. It treats alcoholism as a single disease, even though the emerging evidence indicates that several types of alcoholism probably exist. The DMS-III does include, however, the different types of drinking patterns, continuous and episodic, which should be entered appropriately in the fifth digit of the DSM-III code (p. 17). Also mentioned is the fact that alcohol abuse and dependence tend to run in families and that there is evidence of a genetic factor. Unfortunately, no means for coding familial incidence or familial transmission is yet included.

Some may find it helpful to compare DSM-III with the older criteria published by the National Council on Alcoholism (Criteria Committee, 1972) The NCA criteria include more content relative to the physical complications of alcoholism as well as categories of symptoms that are explicitly labeled progressive. However, since the intent of the Criteria Committee was to prevent overdiagnosis, and because some early symptoms recognized today were not identified at that time, few early symptoms are mentioned (see Sandler, 1980).

The DSM-III, of course, includes the many other psychiatric diagnoses that often coexist with alcoholism, whereas the NCA criteria do not include them. If at all possible, such coexisting diagnoses should be made at the same time as the alcoholism diagnosis so as to ensure adequate treatment (Solomon, 1982). For alcoholics, these other diagnoses often are the affective disorders, anxiety disorders, personality disorders, and schizophrenic disorders, as well as substance abuse disorders other than alcoholism.

Diagnoses specific to alcoholism are found in DSM-III under the categories of substance abuse disorders and organic mental disorders. Misleadingly included under substance abuse disorders (pp. 163–170) is a diagnosis supposedly not indicative of alcoholism, alcohol abuse. The diagnostic criteria for alcohol abuse require a pattern of pathological alcohol use for at least one month, together with impaired social or occupational functioning. Although it does not include symptoms of tolerance or withdrawal, and this category is not considered diagnostic of alcoholism, most experts would agree that this pattern could be alcoholism. The large quantities of ingested alcohol mentioned for this category probably could not be consumed except in the presence of tolerance. If evidence of tolerance or withdrawal is found with assessment, the diagnosis is alcohol dependence instead of alcohol abuse.

Other diagnoses related to alcoholism are found in DSM-III under organic mental disorders (pp. 101–139). These include alcohol withdrawal, alcohol withdrawal delirium, alcohol hallucinosis, and alcohol amnestic disorders. Blackouts and withdrawal may occur relatively early in the alcoholic's drinking career. Blackouts may occur anytime there is a sufficiently high blood alcohol level. Withdrawal occurs when a sufficiently long period of high alcohol intake is followed by a decrease, or cessation, in the amount of alcohol consumed. Even when alcoholics have been drinking heavily they may actually be suffering withdrawal symptoms because of a blood alcohol level that is decreasing.

There are special considerations relative to withdrawal. Although DSM-III stipulates (p. 133) that withdrawal symptoms almost always run a course of five to seven days, the symptoms may continue episodically in what is now being called a "protracted withdrawal syndrome." This syndrome may persist for two years or longer after alcohol intake stops and is characterized by episodic autonomic nervous system lability, various euphoric and dysphoric states, and changes in perceptions of time. The symptoms may be due to the reversible changes in the brain damage and brain atrophy that resulted from alcoholism (Berglund, Bliding, Bliding, & Risberg, 1980; Carlen & Wilkinson, 1980; Ellenburg, Rosenbaum, Goldman, & Whitman, 1980). Which symptoms of withdrawal tend to recur depends on which of the brain structures were damaged (Gross, Rosenblatt, Malenkowski, Lewis, & Broman, 1971). Disturbances in perception and cognition are due to damage of cortical structure and sensory receptors. The affective disturbances are due to limbic system involvement. The disturbances in level of consciousness, clouding of the sensorium, gait disturbances, and nystagmus are due to brain stem disturbances. As work in the neurosciences progresses, the source and effects of the disturbances that appear during withdrawal will become even better identified.

The remainder of the diagnoses found under organic mental disorders involving hallucinosis or seizures sometimes followed by delirium seem to require a well established pattern of pathological drinking that has persisted for years, generally found in older alcoholics. The dementias may be a manifestation of bilateral, diffuse brain damage. This damage is partly reversible over a two-year period of established abstinence, given a favorable family environment with low levels of anxiety.

Major problems in assessment, during and following withdrawal from alcohol, are the central nervous system effects of rising and falling blood alcohol levels, which may be mistaken for other psychiatric diagnoses. The appropriate interventions include: monitoring, assuring the client that these stages are expected and transient but may be recurring, assisting the client to pace himself or herself and focus only on what can be handled now in the present, and encouraging the client to synchronize his or her experiences with others (Eells, 1984). Nevertheless, such symptoms complicate assessment unless baseline data is available about other psychiatric symptoms that preceded the development of alcoholism. Normally, when detoxification from alcohol is complete and abstinence has been maintained for several weeks, other psychiatric diagnoses can be made with greater assurance.

Panic: A Common Problem

Quitkin and Rabkin (1982) have summarized the evidence that shows an association between alcoholism and panic disorder. They further observed that panic disorder occurred in a majority of their alcoholic clients. Panic disorders appear under anxiety disorders in DSM-III (pp. 230–232). However, the panic attacks of many alcoholics occur with less frequency than the DSM-III requirement of three attacks within a three-week period. Nevertheless, many alcoholics do experience them. They are very frightening and, importantly, they often contribute to relapses as the alcoholic turns to alcohol to relieve the symptoms of panic.

Strengths and Limitations of the Model

Referring to Prigogine's model, the disease concept focuses primarily on the individual's internal system. Little attention is given to the conditions that exist between the alcoholic and the environment, except for the environmental influences acknowledged by Pattison et al. (1977) and the familial type of alcoholism described by Goodwin (1979). Even though these external factors impinge heavily upon many alcoholics, their impact is not widely acknowledged by those who subscribe to the disease concept.

One of the important strengths of the disease concept is its very focus on the individual, which leads to a better scientific understanding of the internal processes occurring with alcoholism. Another strength is that its use brings tremendous emotional relief to the alcoholic when the client begins to understand that he or she is not tragically and morally flawed but instead has a disease that can be treated and arrested, if not cured. This belief instills hope. It also implies that it is necessary for the client to adapt to the sick role and comply with the treatment recommended by professionals (or, alternately, by members of A.A.). Finally, it relieves the family of an unnecessary burden of guilt and shame for their part in the alcoholic's illness. It helps them to identify appropriate treatment resources and reduces their blaming behavior toward the client and themselves.

A major limitation of the disease concept is that only the alcoholic family member is labeled as sick when others need help as well. To the extent that patterns in the family and in the environment sustain the addiction, the disease concept, although initially helpful, will eventually prove to be a limited and partial solution. Another major limitation of the disease concept is its evolving nature. Different definitions are given the disease by professionals who espouse the concept but hold different views. This tends to confuse professionals and lay persons alike, since different types of treatment and prevention emanate from the different views. Perhaps the most important implication for the professional role is to stay abreast of the different advances in knowledge that may or may not support the different types of treatment. Major advances relative to the genetic and biological bases of alcoholism may radically change treatment programs in the foreseeable future.

THE DEVELOPMENTAL PSYCHODYNAMIC MODEL

The focus of this conceptual model is the disordered psyche of the alcoholic, which may be either the result of the regressive effects of pathological drinking or the result of poor adaptation in the development of psychic structures (Khantzian, 1982). The assumption is that psychic defenses can be strengthened, developed, or changed through a therapeutic relationship that provides opportunities for awareness, insight, and the practice of new behaviors. The contact with the client is generally long-term. Transference and countertransference issues become important, which implicitly requires that the therapist has sufficiently resolved his or her own views about alcoholism and its related psychic events.

Should There Be a Psychiatric Diagnosis for the Alcoholic?

Often, the developmental psychodynamic view is disparaged by those who promote the disease concept of alcoholism and believe that detoxification, together with continued abstinence, will resolve most emotional problems. This latter view is at least partly correct, as the treatment of alcoholism is complicated by the fact that pathological drinking, in and of itself, can mimic a variety of psychiatric disorders. Thus, the first goal is the establishment of abstinence and assistance in regaining an optimal level of health. However, some alcoholics have other psychiatric diagnoses that preceded their alcoholism (Solomon, 1982). As previously discussed, it is important that any psychiatric diagnoses other than alcoholism are recognized, so that appropriate treatment can be instituted.

Sustained Abstinence and Improvements in Functioning

Studies of alcoholic populations during the first few years of abstinence are beginning to emerge. One example is the longitudinal study carried out by Pettinati, Sugerman and Maurer (1982), whose research subjects included 87 male and 46 female alcoholics admitted to one hospital for treatment. Baseline data on the Minnesota Multiphasic Personality Inventory (MMPI) was obtained on admission and compared with like data at the end of a four-year follow-up period. Additionally, their functioning in the community was assessed yearly on a variety of measures. During their hospitalization, most showed improvements on the MMPI subscale scores, which partly supports the view that detoxification from alcohol alone does result in some improvements in functioning.

Three groups emerged in the Pettinati study. The first group (n = 33), the *completely abstinent,* showed a good level of functioning in the community, and their initial elevations on the depression subscale of the MMPI had returned to normal levels four years later. Additionally, they had fewer rehospitalizations and psychological interventions than the other groups. The association between abstinence and functional improvements partly supports the view that continued abstinence alone may improve functioning. However, we have insufficient data on this population to make that judgement exactly. This group may have been the strongest group functionally anyway, and this characteristic could have enabled them to remain abstinent over the four-year period. Yet a third but unknown variable could have caused both abstinence and a good level of functioning.

The second group (n = 19), the *abstinent with slips,* experienced occasional relapses and did not function quite as well as the first group during the four-year follow-up period. Nevertheless, their initial elevations on the MMPI subscales for depression and psychopathic deviate were within normal range four years later. Again, this data is correlational.

The third and last group (n = 9), the *periodic drinkers,* consistently exhibited a poor level of functioning in their communities. They also showed initial elevations on the psychopathic deviate and hypomanic subscales of the MMPI, which remained elevated at the end of the follow-up period four years later. Even though their subscale scores and level of functioning in the community showed an association, two independent judges failed to predict later psychopathology from their initial subscale scores. Only a few subjects later exhibited other psychopathology that emerged over the study period.

The results of this interesting study are typical of results of other studies that point to apparently different and identifiable types of alcoholics. Although the results have limited generalizability to other populations, they highlight the fact that different groups of alcoholics may require different types of intervention. Those with initially elevated scores for depression seemed to remain abstinent and exhibit a better level of functioning overall. Their needs should not be underestimated, however, given the generally long and difficult period of recovery even for abstinent alcoholics. The group who initially showed depression and psychopathy did not do as well, and the poorest outcome was for those with the combination of hypomania and psychopathy. Minimally, both of these groups appear to need more intensive treatment and more structured environments.

An especially interesting feature of this study is that it introduces, once again, the long-standing question of why some alcoholics can take action in their own behalf in regard to abstinence from alcohol and others cannot. Such deficits in self-care can be subsumed under ego and superego deficits.

Ego Deficits

Khantzian (1982) has developed some special insights about the incapacity of the alcoholic to effectively regulate sets of appropriate defense mechanisms. He identified deficiencies in self-care functions and the regulation of affect resulting from ego deficits. The first involve the individual's external relationships. Outside observers judge the alcoholic's behavior to be reckless and self-destructive, resulting in negative consequences. Khantzian views this type of behavior as the result of failure in vigilance, awareness, cautiousness, worry, and fear that would usually alert an individual to avoid dangerous ways of behaving. This failure in self-regulation is substituted for by ineffective defense mechanisms, namely phobic behaviors, denial, projection, rationalization, and justifications. Little thought or reflection seems to occur relative to the consequence of behavior, and this type of individual usually exhibits an incapacity to delay before acting.

Khantzian (1982) has also described deficiencies in affect regulation involving the ego functions necessary for the regulation of one's internal emotional life. Overwhelming and chaotic internal states are experienced, together with an inability to identify and label inner feelings. Khantzian attributes this primarily to developmental arrest, though it may also be traumatic regression resulting from pathological drinking. Nevertheless, there is a failure to sufficiently differentiate and develop affects that serve as signals and guides to the regulation of behavior. Instead, denial and alcohol ingestion are used to ward off feelings that are experienced as intolerably chaotic.

Importantly, Khantzian relates these disturbances in the structures of the self to the alcoholic's failure to develop and internalize the capacity to care for himself and to nurture and comfort himself appropriately. Instead, what is internalized from others in his early life are pathological parts of the self that are seen as all-good or all-bad. Some of these parts are denied, repressed, and also projected onto others.

Khantzian's ideas about self-care functions have a parallel in some of the activities of Alcoholics Anonymous. New members are often instructed in ways to take care of themselves physically, nutritionally, and emotionally. Congruent with Khantzian's thinking, members are also encouraged to accept what Kurtz (1982) has called one's human limitations, that one cannot control the uncontrollable.

In clinical work with families, one condition is particularly likely to contribute to the disturbed self-care functions and incapacity to regulate personal affect so often found in alcoholics. This condition occurs when a parental problem develops and a child is pressed into service to fulfill the role functions not being carried out by either the drinking or nondrinking spouse. The child who does fulfill these inappropriate adult role functions is often thought of by the parent as a special child. However, while serving as rescuer for the parents, the child is deprived of the natural nurturing he or she would receive as a child. Instead, he or she must function as an adult and often perform a nurturing role toward the parents. Additionally, cut-offs with the extended family system often occur, which further deprives both the child and parents of possible nurturing from grandparents. While forced to play the role of the most responsible one in the family, the child must also heroically attempt to regulate what is a chaotic and nonnurturing household. This task has a heavy cost. While regulating others, this child's own developmental needs are neglected; his or her personal life is out of control. It is this child who often later succumbs to alcoholism and is seen in therapy with the set of symptoms Khantzian describes, particularly the incapacity for self-care and a super-independent posture toward his or her parents.

The Superego

Some of the most important dynamics involving the alcoholic's inner and outer life involve the phenomena of shame. Wurmser (1982) describes shame as the subjective view of a mortally flawed self, which results in abject humiliation, fears of exposure and being seen, and a self-contempt for the weakness of falling short in every way. Wurmser explains that guilt is different, since it limits strength and consists of the subjective fear of retribution from another person one has injured.

According to Wurmser (1981), the feelings of shame are defended against and warded off with many layers of defense, and these layers must be gradually explored in a psychotherapy that results in "cognitive restructuring of current reality and past history" (p. 270). Therapy involves a reeducation of ego functions within a context of superego problems. Wurmser (1982) claims that shame, as a global flaw of the self, is covered over by many defenses including repression, denial, projection, but most prominantly the archaic defense of reversal. Since the individual himself feels weak and shamed, he reverses the humiliation by raging against others, by his contempt for them. Having offered love only to be rejected, the individual seduces others and then rejects them. Having been betrayed, he betrays.

Alcoholic clients who suffer from profound shame, despite years of abstinence, are found to have a two-factored deficiency involving time. One factor takes place in the present: the many reversals and other defenses of denial, repression, and projection that emerge. The second factor took place in the past. The first layer most often takes the form of strong externalization and blaming toward others, which covers a deep shame for having invested oneself by trusting others when they seem to the client not to deserve that trust. As this shame is very gradually exposed and accepted by the therapist, a beginning realization occurs in the client that he or she has been overreaching in blaming and trying to control others. A terrible mortification appears with this important realization. While hurting others he or she also has not lived up to his or her ideal of what he or she should be. Nevertheless, as the therapist listens, it becomes evident to the client that it is acceptable to talk about these things. It is safe; one is not overwhelmed or swallowed up. The boundaries are clearer, and one is lovable. This process occurs again and again as each realization surfaces and it becomes possible to look upon and accept the dark side of oneself.

The second of the two factors is the past life of the client, any exploration of which is mightily resisted at first. Usually the negative parts of oneself, and one or more family members, inhabit this past and are rejected by the client. As the various layers that Wurmser speaks of are uncovered and become resolved to some degree, warm and positive feelings emerge toward the self and the person(s) who had been relegated to the client's past. Finally, there is a shift towards closeness with this person(s), often the client's mother, and the client one day tells the therapist that this person has finally found the client lovable. In this way, the client learns to love both the positive and negative aspects of self.

Strengths and Limitations of the Model

Prigogine (1980) has also commented that systems must have an awareness of the past, present, and future in order to undergo change. The developmental psychodynamic model addresses this through a reconstruction of the client's past life and its integration with the present. The psychic deficits relative to self-care, affect regulation, and shame gradually improve as the alcoholic learns more effective ways of regulating his internal environment and his relationship with his external environment.

Another strength of the model is its value in assisting the client to restructure his psyche and defense mechanisms in appropriately self-protective ways. For the alcoholic who is often labeled self-destructive, this is especially important. Lengthy contact with the therapist provides some assurance of a sufficiently long period of time during which healthier patterns can be internalized. The development of a satisfactorily regulated inner life, promoted during this effort, affords the alcoholic some lasting serenity and peace. The gradual and more optimal reconstruction of the past and its integration with the present is congruent with the approach of Alcoholics Anonymous (Thune, 1977). Finally, interventions are individualized according to the client's needs, as these unfold, and focused attention may be given to the various ways in which the client is attempting new behaviors until self-control becomes effectively established.

The limitations of the model include its length and costliness, not only for the client but also for the therapist who must undergo long, closely supervised preparation in order to do intensive psychotherapy. Also there are questions as to whether the gains in therapy are generalized to the family context. However, the client's verbalizations and the psychodynamics these reveal create ample opportunity for the therapist to monitor these developments. The model does not address the problems relative to overall family functioning. Should there be family problems that create powerful and continuing stresses, the client's gains may be short-lived. Also, this model does not include the education of the client relative to alcoholism, a lack which should be relieved with some appropriate teaching. Finally, an important implication for the professional role is that the setting in which care is provided must be a supportive one in which the resources are made available for the learning entailed in intensive psychotherapy and for appropriate supervision.

THE NEUROPHYSIOLOGICAL MODEL

The neurophysiological model is emerging as very important to alcoholism treatment because of recent findings showing that the brain damage and brain atrophy that occur with alcoholism are reversible to some extent. Particularly, right hemisphere damage seems to be reversible in alcoholics under the age of 40 years (Ellenburg, 1980). Golden, Graber, Blose, Berg, Coffman, and Bloch (1981) also found the left brains of alcoholics to be less dense than the normal brains. Both findings enhance the treatment of alcoholics. Eventually, we may know whether alcoholics possess differences in brain structure and function that precede the development of alcoholism. It begins to appear that Bateson's (1972) thinking, that the alcoholic drinks to correct some type of subjective error in thinking, may have some basis in fact. A basic understanding of right and left hemisphere functioning is necessary to the critique of this model. The reader unfamiliar with this information should first refer to Chapter 3.

The Effects of Alcohol on Brain Lateralization

In order to understand the brain damage associated with alcoholism, it is helpful to review what is known about the general effects of alcohol on the brain. According to Myslobodsky (1976), who reviewed the effects of different drugs, alcohol in mild doses appears to excite the left hemisphere, since it activates speech and produces elation. He cites the Rhodes, Obitz, and Creel, (1975) study, which demonstrated that alcohol at even higher blood levels, sufficient to produce motor and visuospatial difficulties and drowsiness, also produced decreased activity in the right brain hemisphere. We can assume then that alcohol may heighten left brain activity and that the alcoholic drinks to produce this initial effect; however, with declining blood alcohol levels, the alcoholic may show more right brain activity than left. In measuring* the brain dominance patterns of the same alcoholics when they were drinking and when they were sober, it was found that a left brain-dominant pattern shifts to a right brain-dominant pattern within 48 hours after alcohol intake stops. Curiously, this same group of right brain-dominant alcoholics usually engage in a great deal of activity when sober that is related to left brain functioning, such as prodigious reading and occupations that involve computers, language, mathematics, or the law. Perhaps both alcohol and these activities that stimulate the left brain somehow equalize the balance of activity between the right and left brain.

Brain Damage Among Alcoholics

Sandel and Alcorn (1980) categorized as right brain- or left brain-dominant a group of right-handed males who were diagnosed as alcoholics, as well as others diagnosed as depressive, nonparanoid schizophrenic, manic depressive, schizo-affective, and personality disordered (antisocial type). They found that right brain dominance was associated with alcoholism, depression, and nonparanoid schizophrenia; left brain dominance was associated with antisocial type personality disorders; bilaterality was associated with manic depressive and schizo-affective illnesses. Among a small group of sober alcoholics ($n = 12$), Eells (1982) found them to be evenly divided between right and left dominant types; however, continuing data collection on an increasingly larger sample has to date shown the majority of alcoholics to be right brain-dominant. Since it is unknown what proportion of right versus left dominant types are found in the general population, these findings on clinical populations are interesting but speculative.

As for brain damage among alcoholics, the findings generally suggest that right hemisphere damage occurs but is quickly reversible among alcoholics under age 40, who recover both verbal and visuospatial deficits *regardless* of the length of drinking history (Ellenburg et al., 1980). Those over age 40 experience some initial improvement in right hemisphere task performance but this later deteriorates 25 days postdrinking.

Since right hemisphere functions are so often compromised either temporarily or lastingly with alcoholism, these functions are summarized: nonverbal and visuospatial processing, holistic and global problem solving, subjective mood states, emotional judgement, and the comprehension of emotional voice tones and facial expressions. Bradshaw and Nettleton (1981) also include the processing of spatially distributed information and pattern recognition, spatial cognitive mapping of one's surroundings, mapping of exteroceptive body space and body schema, facial recognition, and attention and arousal.

A recent finding of Golden et al. (1981) is that left hemisphere functioning is severely compromised because of a less dense left hemisphere in alcoholics. Deficits in left hemisphere functioning would compromise task performance for, according to Bradshaw and Nettleton (1981), sequential verbal processing, the discrimination of temporal order, sequencing and rhythm, logical thinking, sorting things by categories, the elaboration of detail, and the bilateral fine control of coordination for limbs and fingers.

Still other observers have found frontal lobe impairment that is characterized by poor error utilization, interrupted performances involving sequences and either the loss of a

* The Lateral Eye Movement Index (LEMI) for the measurement of brain dominance can be obtained by writing to the author at the University of Maryland School of Nursing, 655 West Lombard Street, Baltimore, MD 21201.

capacity to plan or to put plans into action, and the impairment of visual scanning (e.g., Goldstein & Shelly, 1982).

When Gudeman, Craine, Golden, and McLaughlin (1977) noted some of these findings, they concluded from a factor analysis of their data on brain function that "the alcoholic is impaired on tasks that require an ongoing integration of time-space in the immediate situation" (p. 39). What seems to be impaired overall is the capacity to integrate the two hemispheres, since the right hemisphere is specialized for space and the left is specialized for chronological time. Following Gudemen's suggestion that interventions be designed to assist the alcoholic with this integration, some intervention strategies of this type were developed (Eells, 1984). These focus on helping the alcoholic to tackle only what can be reasonably accomplished in the present, while gradually developing a broader view of the past, present, and future that can be operationalized in everyday life. This approach is congruent with both Thune's (1977) view that A.A. activities facilitate time integration and the restructuring of time that takes place in different types of psychotherapy. This is a long-term effort that parallels the improvements in brain function during recovery. Also, the integration of space and time is greatly facilitated through interactions with others.

Strengths and Limitations of the Model

The major strength of the neurophysiological model is its capacity to represent the major ways in which humans apprehend their environments. Imbedded in a substrate of structural, biochemical, and other components of the brain, the tasks performed in relationship to the environment range widely from creativity to the ability to use language. When these functions become severely compromised, as with alcoholism, the people affected are seen by others as less than human.

In regard to the Prigogine model, the neurophysiological view addresses the phenomena that occur at the boundary between the alcoholic system and its environment. Both the active alcoholic and the family with alcoholism have frequently been described as systems with relatively closed and impermeable boundaries. Neither permits entry to higher-order input so that growth, development, and change occur. Only the cyclic pattern of addiction remains, until disturbances of sufficient magnitude from inside or outside the system finally push it into crisis. As the neurophysiological model enhances our knowledge of operations at the boundaries of systems, the potentials for intervention expand.

Other strengths of the model include the possibility of integrating knowledge that is now solely psychiatric, psychological, and physiological. Accordingly, the professional role requires a capacity to integrate old and new understandings into the new neurophysiological view.

The severest limitations of the model are those of any new paradigm. Extensive use clinically is necessary in order to assess its validity and practicality. This responsibility is a fundamental component of the professional role.

THE GENETIC, FAMILIAL TRANSMISSION MODEL

There is no longer any question of whether an inherited tendency toward alcoholism exists in families; what is unanswered is a more definitive explanation of its nature. There are many pieces of evidence now that include information about the incidence of alcoholism in populations, mechanisms relative to alcohol at the level of the cell, and responses of certain populations to alcohol ingestion.

Goodwin's (1979) adoption studies show that sons of alcoholics are four times as likely to develop alcoholism when compared to the general population, even when they are adopted out early and raised by nonalcoholic parents. Twin studies also show that identical twins who share the same genetic inheritance have double the rate of alcoholism, as compared to fraternal twins. Based on these results, Goodwin proposed a familial type of alcoholism. Furthermore, Spalt (1979) provided evidence that the genetic nature of inheritance for alcoholism may be an X-linked, recessive gene. He explains that evidence for this occurs when the percentage of affected males, mathematically squared, equals the percentage of affected females. Such proportions of males versus females often are found in clinical populations of alcoholics and in families with alcoholism.

Cellular studies are beginning to provide even more definitive evidence of a genetic origin for alcoholism. According to Obe and Ristow (1979), alcohol has mutagenic characteristics, in that alcohol and its metabolite acetaldehyde induce various chromosomal aberrations. Wartburg (1980) proposes a genetic polymorphism of the liver enzyme deoxyhydrogenase, which normally triggers the metabolism of alcohol. He and his colleagues have postulated nine different phenotypes that are the expression of this genetic polymorphism. One phenotype is the occurrence, in 80% of Orientals, of aversive effects as the result of alcohol ingestion, due to a genetic factor. Another type could be the relatively small population of alcoholics, only about 10%, who develop cirrhosis of the liver. Yet another type could be other groups of persons who experience a different variety of aversive effects from the ingestion of alcohol, notably some groups of women and teetotalers. This data introduces the possibility that in the same family the genetic inheritance may be expressed in different ways, some family members being teetotalers and others being alcoholics of different types.

Finally, Murray and Gurling (1980) summarize many findings that validate the genetic control and regulation of alcohol metabolism. Based on these findings, they propose a genetic model for alcoholism with three components, including: (1) powerful reinforcement effects from alcohol ingestion for the alcoholism-prone, (2) a genetic adaptive mechanism that accounts for the development of physical dependence upon alcohol, and (3) genetic variations in the susceptibility to the pathophysiological effects of alcoholism. On the basis of the emerging evidence, one could conclude that alcoholism appears to be caused more by the forces of nature than by the forces of nurture.

The Multigenerational Transmission Process

The rapidly developing view of the genetic nature of alcoholism does not yet explain why some individuals in families with a presumably equal probability for developing alcoholism in fact sometimes do not. Alcoholism has been known to skip generations in families. The different penetration rates and different expressions of alcoholism can be partly explained by Matsunaga's (1981) model of host susceptibility and host resistance for genetic diseases. He proposes that different variations in susceptibility and resistance may be due to either variations in the latency period required for the disease or inherited tissue resistance that would play a role in the induction phase of the disease. This could explain why some individuals, usually women, in families with a high incidence of alcoholism over generations, experience a later onset of alcoholism than is manifested by some of their male family members. The differences in latency period and tissue resistance could of course be separately transmitted genetically. Genetic factors may also control the progression of the disease once it becomes established. Alcoholics show a wide range of individual differences in the latency, induction, and progression phases of alcoholism, and Matsunaga's model could provide some explanation for these variations.

Another possible explanation for the widely varying expressions of alcoholism in a given family has to do with the emotional processes that prevail, as explained by Bowen (1978).

As adolescents and young adults begin to differentiate a self in relation to their families of origin, the use and abuse of alcohol and other addictive substances provides one mechanism that can be used. The inheritable "strain resistances," which Matsunaga proposes reside in the individual, meet up with the forces toward differentiation that Bowen proposes emerge during the separation from one's family of origin. Those with the strongest inheritance toward alcoholism may find alcohol powerfully reinforcing and choose this alternative in preference to other available alternatives for differentiating a self.

Strengths and Limitations of the Model

Referring back to Prigogine's model, the genetic factors involved with alcoholism represent sets of coherent behaviors that are innate and internal to the system. Of course, the transmission of alcoholism from generation to generation introduces an environmental factor also in that the extended family system is part of the environment and provides inputs to the family system. Long after alcoholics and their families have shut out other environmental forces they continue to be in touch with their extended family systems, which would appear to be the most natural and powerful route to penetrating the boundary of the system with alcoholism. Bowen's family systems theory, of course, makes use of this fact for family interventions.

The strengths of the genetic familial transmission model include its potential for the prevention and interruption of alcoholism through approaches targeted at the family. Genetic counseling, education, and public information are some approaches that could be used. Even better, it may become possible to identify and test individuals who may be prone to alcoholism before it develops. Even this may not work, however, unless the relationship of the family emotional processes to the emergence of alcoholism are addressed.

The limitations of this model obviously include the need for greater understanding of the nature of genetic and familial transmission. When knowledge is forthcoming, it will guide and inform intervention strategies. Until that time, the major implications for the professional role are related to research and to advising individuals and families with alcoholism or the potential for it. Few professionals actually engage in genetic studies at the level of the cell; however, there are other research roles, especially those related to research about families. Additionally, the advising role with families should be vigorously pursued. The knowledge that a genetic and familial transmission of alcoholism exists usually has a very positive effect on them and often considerably relieves the strong tendency to blame each other for the problem of alcoholism. Both individuals and families then become more amenable to therapeutic intervention.

THERAPY FOR A FAMILY WITH ALCOHOLISM

The case of Mary Donovan, a middle-aged alcoholic, is discussed here in order to illustrate the fact that alcoholism affects systems at all the levels previously discussed. These range from the biological levels of the individual to the sociocultural levels of the environment. Intervention at any given level has some effects; however, it is unlikely that any interventions will be successful in the long term until and unless intervention occurs at the level of the family. Alcoholism is a multigenerational process of many interacting levels of hierarchy, interruptable only in that context.

Bowen's Family Systems Theory

Murray Bowen (1978) has developed a theory of family systems therapy that is useful and effective for the family with alcoholism. His theory is utilized in discussing the following case study about the Donovan family. Particular chapters of Bowen's (1978) book which were used include: Chapter 12 "Alcoholism and the Family" (pp. 259–268), Chapter 16 "Theory in the Practice of Psychotherapy" (pp. 337–387), and Chapter 22 "Toward the Differentiation of Self in One's Family of Origin" (pp. 527–547).

Two key concepts of Bowen's theory that are important to this case study are the *differentiation of self* and *emotional cut-off.* According to Bowen (1978) the differentiation of self is at the heart of his theory. Each individual gets from his family of origin a basic level of differentiation, a combination of cognitive and emotional functioning, which he uses in response to his family's emotional process. A poorer level of differentiation means increased vulnerability to high levels of anxiety in the family and is characterized by more emotionality and less use of cognitive functioning. A better level of differentiation means less vulnerability to anxiety and more emphasis on cognitive than emotional functioning, although the two are intertwined. Bowen claims that the level of differentiation is a better predictor of prognosis than the pathological drinking pattern of the alcoholic.

When anxiety runs high in the family intemperate drinking occurs, which then results in even higher levels of anxiety, and so on. The resulting spiral results in impairment of the functioning of one or more family members. Reciprocal over- and under-functioning tend to occur in families with alcoholism, and either type may be alcoholic. The over-functioner's posture, especially in relationship to his mother, is one of super-independence that leads to over-functioning and emotional isolation. This then results in more drinking. The under-functioner is extremely close to his mother and functions less well than the other type in all areas of his life. This is the type of alcoholic who socially deteriorates.

Bowen views alcoholism as only one way in which human beings adapt to the emotional process in their families. Drinking pathologically almost always puts distance between the alcoholic and others and helps him to avoid the over-closeness of fusion (Fogarty, 1977) and its accompanying anxiety.

Yet another mechanism used to manage the emotional process in the family is that of emotional cut-off. *Cut-off* generally is taken to mean the attempt to differentiate by means of physical distance or through the use of internal psychic mechanisms or the use of both (see Bowen, 1978, pp. 382–384 and 535–546). This mechanism, in addition to pathological drinking, is overused in the Donovan family.

The Profile of Mary Donovan, Alcoholic

Mary is an over-functioner, who early on was taught by her parents that she was a special child who could excel and achieve at whatever she tried. Fortunately, this challenge was usually met by a high level of native intelligence and the inculcation of good work habits by her over-functioning mother. Although her father did not work as hard as her mother, he also functioned well at work and at home, except that he was more relaxed and more fun. While Mary's distant mother was always too busy to be bothered very much, her father could always find time to spend with Mary and her younger brother and sister. Her parents frequently argued because of her mother's general dissatisfaction with the father. When they argued, Mary's mother either moved toward the children and became very demanding of them, or would get Mary to do something with her father. Mary's frequent response to her mother's demands was to work harder at school, escape into reading, and dream of the day she could leave home.

Mary's earlier years had been characterized by the avoidance of alcohol because of nameless fears, worry about the alcoholic uncles in her family, and because of the teetotaling habits of both her parents. She hardly ever drank, though once married her husband drank quite a lot. They were divorced after a long course of marital therapy in which Mary was always the one who tried to make the marriage work while her husband did nothing. Her overfunctioning pattern continued into her adult life. After the divorce, she cut-off and moved away from the area where her parents lived, took a new job, and forgot her past. Many restrictions then seemed to be lifted from her life, including any curtailment of her alcohol intake. She began to drink socially and found that she very much enjoyed it. However, within a few months she began to experience some mild anxiety and severe depressions. Her response was to continue drinking with her new friends and to work harder as a double remedy; however, the depressions only increased in intensity and frequency. This downward spiral continued for six years until Mary collapsed physically and mentally. In desperation, she walked into a meeting of A.A. It helped, and she continued to go to meetings. However, she was overcome by the stigma of alcoholism, a family problem she had tried to avoid all of her life. The shame was unbearable, and although she told her parents she dreaded anyone else finding out. She gradually pieced her life back together physically and emotionally. She eventually moved back to the geographic area where her parents lived, with an intuitive sense that there was something back there she needed to resolve. Her progress was interrupted for a time when she experienced a panic attack and drank once again, but for only a few hours. This event was enough, however, to usher in a long period of apprehension that seemed to be affecting her functioning. It was at this point that Mary began therapy. The first priority was to reframe her problem as a family problem and to decrease the level of anxiety in the family system and, of course, for Mary too.

Burning Bridges

In gathering the family history, guided by the use of the genogram, a great deal of information emerged. Both of Mary's parents were teetotalers for very good reasons, which included a heavy incidence of alcoholism over several generations, including their own. Figure 20.1 depicts in the shaded boxes and circles the family members over five generations who have had definite symptoms of alcoholism. Both of Mary's grandfathers had been alcoholics. Three out of five of her father's brothers and both of her mother's brothers were alcoholics. Mary's brother was also an alcoholic, but her sister appeared to have escaped. Only later was she to become aware that both of her sons drank alcoholically and her daughter was addicted to drugs. Mary's family appears to fit the Goodwin (1979) criteria for familial alcoholism.

The other salient feature of the Donovan family was the widespread use of the mechanism of cut-off in attempts to differentiate from families of origin. Many of them had migrated to different parts of the country, especially the alcoholics who had died at an early age. One who needs to burn his bridges in the Donovan family moves very far away. Interestingly, the moves and the onset of addiction often occurred together. During times like this in the family, there was a convergence of emotional forces that seemed to kindle the addiction for those who were vulnerable. Mary herself moved hundreds of miles away from her family and became addicted to alcohol almost simultaneously. During these stress points, why was one particular family member affected and not another? Why Mary?

Mary is an oldest daughter; however, until she worked with her family history she did not know that she was the oldest daughter of an oldest daughter of an oldest daughter. Nor did she know that each of them had run away from home. Mary initially left home to go to college. Then, after her marriage ended, she returned closer to her parent's geographic area and at the same time her alcoholic brother married and moved away. Mary was now the only one left living close to home. She had in fact substituted for her brother.

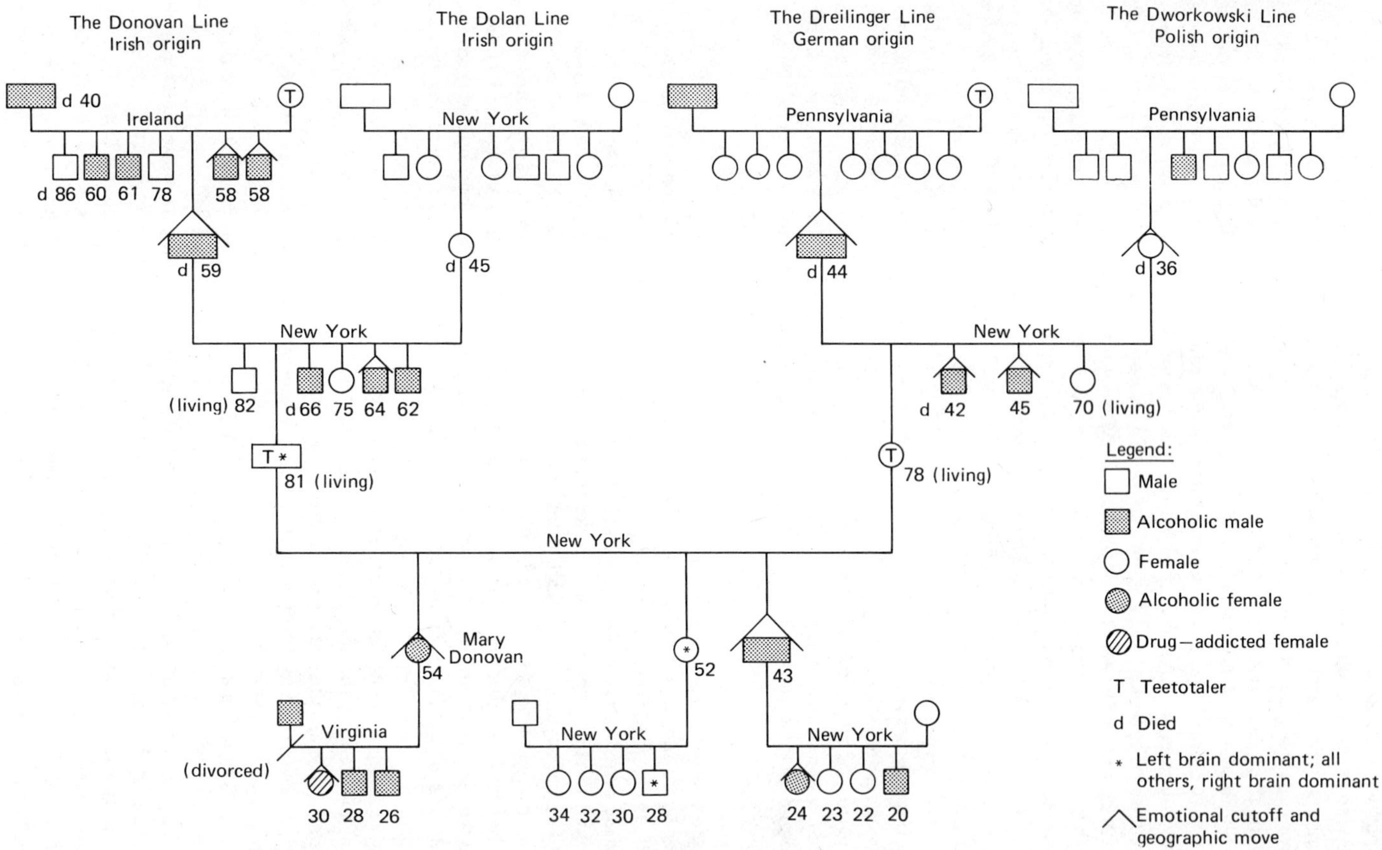

Figure 20.1 The multigenerational transmission process in Mary Donovan's family.

During this time, the relationship with her parents became too intense and uncomfortable. Her parents were in almost constant conflict and she kept getting caught up in it somehow. At this point, she symbolically ran away from home herself by moving away. She remembers almost fleeing with a sense of gratitude to be able to move far away for her new job. However, once she had left, she was desperately lonely for her family and in very frequent touch with her mother.

Perhaps one of the most important features of Bowen's definition of cut-off is the cut-off with the past. One cannot cut off from the past without, at the same time, cutting off one's generational heirarchy. Each of the oldest daughters who ran away did exactly this. The presence of a generational hierarchy introduces options of moving toward other family members both vertically and laterally. With the past and the previous generation cut off, the generational hierarchy of grandparents is lost to the next generation and the possibility of being nurtured by one's parents is also lost. With no pattern, it is difficult to formulate patterns out of one's head alone. For example, how does one learn to be a grandmother when one has had no grandmothers?

At this point in therapy, many toxic issues in Mary's family had been opened up, she had learned a great deal about how family systems work, and her anxiety level in relation to family members had considerably diminished. It was time to take some additional steps by going back into the past, into the family system.

Bridging Cut-offs

One of the most isolated members of her family when Mary began therapy was Mary herself. She was never in touch with her brother or sister; instead, family contacts were always originated by her mother. She was completely out of touch with members of the extended family, but she was very close to her one son who remained at home. The relationship with her former husband was quite hostile and distant.

The first step she tried was moving closer to her mother. Mary initiated conversations and telephone calls; a side benefit was that her father began to relinquish the ideal father picture he had always projected, opened up, and began to tell Mary about some of the aversive conditions of his early life. Trying to get closer to her sister was unsuccessful, and attempts to keep in touch with her brother were complicated by his active drinking and distancing behaviors. A dreadful calm came over the family, a sense of foreboding, and Mary's mother stopped calling her and became quietly remote. However, during this period, her brother sobered up for several months.

The next step she took was to bridge the relationship with her former husband. She wrote him letters about the happenings with their children, contacted her in-laws, and began to explore their family background also. The result was that her youngest son visited his father. Unlike many past visits, this one went very well. The bridge between the two parents had been freeing for the son and his father.

The initial efforts to get closer to her mother had been minimally productive. Mary now decided that this problem had to be resolved in order for her own functioning to remain optimal. She became convinced that if her mother could not bridge her cut-off from her own family, which had now lasted 50 years, she, Mary, would have to do it. Although the story is too lengthy to recount here, Mary traveled back to her mother's hometown, searched for and found her extended family, and then helped her mother to return home as well.

Mary has said that the trip to her mother's hometown was a hunt for her own identity. Discovering the roots of her mother's life gave her roots too. A major taproot had been missing. Many family members were added to Mary's family genogram. Her mother's repressed memories of her childhood came flooding back, and for Mary this elaborated her mother's personality and provided a richer context against which she could more fully understand her mother and herself. She learned that her mother's distance from her had been a wall of defenses holding back a lot of hurt for a frightened woman who had forsaken her past. Mary and her mother had bridged an emotional cut-off that had cost them both dearly over the years.

Not all attempted bridgings of cut-off end as happily as these did for Mary. However, by learning about cut-offs, and surviving the experiences of bridging them, Mary learned some important things about families and cut-offs.

IMPLICATIONS FOR PSYCHIATRIC MENTAL HEALTH NURSING

This chapter has presented important conceptual models being proposed, investigated, and used clinically for the treatment of alcoholism. What model should be adopted for the treatment of active alcoholism? To answer this sweeping question, the alcoholic and his family system can be considered within a time frame of different stages.

The first stage is the time period during which active alcoholism becomes labeled a problem by one or more family members. Most often, the active alcoholic does not see the problem and refuses treatment outright if it is suggested. The most powerful conceptual model at this time is one which is operationalized at the family level with the family member(s) who are motivated to seek help. This family member is most often the nonalcoholic spouse, but it may also be alcoholic parents who are worried about their acting-out adolescent. Family systems theory by Bowen (1978) is the most powerful of the family therapy models because it brings into play the past history of the family, thus reframing the problem as a multigenerational one, which alcoholism most often is. If only one member of the family system can make progress with this therapy model, the rest of the system will benefit. Subsequently, the drinking pattern becomes less intense and the alcoholic is able to enter treatment for his alcoholism. This approach also makes use of the intuitive principle of Al Anon, that the nonalcoholic spouse must "hit bottom," or face the problem first, before the alcoholic does.

The second stage is the time period during which the alcoholic family member accepts the need for treatment of alcoholism and either becomes a member of A.A., enters a detoxification program, or a rehabilitation program, or a combination of these. Almost immediately, the disease concept model is useful to the alcoholic as he or she begins the long education about this illness. For the psychiatric mental health nurse, the neurophysiological model is immediately useful in ascertaining the extent of brain damage and in monitoring its reversibility over the first several weeks and months. It is also useful for teaching the alcoholic and his or her family about the severity of brain damage and that recovery will occur slowly over at least a two-year period. Other psychiatric diagnoses must be made at this time or immediately thereafter. In consideration of these factors, plans should be made with the alcoholic and family for follow-up care. Family therapy should be a requirement made at this time for two reasons: (1) the family's skewed structure and function must be rectified or the alcoholic will drink again, and (2) it provides an opportunity for regular, consistent follow-up during what will be a long period of rehabilitation.

The third stage is the long period of rehabilitation that extends over the next few years. At present, this phase is the most neglected part of the alcoholic's health care. Most alcoholics and their families settle into an uneasy compromise at this point that consists of sobriety punctuated by multiple marital and family problems including divorce, job losses, addiction in the children, and occasional relapse. Even when the alcoholic remains sober and a faithful member of A.A., major family problems persist that require intervention at the family level. Again, the Bowen model for family therapy is the most powerful modality because it appropriately frames the problem by encompassing multigenerational levels. Often the source of stress contributing heavily to the excessive drinking lies in the previous generation; relieving it reduces and finally ends the alcoholic drinking. During this stage, the concepts of the psychodynamic model, including problems with affect regulation, self-care activities, and shame, are also relevant to the alcoholic's rehabilitation. The personality reconstruction that is necessary to long-term sobriety may require intensive psychotherapy for some. Again, the neurophysiological model continues to be useful during this stage, as an aid to understanding the alcoholic's status and recovery of brain function. In regard to operationalizing any of these conceptual models at a given time, the family therapy modality is the first choice and is a requisite in providing a favorable enough family environment so that the recovery of brain function and personality reconstruction may proceed.

SUMMARY

This chapter has illustrated that there are valid conceptual models for intervention in alcoholism with clients and their families but that no one model suffices. There are powerful forces that sustain addiction, whether these are genetic or acquired, familial or individual. Yet, even more powerful forces can be brought to bear to defeat addiction. Some of these forces we know how to orchestrate, notably, the power of a family system. The greatest challenge is the appropriate use of the different models in a timely fashion. Beyond that, the psychiatric mental health nurse must possess the knowledge and courage to impose the necessary conditions each model requires upon the alcoholic system, which otherwise only remains impervious to change.

REFERENCES

American Psychiatric Association. *Diagnostic and statistical manual of mental disorders* (3rd ed.). Washington, D.C.: American Psychiatric Association, 1980.

Ashley, M. J., Olin, J. S., le Riche, W. N., Kornaczewski, A., Schmidt, W., & Rankin, J. G. Morbidity in alcoholics. *Archives of Internal Medicine,* 1977, *137,* 883–887.

Bateson, G. *Steps to an ecology of mind.* New York: Ballantine Books, 1972.

Berglund, M., Bliding, G., Bliding, A., & Risberg, J. Reversibility of cerebral dysfunction in alcoholism during the first seven weeks of abstinence: A regional cerebral blood flow study. *Acta Psychiatrica Scandinavica* [Suppl], 1980, *286,* 119–127.

Bowen, M. *Family therapy in clinical practice.* New York: Jason Aronson, 1978.

Bradshaw, J. L., & Nettleton, N. C. The nature of hemispheric specialization in man. *Behavioral and Brain Sciences,* 1981, *4,* 51–91.

Carlen, P. L., & Wilkinson, D. A. Alcoholic brain damage and reversible deficits. *Acta Psychiatrica Scandinavica* [Suppl], 1980, *286,* 103–117.

Criteria Committee, National Council on Alcoholism. Criteria for the diagnosis of alcoholism. *American Journal of Psychiatry,* 1972, *129,* 127–135.

Eells, M. A. W. Timekeeper-spouses who contribute to equilibrium states in alcoholic family systems. In L. Troncale (Ed.), *A general survey of systems methodology (Vol. 2): Applications to real systems.* Proceedings of the Twenty-Sixth meeting of the Society for General Systems Research with the American Association for the Advancement of Science, Louisville, Kentucky, 1982.

Eells, M. A. W. Psychological aspects of the care of alcoholics. In L. Robinson (Ed.), *Psychological aspects of the hospitalized client* (4th ed.). New York: F. A. Davis, 1984.

Ellenburg, L., Rosenbaum, G., Goldman, M. S., & Whitman, R. D. Recoverability of psychological functioning following alcohol abuse: Lateralization effects. *Journal of Consulting and Clinical Psychology,* 1980, *48*(4), 503–510.

Estes, N. J., & Heinemann, M. E. (Eds.). *Alcoholism: Development, consequences and interventions* (2nd ed.). St. Louis: C.V. Mosby, 1982.

Fogarty, T. Fusion. *The Family,* 1977, *4*(2), 49–58.

Golden, C. J., Graber, B., Blose, I., Berg, R., Coffman, J., & Bloch, S. Difference in brain densities between chronic alcoholic and normal control patients. *Science,* 1981, *211,* 508–510.

Goldstein, G., & Shelly, C. A multivariate neuropsychological approach to brain lesion localization in alcoholism. *Addictive Behaviors,* 1982, *7,* 165–175.

Goodwin, D. W. Alcoholism and heredity. *Archives of General Psychiatry,* 1979, *36,* 57–61.

Gross, M. M., Rosenblatt, S. M., Malenkowski, B., Lewis, E. & Broman, B. *A factor analytic study of the clinical phenomena in the acute alcohol withdrawal syndromes.* Toronto: Addiction Research Foundation, 1971.

Gudeman, H. E., Craine, J. F., Golden, C. J., & McLaughlin, D. Higher cortical dysfunction associated with long term alcoholism. *International Journal of Neuroscience,* 1977, *8,* 33–40.

Jellinek, E. M. P. *The disease concept of alcoholism.* New Haven, CT: Hillhouse Press, 1960.

Khantzian, E. J. Psychopathology, psychodynamics, and alcoholism. In E. M. Pattison & E. Kaufman (Eds.), *Encyclopedic handbook of alcoholism.* New York: Gardner Press, 1982.

Kurtz, E. Why A.A. works: The intellectual significance of Alcoholics Anonymous. *Journal of Studies on Alcohol,* 1982, *43,* 38–80.

Matsunaga, E. Retinoblastoma: Mutational mosaicism or host resistance? *American Journal of Medical Genetics,* 1981, *8,* 375–387.

Murray, R. M., & Gurling, H. M. D. Genetic contributions to normal and abnormal drinking. In M. Sandler (Ed.), *Psychopharmacology of alcohol.* New York: Raven Press, 1980.

Myslobodsky, M. Pharmacologic implications of hemispheric asymmetry. *Life Sciences,* 1976, *19,* 1467–1478.

Obe, G., & Ristow, H. Mutagenic, cancerogenic and teratogenic effects of alcohol. *Mutation Research,* 1979, *65,* 229–259.

Pattison, E. M., Sobell, M. B., & Sobell, L. C. *Emerging concepts of alcohol dependence.* New York: Springer, 1977.

Pettinati, H. M., Sugerman, A. A., & Maurer, H. S. Four year MMPI changes in abstinent and drinking alcoholics. *Alcoholism—Clinical and Experimental Research,* 1982, *6*(4), 487–494.

Prigogine, I., Nicolis, G., & Babloyantz, A. Thermodynamics of evolution. *Physics Today,* 1972, *25*(11), 23–28 and *25*(12), 38–44.

Prigogine, I. *From being to becoming.* San Francisco: W. H. Freeman, 1980.

Quitkin, F. M., & Rabkin, J. G. Hidden psychiatric diagnosis in the alcoholic. In J. Solomon (Ed.), *Alcoholism and clinical psychiatry.* New York: Plenum Medical Book Co., 1982.

Rhodes, L. E., Obitz, F. W., & Creel, D. Effect of alcohol and task on hemispheric asymmetry of visually evoked potentials in man. *Electroencephalography and Clinical Neurophysiology,* 1975, *38,* 561–568.

Sandel, A., & Alcorn, J. D. Individual hemisphericity and maladaptive behaviors. *Journal of Abnormal Psychology,* 1980, *89*(3), 514–517.

Sandler, M. (Ed.). *Psychopharmacology of alcohol.* New York: Raven Press, 1980.

Solomon, J. (Ed.). *Alcoholism and clinical psychiatry.* New York: Plenum Medical Book Co., 1982.

Spalt, L. Alcoholism: Evidence of an X-linked recessive genetic characteristic. *JAMA,* 1979, *241*(23), 2543–2544.

Thune, C. E. Alcoholism and the archetypal past. *Journal of Studies on Alcohol,* 1977, *38*(1), 75–88.

Wartburg, von, J. P. Acetaldehyde. In M. Sandler (Ed.), *Psychopharmacology of alcohol.* New York: Raven Press, 1980.

Wurmser, L. *The mask of shame.* Baltimore, Maryland: Johns Hopkins University Press, 1981.

Wurmser, L. The heavy weight of a thousand unrelenting eyes. Presented to the Boston Psychoanalytic Society, Boston, Massachusetts, September, 1982.

BIBLIOGRAPHY

Miglioli, M., Buchtel, H. A., Campanini, T., & DeRisio, C. Cerebral hemispheric lateralization of cognitive deficits due to alcoholism. *Journal of Nervous and Mental Disease,* 1979, *167*(4), 212–216.

Oke, A., Keller, R., Mefford, I., & Adams, R. Lateralization of norepinephrine in the human thalamus. *Science,* 1978, *200,* 1411–1413.

Pattison, E. M., & Kaufman, E. The alcoholism syndrome: Definitions and models. In E. M. Pattison & E. Kaufman (Eds.), *Encyclopedic handbook of alcoholism.* New York: Gardner Press, 1982.

Smokler, I. A., & Sheurin, H. Cerebral lateralization and personality style. *Archives of General Psychiatry,* 1979, *36,* 949–954.

Tucker, D. M. Lateral brain function, emotion and conceptualization. *Psychological Bulletin,* 1981, *89,* 19–46.

Wexler, B. E. Cerebral laterality and psychiatry: A review of the literature. *American Journal of Psychiatry,* 1980, *137,* 279–291.

UNIT III

ACCOUNTABILITY

PART FIVE SOCIAL CONTEXT

The professional issues surrounding the practice of the psychiatric mental health nurse specialist that arise out of the social context within which the role is practiced are explored in Part Five. If nurses are to practice with accountability, they must face ethical, legal, and professional issues and provide for their continuing professional development. Part Five relates to Standards VII, VIII, IX, and X of ANA's *Standards of Psychiatric and Mental Health Nursing Practice* (1982). However, the discussion goes beyond clinical practice to discuss the social context of that practice.

In Chapter 21 are explored some of the ethical and legal issues that arise within advanced psychiatric mental health nursing practice. A set of six issues are presented that may yield ethical dilemmas and courses of action that follow from various ethical principles are suggested. The six issues discussed are (1) preparation and identification of the specialist as a nurse, (2) relationships with professional colleagues, (3) the relationship with the client, (4) psychotherapy issues, (5) inpatient treatment, and (6) technological advances in practice. Of special interest is the discussion of the complexity of coming to a responsible decision about ethical dilemmas in complex organizational settings. Throughout the discussion, while guidelines are suggested, it is stressed that the final decision maker can only be the individual clinician. By definition, dilemmas do not have easy answers.

Legal issues are of a different order, however. It is stated in Chapter 21 that, unlike ethical issues, legal issues do not present choices. Instead, legal decisions provide a baseline of minimum expectations and agreed upon societal rules. The current status of legal decisions regarding (1) the legal scope of advanced practice in psychiatric mental health nursing; (2) practice, malpractice, and accountability of psychiatric mental health nurses; and (3) the balance between confidentiality and duty to warn is presented. Since the law is in a continual stage of evolution and since laws governing the practice of nursing vary from state to state, the psychiatric mental health nurse specialist must remain alert to changes in the laws that affect his or her practice.

In Chapter 22, some of the issues in the broader health care industry that affect nursing practice, such as health care legislation and financing, regulation and credentialing of nursing and nurses, and maintaining competency and collaborative practice are discussed. The chapter forces the nurse to realize that it is not enough simply to render expert nursing care. There is a context of practice that cannot be ignored because of its effect on psychiatric mental health nursing practice.

Finally, in Chapter 23, the purpose and process of clinical supervision is differentiated from consultation. Clinical supervision is seen as occurring within a relationship where the supervisor has administrative responsibility for the trainee, whereas consultation occurs within a peer or collegial relationship. The process of supervision is described within a stage framework that parallels Lewin's change process. Select issues are discussed that can be expected to arise during supervision, central among them being transference and countertransference.

In Part Five, an attempt is made to assist the practitioner to identify and consider the complexities encountered in the social context of advanced psychiatric mental health nursing.

CHAPTER 21

ETHICAL AND LEGAL ISSUES

Virginia Trotter Betts
Margie Nicks Gale
Joan M. Gibson

Psychiatric mental health nurses (PMHNs) face many legal and ethical dilemmas in their practice. As PMHNs gain increased independence, they take on greater responsibility and accountability. The aim of this chapter is to explore the ethical and legal issues that arise from the advanced practice of PMHNs, including the role of psychotherapist, and to offer guidelines for decision making. Although the PMHN assumes roles in education and research, as well as in practice, this chapter will focus on the arena of clinical practice only.

Ethical and legal dilemmas overlap both theoretically and pragmatically; however, for the sake of clarity, they will be differentiated. The specific issues that pose ethical questions to be discussed are (1) preparation and identification of the specialist as a nurse, (2) relationships with professional colleagues, (3) the relationship with the client, (4) psychotherapy issues, (5) inpatient treatment, and (6) technological advances in practice. The specific legal issues to be discussed include (1) the legal scope of advanced practice in psychiatric mental health nursing, (2) practice/malpractice/accountability, and (3) balancing confidentiality vs. the duty to warn.

MAJOR ETHICAL ISSUES

There is an increasing body of literature in nursing on the topics of ethics in the areas of nursing practice, education, and research. However, according to Aroskar and Veatch (1977), baccalaureate nursing education still tends not to prepare students in the areas of ethics or medical ethics. Therefore, nurses entering graduate programs in PMHN cannot be expected to possess a well grounded background in ethics or nursing ethics. Four documents important to this discussion have been produced by the American Nurses' Association (ANA). These are: *Code for Nurses with Interpretive Statements,* (ANA, 1976a); *Statement on Psychiatric and Mental Health Nursing Practice,* (ANA, 1976b); *Nursing: A Social Policy Statement,* (ANA, 1980); and *Standards of Psychiatric and Mental Health Nursing Practice,* (ANA, 1982). These documents can provide guidelines for consideration of ethical issues in psychiatric mental health nursing advanced practice.

Many ethicists have warned readers not to look for specific answers or even definitive guidelines when dealing with ethics. However, it is attempted in this chapter to clarify available choices and suggest guidelines. The challenge will be to encapsulate ideas that are abstract enough to provide the reader with vision, yet sufficiently specific in content and information to allow the work to be pragmatic.

Ethical Theory and the Function of Professional Codes

While the terms values, morals, and ethics are sometimes used interchangeably, in this chapter they will be defined and used as follows: *value* is, in the broad sense, the worth, goodness, or desirability of something, whether moral or nonmoral, such as tidiness, efficiency, honesty, and compassion. *Morals,* or morality, refer to those traditions of belief about what is right or wrong in human conduct that develop, are transmitted, and are learned independent of rational, ethical inquiry. *Ethics* denotes that branch of philosophy or reasoned inquiry that studies both the nature of and the justification for general ethical principles governing right conduct.

Morality expresses society's basic instructions about what people may and may not do. Ethical theory, on the other hand, describes and justifies such traditions and is often divided into two quite separate areas: scientific and philosophical. The *scientific* branch of ethics gathers and reports accurate empirical information about existing moral beliefs, without evaluating the worth of moral judgments in any way. *Philosophical* ethics moves beyond and either evaluates important moral concepts (for example, freedom, justice, the good) and moral reasoning from a logical as opposed to a psychological perspective or establishes theoretical justifications for what is right and wrong in human actions. These two subcategories of philosophical ethics are known, respectively, as metaethics and normative ethics.

Both scientific and philosophical ethics are useful when developing procedures for resolving concrete ethical disputes and the discussion that follows will focus on an especially useful descriptive theory, Laurence Kohlberg's account of cognitive moral development, as well as on the two main types of normative ethics: Consequentialist theories (Ethical, Egoism, and Utiliarianism) and nonconsequentialist theories (Deontology).

Before doing so, however, mention ought to be made of one component of formalized moral tradition that is not necessarily the product of rational, ethical inquiry but which is, nevertheless, an important repository of and force for the moral beliefs of certain groups: codes of ethics. As Benjamin and Curtis (1981) note, professional codes of ethics are both creed and commandment. They constitute a kind of oath that affirms the highest ideals and standards of the profession and that exhorts individuals always to strive for these standards. As commandment, they provide rules for expected behavior and conduct, and they suggest, usually in general terms, certain ethical principles that professionals ought to consider when determining conduct. Professional codes are taken seriously and form an important expression of a profession's collective identity and mission at any given time. They are limited, however, in their effectiveness as rational tools for analyzing and resolving ethical issues and dilemmas, hence the need for the more systematic, comprehensive, and internally consistent disciplines of scientific and philosophical ethics. For the professional code basic to the nursing profession, see Table 21.1.

Scientific Ethics: A Descriptive Approach to Moral Development

While some would argue that scientific ethics and philosophical ethics (facts and values) have little or nothing to do with each other or that description of the process by which one makes moral judgments has nothing to do with their validity or worth, others such as Kohlberg maintain that there is a connection. Kohlberg argues that moral development is an empirically verifiable process, as well as a prerequisite for sound philosophical reflection about ethical issues (Kohlberg, 1976a,b, 1983). His *theory of cognitive moral development* built upon the developmental work of Piaget. Just as Piaget showed that thinking occurs as a psychological developmental process that moves in sequential stages, so has Kohlberg argued that moral reasoning is developed. His work sheds light on the process, rather than the content, of moral reasoning and behavior and his perspective emphasizes the structure of thinking as opposed to the judgemental perspective of the goodness or badness of

Table 21.1 Code for Nurses

1. The nurse provides services with respect for human dignity and the uniqueness of the client unrestricted by considerations of social or economic status, personal attributes, or the nature of health problems.
2. The nurse safeguards the client's right to privacy by judiciously protecting information of a confidential nature.
3. The nurse acts to safeguard the client and the public when health care and safety are affected by the incompetent, unethical, or illegal practice of any person.
4. The nurse assumes responsibility and accountability for individual nursing judgments and actions.
5. The nurse maintains competence in nursing.
6. The nurse exercises informed judgment and uses individual competence and qualifications as criteria in seeking consultation, accepting responsibilities, and delegating nursing activities to others.
7. The nurse participates in activities that contribute to the ongoing development of the profession's body of knowledge.
8. The nurse participates in the profession's efforts to implement and improve standards of nursing.
9. The nurse participates in the profession's efforts to establish and maintain conditions of employment conducive to high quality nursing care.
10. The nurse participates in the profession's effort to protect the public from misinformation and misrepresentation and to maintain the integrity of nursing.
11. The nurse collaborates with members of the health professions and other citizens in promoting community and national efforts to meet the health needs of the public.

SOURCE: American Nurses' Association. *Code for Nurses with Interpretive Statements.* Kansas City, MO: American Nurses' Association, 1976, p. 3. Reprinted with permission.

decisions. According to the theory, the word *cognitive* refers to the structural processes of thinking that reflect moral reasoning. The term *moral* refers to decisions that are made that involve universal values such as the sanctity of life and the need for authority and their conflicts (Guidance Associates, 1976). While Kohlberg's theory, as any theory, has its critics (Gilligan, 1978; Omery, 1983), many nurses have found his framework especially useful so it will be referred to in the discussions that follows.

Table 21.2 delineates the levels and stages in Kohlberg's theory of moral development: the preconventional level in moral reasoning (Stages 1 and 2) that focuses on the direct consequences of actions to the individual (punishment, reward, or exchange of favors); reasoning at the conventional level of moral development (Stages 3 and 4) that centers on loyalty and the need to actively maintain support and justify the social order; and, finally, the postconventional, or principled, level (Stages 5 and 6) that focuses on moral reasoning that is valid according to principles to which the individual subscribes.

Kohlberg argues that people can understand arguments at their own stage, at all stages beneath their own, and sometimes at one (and occasionally two) stages above their own. They generally prefer the highest stage of thought they can comprehend. Therefore, educators in ethics must begin at the level of the learners and provide an environment that is conducive to the learner's ability to attain higher stages of reasoning and understanding. Deliberate attempts to facilitate stage change through educational programs have been successful. While moral education has largely been researched in primary education, it is beginning to be studied in higher education as well (Guidance Associates, 1976).

Table 21.2 Levels and Stages of Moral Development

The Preconventional Level (Stages 1 and 2)

At this level, the power of authority figures or the physical or hedonistic consequences of actions, such as punishment, reward, or exchange of favors determine moral judgment. The level has the following two stages:

Stage 1: The Punishment and Obedience Orientation At this stage, the physical consequences of doing something determine whether it is good or bad. People at Stage 1 think about avoiding punishment or earning rewards, and they defer to authority figures with power over them.	Stage 2: The Instrumental Relativist Orientation At Stage 2, moral judgment leads to action that satisfies one's own needs and sometimes meets the needs of others. Stage 2 thought often involves elements of fairness, but always for pragmatic reasons, rather than from a sense of justice or loyalty. Reciprocity, a key element in Stage 2 thought, is a matter of "you scratch my back and I'll scratch yours."

The Conventional Level (Stages 3 and 4)

People at this level value maintaining the expectations of their family, group, or nation for their own sake and regardless of immediate consequences. People at the conventional level show loyalty to the social order and actively maintain, support, and justify it. This level has the following two stages.

Stage 3: The Interpersonal Sharing Orientation At this stage, people equate good behavior with whatever pleases or helps others and with what others approve of. Stage 3 people often conform to stereotypical ideas of how the majority of people in their group behave. They often judge behavior by intentions, and they earn approval by being "nice."	Stage 4: The Societal Maintenance Orientation Stage 4 thought orients toward authority, fixed rules, and the maintenance of the social order. Right behavior consists of doing one's duty, showing respect for authority, or maintaining the given social order for its own sake.

The Principled Level (Stages 5 and 6)

At this level, people reason according to moral principles which have validity apart from the authority of the groups to which the individuals belong. This level has the following two stages.

Stage 5: The Social Contract, Human Rights, and Welfare Orientation People at Stage 5 tend to define right action in terms of general individual rights and standards which have been examined critically and agreed upon by the society in a document such as the Declaration of Independence, rather than unquestioningly accepting authority as in Stage 4. Stage 5 thinkers stress the legal point of view, but they emphasize the possibility of changing laws after rational consideration of the welfare of the society. Free agreement and contract bind people together where no laws apply.	Stage 6: The Universal Ethical Principle Orientation At Stage 6, people define the right by the decision of their conscience guided by ethical principles such as respect for human personality, liberty compatible with the equal liberty of all others, justice, and equality. These principles appeal to logical comprehensiveness, universality, and consistency. Instead of being concrete rules, they are abstract ethical principles.

SOURCE: Guidance Associates, Inc. Teacher training in values education: A workshop. *Leadership Manual,* Handout 3. New York: Harcourt, Brace & Jovanovich, 1976. Reprinted with permission.

Philosophical Ethics

While scientific theories neither evaluate nor provide guidelines for resolving concrete moral disputes, philosophical ethical theories do whether, as in the case of metaethics, by recommending changes in our understanding of important ethical concepts such as beneficence (the duty to do good for others), autonomy (the right to self-determination), and justice (the obligation to treat like cases in like fashion and always to strive for fairness) or by developing normative ethical theories for clarifying, structuring, and ultimately justifying individual ethical decisions. Normative theories are usually divided into two types: Consequentialist (or Teleological) ethical theories and Nonconsequentialist (Deontological) ethical theories.

Consequentialist ethical theories argue that an act is judged right or wrong solely on the basis of the value of its consequences. For example, an *ethical egoist* argues that an act is right if it produces the greatest amount of good for him- or herself, while a *utilitarian* requires that the balance of good be computed for the greatest number of people. Despite their differences, these consequentialists focus on the effects of actions, and find insignificant any notion that the intrinsic value of actions matter. Nonconsequentialist ethical theories, on the other hand, are theories of obligation that may, as in the case of *act deontology,* argue that individual actions are intrinsically right or wrong and may be discerned as such through intuition or, as with *rule deontology* (for example, Kantianism), argue for the intrinsic worth of general rules or principles when evaluating classes of actions. The duty to promote the principles of autonomy, beneficence, and justice is a position common to contemporary deontologists examining medical ethical issues.

Impact of Ethical Theories on Nursing

A number of nurse educators (Davis & Aroskar, 1983; Kelly, 1981; Krawczyk & Kudzma, 1978; Mahon & Fowler, 1979; Munhall, 1982) have used Kohlberg's model as a framework for understanding ethical issues in nursing. Nursing research has also used Kohlberg's theory to look at nurses' moral reasoning. Ketefian (1981) found that the level of moral reasoning is positively related to moral behavior when using the ANA *Code for Nurses* (1976a) as the standard for moral behavior. This same study, also supported by Crisham (1981), found that increased formal education is positively correlated with higher levels of moral reasoning and more accurate moral behavior. Experience with previous deliberation about real life nursing dilemmas was another important factor in higher levels of moral reasoning. However, increased experience in the hospital milieu tended to have a negative effect on the level of moral reasoning.

While the principles of beneficence and justice are important in assessing and resolving ethical issues, the principle of autonomy has come to dominate discussions. A comprehensive discussion of this concept may be found in Dworkin (1976), Gadow (1983), Lumpp (1979), and Beauchamp and Childress (1983).

Although the discussion of autonomy in medical ethics usually is in reference to the autonomy present and encouraged on the part of the patient or client, autonomy begins with the autonomy of the health care provider who is in a relationship with the client. Because PMHN specialists envision their role to be more autonomous, they have the ability to encourage and foster the parallel process of autonomy for their clients. The autonomy principle can be seen as analogous to the principle of liberty, one of the ten universal moral issues identified by Kohlberg.

What do these findings mean for the PMHN? In general, it means that masters and doctorally prepared PMHNs should be in a better position to make moral and ethical decisions. This does not mean that they always do, however. Since these specialists are often in the position of being in a more independent practice, it would seem that improved ethical decision making is necessary for their professional development.

ETHICAL ISSUES IN PRACTICE

This section will focus on ethical issues encountered in clinical practice by PMHNs prepared at the masters and doctoral levels. It assumes that the reader already has knowledge of the ethical issues for the generalist psychiatric nurse. A good resource for a basic review of ethical issues for the generalist is given by Haber, Leach, Schudy, and Sideleau (1982) and Wilson and Kneisl (1983). This discussion will use the ANA *Code for Nurses* (1976a), Kohlberg's theory, and three philosophical theories as approaches to the moral dilemmas.

There are six general areas of practice that will be discussed. These areas include (1) preparation and identification of the specialist as a nurse, (2) relationships with professional colleagues, (3) the relationship with the client, (4) psychotherapy issues, (5) inpatient treatment, and (6) technological advances in practice. Some of the above issues overlap, but the practical aspects and content of each issue make them distinct.

Preparation and Identification of the Specialist as Nurse

One of the most important questions the PMHN has to ask him- or herself is, "Who am I?" The allure of becoming a psychotherapist and being seen as an equal colleague of other mental health professionals has too often led to the blurring of the role of the PMHN as a nurse. Although PMHNs engage in the practice of psychotherapy with individuals, groups, and families, the primary identification must be within the discipline of nursing. A distinction between an interdisciplinary and a multidisciplinary approach to mental health care will be made in this chapter, as well as a recommendation of the latter.

An interdisciplinary approach assumes that people from different disciplines can be interchanged. The multidisciplinary approach assumes that people in various disciplines have some aspects of a role that are interchangeable but that people maintain the uniqueness of certain role tasks. The following is an example of the problems encountered when the nurse's role is blurred.

Two graduate students in a mental health nursing program were presenting a family therapy case to a consulting psychologist. A 15-year-old female who was a member of the family was pregnant and had been seen at a public clinic and diagnosed as probably pretoxemic. During the previous session, the young woman had been eating salted potato chips and the students reported this action. When asked by the consulting psychologist what the nursing action would be in relation to the risk for this pregnant female, one of the graduate students responded, "I'm not a nurse any more, I'm a family therapist." In this example, the nurses were not using their unique background and offering their special skills to this family in therapy.

Using an egoist ethical approach, perhaps the nurses found the role of family therapist more rewarding and more interesting than the role of nurse. However, can the nurse take the hat of the registered nurse on and off and become just a family therapist any more than a registered nurse can take off the hat of nurse and become a lay midwife? Historically, the answer to the latter has been no. Using the *Standards of Psychiatric and Mental Health Nursing Practice* (ANA, 1982), the answer would also be "no." In the name of the principle of beneficence and implying a deontological duty to act accordingly, Standard V (ANA, 1982, pp. 6–7) states: "The nurse intervenes as guided by the nursing care plan to implement nursing actions that promote, maintain, or restore physical and mental health, prevent illness and effect rehabilitation." The accompanying rationale clearly identifies a value basic to the profession: "Mental health is one aspect of general health and well being. Nursing actions reflect an appreciation for the hierarchy of human needs and include interventions for all aspects of physical and mental health and illness" (p. 7). Although there is leeway in how health care needs are to be specifically met, it does state that the nurse is accountable for making sure that the total client needs are met. Therefore, the physical health of clients is still the responsibility of the PMHN and the unique perspective and abilities of the PMHN are enhanced.

Another issue that emerges when the nurse asks "Who am I?" deals with professional autonomy: the need for peer review and understanding the individual limitations of the nurse. The need to maintain professional competency as a nurse is addressed in Standards VII, peer review, and VIII, continuing education (ANA, 1982, pp. 15–16). One way for the PMHN to show evidence of peer review is to undergo the formal certification process in his or her specialty area offered through ANA. As a long-term goal, the PMHN should be committed to the ongoing pursuit of new knowledge to ensure his or her own professional growth.

Relationships With Professional Colleagues

A second major area that may produce conflict for the PMHN is in relationships with professional colleagues and other agencies. The two problems to be addressed here are accepting the client already engaged in therapy with another professional and the nurse's need for continuing consultation.

Accepting Another Professional's Client

The PMHN may find him- or herself faced with a client requesting services who is already engaged in therapy with another nurse or mental health colleague. Presently, there are no standards or guidelines in the *Code for Nurses* (ANA, 1976a) to guide the nurse's behavior in these situations. However, other professions have included in their code of ethics statements about behavior relating to duties to other professional colleagues. Although nurses owe respect and consideration for the professional autonomy of their colleagues, the primary concern is beneficence and serving the client's needs. It is recommended that the nurse use the clinical therapeutic focus as a guide. If the client has unmet, unresolved conflict with a former therapist, the nurse might encourage the client to work it out and possibly return to that therapist for continued care. If the nurse cannot reconcile a resolution of a break in the relationship between the client and a former therapist, then the nurse should facilitate the best transition possible for continued care.

PMHN's Need for Ongoing Professional Consultation

The need for consultation from professional nurse colleagues is essential to the ongoing development and maintenance of competence in nursing. This position is supported by the *Standards of Psychiatric and Mental Health Nursing Practice* (ANA, 1982, pp. 15–16) and the *Code for Nurses* (ANA, 1976, p. 13). Although the PMHN may receive consultation from professional colleagues in other disciplines of mental health, there is no substitute for ongoing consultation from professional nurse colleagues. The practice of nursing has a unique focus that can best be addressed by other nursing colleagues who share that perspective.

The Relationship With the Client

Initiating Therapeutic Relationships

The first issue that emerges for the nurse and the client is that of accepting the client into a therapeutic relationship. The question arises, "what are valid and invalid reasons for accepting or not accepting a particular client?" The first article in the *Code for Nurses* states: "The nurse provides services with respect for human dignity and the uniqueness of the client unrestricted by considerations of social or economic status, personal attributes, or the nature of health problems" (ANA, 1976a, p. 3). This definition could place the nurse in private practice in the moral dilemma of whether he or she should give away services to meet society's economic need and thus be unable to maintain the autonomy of private practice owing to insolvency.

This question was addressed by Hoeffer (1983). The moral dilemma is that of individual autonomy, or liberty, of the nurse versus the distributive justice of health care for the public. Hoeffer acknowledges that private practice has a special appeal to nursing but counters that the principles of distributive justice would demand alternative models for provision of nursing mental health services. She offers three alternative models that include nurses' participation in health maintenance organizations, social/health maintenance organizations, or community nursing centers. She concludes that while the private practice model may be attractive to nurses, it does not have the greatest positive impact on mental health care delivery, implying a utilitarian analysis that the greatest good will not be available to the greatest number of people.

There are other choices to consider. First, professional nurses could reevaluate the statement in the *Code for Nurses* in reference to the economic circumstances of clients. This route has been taken by other health care professionals who have changed standards in their code of ethics that they felt detracted from the autonomy of the individual members (Bursten, 1980). Second, the nurse's private practice could be envisioned as a whole in which the principle of offering services to all socioeconomic groups is maintained. To continue to offer services and maintain a certain level of autonomy, the nurse could offer a specific percentage of services on a sliding scale to clients without sufficient resources for the full fee and/or offer consultative services to a public agency such as a community mental health center. An argument could be made for this approach using deontological theory in that it allows for the maintenance of autonomy of the nurse while also serving the principle of beneficence by meeting the community's need for health care.

There are other situations that demand that the nurse make a decision about the appropriateness of accepting a client. It is not unusual for a client to seek mental health services when wanting to gain custody of a child currently in the guardianship of a spouse. The client's goal is to develop testimony for litigation. If it is clear that the seeking of services, specifically, will draw the nurse into the courtroom and legal proceedings, he or she should ask, "Is it ever right to knowingly go into a therapeutic relationship which is for the sole purpose of proceedings?"

A third situation arises in accepting a therapeutic relationship with a client who may be potentially assaultive and/or does not authorize release of information from previous health care providers. The nurse must decide if the setting in which the therapeutic relationship exists would be safe on an ongoing basis for both the nurse and the potentially assaultive client. If the answer is no, it is incumbent upon the nurse to refer the potential client to a more suitable individual or agency.

While the issues of ability to pay and potential violence on the part of the client have been phrased in terms of the decision to accept a client, these can certainly emerge during therapy as well. We recommend that the nurse take advantage of consultation to help ensure that, whatever course of action is decided, the client will receive adequate services in a setting that will meet his or her needs.

Informed Consent on PMHN Scope of Practice

A second ethical issue centering on the overall relationship with the client is that of providing complete information to the client about the limitations of practice and privilege of the

PMHN. The scope of the nurse's practice varies from state to state. Therefore, nurses must know their legal limitation of privilege and confidentiality as well as be aware of their own individual limitations in knowledge and skills.

Nurses may be reluctant to share a complete informed consent because it may be seen as compromising their autonomy by limiting the scope of practice in which they engage. For example, a nurse-client relationship does not have privileged communication in most states, although in many states psychiatrists and psychologists do have privileged communication with clients. Privilege is the status that is afforded the client to maintain privacy and belongs to the individual, not to the professional. In most states, the PMHN is bound to protect the confidentiality of the client but is not afforded the privilege in the nurse-client relationship to protect that confidentiality. Therefore, the PMHN's client has no claim to privilege in a court of law. A client informed of this may then choose to seek psychotherapy from a psychiatrist or psychologist instead of a nurse. Another example is that the nurse may be limited in third-party reimbursement and thus his or her services may be more expensive to the client than the psychiatrist's or psychologist's services, which can be fully reimbursed by most insurance companies. It is incumbent upon the nurse to fully inform his or her clients that alternative services are available. Giving full informed consent does not, however, preclude the nurse from sharing reasons why he or she may provide higher quality services than other mental health professionals.

Acceptable Professional Behavior

A third client relationship issue is the nature of professional vs. social behavior between the client and the nurse. Because psychiatric mental health nursing demands that nurses assume many roles during a therapeutic relationship with the client (counselor, educator, and often surrogate parent), the nurse must learn very early to separate the professional nursing role and the social relationship roles that are practiced in helping the client learn how to relate to other people. Therefore, the issue of whether the nurse and the client become friends during or after therapy is a central issue. Although this question has both ethical and therapeutic components to it, the former shall be addressed here.

The ethical stance of the nurse must be the duty to see that the client's needs are to be met first in the therapeutic relationship. The nurse must meet his or her personal needs for friendship outside of the professional and therapeutic setting in which he or she works. Although the decision not to initiate a friendship between nurse and client during therapy is a common standard, the question of developing a friendship after therapy is formally terminated is a grayer area.

Standards for acceptable professional behavior in the area of sexual contact and sex therapy with clients is a topic widely discussed by mental health professionals. There is no mention of sex therapy, specifically, in the *Standards of Psychiatric and Mental Health Nursing Practice* (ANA, 1982). While not all PMHNs have acquired the knowledge and skills to do sex therapy, the PMHN is in a unique position to do so because of his or her extensive background in the biological sciences. A code of ethics is provided for sex therapists by the American Association of Sex Educators, Counselors, and Therapists (AASECT). The AASECT *Code of Ethics* (1980) provides the following guidelines for acceptable professional behavior:

> Section 3: 7. It is unethical for the therapist to engage in sexual activities with a client.
>
> 8. Procedures involving nudity of either the client or the therapist or observation of client's sexual activity go beyond the boundaries of established therapeutic practice and may be used only when there is good evidence that they serve the best interest of the client.
>
> 9. Client nudity during a physical examination by a licensed physician, nurse, or physician's assistant is not prohibited or unethical.

> 14. Although controversial, the use of partner surrogates in sex therapy may be an ethically permissible way of establishing a therapeutic environment, when conducted in a responsible manner. If partner surrogates are to be used at all, it should be understood that the partner surrogate is not a sex therapist; surrogates should understand that their role is not that of sex therapist or psychotherapist; and sex therapists working with partner surrogates must exercise diligence and concern for protecting the dignity and welfare of both the surrogate and the client.
>
> (AASECT, 1980, pp. 7–8)

Bouhoutsas, Holroyd, Lermann, Farer, and Greenberg (1983) gathered data about sexual contact between patients and psychotherapists by means of a survey. They report that (1) patients are not seductive, (2) sexual intimacy during therapy does fall below the community standard of practice, and (3) sexual intimacy with patients is harmful rather than beneficial. Some of the harm reported included increased depression, lack of motivation, impaired social adjustment, significant emotional disturbance, suicidal feelings or behavior, and increased drug or alcohol use. Eleven percent of the cases were hospitalized and 1% committed suicide. Yet they found that patients were reluctant to report this behavior even when they recognized that it was either illegal or unethical.

What is the impact of these data on the role of the PMHN in the conduct of psychotherapy and sex therapy? The minimal standard of care is that the therapist not engage in sexual activity with a client. There is also the question of what action to take when knowledge of such conduct on the part of a colleague comes to the nurse's attention. If this knowledge is gained within a therapeutic relationship with a client, the issue of confidentiality must be considered. When a release from the client is obtained, PMHNs are bound first to confront the mental health colleague involved in an attempt to clarify and resolve the issue. If this action is not successful, the PMHN should follow with a report to the appropriate professional ethics committee and/or licensing board.

Psychotherapy Issues

The fourth major area of ethical issues focuses on the nurse's role in psychotherapy. The two specific issues to be examined here are informed consent and cases that involve suicidal and homicidal clients.

Informed Consent

Entering into a therapeutic relationship with a client who has given informed consent for the treatment is not always easy to accomplish. Ethical consideration for informed consent with the use of behavior therapy and in the treatment of individuals of vulnerable groups will be discussed.

BEHAVIOR THERAPY. The term behavior therapy is used broadly here to include the many techniques and approaches that directly affect a change in behavior as an outcome. Although the goal of all psychotherapy is to effect some change in behavioral outcome, the common theme will be the question of informed consent or complete knowledge of the client of the process in which behavior is ultimately changed. This issue arises not only in individual therapy, but in marriage, family, and group therapies as well. Several examples in which PMHNs might be engaged would include behavior modification, hypnotism, the use of paradoxical intentions, or techniques of neurolinguistic programming. The ethical conflict that could be seen to occur centers on autonomy, or liberty, versus quality of life and/or the public welfare.

Excellent guidelines for the optimum preservation of autonomy when dealing with behavior control have been proposed by Gerald Dworkin (1976). Though these guidelines take the form of general considerations rather than specific actions, they provide ideas that promote self-reflection on the part of the therapist. Perhaps one of Dworkin's most piercing comments is that "autonomy is in greater danger from manipulative methods of influence than from those outright assaults on the individual associated with the notion of brainwashing and psychosurgery" (1976, pp. 26–27). Briefly, Dworkin states:

1. Methods of influence should be used that support the self-respect and dignity of the individual client. The therapist and the client should ideally be seen as equals in this process.
2. Do not use destructive means that will inhibit the individual's rational reflection on his or her own interests.
3. The fundamental ways in which the person identifies him- or herself as an individual should be maintained.
4. Avoid methods of influence that have a strong reliance on deception or on keeping the individual ignorant of relevant data.
5. Methods of influence that are not specifically intrusive are preferable to those that are.
6. The concept of temporality of the intervention should be considered. Interventions that have reversible outcomes would be preferable to those that do not. Also, the rapidity of change would be included for consideration.
7. Methods that require the active participation of the individual, or that work through the cognitive and affective processes, are preferable to those that short circuit motivation and decision making of the individual.

The crux of the controversy over behavior therapy, whether using it in the mode of individual or any other therapy, is defining the conditions of informed consent. There are generally four types of consent given in reference to health care. The first one is known as *implied consent,* in which a person implies that he or she has given consent for a minor procedure. An example would be a consent to have blood drawn or consent to give a urine sample. The second form of consent is *presumed consent.* In this case, it would be presumed that if the client were able, he or she would give consent. An example would be a comatose patient who has been in an accident and is facing surgery and/or needs emergency services. It is presumed that a comatose patient, if alert, would give consent for the needed treatment. A third form of consent is *vicarious consent,* or *proxy consent,* and is given by a parent or guardian on the part of another party. This consent might be given for children, prisoners, mentally handicapped, and the elderly. The last type of consent is the truly legal *informed consent,* in which the client has full knowledge and gives consent after being sufficiently informed of the nature, purpose, and attendant risks involved in the procedure. The three elements required for a legal informed consent are (1) the patient must have legal capacity to give the consent, (2) the consent must be voluntary, and (3) the patient must have sufficient knowledge of the procedure and risks to give the consent (Rada, 1982).

VULNERABLE GROUPS. As difficult as it can be to decide the parameters of ethical mental health care for adults, the issues become even more complex when the client is a child, prisoner, mentally handicapped, or elderly person. Do these individuals have the capacity and/or the freedom to choose? One must consider, "Do they have the legal capacity and competency to give consent?"; if so, then informed consent must be obtained. However, if the client is deemed incompetent, then vicarious or proxy consent from a guardian must be solicited.

The ethical issue here hinges on what constitutes competency on the part of this group of individuals. Given that the individual possessed the cognitive emotional capacity to understand the nature, purpose, and attendant risks involved in treatment or any procedure, would the individual choose to exercise the freedom and autonomy to refrain from giving consent?

This particular group of individuals as clients and potential research subjects has been seen as particularly vulnerable and has been treated and considered with care in ethical standards for research purposes. However, further consideration should be given for the autonomous decision making of each of these individuals in providing informed consent for treatment purposes.

The Potential of Violent Behavior

A most complex ethical issue involves psychotherapy with the client who is potentially suicidal or homicidal. Although both of these clients present with potentially assaultive behavior to themselves or others, and therefore raise the issue of life, they will be discussed separately.

POTENTIAL SUICIDAL BEHAVIOR. Fromer (1981) has provided an excellent review of the historical and religious basis for the current view of suicide in this country. She specifically addresses the philosophical basis for nursing intervention that usually hinges on the principle of beneficence—specifically nonmaleficence: "first, do no harm." Further interpretation of this maxim explores the conflict of the autonomy of the patient vs. the sanctity of life. As Fromer views it, the moral dilemma of suicide asks the question, "When, if ever, is it morally permissible to restrain someone in emotional despair from killing himself?" (1981, p. 2). Fromer's discussion includes a distinction among the terms morally wrong, morally blameless, and morally incorrect acts. These terms are used to differentiate various etiologies of suicide ranging from the terminally ill patient with intractable pain who rationally decides on suicide, the temporarily distraught and irrationally depressed patient who contemplates suicide, and the angry, manipulative patient who contemplates suicide as revenge against friends and relatives. Fromer favors the view that autonomy must be maintained and fostered in the patient and therefore offers the recommendation that the patient be detained from committing suicide for a period of not more than 24 hours. This recommendation follows her assertion that "suicide should always be a fully autonomous decision; therefore, the only permissible temporal or physical restraint that can be placed on a suicidal person are those that are productive of the goal of autonomy" (Fromer, 1981, p. 6).

Many PMHNs will object to this recommendation. Fromer offers this as an alternative to the automatic protective reaction that most nurses have in response to suicidal attempts by their patients. Certainly, the clinical issue of siding with the healthy part of the patient is also closely tied to the ethical stance of fostering autonomy on the part of the patient. Fromer's recommendation for further research in this area is indeed warranted. This research would include an assessment of PMHNs' philosophical stance on suicide, followed by case studies documenting the outcomes of their interactions and interventions with suicidal patients.

POTENTIAL HOMICIDAL BEHAVIOR. The ethical dilemma involving the duty to warn a potential victim of a homicidal client in psychotherapy was highlighted in the landmark case of *Tarasoff v. Regents of the University of California* in 1976. Briefly summarized, this case involved a young man who was an outpatient in psychotherapy at a university counseling center. The client admitted to his psychotherapist that he intended to harm and kill his former girlfriend, Tatiana Tarasoff. The psychotherapist, predicting potential harm to the victim, notified campus security who picked up the client, detained him for a short while, but determined he was not a potential threat to Ms. Tarasoff and let him go. No further action was taken and two months later the client did, indeed, kill Ms. Tarasoff. Subsequently, her parents sued the therapist and the California State Board of Regents, who were responsible for overseeing the counseling center. Additional details of this case can be found in many journal articles and law review references such as Wise (1978), Kjervik (1981), and Dix (1981).

Although the Tarasoff case has become synonomous with the term "duty to warn," this is truly a misnomer. Actually, the case created a new duty of *care* for the psychotherapist that involves the consideration of the client's potential homicidal danger to a third person. In the event of potential harm, the therapist must act to prevent harm to the third party. Thus, more broadly viewed, this prevention of harm may include a duty to warn the potential victim but does not absolutely and necessarily include a duty to warn the potential victim. Because of the controversy surrounding the elements of the Tarasoff and other related cases, let us examine the identifying characteristics that categorize this problem among true ethical dilemmas as defined by Curtin (1982).

The focus of the dilemma includes three areas: (1) the confidentiality between therapist and client, (2) the therapist's duty to the general public, and (3) the therapist's difficulty in predicting dangerousness (Kjervik, 1981, p. 13). A general standard of care (the therapist must *act* in order to prevent harm to the third party) must be adhered to by professionals, including nurses. This does not release the PMHN from further consideration of additional aspects of this ethical dilemma.

A survey conducted by Wise (1978) which assessed psychotherapists' behavior, prior to the Tarasoff case, when faced with the conflict between confidentiality and potential harm to victims indicated that well over 50% of the respondents were already taking a course of action to protect the victim from harm before a legal standard of care had been established. Additionally, not only have psychotherapists engaged in such action on their own, they have also identified many other alternatives than simply to warn a potential victim. Dix (1981) has identified well over 17 possible actions to be taken to protect the potential victim from harm, given the specific type of harm predicted and the circumstances of the individual situation. Generally speaking, then, the suggested standard would minimally include ascertaining (1) what is the nature of the dangerous homicidal threat, (2) what does it mean knowing or having to know about the danger, and (3) what does the PMHN do when confronted with a psychiatric patient who threatens to harm another person? Thus it would be wise for the PMHN faced with a potentially assaultive client (1) to seek consultation to confirm the nature of the potential harm and prediction of violence and (2) to make a concerted effort to identify many alternatives that would meet the particular clinical situation beyond just the narrow view of "duty to warn the potential victim." Since there is currently only one published study on the impact of Tarasoff on the clinical work of psychotherapy, there is a great need for continued research and dissemination of that work to the professional community (Rada, 1982).

Inpatient Treatment Issues

The fifth major area of ethical issues for the PMHN is that involving inpatient psychiatric hospitalization. Perhaps the unique and common theme of most ethical issues that occurs for psychiatric inpatients is that of autonomy. While the issues faced by the generalist and the specialist in psychiatric nursing in inpatient settings are the same, the specialist is expected to demonstrate a leadership role. This leadership role includes the ability to facilitate ethical decision making in a complex organization such as the hospital. Ethical decision making that includes work with a team of health professionals is almost always more complex than that between the client and the nurse in an outpatient setting. The list of possible, but not exhaustive, specific issues encountered in an inpatient setting include (1) the right to receive treatment, (2) the right to refuse treatment, (3) electroconvulsive therapy, (4) hospitalized children and adolescents, (5) incompetent practitioners, (6) the release of potentially violent patients, and (7) "new psychiatry" somatic therapies. Each one of these issues ultimately involves the autonomy of the individual seeking treatment.

Since space does not permit a discussion of each of these issues, a model will be offered by which the PMHN can facilitate ethical decision making in complex systems. The following model has been developed by Leah Curtin (1982).

Step 1: As much data as possible are gathered relevant to the ethical issue at hand. The information should be as accurate as possible.

Discussion: Kohlberg's notion of the cognitive element of moral decision making is obvious here. The person who has a greater ability to engage in critical analysis will be able to gather more pertinent, accurate, relevant data.

Step 2: The specific components of the ethical problem, situation, or dilemma are identified. Three characteristics must be met to determine that this is indeed an ethical dilemma. They are (1) the issue could not be resolved simply by further understanding of scientific data; (2) the problem is "inherently perplexing"; and (3) the resolution to the dilemma will have implications that affect many areas of human concern. Also at this stage, the analysis of the problem includes a thorough understanding of what the true conflict is.

Discussion: Again, the need for cognitive ability to differentiate and sort data is essential in this step. Also key is the distinction that a true moral dilemma exists. An understanding of basic ethical principles would be needed at this stage. Is this an issue of autonomy/liberty vs. property or is this a dilemma of autonomy/liberty vs. life? It is very important to identify a moral dilemma as opposed to a mere conflict of nonmoral values. Remember that a value may be in the realm of tidiness and efficiency whereas true moral dilemmas deal with one or more of the following ten issues: punishment, property, roles and concerns of affection, roles and concerns of authority, law, life, liberty, distributive justice, truth, and sex (Kohlberg, 1976a).

Step 3: The identification of all individuals involved in the ultimate decision making of the moral dilemma should be done in this step. Additional key factors include how these individuals are linked together, what is the power of each, and what is their commitment to this particular situation.

Discussion: This step is very important in the institutional setting. There are usually more people involved in the decision about a moral dilemma than is realized. Because this step takes time, thought, and effort, it is too often omitted.

Step 4: The possible courses of action and alternative options available must be projected as accurately as possible.

Discussion: The PMHN must use this step as the opportunity to project a wide range of possible courses of action. When possible, brainstorming and the solicitation of possible actions from all the individuals identified in Step 3 should occur. This is the opportunity to use creative problem solving instead of locking oneself into a rigid set of rules or patterns.

Step 5: Reconciliation of the facts and values must occur. This means that the principles that have been identified in Step 2 must be considered in light of the options presented in Step 4, yet this must be done by all of the persons included in Step 3. It is readily apparent how complex is the task in Step 5.

Discussion: In this step, the various reasons why people propose specific courses of action must be examined. In a given group, one person may use principles of law to make a decision, another may use a professional ethical code, while still another may use duties and rules that are identified as universal principles. Disagreement over the rationale, however, does not mean all these individuals necessarily disagree on the recommended action. The overriding question that needs to be addressed is, "Who should make the decision and whose autonomy supercedes the autonomy of others making the decision?"

Step 6: Resolution occurs in this step. This step does not necessarily mean that a true solution always occurs, but this does propose the notion that every dilemma and every situation will be resolved somehow at some time.

Discussion: In many cases, the resolution may occur by the parties choosing not to take a plan of action at all. This, of course, is a form of passive decision making. Perhaps this is because a true ethical dilemma often requires making a choice between two equally unappealing actions and responsible decision making in a complex organization is very complicated.

Step 7: Develop a plan for action.

Discussion: As with all nursing plans, this plan should be as clear and specific as possible. All parties who will carry out the plan should be involved in its development and in providing feedback on how the plan will be implemented. (Reprinted with permission from Curtin, L., & Flaherty, M. J. (Eds.), *Nursing Ethics: Theories and Pragmatics.* Bowie, MD: Robert J. Brady Company, 1982.)

Curtin's model is similar to the process of problem solving. It offers more than a simple problem-solving approach, however, in that it specifies both the cognitive, ethical, and moral components of a true ethical dilemma. There is a great need for empirical evaluation of the use of such a model in the inpatient setting. Both the implementation of this process and the evaluation of it through research are within the scope of the role of the PMHN.

Dilemmas Involving Technological Advances in Practice

Every specialty in the health sciences is faced with the task of addressing ethical dilemmas involving technological advances used in the area of practice. Psychiatric mental health nursing is certainly no exception to the challenge. The possible technological advances posing dilemmas may include such activities as computerized psychosocial assessment, therapy sessions, and patient records; audio-video recording and playback; and the use of biofeedback techniques. These technological advances pose two possible threats to clients. One is the threat to the protection of confidentiality with the use of computerized records and the use of audio-visual recording equipment. Methods to assure confidentiality with the use of this technology should be anticipated and instituted (Fowler, 1983). The second threat to the client is the possibility of being treated as an object rather than being treated as a seeker of mental health services. Further discussion of the importance of maintaining the subjectiveness of the client are offered by Dworkin (1976) and Gadow (1983).

MAJOR LEGAL ISSUES

In reviewing the ethical portion of this chapter, it is clear that a knowledge of ethics will enhance psychiatric mental health nursing's (PMHN) ability to make choices and delineate multiple options for practice. Legal knowledge is less a framework for options and more a baseline for minimum expectations and agreed upon societal rules. Thus, although the law does evolve and change, the remainder of this chapter will focus on aspects of advanced psychiatric mental health nursing that are delineated by legal rules and precedents.

The areas that will be discussed are (1) the legal scope of advanced practice in psychiatric mental health nursing; (2) practice/malpractice/accountability issues of PMHN; and (3) the balance of confidentiality vs. duty to warn by PMHNs. This is a list of timely and crucial legal issues for the PMHN.

Scope of Practice

Nursing as a profession is given effect and recognition through state law. Nurse practice acts in each state regulate entry into the profession and statutorily define the scope of nursing practice in that state. A variety of economic, political, social, and professional issues impact on the state regulation of nursing practice and the implications of such regulation must be recognized.

Currently, three major patterns of nurse practice acts have emerged: regulatory acts, expanded definition acts, and delegatory acts. Some statutory language recognizes advanced practice per se while in many acts it is not acknowledged (Bullough, 1980). Despite differences in the law, PMHNs must define, limit, or fit their practice within the particular language of the particular nurse practice act in the state in which they practice.

Expanding Scope of Practice

Certainly the knowledge base and practice competence of PMHN has evolved beyond many states' statutory recognition of nursing. Since the ANA published the *Statement on Psychiatric and Mental Health Nursing Practice* in 1976, there has been a national recognition within the profession of what constitutes the specialty of advanced psychiatric mental health nursing. The "psychiatric mental health nursing specialist is distinguished by graduate education, supervised clinical experience, depth and amount of knowledge, competence and skill in the practice of psychiatric and mental health nursing" (ANA, 1976b, p. 10). In the same publication, there is recognition that there may be various settings in which nurses may practice psychiatric mental health nursing as well as perform many functions. "Two principal arrangements for psychiatric mental health nursing are: organized settings and self-employment settings. Nurses who work in organized settings can be remunerated on either a salary basis or a fee for service basis" (ANA, 1976b, p. 7). Self-employed psychiatric mental health nurses may gain their compensation for their services through either third-party payments or direct client fees.

Practice Challenges

The *Statement on Psychiatric Mental Health Nursing Practice* (ANA, 1976b) seems consistent with the *Standards of Psychiatric and Mental Health Nursing Practice* (ANA, 1982) and *Nursing: A Social Policy Statement* (ANA, 1980). However, as nurses increasingly seek independent and autonomous practice roles, that is, a fee for service practice, legal challenges are sure to arise in increased frequency and depth. It seems clear that as nurses begin to compete economically with psychiatrists, clinical psychologists, and psychiatric social workers for some of the direct reimbursement or third-party reimbursement monies in the mental health system, these other professions will question nursing's qualifications to practice psychotherapy, crisis counseling, family therapy, and the like.

The public purpose of any state regulatory act is to protect the safety of consumers and promote the public welfare. The public and all consumers should be protected from unscrupulous individuals who advertise and offer services for which they have no expertise. However, other professionals are most interested in being protected from economic competition for clients and these professionals actively support legislation that limits nursing practice to the generalist level as well as locally instituting legal challenges of advanced nursing practice through various state regulatory/licensing boards. Currently, nurses with advanced preparation and expertise in various nursing specialties are involved in an increased number of lawsuits (*Sermchief et al. v. Gonzales et al.*, 1983; *Nurse Midwifery Associates et al. v. B. K. Hibbet et al.*, 1983) whose outcomes will directly affect the future of nursing as an autonomous, accountable profession with definite rights to advanced practice.

Strategies for Right To Practice

If or when PMHNs are challenged in their right to practice, some preplanned strategies would seem effective to employ. One strategy would be to have the prior backing of the State Board of Nursing for their practice and to know the Board will interpret the State Nurse Practice Act as including the many activities of psychiatric mental health nursing within its definition. The State Board of Nursing needs to be a strong voice that supports rapidly expanding nursing knowledge and expanded practice capabilities.

A second approach would be to seek support from the state nursing association and directly from ANA. A nurse whose practice is guided by the ANA *Standards of Psychiatric and Mental Health Nursing Practice* and the *Statement on Psychiatric and Mental Health Nursing* should receive guidance and assistance from the professional organization.

A third approach would be to retain immediately legal counsel capable of advocating professional practice issues. Appropriate, assertive responses to challenges in many cases decreases the likelihood of formal actions being filed and increases the recognition of PMHNs as practitioners with protected rights.

An excellent example of an appropriate response to a challenge in practice is as follows. A certified practitioner of psychiatric mental health nursing in New Jersey was challenged by the state attorney general's office following queries by the boards representing medicine and clinical psychology as to her ability and authority to perform psychotherapy. Strong positive response on the part of the New Jersey Board of Nursing, the Society for Certified Clinical Specialists of the New Jersey State Nurses' Association, and by the individual nurse and her attorney that her practice of psychotherapy is an accepted activity of advanced nursing practice in New Jersey resulted in a successful resolution of this challenge without formal litigation (Corn, 1978). It would seem that nurses can learn from this experience that (1) challenges to nursing practice will occur; (2) such challenges must be met assertively and appropriately; and (3) such challenges can result in successful resolution with unified support within nursing. However, not all challenges will be rebutted so successfully. It is, therefore, imperative that all nurses maintain current knowledge in case law on scope of practice as it evolves.

Practice/Malpractice/Accountability

Protection

Despite the enormous proliferation of malpractice actions against health care providers in the last 15 years, nursing, as well as other mental health professions, have been somewhat protected. Nursing has been protected in that plaintiffs have recovered money damages from physicians or from employing agencies rather than from the nurse. However, as nurses become more visible as a group of autonomously practicing professionals, there will be an increased number of law suits in which the nurse will be named directly as defendant. Likewise, as the education and expertise of the nurse increases, an increased standard of care will be applied (Campazzi, 1980).

Mental health professionals have also been protected from the proliferation of malpractice suits owing to lack of specificity of harm and the reluctance on the part of some juries and courts to consider emotional harm and to understand psychiatric injury. The three types of cases most likely to result in successful malpractice litigation in the mental health field are (1) failure to take action to prevent suicides, (2) sexual relations with clients, and (3) the use of untried therapeutic measures with poor results (Schultz, 1982).

Malpractice Actions

Malpractice comprises specific kinds of negligence actions with the prerequisite that the defendant be a person who has special knowledge and skills and, through the defendant's practice of his specialty, injury to the plaintiff arises. For a patient plaintiff to recover money damages from a nurse defendant in a malpractice action, all elements of negligence must be made out in a court of law (Prosser, 1971, p. 143).

The elements are as follows: (1) there exists between the nurse and the client a duty to use due care; (2) there is a failure on the nurse's part to meet the standard of care that results in a breach of duty owed; (3) there is a foreseeability of harm in not meeting the standard of care; (4) the failure to meet the standard of care directly or proximately causes injury to the patient; and (5) the patient must prove his injuries.

There are no recorded cases on appellate review of malpractice actions against PMHNs, but successful actions have been maintained against psychiatrists and clinical psychologists (Cohen, 1979). It is only a matter of time and increased consumer/attorney recognition before such actions will be filed against PMHNs. Therefore, PMHNs need preventive strategies to decrease suits/recoveries for malpractice.

PRIMARY PREVENTION STRATEGIES. Lawsuits are filed by dissatisfied, angry, and injured clients. Prevention activities of the nurse to reduce the incidence of such filings include (1) giving personalized, concerned care, (2) including the client and significant others in health planning and treatment, (3) meeting the needs of the client, not the nurse, in relationships, and (4) demonstrating the nurse as a capable, knowledgeable professional.

PREVENTION OF MONETARY RECOVERY. Even these approaches will not always prevent malpractice actions from being instituted. Therefore, the nurse who is sued must be able to rebut malpractice accusations. This is done by proving the nurse met or exceeded the standard of care in the given situation. The "reasonable man" standard of care used in malpractice actions is one of peer reasonableness and will be developed by expert testimony on both sides. Thus, knowing and practicing what other PMHNs would find minimum or safe care is quite important,

Reading, continuing education, national/regional meetings, and "keeping up" in general is important for validating nursing practice. Also, introducing the ANA *Standards of Psychiatric and Mental Health Nursing Practice* would be a helpful documentary production to demonstrate to the jury that national clinical standards were met in the instant case. However, to be useful, such an introduction would mandate that the nurse had used the standards not only in practice but also in documentation of care planning and all aspects of record keeping.

Juries are most responsive to professions and professionals who demonstrate accountability and concern for consumers. Nursing is the first profession to develop clinical standards of practice. These standards, implemented through practice and proved through quality assurance programming, are capable of being evaluated in court and are a major step in securing the public trust in nursing at both the generalist and specialist levels. Licensure, certification, and clinical supervision appropriate to the practice setting and case complexity are other elements for demonstrating PMHN's quest for accountable, responsible practice. Acts that demonstrate accountability are supportive rebuttal to malpractice allegations.

Balancing Confidentiality and the Duty To Warn

From the earliest days of their educational experience, nurses acknowledge that data generated about a client from any source are confidential. Professionally and ethically, nurses are bound to use client data for the enhancement of care rather than for the purposes of voyeurism, titilation, or gossip. This is especially important in mental health settings owing to the continuing stigmatization of mental/emotional clients and their problems in our society.

Statutory privilege that prevents a professional from being required to divulge client information under oath rarely extends to nurses, although statutes differ on a state by state basis. In the absence of a statutory privilege on communication for nurses, PMHNs should carefully weigh the types of information shared in nurse-client relationships, especially if criminal or civil litigation appears to be a probability.

Following the decision in *Tarasoff v. the Regents of the University of California* (1976), all counseling/therapy disciplines are rethinking their duty for confidentiality. Prior to Tarasoff, there was a strong belief that both ethically and legally the communications between therapist and client were privileged and the confidentiality should be maintained at all cost. The decision in Tarasoff changed the principle to indicate that the legal duty to maintain client confidentiality to promote the therapeutic relationship is cut off when the protection of the public safety is at issue. Thus, therapists working with clients who have violent tendencies, violent ideation, and somewhat clear plans to do harm to a third person have now an affirmative legal duty to act to prevent the violence if at all possible (Kjervik, 1981).

Many therapeutic strategies can be employed by PMHNs when an assessment of potential violence is made. Voluntary admission of the client to a hospital, involuntary commitment, notification of law enforcement officers about the threat, and notification of the potential victim or the family are among the choices available. Such a mandate of the duty to warn or to protect third persons clearly indicates that PMHNs must be aware of the potential for violence and characteristics of clients with whom there is likelihood that violent threats might be carried out. Foreseeability of the plan, victim, methodology, and intent to do harm is usually the standard that will be applied. With an assessment of dangerousness, the standard of care for the nurse therapist is based on what the reasonably prudent nurse acting in the same or similar circumstances would do. It is important that the method of warning the potential victim is one that will be both effective and also least harmful to the client (Kjervik, 1981).

SUMMARY

The PMHN faces the increasing challenge of ethical dilemmas as the role of psychiatric nurse is expanded and enhanced. Kohlberg's theory of cognitive moral development was presented as a prerequisite to understanding moral reasoning and three ethical theories from philosophy were briefly described as foundations for ethical decision making. Six areas of practice were discussed using the ANA *Code for Nurses* and the ANA *Standards of Psychiatric and Mental Health Nursing Practice* as guidelines.

Legal issues impacting on the PMHN also abound. The law is evolving as is the discipline of nursing, and the law will dynamically impact on the discipline in the years ahead. Three legal issues were the focus of this chapter: scope of practice for the PMHN, malpractice and accountability, and the competing need for confidentiality and the duty to warn. Continued sharing of confrontations, litigated cases, and positive solutions in the legal sector are important to the growth and development of psychiatric mental health nursing as an advanced specialty.

REFERENCES

American Association of Sex Educators, Counselors, and Therapists (AASECT). *Code of ethics.* Washington, DC: AASECT, 1980.

American Nurses' Association. *Code for nurses with interpretive statements.* Kansas City, MO: American Nurses' Association, 1976a.

American Nurses' Association. *Statement on psychiatric and mental health nursing practice.* Kansas City, MO: American Nurses' Association, 1976b.

American Nurses' Association. *Nursing: A social policy statement.* Kansas City, MO: American Nurses' Association, 1980.

American Nurses' Association. *Standards of psychiatric and mental health nursing practice.* Kansas City, MO: American Nurses' Association, 1982.

Aroskar, M., & Veatch, R. M. Ethics teaching in nursing schools. *Hastings Center Report,* 1977, *7,* 23–26.

Beauchamp, T. L., & Childress, J. F. *Principles of biomedical ethics* (2nd ed.). New York: Oxford University Press, 1983.

Benjamin, M. & Curtis, J. *Ethics in nursing.* New York: Oxford University Press, 1981.

Bouhoutsas, J., Holroyd, J., Lermann, H., Farer, B., & Greenberg, M. Sexual intimacy between psychotherapists and patients. *Professional Psychology: Research and Practice,* 1983, *14,* 185–196.

Bullough, B. *The law and the expanding nursing role* (2nd ed.). New York: Appleton-Century-Croft, 1980.

Bursten, B. Medical responsibility in institutional settings. *American Journal of Psychiatry,* 1980, *137,* 1071–1078.

Campazzi, B. Nurses, nursing and malpractice litigation. *Nursing Administration Quarterly,* 1980, *5,* 1–18.

Cohen, R. *Malpractice.* New York: Free Press, 1979.

Corn, F. Regional News, *Pacesetter,* American Nurses' Association, 1978, *3(2),* 4–5.

Crisham, P. Measuring moral judgement in nursing dilemmas. *Nursing Research,* 1981, *30,* 104–110.

Curtin, L. No rush to judgment. In L. Curtin & M. J. Flaherty (Eds.), *Nursing ethics: Theories and pragmatics.* Bowie, MD: Robert J. Brady Co., 1982.

Davis, A., & Aroskar, M. A. *Ethical dilemmas and nursing practice* (2nd ed.). New York: Appleton-Century-Croft, 1983.

Dix, G. E. Realism and drug refusal: A reply to Appelbaum and Gutheil. *American Academy of Psychiatry and Law,* 1981, *9,* 180–198.

Dworkin, G. Autonomy and behavior control. *Hastings Center Report,* 1976, *6,* 23–28.

Fowler, R. D. Ethical practice. *Psychiatric Systems Dialogue,* 1983, *20,* 5–6.

Fromer, M. J. The suicidal client: Philosophical bases for nursing intervention. *Nursing Law and Ethics,* 1981, *2,* 1–8.

Gadow, S. Existential advocacy: Philosophical foundation of nursing. In C. P. Murphy & H. Hunter (Eds.), *Ethical problems in the nurse-patient relationship.* Boston: Allyn & Bacon, 1983.

Gilligan, C. In a different voice: Women's conceptions of self and of morality. *Harvard Education Review,* 1978, *47,* 481–517.

Guidance Associates. Teacher training in values education: A workshop. *Leadership manual.* New York: Harcourt, Brace & Jovanovich, 1976.

Haber, J., Leach, A., Schudy, S., & Sideleau, B. *Comprehensive psychiatric nursing* (2nd ed.). New York: McGraw-Hill, 1982.

Hoeffer, B. The private practice model: An ethical perspective. *Journal of Psychiatric Nursing and Mental Health Services,* 1983, *21,* 31–37.

Kelly, L. *Dimensions of professional nursing* (4th ed.). New York: MacMillan Publishing, 1981.

Ketefian, S. Moral reasoning and moral behavior: Among selected groups of practicing nurses. *Nursing Research,* 1981, *30,* 171–176.

Kjervik, D. The psychiatric nurse's duty to warn potential victims of homicidal psychotherapy outpatients. *Law, Medicine, and Health Care,* 1981, *9,* 11–16.

Kohlberg, L. The cognitive-developmental approach to moral education. In D. Purpel & K. Ryan (Eds.), *Moral education, It comes with the territory.* Berkeley, CA: Phi Delta Kappa, 1976a.

Kohlberg, L. Moral stages and moralization: The cognitive developmental approach. In J. Lickona (Ed.), *Moral development and behavior.* New York: Holt, Rinehart & Winston, 1976b.

Kohlberg, L. *Recent research in moral development.* New York: Holt, Rinehart & Winston, 1983.

Krawczyk, R., & Kudzma, E. Ethics: A matter of moral development. *Nursing Outlook,* 1978, *26,* 254–257.

Lumpp, S. F. The role of the nurse in the bioethical decision-making process. *Nursing Clinics of North America,* 1979, *14,* 13–21.

Mahon, K. A., & Fowler, M. D. Moral development and clinical decision-making. *Nursing Clinics of North America,* 1979, *14,* 3–12.

Munhall, P. Moral development: A prerequisite. *Journal of Nursing Education,* 1982, *21,* 11–15.

Nurse Midwifery Associates et al. v. B. K. Hibbett et al. Federal District Court of Nashville, No. 82–3228, 1983.

Omery A. Moral development: A differential evaluation of dominant models. *Advances in Nursing Science,* 1983, *6(1),* 1–17.

Prosser, W. *Law of torts* (4th ed.). St. Paul, MN: West Publishing Co., 1971.

Rada, R. T. Forensic psychiatry: Overview of current issues. *Audio Digest Psychiatry,* 1982, *11,* 11.

Schultz, B. M. *Legal liability in psychotherapy.* Washington, DC: Josey Bass, 1982.

Sermchief et al. v. Gonzales et al. Supreme Court of Missouri, No. 64692, 1983.

Tarasoff v. Regents of University of California. 551 P2334, 1976.

Wilson, H. S., & Kneisl, C. R. *Psychiatric nursing* (2nd ed.). Menlo Park, CA: Addison-Wesley, 1983.

Wise, T. P. Where the public peril begins: A survey of psychotherapists to determine the effects of *Tarasoff. Stanford Law Review,* 1978, *31,* 165–190.

BIBLIOGRAPHY

Andrews, S., & Hutchinson, S. A. Teaching nursing ethics: A practical approach. *Journal of Nursing Education,* 1981, *20,* 6–11.

Carroll, J. L., & Rest, S. R. Moral development. In B. Wolman (Ed.), *Handbook of developmental psychology.* Englewood Cliffs, NJ: Prentice-Hall, 1982.

Gadow, S. Advocacy nursing and new meanings of aging. *Nursing Clinics of North America,* 1979, *14,* 81–91.

Jametown, A. The nurse: When roles and rules conflict. *Hastings Center Report,* 1977, *7,* 22–23.

King, E. C. *Affective education in nursing.* Rockville, MD: Aspen Systems Corp., 1984.

Kohlberg, L. *Recent research in moral development.* New York: Holt, Rinehart & Winston, 1983.

L'Abate, L. (Ed.). *Values, ethics, legalities and the family* therapist. Rockville, MD: Aspen Systems Corp., 1982.

CHAPTER 22 PROFESSIONAL ISSUES

Maureen L. Boshier

Professional issues regarding nursing practice are as varied, complex, individual, collective, and simple as any of the concepts that form them. As a member of the nursing profession, it is not at all unlikely that the nurse will experience feelings similar to those expressed by Lewis Carroll's heroine, Alice, who did indeed think she knew who she was that morning but after wandering through Wonderland, was not at all sure.

This chapter is designed to focus attention on some of the critical "out of nursing" but "part of nursing" issues that impact on practice. These issues include health care legislation and financing, regulation and credentialing of nursing and nurses, maintaining competency, and collaborative practice.

It is not feasible for anyone who intends to practice nursing to remain uninformed regarding the parameters of health and practice regulation. The master's-prepared psychiatric mental health nurse must determine the ways and means for practice and this process will be influenced by a number of the major issues that shape the health care work force. The issues include the size of the needed pool of providers, including who is recognized as a reimbursable provider of mental health care services, and how much traffic the market can bear, the distribution of providers throughout the community, and, in the face of decreasing revenues and increasing costs, which providers will be identified as survivors in the health care market.

It is with this in mind that an overview of where psychiatric mental health nursing has been and what it will need in order to keep moving ahead is presented to provide a helpful perspective and, hopefully, a conceptual framework from which the reader may progress. Certainly, all the issues cannot be addressed in this chapter, but perhaps the overview presented will stimulate thinking, questioning, and pondering by the individual of the issues identified, as well as others to be resolved.

AN OVERVIEW: GOVERNMENTAL HEALTH PLANNING POLICY

Any time legislation is enacted that impacts on the health care of the community, be it via state or federal action, a corollary impact on nursing and its role in providing health care must be expected. Hopefully, in recognizing this fact, nurses will not just expect an impact but will anticipate this impact by becoming knowledgeable, expert participants in the political process that results in the formation of health care policy. Following is an overview of some of the significant pieces of federal legislation that have charted the course and led to the formation of the present day health care policy in this country.

The ongoing role of the federal government in health care policy formation was established in the 1930s. In 1932, a committee was formed to address rising health care costs and unequal distribution of health care services. The 1935 Social Security Act contained provisions to provide funds to states to finance some basic health care programs in maternal/

child health, communicable disease control, and the training of public health personnel. The Federal Security Agency, formed in 1937, had five components: U.S. Public Health Service, the Social Security Administration, the Office of Vocational Rehabilitation, the U.S. Children's Bureau, and the Food and Drug Adminstration. Until this time, governmental involvement in health care had been more limited.

The depression of the 1930s focused attention on the urgent need to provide coverage for health care costs of the nation through some form of national funding. In 1946, a proposal by President Truman called for payment of medical costs through compulsory insurance premiums and general revenues. This proposal was supported by the American Nurses' Association, the National League for Nursing Education, and the National Organization for Public Health Nursing. President Truman's proposal was adamently opposed by the American Medical Association, which launched a massive public education campaign to inform the public about the dangers of socialized medicine and the socialization and governmental control of American life (Kalisch & Kalisch, 1982). The resulting compromise legislation became commonly known as the Hill-Burton Act, which provided funds for hospital construction. The stage had been set for recognizing the influence of the organized, financially supported efforts of the American Medical Association.

The involvement of the federal government in health care continued to grow in the decades after World War II. The 1950 amendment to the Public Assistance Title of the Social Security Act provided for sharing of health care costs by the federal government. The Kerr-Mills Bill of 1960 increased federal monies for the health care of the aged and those considered medically indigent. The debate on the enactment of legislation to provide national health insurance never really ceased. In 1965, Medicare and Medicaid legislation was enacted to fund health care for the elderly and the poor. Concomitantly, the federal government enacted legislation to provide quality control over services provided through Medicare and Medicaid. The legislation was also meant to oversee costs and access to services with the Regional Medical Program Act and the Comprehensive Health Planning and Public Health Services Act. A strengthening amendment to the Social Security Act in 1972 called for the establishment of Professional Standards Review Organizations to assure that services provided under Medicare and Medicaid were necessary, appropriate, and were procured in the most appropriate facility. The Health Maintenance Organization Act of 1973 amended the Public Health Services Act and called for the Department of Health, Education, and Welfare to develop alternatives to traditional forms of health care delivery and financing by establishing a federal demonstration project. Still, the issues addressed in these laws were primarily related to medicine (physicians) and health care facilities (hospitals) and not to nursing.

The National Mental Health Act, signed into law by Truman in 1946, authorized the establishment of the National Institute of Mental Health with an appropriation to launch a national mental health program beginning in 1947. The National Health Planning and Resources Development Act of 1974 underscored public awareness of inadequate, ineffective, and poorly distributed health care resources. For those concerned with mental health care it further emphasized the issues of linking national mental health concerns to statewide health systems agencies, cultivation of skills in mental health policymaking on all levels of governance and earmarking monies for mental health planning and resource development.

In 1975, the Health Planning and Resources Development Program was implemented in an attempt to incorporate health planning in health legislation. The program called for a network of Health Systems agencies and State Health Planning agencies to issue certificates of need to control the number and types of health facilities constructed. These constraints were an attempt to limit expenditures and duplication of services. Although the pool of nurses prepared at the master's level had begun to increase at this time, no general planning for utilization of these nursing specialists was incorporated in addressing the tasks identified by this legislation. In part, this may be due to the fact that the concepts of autonomy of nursing practice and the potential expansion of nursing services have not been formally established in the minds of the public, the profession, and the policymakers. These circumstances persist, despite national studies such as the 1970 *An Abstract for Action* by the National Commission for the Study of Nursing and Nursing Education that have called for improving the delivery of health care services through better utilization of nursing expertise and nursing roles.

Federal involvement in regulating and funding health care continues as the issues of health care costs, delivery of services, resources, and demands are highlighted by consumers, policymakers, and providers. At present, there does not appear to be a cohesive, coherent national policy regarding mental health issues. The focus for policy development in this area appears to have come from the National Commission on Mental Health. Professional groups involved with psychiatric mental health care hopefully will begin conveying their views to the public and the policymakers so that the development of a useful national mental health care policy will be forthcoming. Although nurses are consumers and providers, they need also to become policymakers. It is astounding that so many crucial pieces of health care legislation were developed, proposed, and passed with so little input from and recognition of nursing. Senator Inouye of Hawaii has been quoted as saying, "You nurses, you can have whatever you want, you can control the health care system, you have more power than any other group, including all the oil lobbyists, but you will go to your graves with 'docile' written on your tombstones" (Lang, 1983).

The Political Process

Gaining access to policy formation begins with participation in the election of a candidate and involves the candidate's stand on issues and his or her placement and involvement with legislative committees. Obviously, the nurse should have personal and professional interest and input into this process. Examination of the activities of elected officials at state and federal levels clearly identifies the powerful policymakers. Without question, decisions are made with or without input from nursing. The goals of the nursing profession can become translated into policy only with personal involvement and the risk-taking required to affect the process on many levels. Often, this is time consuming and tedious. However, planning and implementation of policy occurs when the interests of a group are unified and expressed to the public, the local political bodies, and the national policymakers. Initial areas of inquiry will involve examination of policymaking at the state level regarding who is consulted when health planning, reimbursement issues, or health and nursing statutes are drafted. If policymakers are not educated to seek out nursing expertise, it is not unusual to expect that it will be medical and /or hospital expertise that will be utilized, as these groups have long been considered the experts in health care definition.

Public support and attention to an issue by a large segment of the population succeeds in placing that issue on a policymaking agenda. Strategic use of the media is an asset in impressing the public and the policymakers with the urgency of an issue and its need for public attention. Professional nursing organizations provide a means whereby the nurse can make a knowledgeable impact on policymakers. Yet these organizations and groups and nurses need to display cohesiveness in presenting a unified, thoughtful, and intelligent approach to an issue for consideration by policymakers. It is regrettable that although there are numerous professional nursing groups with which the nurse can affiliate, there are far too many nurses who do not avail themselves of this opportunity. There are approximately 21 nursing specialty organizations in addition to the American Nurses' Association and the National League for Nursing and their respective subgroups. Of the 1.7 million nurses in this country, probably less than 25% belong to a nursing organization. According to statistics compiled by the American Nurses' Association in January 1983, 354,940 nurses belong to nursing organizations. Unquestionably, the absence of a unified voice for nursing promotes vulnerability to attack by those who are opponents to nursing goals and values. The American Nurses' Association's Council of Specialists in Psychiatric and Mental Health Nursing has approximately 676 members, although it is estimated that there are probably some 6,000 master's-prepared psychiatric mental health nurses. Membership in this council provides, among other things, an opportunity for specialists to work toward professional, political, and educational goals and to interact with the Joint Commission on Inter-professional Affairs (JCIA). The JCIA, founded in 1974, has representatives from the American Nurses' Association, the American Psychological Association, the National Association of Social Workers, and the American Psychiatric Association. This group meets three times a year to address legislature, reimbursement, education, and patient care issues related to mental health.

Balancing diverse nursing goals and values within a cohesive framework is no easy task. However, professional growth is severely impeded and is also manipulated by those who would limit nursing influence. All too often strong, conflicting, and vocal detractors of the profession come from the ranks of the nursing profession itself. This situation can only be ameliorated through educating nurses to the political process and involving them in the process. If united, the nursing profession has the numbers to influence decision making, design parameters for practice, and write policy. For nursing to survive, there is no way around involvement in politics and policymaking. Ultimately, success will rest with what nursing can do, and does do, for itself.

Health Care Payments

The rigorous attention to cost containment in health care creates an interesting set of circumstances for nursing. Health care financing and even health planning has not addressed nursing services as a specific entity in the health care picture. Current trends to find the means to provide quality care in new ways could be an opportunity for nurses to practice in a more prominent way.

Most individuals' health care costs are paid for by a third-party payer/health care financer, which is to say a commercial, governmental, or a nonprofit prepaid program commonly called health insurance. Payments may be made based on the fee charged for the service or by paying a fixed amount of money to those responsible for providing the health care.

Blue Cross and Blue Shield, established as a nonprofit, tax-exempt, prepayment insurance company during the 1930s, and presently a major health care financer, today administers, depending on geographic area and local policy, state health care programs such as Medicare, Medicaid, and the Civilian Health and Medical Program of the Uniformed Services (CHAMPUS). The majority of the board of directors of this company is composed, by law, of physicians and hospital administrators. This board makes the decisions regarding the allowable services and fees to be reimbursed and which providers will be reimbursed. Traditionally, the physician and the hospital have been the identified reimbursable providers. The exclusion of certain services for reimbursement and the exclusion of certain procedures from reimbursement eligibility affects those who are not physicians. The Rural Health Clinics Act of 1977 made it possible for nurses to receive direct payment for services through Medicare and Medicaid in rural areas. In 1979, in selected geographic areas, a pilot project for reimbursement of master's-prepared clinical specialists in psychiatric mental health nursing was provided through CHAMPUS. Despite these efforts, reimbursement for nursing services, both inpatient and outpatient, has been limited and never universally established.

The ANA's (1983a, b) *American Nurse* reported in May and June 1983 that West Virginia and Washington are the only two states that allow direct third-party reimbursement for registered nurses performing services within their scope of practice. Seven other states include nurse midwives among those eligible for third-party payment: Alaska, Maryland, New Jersey, New Mexico, New York, Pennsylvania, and Utah. Four states have determined that nurse practitioners are eligible for reimbursement: Montana, Maryland, Mississippi, and Oregon. Only California provides for reimbursement of psychiatric nurse specialists—nurses holding a master's degree with two years experience in the field. Most state laws with reimbursement provisions call for payment only if services are reimbursable when provided by physicians or other health care personnel. It is encouraging that momentum for providing reimbursement of nursing services by health insurers appears to be building. In 1983, enabling legislation was introduced in Maine, Massachusetts, Minnesota, New Jersey, New York, Pennsylvania, and Texas, in addition to laws passed in Montana and West Virginia.

The rapidly rising cost of health care has everyone's attention. It is contended that when an individual is insured, more can be afforded in paying for physician fees and services. If the health care financer is Medicare or Medicaid, the payment has been for those costs that are determined as "allowable" or necessary to the service. In addition, payments are also made on a retrospective basis, that is, the historical cost of the service. This method does not account for those costs that are required to operate the facility. Thus, for the facility to meet its full financial responsibility, the cost difference has to be shifted somewhere which is usually to the self-pay and the commercial insurance clients. To address this problem and the problem of the soaring cost of health care in general, a prospective payment mechanism for acute care hospitals was proposed by the top officials in the Department of Health and Human Services. Prospective payment means fixing the level of payment before services are provided based on a patient's diagnosis and the rate and type of discharge.

It should be noted that this proposal continues to include nursing care costs in an aggregate sum along with room, board, and maintenance costs. Grouping together these charges makes it more difficult to determine necessary cost containment efforts applicable to nursing in an equitable and realistic fashion. Congress has approved a Medicare prospective pricing plan for most inpatient services as part of the Social Security amendments of 1983. This plan sets pricing for each Diagnosis Related Group (DRG) and puts the hospital in the position of covering the differences between average costs, for length of stay and use of services, and the actual DRG prices. This action is intended to provide an incentive to hospitals to manage costs within available revenues. It is also intended to involve the physician in managing patient services such as those related to discharge and services ordered. Again, the plan does not specifically address nursing care costs. Prospective pricing applies to all hospitals except children's, psychiatric, rehabilitation, and long-term hospitals. This action should serve as a red light to psychiatric mental health care providers in terms of preparing for similar events in their field. Further, the Tax Equity and Fiscal Responsibility Act (TEFRA) enacted in September 1982 discontinued nursing salary cost differential, required employers to continue insurance coverage for workers over age 65, and substantially reduced reimbursement for such providers as radiologists and pathologists. It is readily apparent that this act impacts on hospital costs and financing in a significant way. This is the first attempt, through legislation, to limit significantly fees that are recovered by physicians.

Psychiatric units in general hospitals will be reimbursed on the basis of retrospectively determined costs subject to a cost-per-case limit on allowable rate of increases established by TEFRA.

The true consequences of TEFRA and prospective reimbursement will not be immediately known. There is no question that these measures will change the traditional financing of health care. It is to be expected that similar plans will be forthcoming from the prepaid, nonprofit, and commercial insurance companies as well.

It is also of interest that a measure to prohibit the Federal Trade Commission (FTC) from applying the restraint of trade statutes to the regulation of the health professions narrowly missed adoption. This proposal was strongly supported by the American Medical Association but was opposed by the American Nurses' Association, the American College of Nurse Midwives, and the National League for Nursing. Their opposition was based on the fact that such legislation would continue to limit consumers' access to health care providers other than physicians. Reauthorization of the FTC and the exemption of professionals from FTC jurisdiction will again be debated by the 98th Congress.

Increasing consumer demands for participation in health care delivery can create opportunities for nurses because of their knowledge of the health care system, their assessment abilities, and their willingness to be directly accessible to the consumer. Competition and the potential to reduce health care costs via competition and unrestricted entry into the health care system cannot occur without third-party reimbursement for all licensed professional providers.

It appears evident that the trend in reimbursement by health care financers will be geared toward costs rather than services. The task of reducing costs while maintaining the quality and accessibility of health care services is being addressed on all fronts by policymakers, health care financers, and providers. Nursing participation in this task and the legislative focus of the nursing profession should be on the policies that address Medicare and Medicaid programs, prospective reimbursement, and health care financing. Indeed, one of the ANA legislative practices for the 1980–1982 biennium has been to define nursing's interests in the developing competition strategies in the health care industry.

The current practice of including nursing costs into generally nonitemized costs such as room rates prevents identifying the cost of nursing services. It also contributes to the lack of an available cost reimbursement structure for nursing services. Cost containment efforts will necessarily address identifying appropriate, high quality care, predicting and controlling costs, discouraging the unnecessary use of services, and providing a wider range of services in other than hospital settings. These efforts will also consider better consumer education in the areas of prevention and health maintenance. Health care, which is not necessarily the same as medical care, will have to be based on consumer needs. A health care focus can, utilized appropriately, contribute to the autonomous, more far-reaching provision of nursing services. Nursing expertise is unequivocally based on patient/consumer need but must be clearly identified as such to the public, the policymakers, and the health care financers. As the health care picture changes, nursing will need to be ready with (1) identifiable standards of practice and mechanisms for monitoring practice, (2) identifiable advanced practice credentials, and (3) proof of efficiency of services regarding quality and cost savings. This will require the collection of data to demonstrate the efficacy of reimbursement of the costs of providers who are other than the traditional physician and hospital. Health care financers are examining costs and seeking ways to limit numbers of eligible providers, as well as types of providers, and this can certainly affect the practice of master's-prepared psychiatric mental health nurses. Employers who pay employees' health insurance premiums are asking health care financers to justify the factors considered in determining premiums. This position also focuses the financers on addressing reimbursement from the standpoint of cost-effective care.

The potential adverse impact of this trend on the practice of master's-prepared nurses can be circumvented. One possibility is if eligible nurse providers can develop a cost reimbursement proposal that is attractive to the health care financer. To be attractive, such a proposal would need to demonstrate that nurses can provide high quality, cost-effective, affordable care that addresses health maintenance and so reduces the higher cost of hospitalization. The proposal would need to ensure that the care is delivered by credentialed nurses who meet standards of practice and are able to be self-monitoring in terms of their practice. The traditional ways of delivering health care are rapidly changing. Now is the right time for new ideas.

There may be several ways to develop and implement such a plan for reimbursing nursing costs. One possibility is a proposal that strongly indicates the expected outcome to be cost saving when services are delivered by master's-prepared nurses. The proposal could be presented to a health care financer for funding as a pilot project to demonstrate and document cost savings. If successful, the proposal could be considered for inclusion as an established part of reimbursable costs. The provider reimbursement manager or provider relations' representative of an insurance company or health maintenance organization is the contact person for such a proposal. In selecting an organization with whom to initiate such a discussion, one would need to evaluate the financer's commitment to subscriber education, research, and development. Do they employ an educational specialist who provides subscriber education on health maintenance? Do they employ statisticians who analyze cost-appropriate and cost-effective utilization of services?

Such a proposal would need to consider the following factors: demonstration of the potential and actual demand for specialized knowledge, skills and services and demonstration of the cost benefit of services in the areas of prevention, health maintenance, and treatment. This action would initiate reliable access for the master's-prepared psychiatric mental health nurse into the health payment system, since the health care financers are on the move to address the issues identified above.

Obviously, the outcome of any policies that will address reimbursement of health care costs will be influenced by cost containment efforts, the special interests of powerful providers such as physicians and insurance companies, and the public demand for services. The challenge to nursing to become a visible part of this picture could not be clearer.

OVERVIEW: THE PHILOSOPHY AND FUNDING OF NURSING EDUCATION

Gaining perspective on the path traveled, to determine the path ahead, can be a useful experience. It is fascinating to note that as far back as the 1800s, when nursing education programs were first established, the particulars of nursing education, its structure and design, have been directly influenced by physicians and hospital administrators. Then, as now, nonnursing persons with vested interests in the definition of nursing practice argued against providing nursing education in affiliation with schools and universities on the ground that there was no need to prepare unnecessarily overeducated nurses. However, nurses are assuming more responsibility and accountability within the health care system and the need for preparation at the baccalaureate and master's level in nursing is abundantly clear. To meet the opportunity and requirements for a broader scope of practice, master's level education is necessary.

Although they are the largest group of health care professionals, nurses seem to continue to be required to justify the stands they take and their delineation of the roles they choose. Indeed, for a variety of reasons, including the dissension in the nursing profession itself, the definition of the nursing role is sometimes not self-determined.

Nursing Education

Basically, the parameters for nursing practice are derived from nursing education. A variety of professional nursing organizations have been involved in setting the standards for nursing education. In 1932, the Collegiate School of Nursing, although not an official accrediting body for nursing education, provided the initial impetus for many of the policies established in higher education. The National League for Nursing Education, formed in 1939 and now known as the National League for Nursing, is accepted as the official professional organization that sets standards for nursing education and accredits nursing programs.

The direction in nursing today, both in education and in practice, appears to be shifting toward a separation of nursing from the influence and limits of hospitals and physicians and into a broader range of services and expertise provided to the public. The *Abstract for Action* published by the National Commission for the Study of Nursing and Nursing Education in 1970 clearly recommended the restructuring of nursing roles, nursing education, and the enhancement of care by utilizing nursing expertise and recognizing nursing as a full profession. Since 1923, in the majority of the surveys and studies written, the requirements for nursing education have unequivocably recommended the collegiate setting for preparing nurses. Such recommendations and observations, although frequently stated in the literature, have yet to be fully established by the nursing profession.

Funding Nursing Education

Certainly, trends in nursing education influence the philosophy of practice. In addition, however inappropriately, the availability of funding sources influences the enrollment patterns and the selection of an educational program by an individual. If nursing's educational programs do not emphasize the attainment of advanced degrees and if the marketplace and those practicing nursing do not emphasize the advanced degree as well, the advancement of the nurse and the practice of nursing will stagnate. More specifically, if undergraduate nursing does not expose the student to the general practice of psychiatric mental health nursing, can it be expected that advanced preparation will be sought in this area? Of some concern, in the associate degree and baccalaureate degree nursing curricula, is the emphasis on an integrated curriculum that may lack explicit exposure to psychiatric nursing experience. Master's-prepared psychiatric mental health nurses themselves fostered the integration of psychiatric mental health concepts into basic curricula. Retrospectively, it seems necessary to provide students with good psychiatric nursing experiences to stimulate their interest in the selection of psychiatric mental health nursing as a specialty. Trends have been identified in decreasing enrollments of psychiatric mental health master's programs which is cause for concern (Mitsunaga, 1982).

It is self-evident that nursing education involves cost. Yet the history of federal funding for nursing education clearly indicates that relying on the availability of such funding is not reasonable for nursing education.

The basic piece of federal legislation relative to nursing education is the Nurse Training Act of 1964, which was amended to continue funding until the present. Monies actually available under this legislation have undergone many challenges resulting, at present, in a very limited allocation that has required extensive political activity to maintain continued availability of even this limited funding. The Nurse Training Act will come up for reauthorization in 1984. The trend of policymakers to fund nursing based on numbers of nurses produced, instead of from the perspective of developing all aspects of quality nursing care, can be considered a dangerous, well-established practice that needs reversal. Only by reversing this trend will the advancement of nursing through advanced degree education become a stronger reality. The 1983 Institute of Medicine study (IOM), entitled *Nursing and Nursing Education: Public Policies and Private Actions,* was mandated by Congress via the amendments to the Nurse Training Act in 1979. This study indicates no need to continue federal support to increase the overall supply of generalist nurses but recommends expanded federal support of fellowships, loans, and programs at the graduate level to increase the numbers of nurses with advanced degrees. The IOM study also recommends establishing an organizational entity at the federal level to place nursing research in the mainstream of scientific investigation. Research is definitely a requirement for strengthening and defining practice. However, nursing research has received only five million dollars in federal funding as opposed to three billion dollars in funding for biomedical research (Kalisch & Kalisch, 1982, p. 199). Extensive research is required to identify nursing actions, to test nursing actions, and to identify outcomes, the necessary knowledge to improve practice.

The most significant piece of legislation in the development of psychiatric mental health nursing as a specialty was the National Mental Health Act of 1946. The activities of the Psychiatric Nursing Education Branch of the National Institute of Mental Health (NIMH) have included the administration of traineeships for graduate nursing education in psychiatric mental health nursing. However, in keeping with the trend evidenced by the administrations of Nixon, Carter, and now Reagan, clinical training funds, budgeted requests and allocation of funds are beginning to be severely limited as well. At present there is some debate as to whether or not those committed to master's-prepared psychiatric mental health nursing ought to be putting political energy into maintaining/increasing NIMH funds or to securing Nurse Training Act monies. The fickleness of federal support for nursing education is well known. Funding is usually based on head counts and shortages rather than on an assessment of what educational preparation benefits the public and the greatest needs of the health care delivery system. In the wake of the Institute of Medicine report that advocates increased financial support of advanced educational preparation in nursing, NIMH funds usually provided for graduate education need to be maintained and increased through well-placed political pressure.

Perhaps in this present era of health care reform, efforts to restore funds can be mobilized. The role of the graduate-prepared psychiatric mental health nurse could be emphasized as a way of addressing the inequitable and ineffective provision of health services and the remarkable escalation of health care costs in traditional health care settings.

PROFESSIONAL DEVELOPMENT

The scene involving resources has been explored and the allocation of resources and the policies influencing their allocation have been identified. Next, the nursing profession itself will be discussed. The socialization of nursing, the specific regulatory/credentialing components of nursing practice, maintaining competency, and the utilization and collaboration of master's-prepared psychiatric mental health nursing specialists with other providers of mental health care services will all be considered.

The Socialization of the Nursing Profession

Socialization implies an internalization of values that results in appropriate behaviors. Many argue that the socialization of the nursing profession has been strongly influenced by values perceived to be part of the traditional female role: subservience, an orientation to serving others, a lack of career orientation, commitment and willingness to maintain, at all costs, a status quo. As the majority of nurses are women, it is also argued that the nursing profession will have difficulty resocializing members who have a long history steeped in traditional female values and roles. It is also said that nursing education fosters maternalistic values and may not facilitate an orientation to career planning. In keeping with patterns evidenced by oppressed groups, for example, slum dwellers who riot and destroy their own neighborhoods, the nursing profession is sometimes judged as engaging in lateral attacks on problems rather than using hierarchal attacks. This approach results in unchanged, mostly ineffective, decision-making actions. It is useful to explore the cultural and personal values that shape one's concept of self and one's behavior. Confidence, assertiveness, and independence, the characteristics that promote successful professional achievement, need to be emphasized without unconscious impediment. Because socialization influences choice and action, a connection appears to exist between the state of today's nursing profession, lack of unity, autonomy, power, and definition and the fact that nursing is a predominantly female profession.

However, resocialization occurs and reoccurs through life and/or a career. Advances or changes are made in one's education, work setting, status, role expectation, role definition, and performance. Indeed, a case can clearly be made for the resocialization of nursing by facilitating graduate education. Such education expands learning and expertise and advances practice by developing higher levels of nursing competence in many areas including research, practice, teaching, and consultation. The master's-prepared nurse is more able to conceptualize, articulate, and define positions and supporting rationale. She or he can critically analyze situations using organizational and clinical theories and assume and define new nursing roles. Advanced education assists in facilitating change in self to promote growth and the development of roles in new and traditional health care settings. A clearer delineation of levels of competence and practice becomes possible. Collaboration instead of competition can be modeled and the breaking down of preconceived notions about nurses and nursing roles can be enacted. Master's-prepared specialists accomplish this task on the basis of their broader base of preparation for practice and by practicing nursing as experts. Their effectiveness has been demonstrated through intelligent interpretations and effective communications, beginning skills in research, service as consultants to other nurses, provision of new interventions for health care problems, and carrying their own caseload. The public, the nursing profession, and allied professions need to be educated to the fact that master's-prepared nursing practice can provide enhanced skills and improved patient outcomes.

Utilization of Master's-Prepared Psychiatric Mental Health Nurses

Nurses are the major category of professionals employed in psychiatric mental health facilities. Although it is difficult to determine distribution based on academic preparation, the U.S. Department of Health and Human Services (1981) *Source Book-Nursing Personnel* estimated that there were perhaps 6,000 master's-prepared psychiatric nurses.

Vaughn (1983) in an article in the October 1983 issue of *Nursing and Health Care* indicated there were 154 master's programs in nursing in 1982. Two-thirds of these programs were publicly supported. Overall enrollment in master's programs has continued to increase since 1961 with 17,085 enrollees in 1982. The majority of students were in advanced clinical practice fields. In the 1981–1982 academic year, 5,193 master's-prepared nurses graduated and 15.2% of those graduates were specialists in psychiatric mental health nursing. The number of master's-prepared graduates has not kept up with the number of enrollments because of the increased number of students enrolled in part-time study, which prolongs program completion time.

Employment opportunities for master's-prepared psychiatric mental health nurses include such varied settings as academia, administration, interdisciplinary community health teams, hospitals, private practice, and governmental agencies. Frequently, master's-prepared psychiatric mental health nurses need to define their role, scope of practice, and specific provider benefits to potential employers and clients alike. In some instances, positions for social workers, psychologists, and other counselor/therapist positions can be effectively and productively filled by psychiatric mental health nurses with master's preparation who avail themselves of the opportunity to provide prospective employers with detailed schemes for utilizing their expertise. Most hospitals have an easily identifiable client population for the master's-prepared psychiatric mental health nurse in terms of patients, families, nursing, and other staff members who could utilize the educational, consultative, and treatment services of these experts.

In developing a practice role, master's-prepared psychiatric mental health nurses should consider several factors. They need to identify their scope of knowledge, skill, and expertise available to clients, as well as their individual interests, strengths, and weaknesses. It is important to identify the client population selected for service. Their presentation of the cost benefits of their specialized service and expertise to the public and to employers or financers is enhanced when they emphasize the manner in which their expertise strengthens existing services and adds unique dimensions to services because of nursing knowledge. Competition from professions such as psychiatry, psychology, and social work may become more rigorous because of the redetermination of health care financing. However, master's-prepared psychiatric mental health nurses, by nature of their general and specialized nursing preparation, can consider themselves well equipped to claim a place in the spectrum of health care services.

External Regulation of Practice

Not to be overlooked in planning for practice are the external regulations of Nursing Practice Acts and the Regulations and Policies of State Boards of Nursing. Licensure is essentially a governmental agency's granting of permission to practice to an individual who has met minimum standards of competency. The goal of such governmental action is to insure that public health safety and welfare will be protected. Licensure laws externally regulate the profession in that they are mandated by the legislature on behalf of the public. These laws are differentiated from the internal or intraprofessional structures for practice that may be promoted by a non-lawmaking professional organization.

The first professional group to establish criteria for practice in the law was medicine. This early step contributed to establishing the control of medicine over the arena of health care—an example, once again, of the early bird getting the worm.

Nursing leaders of the 1900s believed licensure laws to be necessary to prohibit untrained nurses from practicing, thus protecting the public and upgrading and standardizing the preparation of nurses. The first Nursing Practice Acts came into existence in 1903 and, by 1950, all states had such legislation. All of the acts generally contained a definition of nursing, requirements for licensure as a nurse, and provisions for addressing violations of the law. In addition, nursing statutes have also addressed requirements for nursing education programs and advanced nursing practice. Rapid changes in the field of nursing require drafting of practice acts that are comprehensive but flexible in nature. Changes in state nursing laws must be made by legislation. Regulations promulgated by boards of nursing are often handled in public hearings and do not require legislative approval, provided the law grants such authority to the Board. Professional organizations are frequently involved in the promulgation of nursing laws and regulations and such legislation should reflect the standards of the profession in meeting the goal of protecting the public.

Suggested formats for nursing legislation can be and have been proposed by professional organizations, as well as organizations composed of regulatory boards. For example, two documents published by the American Nurses' Association in 1980 address nursing legislation and the definition and scope of nursing practice from a national perspective: *Nursing Practice Acts: Suggested Legislation* (1980b) and *Nursing: A Social Policy Statement* (1980a). The Social Policy Statement discusses the "Social Context of Nursing," "The Nature and Scope of Nursing Practice," and "Specialization in Nursing Practice." The American Nurses' Association's "Suggested Legislation" document covers such areas as "Policy Decisions," "Rules and Regulations," "Legal Regulations of Nursing Practice," and a series of articles for Nursing Practice Act Legislation. Hence, both documents create a framework for addressing nursing practice and nursing legislation in a comprehensive yet flexible manner.

In June of 1979, the National Council of State Boards of Nursing (NCSBN) became a free-standing organization after having been part of the American Nurses' Association since 1945. This action occurred because nursing leaders involved with governmental regulatory agencies questioned the funding and support of state government employees, that is, State Boards of Nursing, by the professional organization which they were responsible for regulating. In addition, public concern and criticism was increasing regarding an apparent collision between regulatory boards and professional societies that could result in promoting economic advantages for the profession being regulated. Conflict of interest charges and questions about regulatory board activities resulted in state laws requiring open meetings and advance public notice of meetings of boards and also periodic reviews (Sunset law) of the operation and function of regulatory boards. Nursing leaders sitting in administrative or appointed positions in regulatory agencies are public servants and cannot appear to be dictated to by lobbyists or representatives of the profession. As regulatory work is demanding and stressful, there is a need for a resource for problem solving and discussion. A free-standing NCSBN fulfills this need along with meeting the obligations of the National Council. In keeping with its goal to assist member boards in their work with regulation and legislation, in 1982 the Nursing Practice and Standards Committee of the NCSBN presented a *Model Nursing Practice Act* to the delegate assembly. This document was then adopted as a guide for use when considering changes to State Nursing Practice Acts.

National Council of State Boards of Nursing membership consists of members and executive staff of Boards of Nursing, whose goals include achieving uniformity in licensure standards and regulatory policies and procedures for the licensure examination. The NCSBN Model Act was developed by professional nurse employees or members of regulatory agencies, that is, State Boards of Nursing. In contrast, the previously mentioned documents, *Nursing Practice Acts: Suggested Legislation* and *Nursing: A Social Policy Statement,* were developed by a professional nursing organization, the American Nurses' Association.

The Model Act grew out of attempts by many states and territories to respond to changes in nursing practice by updating acts to be more comprehensive and consistent. The Model

Act serves as a guideline to legislation and has been provided so that nursing legislation can be patterned on standards that reduce ambiguity but contain essential provisions in uniform language. Hopefully the outcome will be a common nationwide understanding of the legal practice of nursing. The Model Act of the National Council of State Boards of Nursing is a resource to state regulatory agencies who must maintain, in the public eye, some distance from overt control by the professional association. The NSCBN Act was developed utilizing the American Nurses' Association document on legislation as a reference, as well as a variety of other sources. This document brings a different perspective to its proposed articles for legislation because it was developed by numbers of regulatory agencies and consideration was given to distinguishing between statutory and professional definitions of nursing practice.

CREDENTIALING

As previously stated, legislators have been voicing increasing concern over the plethora of laws that govern the health care professions. Regulatory boards have been criticized for being more responsive to the needs of the profession than the needs of the public. They have also been accused of protecting the profession by restraining trade and competition, meanwhile overlooking the violators of the law within the professional ranks. On the one hand, unregulated practice can endanger the safety of the public but, on the other hand, restrictive legislation can create barriers to practice and dilute competition. There is a delicate balance to enacting legislation that bears directly on the protection of the public while allowing for expansion of practice.

In some states, legislation has been sought to define the credentials and roles for advanced practitioners of nursing. This action was motivated, in some instances, by the nurse specialists themselves, who felt that legislation was a definitive means for establishing practice rights and removing potential legal challenges. The public does need standards by which to assess the practice of those who claim to be specialists.

Credentialing by the Profession

The recognition of expanded role, advanced practice, or specialization in nursing marks an advance for the profession. However, the delineation of such roles and the credentialing of such nurses poses complicated issues for nursing. The concept of specialization implies the narrowing of focus to a specific area of knowledge, practice, and expertise based on education and training. However, in some settings, this specialization is predicated on practical experience rather than on advanced formal education and supervised clinical practice. The American Nurses' Association supports specialty practice based on graduate education and certification for practice obtained through the professional organization. The Association's stand is based on the rationale that the profession is obligated to identify and should provide the means for identifying, within nursing and for the public, those nurses who can be considered specialists. However, there are at least twenty-one nursing specialty organizations that do not affiliate with the American Nurses' Association that have created their own standards for credentialing and practice in specialty areas. A large number of these groups do not require graduate degrees for certification. The waters are murky in terms of which professional group is the authority for identifying specialists and the standards for credentialing. The American Nurses' Association (1980a) document *Nursing: A Social Policy Statement* states that graduate education is the basic requirement for a specialist in nursing practice. Yet certification examinations offered by the American Nurses' Association, not to mention all the other groups, do not uniformly require at least a master's degree prior to the examination for certification. Certification, for the generalist nurse who has a certain amount of experience, is provided in addition to certification of the nurse called a clinical specialist who holds a master's degree and has practice experience. The American Nurses' Association, for example, provides certification examinations for the generalist and the specialist in psychiatric and mental health nursing. As of May 1982, there were approximately 717 American Nurses' Association-certified nurses with master's degrees and specialization in adult psychiatric mental health nursing and an additional 66 certified nurses with master's degrees and specialization in child and adolescent psychiatric mental health nursing. There were also 679 nurses with American Nurses' Association certification as psychiatric and mental health nurses. This dual level of American Nurses' Association certification is also true for other clinical specialties, such as medical-surgical nursing. Most individuals do not know what a certification process does or who it really serves. Dual levels of certification can be confusing to the profession and the public alike. If licensure indicates compliance with minimal standards for competence and if certification at the generalist level and at the graduate level are offered by a professional agency, the question of what certification means to practice must surely be clarified.

The External/Internal Control of Practice Dilemma

In the absence of a clear-cut understanding of certification provided by the profession, the public and sometimes the profession as well turns to the law for uniform credentialing standards and protection. Although it is argued that licensure by a law should only address minimum standards for basic generalized practice, regulatory agencies do become involved in regulating specialist practice as well. As previously indicated, in some instances, nurses may be set forth as "specialists" based on experience in a particular area of nursing. Boards of Nursing may be asked to determine how nurses may practice under a given nursing practice act in roles that are more advanced than those of the new graduate. In these cases, the definition of advanced practice may be based not on formal education but on the acquisition of new skills and information gleaned from the work setting. A case in point would be the practice of nurses in emergency departments, intensive care departments, and perhaps even psychiatric units. Nurses may learn new skills that emanate from the nursing domain and also be approached to assume responsibility and skills that have traditionally been considered medical practice. Generalist certification could be an answer to some of these issues but not all. The issue remains of stressing the importance of utilizing master's-prepared specialists versus experienced generalists so that the resulting quality of practice is raised.

Nonetheless, master's-prepared psychiatric mental health nurses must be licensed in the state in which they practice and must, therefore, know the regulatory parameters of their Nursing Practice Act. In accepting the role of a specialist and practicing as such, the risks for litigation increase and familiarity with the standards applicable to practice is essential. In New York on October 5, 1983, the American Society of Law and Medicine sponsored a conference, entitled "Legal Controversies in Nursing," at which Barry Gold, J.D., LL.M., the chairman of the New York State Bar Association's Committee on Mental and Physical Disabilities gave an opening speech. Mr. Gold identified three societal trends that will increase the number of cases litigated against nurses: the changing role of nursing practice, increased expectations by health care consumers of the nature of health care delivery, and increased tendencies on behalf of consumers to challenge disputes in court. Mr. Gold noted that, currently, nursing malpractice insurance rates are low and nurses are named in only

0.7% of all malpractice cases. In this society, however, professional growth means increased risks and nurses must insure that they practice according to specified standards of practice.

Certification through a professional organization is a voluntary procedure that does not prohibit others from providing services in the specialty arena, and it does not provide or supercede the authority of nursing law. As the profession advances, the question of who can legitimately be called a specialist is also being advanced. The roles for nurses are still evolving and the differentiation of levels of practice and the connection between education and practice requires demonstration and support from research, which can also provide a clear nursing practice definition. Undeniably, research can provide data for clinical, administrative, organizational, and policy decisions. It can also provide the data necessary for classifying clients, nursing interventions and their outcomes, and for describing the structure, process, and outcomes of nursing care (Lang, 1983).

Psychiatric Mental Health Nursing: Credentialing by the Profession

Master's-prepared psychiatric mental health nurses are generalists by virtue of their baccalaureate preparation and licensure, and specialists by virtue of their master's degree and certification state and/or professional. Basic standards for practice and a Code of Ethics have been published by the American Nurses' Association. The certification process provided by the American Nurses' Association is intended to document the qualifications of the clinical nurse specialist who provides care in a defined specialty area of practice. It is also hoped that certification can be utilized as a basis for receiving third-party reimbursements and occupational status in practice and employment.

In 1966, five divisions on practice were established in the American Nurses' Association: Community Health Nursing, Geriatric Nursing, Psychiatric and Mental Health Nursing, Medical-Surgical Nursing, and Maternal and Child Health Nursing. The overall purpose of these divisions is the advancement of nursing practice by providing forums for discussion of common issues and developing statements of standards of nursing practice and mechanisms for certification. In addition to the Division on Psychiatric and Mental Health Nursing, a Council of Specialists in Psychiatric Mental Health Nursing was formed in 1974 to recognize the master's-prepared specialist. The Council developed criteria for certification, addressed legislation affecting advanced practice, and provided a forum for critical examination of issues that will increase psychiatric nursing's impact on health care, professional education, and political systems. The impressive goals of the Council for the 1982–1984 biennium include defining the scope of practice by refining the concepts in *Nursing: A Social Policy Statement;* developing a model peer review system; sharing information about research, education, clinical practice, health legislation, and political strategies; recognizing excellence in research, scholarship, and practice; pursuing varied payment mechanisms; interacting with consumer groups; establishing a network of specialists; and determining the supply, distribution, and utilization of specialists in psychiatric mental health nursing. If such goals can be successfully addressed, an action plan for practice will be forthcoming. These goals are important to anyone who practices; participation in meeting them is crucial.

Standards Which Are Applied to Practice

The Division on Psychiatric and Mental Health Nursing published in 1973 and revised in 1982 the *Standards of Psychiatric and Mental Health Nursing Practice.* These standards attempt to fulfill the profession's obligation to provide a means for improving the quality of care, to monitor standards of practice, and to self-regulate the profession. These standards, if called to bear when an examination of practice occurs, will most probably be used in conjunction with the State's Nursing Practice Act, the American Nurses' Association's *Code for Nurses With Interpretive Statements, Nursing: A Social Policy Statement*, and the American Nurses' Association's Statements on Nursing Practice and Psychiatric Mental Health Nursing Practice. These are the standards by which an individual nurse's practice may be judged. Therefore, intimate familiarity with these documents is essential. The permissible area of practice is usually defined by the licensing statute and a statute may or may not deal with specialty roles. However, statutes have been utilized to differentiate between physician and nonphysician activity. Many nursing statutes have attempted to address this issue by using language that permits more autonomous nursing functions. For example, some statutes differentiate between dependent, independent, and interdependent nursing acts, as well as define criteria for expanded, advanced, or specialty practice. For example, see the nursing statutes of Idaho, South Carolina, or Nebraska. Generally, liability in practice can be incurred if one practices medicine without a license or assists someone else to practice medicine without a license by delegation. Additionally, one is liable if the duty to refer a client whose problem is beyond the provider's area of knowledge, skill, or capacity for treatment with reasonable success is violated. These issues pose grey area problems for the master's-prepared psychiatric mental health nurse which require consultation. The legal tenet "to do no harm" applies to nursing practice. Nursing statutes are implemented on the basis of delegated authority granted by the legislature. Each state legislature, as the representative body of the citizens, determines practice parameters.

Philosophically, licensure should provide for basic, minimal entry level credentialing and the professional societies should provide the credentialling for advanced/specialty/practice. Licensure laws currently do define the basic entry into practice requirement but also address advanced practice criteria as a result of a public need to know how to identify nursing specialists. The needs of nursing specialists themselves to have their practice recognized by an authoritative source and the present lack of uniformity among the credentialing standards set by the professional nursing societies have also pressured regulatory boards to set criteria for advanced practice. As nurses' practice will be judged by the nursing laws and the nursing standards set by the professional societies, a need to be cognizant and familiar with all standards is evident.

Maintaining Competency

It is commonly accepted that continued learning and the maintenance of a current knowledge base are requirements for practice. Some nursing statutes address these items by requiring continuing education and actual practice in order to retain a nursing license. The public is aware that completing an educational program is only part of the picture and so have become intolerant of those who do no more than graduate from a program of study, hence the legal requirements for continuing education and actual practice for relicensure.

In examining what is considered to be societally acceptable for practice, the following criteria are identified:

1. Academic preparation (degrees)
2. Licensure
3. Voluntary (or mandatory) certification of skills and knowledge
4. Monitoring of practice competency by mandatory peer review, continuing education, periodic examinations, scholarly activity, or audits

It is recommended that master's-prepared psychiatric mental health nurses plan a system for evaluating their work, which will measure and describe the effects of their care by formulating criteria, collecting data, analyzing the data, and planning remedial action. The information obtained in evaluation can provide the basis for good decision making, which will be reflected in good patient care outcomes. The evaluation process could include the use of multiple resources such as chart audits, peer review, consultation, or supervision. An analysis that examines such factors as services utilized, manpower hours, cost of services, quality of services based on outcomes, and benefits to the community would be similar to the criteria utilized in Medicare and Medicaid reviews and reviews done by the Joint Commission on the Accreditation of Hospitals. Learning the system means learning the marketplace that provides an entree to policymakers, financers, and quality control surveyors. Decisions about practice must mediate such factors as government regulations, political pressure, public receptivity, patient reactions, costs, legal opinions, and professional philosophy. Consumers are demanding greater accountability, quality control, and protection when utilizing health care services. Continuing competency is one of the issues that must, therefore, receive the attention of the providers. It is a step in the right direction when we influence change in the system, rather than waiting for changes to influence us. By firmly establishing and utilizing standards of care and requirements for continued competency, we respond to the public demand for accountability, monitoring practice, and insuring quality care.

Collaboration Versus Competition

Mental health is one practice area in which it has been somewhat easier for nurses to establish themselves in collegial relationships. Perhaps this is because of the less absolute nature of the knowledge base and the natural fit of nursing knowledge and practice into the care requirements of the client group. It also appears that the fight for "owning the patient" has been less intense in this area, although this may change with reversals in health care financing and the efforts of medicine to control health care practice.

When professionals work together on solving a problem, the improved outcome and the benefit of the patient can become the goal and there is less need for dominance. For some, interdisciplinary collaboration poses a threat to autonomy and recognition of their expertness in their specialization. When priorities and responsibilities are negotiated by the collaborators, the specialization of each is more readily apparent and forms the center of the contribution each makes to the problem. Each discipline can be considered unique in the perspective brought to bear on the issue being considered. Given the traditional role of nursing, collegiality might be a concept that needs to be fostered in graduate education so that it can be implemented in practice. It would also be useful to have collaborative and independent practice information more widely disseminated through the literature.

SUMMARY

Graduate education prepares the psychiatric mental health nurse to practice as a psychotherapist with individuals, groups, families, and couples by making assessments, diagnostic formulations, and providing treatment and disposition. In addition, the master's-prepared psychiatric mental health nurse's degree of knowledge and skill provides a basis for consultation, teaching, and research. Barriers to practice can be outlined as follows:

1. Regulations and laws that may limit scope of practice

2. Health care financing mechanisms that do not recognize nurses as eligible providers
3. The lack of a generally accepted method for credentialing or certifying nurses as providers
4. The lack of sufficient research data that support the utilization of master's-prepared nurses to increase the quality of care and improve patient outcomes so that employment and financing issues are resolved
5. The efforts of organized medicine to limit access to care to providers who are physicians
6. The lack of education of the consumer and employer regarding the benefits of effective utilization of master's-prepared nurses
7. The lack of differentiation in the marketplace between levels of nursing practice as linked to nursing education
8. The limited availability of financial resources for increasing the numbers of nurses in advanced degree programs
9. The limited availability of funding for nursing research
10. The great competition for any available health care funding and the increasing demands on the distribution of limited resources

The solution is to become involved—become knowledgeable about professional issues that affect practice by analyzing the facts and identifying the trends in standard setting and policymaking. One of the most effective means for communicating nursing knowledge and experience to those who legislate policy is through one's own involvement in politics. Become visible to the public, the policymakers, and the profession. Formulate some basic tenets for professional life, which might include the following.

1. Self-taught or experienced knowledge of the systems that beget laws and regulations for licensure, health care policy, and health care financing
2. Identification of ways to establish personal involvement in the governmental body's committee system to establish how and when information should be channelled to have maximum effect
3. Knowledge of the political goals of the local and national nursing organizations and participation in meeting them, especially in the area of promoting reimbursement, nursing autonomy, and additional funds for nursing research
4. Knowledge of one's obligations and responsibilities under the state licensure laws; participation in the promulgation of laws that protect the public but support the growth of nursing as a profession
5. Knowledge regarding the trends in health care delivery by studying financing patterns and marketing information; becoming flexible and alert to providing services that are needed and demanded
6. Development of a personal definition for practice that encompasses one's skills, strengths, expertise, and interests
7. Fostering awareness that the master's-prepared psychiatric mental health care nurse is the best-prepared individual in the field to provide mental health care services because of extensive care experience, knowledge of principles of nursing, medicine, public health, mental health, and community health, and preparation that focused on prevention and health maintenance

All in all, this is the most exciting time to be practicing nursing as nurses are more aware, more independent, and more prepared to assume autonomy and to provide nursing services to a public ready for change. Nurses will, however, have to seize and utilize this moment themselves.

REFERENCES

American Nurses' Association. *Nursing: A social policy statement.* Kansas City, MO: American Nurses' Association, 1980a.

American Nurses' Association. *Nursing practice acts: Suggested legislation.* Kansas City, MO: American Nurses' Association, 1980b.

American Nurses' Association. West Virginia law requires RN reimbursement. *American Nurse,* 1983a, *15,* 8.

American Nurses' Association. Nurses eligible for direct payment in 13 states. *American Nurse,* 1983b, *15,* 1.

Institute of Medicine Health Care Services Division, Nursing and Nursing Education Committee. *Nursing and nursing education: Public policies and private actions.* Washington, DC: National Academy Press, 1983.

Kalisch, B. J., & Kalisch, P. A. *Politics of nursing.* Philadelphia: Lippincott, 1982.

Lang, N. Nurse-managed centers, will they survive? *American Journal of Nursing,* 1983, *83,* 1290–1293.

Mitsunaga, B. K. Designing psychiatric/mental health nursing for the future: Problems and prospects. *Journal of Psychiatric Nursing and Mental Health Services,* 1982, *20(12),* 15–21.

National Commission for the Study of Nursing and Nursing Education. *An abstract for action.* New York: McGraw-Hill, 1970.

United States Department of Health and Human Services, Bureau of Health Professions. *Sourcebook—Nursing personnel.* Hyattesville, MD: United States Department of Health and Human Services, 1981.

Vaughn, J.C. Educational preparation for nurses—1982. *Nursing and Health Care,* 1983, *4,* 460–464.

BIBLIOGRAPHY

Aiken, L. (Ed.). *Health policy and nursing practice.* New York: McGraw-Hill, 1981.

Aiken, L. *Nursing in the 1980s: Crisis, opportunities, challenges.* Philadelphia: Lippincott, 1982.

Aiken, L. Nursing's future: Public policies, private actions. *American Journal of Nursing,* 1983, *83,* 1440–1444.

American Nurses' Association. *Code for nurses with interpretative statements.* Kansas City, MO: American Nurses' Association, 1976.

American Nurses' Association, Division on Psychiatric and Mental Health Nursing Practice, *Standards of Psychiatric and Mental Health Nursing Practice.* Kansas City, MO: American Nurses' Association, 1982.

Archer, S. E., & Goehner, P. A. *Nurses: A political force.* Monterey, CA: Wadsworth, Health Sciences Division, 1982.

Balent, J., Menninger, K., & Hurt, M. Job opportunities for master's prepared nurses. *Nursing Outlook,* 1983, *31,* 109–114.

Blake, P. The clinical specialist as a nurse consultant. *Journal of Nursing Administration,* 1977, *7,* 33–36.

Brill, E. L. *Foundations for nursing.* New York: Appleton-Century-Crofts, 1980.

Bullough, B. (Ed.). *The law and the expanding nursing role.* New York: Appleton-Century-Crofts, 1975.

Chaska, N. L. *The nursing profession: A time to speak.* New York: McGraw-Hill, 1983.

Crabtree, M. S. Effective utilization of clinical specialists within the organizational structure of hospital nursing service. *Nursing Administration Quarterly,* 1979, *3,* 1–11.

Davis, A. J., & Aroskar, M. A. *Ethical dilemmas and nursing practice* (2nd ed.). New York: Appleton-Century-Crofts, 1983.

DeSantos, G. Power, tactics and the professionalization process. *Nursing and Health Care,* 1982, *3*(1), 14–17.

Diers, D. Nursing reclaims its role. *Nursing Outlook,* 1982, *30,* 459–463.

Donnelly, G. F., Mengel, A., & Sutterly, D. C. *The nursing system, issues, ethics and politics.* New York: Wiley, 1980.

Ellis, J. R. *Nursing in today's world: Challenges, issues, trends.* Philadelphia: Lippincott, 1980.

Fagin, C. M. Psychiatric nursing at the crossroad: Quo vadis. *Perspectives in psychiatric care,* 1981, *19*(3, 4), 99–106.

Griffith, H. Competition in health care, what will it mean for nurses? *Nursing Outlook,* 1983, *31,* 262–265.

Ham, L. M., & Chamengs, P. A. Nursing history: Our wasted asset. *Nursing and Health Care,* 1983, *3,*(8), 434–437.

Herkimer, A. G., Jr. The impact of third party payers on hospital rates and the bottom line. *The Health Care Supervisor,* 1983, *1–2,* 1–10.

Kalisch, P. A., & Kalisch, B. J. *The advance of American nursing.* Boston: Little, Brown, 1978.

Kalisch, P. A., Kalisch, B. J., & Titus, S. *Nursing involvement in the health planning process.* Hyattesville, MD: Health, Education, and Welfare, Bureau of Health Manpower, Division of Nursing, 1977.

Keenan, T., Aiken, L., & Leighton, E. C. *Nurses and doctors, their education and practice.* Cambridge, MA: Oelgeschlager, Gunn & Hain, 1981.

Kelly, L. Y. *Dimensions of professional nursing.* New York: MacMillan, 1981.

Koltz, C. *Private practice in nursing: Development and management.* Germantown, MD: Aspen Systems, 1979.

Lancaster, J., & Lancaster, W. (Eds.). *Concepts for advanced nursing practice: The nurse as a change agent.* St. Louis: C. V. Mosby, 1982.

Lynch, M. L. (Ed.). *On your own: Professional growth through independent nursing practice.* Monterey, CA: Wadsworth, Health Sciences Division, 1982.

Lysaught, J. P. *Action in affirmation: Toward an unambiguous profession of nursing.* New York: McGraw-Hill, 1981.

Mayers, M. C., Norby, R. B., & Watson, A. G. *Quality assurance for patient care nursing perspectives.* New York: Appleton-Century-Crofts, 1977.

Miller, J., & Paulsen, S. Should there be a national organization of directors of graduate programs in psychiatric mental health nursing? (Point/Counterpoint). *Perspectives in Psychiatric Care,* 1980, *18(3),* 118.

Morris, K. H., & Schweiger, J. A. *Clinical nurse specialist role creation:* An achievable goal. *Nursing Administration Quarterly,* 1979, *3,* 67–75.

Muff, J. (Ed.). *Socialization, sexism and stereotyping: Women's issues in nursing.* St. Louis: C. V. Mosby, 1982.

Mundinger, M. O. *Autonomy in nursing.* Germantown, MD: Aspen Systems, 1980.

Murchinson, I., Nichols, T. S., & Hanson, R. *Legal accountability in the nursing process* (2nd ed.). St. Louis: C. V. Mosby, 1982.

Narrow, B. W. *Fundamentals of nursing practice.* New York: Wiley, 1982.

National League for Nursing. Papers presented at the 16th Conference of Council of Baccalaureate and Higher Degree Programs, Philadelphia, November 1976. Publication 15–1659. New York: National League for Nursing, 1976.

National League for Nursing. *Emergence of nursing as a political force.* Publication 41–1760. New York: National League for Nursing, 1979a.

National League for Nursing. *Health care in the 1980s. Who provides? Who plans? Who pays?* Publication 52–1755. New York: National League for Nursing, 1979b.

National League for Nursing. *Developing the functional role in master's education in nursing.* Presented at the workshop, Developing the Functional Role in Master's Education in Nursing, Dearborn, Michigan, April 1980.

National League for Nursing. *Increasing our visibility: Toward a stronger public image for nursing.* Publication 16–1914. New York: National League for Nursing, 1982a.

National League for Nursing, Division of Research. *Nursing data book 1981.* New York: National League for Nursing, 1982b.

National League for Nursing. *Who's shaping health care?* Publication 52–1871. New York: National League for Nursing, 1982c.

Nursing Practice and Standards Committee. *Model nursing practice act.* Chicago: National Council of State Boards of Nursing, 1982.

O'Rourke, K. A., & Barton, S. R. *Nurse power unions and the law.* Bowie, MD: Brady, 1981.

Pennington, E. A. *Interdisciplinary education in nursing.* Publication 15–1877. New York: National League for Nursing, 1981.

Schmidt, M. S. Why a separate organization for state boards? *American Journal of Nursing,* 1980, *80,* 725–726.

Styles, M. M. *On nursing: Toward a new endowment.* St. Louis: C. V. Mosby, 1982.

Turnbill, E. Health care issues as an interdisciplinary course. *Nursing Outlook,* 1981, *29,* 42–45.

Wecht, C. H. *Legal medicine 1982.* Philadelphia: W. B. Saunders, 1982.

Yura, H. *Nursing leadership: Theory and process.* New York: Appleton-Century-Crofts, 1981.

CHAPTER 23 CLINICAL SUPERVISION

Deane L. Critchley

Traditionally, supervision in the mental health professions has been an essential element and a principal method of training to develop psychotherapeutic skills. Discussion of clinical supervision is limited in the nursing literature.

In this chapter the role of clinical supervision is discussed in psychiatric mental health nursing, its characteristics, purposes, and stages. Next, the chapter is focused on how the issues of transference and countertransference affect supervisee development. Then supervisory issues that arise when the supervisee's client is chronically ill or violent or self-destructive are dealt with. In the final section of the chapter, how to help the supervisee learn to be a supervisor and when to terminate the supervisory relationship are discussed.

Clinical supervision in psychiatric mental health nursing is derived from the traditional nursing practice of monitoring the work of others via modeling, discussions, and general oversight combined with the knowledge of process that came initially from psychoanalysis.

One of the chief contributions of psychoanalytic theory has been the understanding of intrapsychic processes including transference and countertransference. Together these two approaches (the traditional and the psychodynamic) provide an understanding of the environmental and intrapsychic factors that need to be integrated to achieve clinical competence.

Clinical supervision is an important educational and maturing process for clinicians. This is true for psychiatry, clinical psychology, social work, and psychiatric mental health nursing. Clinical supervision is a process that enhances teaching and learning for those involved.

OBJECTIVES OF CLINICAL EDUCATION

There are generally three major objectives in the clinical education of mental health professionals. These objectives include acquisition of factual knowledge and theoretical concepts. A second objective is the achievement of competent use of interpersonal helping skills such as empathy and specific intervention techniques. The third objective is enhanced personal self-knowledge about one's own current, ongoing life experiences, as well as an awareness of how one's previous life experiences affect one's present interactions.

Clearly, there are a variety of methods by which these objectives can be met. Didactic coursework, skill training via practicum experiences, simulation, videotaping, role playing, and forms of group supervision, as well as individual supervision, are all important learning tools. One needs to remember that a characteristic of any type of supervision is its focus on understanding nonverbal behaviors that are seen as equally important as verbal responses. The essence of supervision is to help the supervisee to become more therapeutic with others rather than to teach a myriad of skills and techniques in order to "do therapy."

Often an important adjunct to supervision is personal therapy. Most effective therapists become aware that all human beings have some conflicts that interfere with their therapeutic relationships with clients. Such concepts as tact, timing, or dependence, to name only a few, take on new meaning after experiencing one's own therapy. Additionally, therapists usually have a better sense of what they themselves mean to a client after having experienced a similar alliance with their own therapist. Finally, therapists who are familiar with their own personal issues are in a better position to distinguish between what is happening with the client and what is happening within themselves.

Supervision also functions as a support system for those providing care. It is an essential element in therapeutic relationships. One must care about oneself and experience being cared for before one is able to give care to others. All psychiatric nurses who engage in clinical work experience some degree of emotional stress. There are stresses associated with such client behaviors as hopelessness, manipulation, and self-destruction. Stress is evoked simply by listening to the troubles of another human being. Stress is inherent in the intimacy and responsiveness required of the nurse who is part of a therapeutic relationship. Thus, supervision provides the nurse with a clinical support system and contributes greatly, if indirectly, to the quality of nursing care.

Ideally, in supervision the supervisor places his or her skills, competence, knowledge, and empathy in the service of the supervisee. Both supervisor and supervisee bring varying amounts of personal maturity, knowledge, and understanding to the relationship. Lack of information and misinformation, as well as anxiety, however, lead many to discount or negate the value of supervision.

Many psychiatric nurses who find themselves in supervisory roles do so realizing they have never had formal preparation as supervisors. Often clinical supervision is confused with therapy, which contributes to both a misunderstanding and a mistrust of the supervisory process. Clinical supervision requires a consistent relationship over sufficient time to permit the process and issues to develop. Supervision should neither be hurried nor abbreviated. When one tries to do either, frustration and disappointment result. Regardless of the type of supervision used, the supervisory techniques emphasized or the treatment modalities being supervised, clinical supervision can provide the arena in which the supervisor and the supervisee can integrate theory and didactic knowledge with empathic understanding of clinical process.

SUPERVISION AS AN ORGANIZING FRAMEWORK

Clinical supervision can be structured as a means of organizing data critical to understanding the concepts and behaviors within the therapeutic process. Clinical supervision can provide a means of describing and analyzing observations within a particular conceptual framework.

For example, if one uses a developmental framework, then cognitive, affective, motor, and psychosocial components can be described with increasing precision. The task of clinical supervision is to integrate this conceptual process with an empathic understanding of the client as a human being. Using this approach also makes it possible to examine how the behavior of the supervisee has influenced the observations, their interpretations, and the overall quality of the interactions.

One caveat needs to be repeated here. As we have learned in both Chapters 2 and 4, any theoretical framework has possible disadvantages. While it serves to organize data in a logical fashion, one can also distort the data in order to make them fit a particular theory. Overrigid adherence to a framework may distort one's perceptions and lead to distortions of the behavioral data. Despite these dangers, one needs some means of looking at complex, multiple behavioral elements in a way that permits one to identify antecedents, connections, and meanings. At this stage of psychiatric mental health nursing development, the use of appropriate conceptual frameworks is the most likely means of achieving this purpose.

Definitions of Supervision

There are probably as many definitions of supervision as there are people who engage in it. Certainly there are differing definitions between and among disciplines. Supervision can be technical or administrative or an intensive clinical therapeutic process. Often those who speak of supervision fail to clarify the type to which they are referring. Such an omission leads to confusion. Discussions may seem to be totally contradictory when, in fact, they involve totally unrelated supervisory processes.

Clinical supervision has been described from many perspectives. Gaoni and Newmann (1974) describe a four-stage developmental model for the supervisor-supervisee relationship. They see the relationship progressing initially from that of teacher-pupil, to an apprenticeship focusing on the client, to a focus on personality issues and increased self-awareness of the trainee, and, finally, to mutual consultation.

One approach to supervision focuses on its therapeutic aspects. This view holds that the supervisee illustrates, in her or his relationship with the supervisor, the client-trainee relationship. Additionally, the way in which the supervisor responds to the trainee illustrates or models ways to respond to the client. This approach operates on the assumption that pointing out transference and countertransference problems will help resolve them. The basic premise behind this approach is that it stimulates the trainee to increased self-reflection.

A second view of clinical supervision holds that it is aimed primarily at changing attitudes. This position holds the supervisor's attitude to be critical to the process and that the process can open new horizons to the trainee. This view, even though it recognizes that the trainee is not the client, still holds that a "parallel process" occurs between treatment and supervision.

Hora (1957) has described such a process wherein the supervisee identifies with the client and in the supervisory relationship behaves in such a manner as to elicit emotions in the supervisor that the therapist has previously experienced with the client. Similarly, research by Muslin, Burstein, Gedo, and Sado (1967) indicates that the data given by therapists to their supervisors, at least in the early stages, reflect therapist needs rather than client difficulties.

One must be sensitive to a built-in hazard with this approach. If one believes the trainee inevitably recreates the therapist-patient interaction with his or her supervisor, then the supervisor may think he or she can illustrate with the trainee the supervisor's style with clients. Obviously, the supervisor needs to look for clues of stress revealed by the nurse in the way the session is reported. However, when the supervisor focuses primarily on the supervisee, the client is lost to sight, and the supervision evolves into personal therapy for the supervisee.

Haller (1976) defines supervision as a "process whereby a therapist, frequently, but not always a relative beginner, is helped to become a more effective clinician" (p. 36). The discussion of supervision in this chapter is based on the following definition. Supervision is an intensive, interpersonally focused professional function in which one person who is hopefully skilled, knowledgeable, and empathic is designated to facilitate the development of clinical therapeutic competence in another person.

Supervision Contrasted with Consultation

At this point, it is perhaps useful to distinguish briefly between clinical supervision and consultation. In clinical supervision, administrative responsibility for the trainee is given to the supervisor who thus, by definition, can hold the supervisee responsible, that is, accountable for his or her clinical work. Additionally, one member of the dyad serves to facilitate the professional development of the other. The supervisor serves as a provider of theoretical knowledge and therapeutic techniques, validates the use of the nursing process, and supports the working through of transference and countertransference reactions. This delegation of authority to one member, the supervisor, is essential to meet the goals of the supervisory process. In contrast, when this authority dimension is absent, then the process is not supervision but consultation. Typically, consultation denotes a peer or collegial relationship and the consultee is free to use or not use the outcomes of the consultation. A more detailed discussion of the consultative process can be found in Chapter 17.

Supervision then attends to three basic functions: (1) to monitor the welfare of the client, (2) to promote the supervisee's professional growth, and (3) to evaluate the supervisory process and the resultant learning of the supervisee.

Supervision is made up of several components: the supervisor, the supervisee, the relationship between them which is a vital aspect of the supervisory process, and the context within which the supervision occurs, that is, the professional setting, for supervision does not occur in a vacuum. Another relevant component, although an indirect one, is the relationship between the trainee and the client.

Supervision Contrasted with Therapy

While there are some competencies that are common to both a good therapist and a good supervisor, there are others that are quite different. Despite the fact that there are to a certain extent common skills and common goals involved in therapy and supervision, it is important to remember that the goal of supervision is not therapy for the supervisee. The goals of supervision are to help the supervisee develop greater clinical competence through the discussion of issues encountered in therapeutic work and to catalyze the nurse's creative and therapeutic use of self.

In contrast, the purpose of therapy is to help clients to understand themselves better and to recognize those conflicts that are manifested in disturbing behaviors and ultimately to change toward growth and increased autonomy.

Therapy is based in almost all cases on the client's recognition of a problem and seeking assistance to deal with the problem. Thus, therapy is an acknowledgment and explicit agreement by the client of a problem and an interest in alleviating the problem. Consequently, there is an understanding that issues of personality, life-style, and destructive behaviors are critical to the work of therapy.

Supervision, on the other hand, is often required rather than chosen, as for students in clinical work. There is no explicit agreement around the need for supervision. Initially, the supervisee typically has only an intellectual acceptance of the idea that supervision can in some vaguely understood manner contribute to one's growth and competence as a clinician.

The aim of supervision is the teaching of psychotherapeutic skills. The goal of therapy is to help the client to function more effectively in all areas of life. The goal of supervision is to deal with the supervisee's problems in the supervisory and therapeutic relationships only to the extent that they are affecting the nurse's ability to learn from the supervisor and be effective with clients.

Other critical differences between therapy and supervision include the following. First, the supervisor needs to permit the supervisee autonomy in treating the client whenever appropriate. While the same need exists in the therapist-client relationship, it is highlighted in the supervisory process. Second, a supervisor has the responsibility to evaluate the supervisee according to some predetermined external standards as set forth by a graduate program, an agency, or through certification or credentialing. This characteristic is certainly not one that appears commonly in the context of counseling or therapy. Third, a supervisor serves as a role model. As part of this role, he or she needs the ability to determine when to explore personal issues. This is not a decision a counselor or therapist needs to address.

Supervision as Modeling

The supervisory process is most effective as a learning model when the supervisor keeps clearly in mind that the trainee is not the client. The best modeling of the therapist role occurs when the supervisor focuses on assisting with specific problems that arise in carrying out the psychotherapeutic task. In other words, the supervisor can best demonstrate how to take responsibility for providing help by in fact providing help. This process does not mean that the supervisor answers all questions or provides all the necessary information. Rather, the supervisor points out "blind spots" and raises pertinent questions for the supervisee to think about and reformulate for further discussion. An equally important task is to help the supervisee refine the ability to observe more closely and to describe more exactly both the client's and his or her own behaviors as part of an interactive process. The supervisor is an active participant in an affectively charged learning process the focus of which is learning and personal growth.

Supervision, like the nursing process, uses problem solving as its basic methodology. Through problem solving, the supervisee learns that one cannot do therapy to someone, but that one can work together to find solutions that are helpful.

One of the tasks of supervision is to help the trainee explore ways of adjusting social and professional roles. For example, to point out how a client is making inappropriate demands on the therapist may help him or her to change a social response into a professional one. Or, together they may identify varieties of therapist responses that are all reasonably therapeutic. In this way, supervision can help supervisees to reshape continually their images of the client and to shift their own mental sets appropriately. If the supervisor focuses on the interactive nature of the therapist-client relationship, then the constant changes in both the client and the therapist are kept in awareness. Thus, therapist interventions can change correspondingly.

This model of supervision identifies three stages of supervisee development and several developmental issues for the supervisee that need to be addressed during the supervisory process. It is also based on the premise that professional development is continuous and ongoing throughout one's professional career. An important characteristic of a stage model is that an individual may be at several different stages concurrently, depending on the issue involved. As the knowledge and skill of both supervisee and supervisor increase, stages and issues may be worked through in greater depth.

Stage One

This stage of the supervisory relationship is often termed the "honeymoon stage" and has certain distinct characteristics. One of these can be termed unawareness. Beginning supervisees often exhibit a naive lack of awareness of any difficulty or deficiency in a specific area or in regard to important issues, either in themselves or in the client. The supervisee wants to be helpful to the client and believes that because of his or her attention and concern, the client is getting better. The more experienced supervisee often experiences a blind spot in relation to issues of resistance. This lack of awareness of being stuck is often accompanied by a deceptive sense of stability or security. The stage is also characterized by a tendency toward simplistic "black and white" thinking. The supervisee may seem particularly obtuse to the impact of his or her behavior on the client or supervisor. Often at this stage, the supervisee views the supervisory process with little interest. One might describe the supervisee's "stuckness" in old patterns of thought and behavior as being "frozen" in the same sense that Lewin (1948) has described it in his description of the change process. The supervisee often exhibits a low self-concept, resulting in overdependence on the supervisor for direction. Commonly, supervisees in this stage may idealize the supervisor as an omnipotent and omniscent figure or, because of their level of unawareness and sense of security, may view the supervisor as unnecessary. During this stage, the disregard of the supervisor is more neutral than in the second stage when hostility or defensiveness is more characteristic.

This stage provides a certain measure of genuine security for the supervisee as he or she may remain at this level with certain issues while moving on to other stages when dealing with other issues. Supervisors often engage in mutual goal setting with the supervisee. It is important to remember in terms of the characteristics of the stage that the supervisee should not exercise total or, at some points, even primary input into setting the goals since their awareness or understanding of the areas needing development is limited.

Frequently, during this beginning phase a degree of "testing" occurs, that is, presenting an "insolvable" problem to be solved. For example, a nurse working with a severely burned child asked how she could make the child forget his condition and be happy. Obviously, the problem as stated is impossible to accomplish. The problem needs to be redefined more appropriately in terms of how to help reduce the child's anxiety so that the pain is more bearable. It is during this stage, also, that the supervisee is striving to identify the supervisor's style whether critical, hostile, or supportive, while the supervisor is trying to assess the supervisee's sensitivity to criticism and openness to exploration of the self.

During stage one, the supervisor needs to assess the supervisee's capacity for learning and for empathy with someone who is in pain. The assessment needs to include whether supervisees are likely to use the client relationship to fulfill their own needs for power or positive regard. Are supervisees able to view themselves in any way objectively or are they so well defended against self-awareness that any comment is taken as criticism? Are supervisees able to see that the purpose of sensitively made comments is to promote self-observation and growth?

Stage Two

During the second stage, a marked shift occurs. The characteristics of this stage include instability, disruption, confusion, and conflict. To use Lewin's analogy, "unfreezing" occurs in the supervisee's attitudes, emotions, and behaviors. His or her traditional ways of viewing self and others becomes loosened and open to new ideas. Initially, however, the supervisee's attitude toward him- or herself reflects a general confusion and vacillation between a sense of failure and incompetence to feelings of great ability and expertise. A sense of failure is exacerbated as the client's problems surface and the supervisee's anxiety rises as he or she realizes the client is not better.

During this stage, the supervisee begins to realize that the supervisor cannot provide the ultimate answers. This realization usually generates disappointment and anger. The supervisor is alternately seen as all-knowing or as incompetent and inadequate because of his or her failure to "come through" when needed. At times, the supervisor is perceived as deliberately withholding information. It is crucial for the supervisor to understand the characteristics of the stage rather than to take the supervisee's anger and hostility personally. The use of humor can be an effective means of reducing anger and resentment. The value of the second stage is that it is here that the learning of new behaviors begins. Despite its outward manifestations, it is an optimistic growth-producing period. Existing patterns of behavior have been challenged, leaving room for new learning to occur. Hopefully during this stage the nurse practices problem solving with the guidance and direction of the supervisor.

One finds little research on the supervisory process in the literature. One of the few studies by Doehrman (1976) underscores the characteristics found in the second stage of the supervisory process. Doehrman found that tension in the supervisory relationship is inevitable, but when understood and used properly it promotes the supervisee's personal growth. Learning to be therapeutic inspires anxiety and resistance in the learner related to the perceived need to change. These actions are expressed in the supervisee's characteristic behaviors for resisting authority. Ways of resisting help in supervision are closely related to difficulties in giving help to clients. Insights into these resistances will also provide insight into the problems encountered as a therapist. Deprived of these insights, the supervisee cannot grow as a therapist. There will be no learning, no change, and the status quo will be preserved.

Stage Three

The transition from the second to the third stage is generally welcomed by both the supervisee and the supervisor. It can be described as the calm after the storm. Characteristics include a reorganization and integration and a new cognitive understanding. Stability reoccurs, this time based on an awareness of uncertainty and an ability to monitor constantly one's therapeutic work. Again, in terms of Lewin's concept, it can be described as "refreezing," in which new integrated learning takes on a new and different form. This stage represents the possibility of assimilating the intense emotional factors that were churned up during the previous stage and to integrate them into a new conceptual understanding. During this stage, the supervisee acquires a more solid, realistic self-view and a basic acceptance of both his or her strengths and weaknesses. The supervisee is neither frightened by nor feels guilty for his or her less effective skills. There is confidence that these areas can and will develop. Additionally, the supervisee acquires a more realistic view of the supervisor. Expectations for supervision are more in line with what is possible. The supervisee takes more active responsibility for the content and process of the supervision. This stage, like stage one, is stable; however, the stability is far more flexible and permits continued growth.

Varieties of Supervision

The process of supervision requires the nurse to record his or her interactions with the client. This can be done through written process notes or audio or videotapes. By far, the most accurate and complete information is provided by videotapes. Use of videotapes permits exploration of nonverbal behaviors most readily. Observation and understanding of nonverbal behaviors is probably one of the most difficult tasks for a therapist to learn. Videotapes permit repeated, joint observation of the interactions. They also provide the data necessary for examination of minute components of the total behavioral sequence that can give meaning to previously unexplained behavior.

Learning to record in writing, as in process notes, both verbal and nonverbal aspects of the interaction is very difficult. It requires constant encouragement for the supervisee to move from recording the client's verbal communication to recording the client-therapist verbal communication, let alone nonverbal behaviors. However, with any method, the nurse analyzes the data, extracts themes, and identifies problems relevant to the therapist-client relationship. The supervisee then reviews the literature, draws inferences, evaluates the interventions used, and formulates plans for the next session. During supervision, this information is shared and feedback is received.

A controversial point is whether the supervisor should enter therapy sessions under special circumstances such as when the client's behaviors are intimidating the therapist or when no movement has occurred in therapy for a long time. Supervisors who have experienced such supervision as helpful in their own learning are more comfortable in offering it to a supervisee as a choice for learning rather than as a statement of the therapist's incompetence.

Another form of participant supervision occurs most frequently in milieu settings. The supervisor may find it helpful to observe an interaction between the supervisee and the client in order to understand the impact of other clients and staff on the therapist-client interaction. A supervisor may also demonstrate a particular intervention with a client if this is not threatening to either the supervisee or the supervisor. It is helpful, too, if the intervention is likely to be successful. This kind of participant supervision may be especially effective because the supervisor is a less involved person who can look at the client's behavior more objectively.

Supervision of Different Treatment Modalities

All psychotherapeutic work with clients, be it individual, couple, family, child, group, or any other modality, requires interpersonal learning with a senior clinician skilled in that particular therapy. Clinical supervision can provide the arena for such learning.

As more people become involved as clients in any therapeutic situation, the more complex the interactions become. Psychopathology as well as integrative capacities may be expressed differently in a group setting than in an individual one. In addition, the therapist needs to learn the ways in which conflicts are expressed in groups such as families. Therapists need also to understand dynamics such as alliance and splitting as they occur in these situations.

There are special problems involved in psychotherapeutic work with children and adolescents both individually and in groups. Psychotherapeutic work with these or any special client population requires supervision from individuals with particular expertise in the field.

There are numerous approaches to family therapy that, while they may have differences, all use similar principles of intervention. Therefore, supervision from an experienced family therapist will be helpful regardless of his or her theoretical orientation. Frequently in family therapy, cotherapists are used, which means the supervision should include both therapists. The supervisory process can then deal, as well, with the viscissitudes of collaboration.

Successful family therapy calls for more refined observational skills and understanding more complex transference and countertransference phenomena. Therefore, it is difficult to provide supervision of this modality unless one has had supervised experience and is a competent family therapist.

Supervisors of group therapy can only be effective in supervising work with groups in which they are knowledgeable of the developmental issues and psychopathology involved. For example, psychotherapeutic work with groups of adolescents requires specialized approaches. Of course, this can be said about working with any particular developmental population. Since group therapy is finding wide application with specialized groups such as substance abusers and pregnant adolescents, it is necessary to prepare not only competent clinicians but also competent supervisors.

Two other areas requiring specialized expertise are psychotherapy with children and adolescents. Unfortunately, there are relatively few nurses who have the necessary educational background to work effectively in these areas. Many nurses have clinical experience with these age groups. However, they have not usually had clinical supervision from someone who has both the academic and clinical backgrounds necessary to help another learn the essential skills. Without this kind of supervision to make one a competent clinician, it is difficult to help others acquire the knowledge and skills required.

The particular areas mentioned above require specialized competencies. Currently, there are a lack of professionals prepared to supervise others in these treatment approaches. The question arises then whether a nurse need always be supervised by another nurse. The more inexperienced the nurse-trainee, the more important it is that supervision provide a role model of the discipline. With more experienced nurses who are seeking specialized learning and are secure in their professional identity, the supervisor need only have expertise in the particular field of interest. However, an extended period of supervision with a member of one's own discipline is always helpful.

ISSUES IN SUPERVISEE DEVELOPMENT

As mentioned previously, when one works with a supervisee, one may note the recurrence of a particular issue again and again. As one gains experience as a supervisor, one also begins to note the recurrence of a particular issue or issues with most of the supervisees with whom one works. There seem to be a number of basic issues that nurses, along with other mental health professionals, inevitably encounter during their professional development.

Developing a knowledge of these issues permits the supervisor to identify more quickly the core theme without being distracted by the content of the situation. The identification of such issues also permits the supervisor to anticipate or even to encourage the emergence of certain themes. Finally, such an awareness increases the supervisor's ability to conceptually tie together apparently unrelated occurrences and to determine a possible therapeutic rationale.

Issues that have been identified as important to wrestle with during one's professional development involve competence, emotional awareness, empathy, autonomy, professional identity, self-worth, self-determination, respect for individual differences, and professional ethics, to name only a few. Generally, each of these issues will need to be dealt with at some point during the supervisory process. The following discussion will deal with the particularly important issues of transference and countertransference.

Transference and Countertransference

Two issues of particular importance are those of transference and countertransference. In supervision, one needs to deal with the client's projection on to the therapist of both good and conflicted aspects of old relationships. One needs also to deal with the anxieties evoked in the therapist by the client, anxieties that are aroused owing to the therapist's own unresolved conflicts.

Transference

It is necessary for the supervisor to help the supervisee understand that the client's projections on to the therapist, while unreal, are vital parts of the therapeutic process. Thus, positive transference is part of the motivation to trust the therapist, to view her or him as a benign and helpful parent, and to begin the work of therapy. When positive transference is diminished or lacking, as with clients who have never developed trust, then the client's view of the therapist from the outset may be a hostile one. Supervision helps the supervisee become aware of the evidence of positive transference in the client's behavior and how it may be used to further treatment.

The client's negative transference causes him or her to attribute to the therapist such feelings as being noncaring, hostile, critical, or dissatisfied with the client's progress. Supervision can help to identify the negative transference expressed in the client's behavior. Recognition of these behaviors reinforces the supervisee's understanding that the behaviors are projections from the client's past experiences rather than the results of therapist responses. Recognition that it is the reduction of negative transference attitudes in clients that lead to more integrated behavior is a major part of the work of therapy and of supervision.

Countertransference

Countertransference attitudes and feelings in the therapist are elicited by client behaviors that bring into awareness experiences out of her or his past. While positive countertransference is rarely discussed, its presence helps to consolidate the therapeutic relationship. The anxiety aroused by negative countertransference is generally the most difficult for the therapist to recognize and resolve. Negative countertransference represents unresolved early conflicts. While it may initially be difficult for the supervisee, discussion of these feelings in supervision permits an understanding of client behaviors that have elicited the feelings. Understanding the negative countertransference provides important data about the present manifestations of the client's unresolved conflicts with past significant figures. While the supervisor does not make interpretations to the supervisee, questions can be raised. "What is it in the client that makes you uneasy?" Certain feelings such as anger, helplessness, placating and obsequiousness, and passive-aggressive behavior all make one uneasy. The supervisor can identify the origins of such behavior in most people and can help the supervisee to identify the origins of her or his own feelings as well as possible interventions. When this happens, it often has dramatic results. As these are complex issues, the following illustration may help clarify these points.

A psychiatric nurse was treating an isolated, fearful and suspicious woman who had no support system other than a few members of her church group. The client, Anne, had no car and a phobia about using the bus. Her phobia not only restricted her movement in general, but also interfered with her therapy appointments.

Initially, the nurse was overwhelmed by the client's helplessness. Every suggestion the nurse offered to assist Anne to keep her appointments was countered with numerous statements that it would not work and that she (the client) just could not do it. The nurse felt increasingly helpless and angry.

As she dealt with her own feelings in supervision, the nurse was able to understand and empathize with the intensity of her client's panic and hopelessness. She was then able to offer to help Anne learn to use the bus system between her home and the clinic. On a regular basis for several weeks, she first drove Anne along the bus route she would take to come to the clinic and then rode the bus with her until Anne had the courage to make the trip alone.

The interactions between the two during these "lessons" were, of course, the therapeutic process aimed at reducing Anne's helplessness. The client's increased ability also enhanced the nurse's sense of effectiveness. The nurse's willingness to step outside the traditional therapist role demonstrated her concern to Anne and greatly facilitated the therapeutic relationship. However, it was not until the nurse was able to use the supervisory process to look at the feelings Anne aroused in her that she was able to sensitively and accurately identify both Anne's needs and her fragility. Once this happened, the nurse was able to develop creatively a means of helping Anne through the therapeutic relationship.

During this process, the nurse became aware of her own anxieties that stepping out of the traditional therapist role would increase the client's dependence on her. Discussing her fears in supervision increased her self-awareness of her own dependency needs. This awareness led, in turn, to a fear of rejection by the supervisor if she expressed her needs. The nurse was also able to recognize a fear she and the client shared. This feeling was that giving into dependency would result in regression and that it would be impossible to regain independent functioning.

In such a situation, the supervisor needs to explore at length with the supervisee the client's dependency needs, their origins, and possible interventions. Exploring the etiological issues and interpersonal processes by which such needs are expressed in behavior as well as the areas of effective, independent functioning increased the nurse's understanding and comfort about the client's dependency. In turn, the nurse was then able to deal with her own dependency needs. She could then permit the client's increased dependency as a first step toward greater independence. Supervision assisted the nurse to acquire greater awareness of how her fear of her own dependency needs was interfering with the therapeutic work with the client. Supervision did not, however, attempt either to provide therapy or to "meet" the supervisee's dependency needs.

One of the most difficult yet important tasks of supervision is to identify those individuals who as therapists are fearful of becoming aware of their own and others' feelings. These individuals tend to use power and coercion to make clients change. As therapists, they seek to solve their own problems through solving others' problems. To become clinically competent, these individuals must be strongly urged to have personal therapy.

Therapeutic Implications of Supervision

Differences between supervision and therapy have been discussed earlier in the chapter. It is important to note that effective supervision, while not therapy, can be therapeutic. Therapy has been defined previously as an explicit agreement to work together with the client to resolve specific problems. Supervision is not based on the same premise. It can be therapeutic, however, if by therapeutic one means relief of emotional discomfort and personal growth. As both Sullivan (1954) and Szurek (1950) have described, a variety of experiences with people such as teachers or mentors can contribute to personal growth by providing models for identification and thus can be seen as therapeutic.

A major determinant of whether supervision is also therapeutic is the conscious effort of the supervisor to be authoritative rather than authoritarian. Authoritarian behavior is designed to benefit only the authoritarian person. Authoritative behavior is designed both to problem solve and to contribute to another's personal and professional growth. To the extent that the supervisee identifies with the authoritative attitudes and behaviors of the supervisor, this permits one to behave similarly with clients and others and to recognize one's own personal growth.

Crisis Supervision

Ideally, if there is continuity of supervision, there will be few situations arising that require extra supervision. On the other hand, just as the client needs to test the therapist's willingness to recognize special needs, real or unreal, the same dynamics hold for the supervisee. In addition, actual emergencies can occur. Supervision around a crisis is an opportunity for learning. As such it is part of the supervisor's professional responsibility to be available for such work.

Unfortunately, in many settings the demand of the technical procedures or routines take precedence over affective learning. Supervision may only occur around crises. If supervision is only intermittent, it is difficult to help the supervisees define for themselves assets and strengths as well as areas for growth. Under such conditions, it is especially difficult to develop a nonhostile yet questioning atmosphere. Such crisis-oriented supervision is usually technical rather than process oriented and tends to exaggerate the negatives of behavior rather than the excitement of continued learning in self-understanding and understanding others.

The following section discussing the supervisory aspects of special clinical issues illustrates emergent situations that can occur and may call for additional supervisory sessions.

SPECIAL CLIENT POPULATIONS

There are a number of extremely difficult client populations that pose particularly difficult therapeutic and supervisory problems. The therapeutic problems with such populations are discussed in Parts Three and Four of this book. Examples of supervisory issues related to work with some of these populations will be discussed here.

Chronic Mental Illness

When working with the chronically mentally ill, one has to deal with one's own discouragement that frequently accompanies such work. Discouragement often arises from the lack of manifest therapeutic progress and the difficulty in recognizing the tiny increments of change. Such discouragement inhibits a task-oriented approach aimed at helping the client achieve behavioral change no matter how small. These feelings are grist for the mill in supervision and can also help the supervisee better understand the intensity of the family's frustration and discouragement with the client. The nurse can use the techniques learned through supervision to help the family recognize its role in promoting change in the client's behavior.

Chronic Physical Illness

Chronic physical illness creates special problems because it interferes with development and healthy adaptation. Interference occurs from the realistic limitations of the disease. It occurs also from reinforcement of dysfunctional behaviors and avoidance of difficult and anxiety-producing yet growth-promoting experiences. Supervision of psychotherapeutic work with such clients needs to acknowledge the natural sympathies and protective feelings of the therapist, the family, and of other helping individuals involved in the client's life.

Discussion of the presence, origin, and meaning of such feelings allows the supervisee to support yet encourage clients to strive toward their full potential. It also promotes insight into the anger the therapist can feel when he or she believes the client is "not trying."

Such clarity in supervisees enables them to be more clearly reality oriented with the client, the family, and other helping people. This type of reality orientation looks at the real limitations imposed by the illness and the clients' perception of the limitations that prevent their living more fully.

A common therapeutic dilemma occurs when the client exhibits noncompliance with the therapeutic regimen. Among the dynamics involved in noncompliance are self-destructive tendencies and a need to control others as a response to feelings of helplessness. Often, noncompliance is an indication that the health professionals have failed to establish a helping relationship with clients or to recognize their feelings of anxiety, helplessness, hopelessness, fear, anger, and grief that the disease has precipitated.

Part of the supervisory task is to help the supervisee deal with all the participants in the client's environment. The intensity of feelings expressed by so many, in addition to the client's behavior, can be experienced as overwhelming by the therapist. Noncompliance may also reflect a conspiracy by the family because of their own difficulty in being firm and in not having clear and realistic expectations of the client's capacity for progress. The supervisor's clarity about the client's capacities encourages supervisees to clarify their own feelings and thus be able to maintain reality orientation with client and family.

The anger many of these clients express both covertly and overtly is extremely difficult to experience without personalizing the feelings. As one who is trying to help, the anger often seems unjustified.

The kinds of clinical tasks expected of nurses in burn units, oncology units, psychiatric units, indeed any area where life-shattering or life-threatening illness occurs, are well known. At times, the clinical responsibilities arouse feelings of anguish, despair, or futility that, if not resolved, can seriously compromise the quality of care nurses give. The following illustration deals with some of the supervisory issues involved when the supervisee works with a chronically ill client.

In a hospital setting, a nurse was working with a 16-year-old boy with severe ulcerative colitis. She went to her supervisor to discuss the fact that he was refusing to take the necessary fluids. Initially, the supervisor saw the nurse on an irregular basis. The discussions focused on increasing the boy's fluid intake. However, the boy's refusing behavior continued and his physical condition dramatically worsened. The supervisor began to see the nurse daily and went to see the boy for herself. As soon as she met him, the supervisor realized, at first hand, the angry, rejecting nature of the boy's behavior even toward her, an unknown. This encounter gave her clues about the relationships between the nurse and the boy and the intensity of the boy's anger and rejection toward all personnel. From this point, the supervisor was able to be more helpful to the nurse. Together they were able to clarify the nature of the boy's anger expressed toward everyone as a defense against the fear that no one could really care about anyone as "nasty" as him, "nasty" both because of his offensive behavior and his frequent, uncontrollable loose bowel movements. As the nurse began to understand the motivation behind the boy's behavior, she no longer experienced it as a personal attack. Her understanding permitted her to see the boy's fear and pain and to respond more appropriately. It is quite probable that if the supervisor and the nurse had had an established supervisory relationship, the nurse would have been helped to examine her relationship with the boy on an ongoing basis rather than after the crisis had occurred. Such a process would not only have contributed to the supervisee's learning but may well have diminished the intensity of the crisis.

Excitement in learning about oneself and others is most likely to happen when one is supervised by someone who has experienced firsthand the supportive, growth-producing aspects of supervision. Within the context of such a relationship, crises can be seen as special opportunities for learning and growth.

Violent and Self-Destructive Behavior

One of the most anxiety-provoking situations for both supervisor and supervisee is the threat of self-destructive or violent behavior by a client. Anxiety aroused by such a threat may interfere with the understanding that such behaviors are a call for help. This same anxiety often makes the therapist feel responsible for the client's life and behavior despite knowing in reality that the client is ultimately responsible. Unless the supervisor understands and controls his or her own anxiety, it will contribute to the supervisee's anxiety and feelings of helplessness. Recognition of these feelings facilitates the supervisee's understanding of the disengagement from the client by some family members. Life-threatening behavior presents a real test of the supervisor's capacity to help the supervisee.

Violent clients also present difficult supervisory problems as clinical specialists' knowledge of the law mandating therapists to report serious threats of violence involving others to appropriate agencies and to the individual threatened is critical. Despite this, therapists tend to deal with their own fear and anxiety by minimizing the seriousness or evidence of intent to do violence. It is critical for the supervisor to help the supervisee understand that failure to be open and honest with a violent client about the fear the threats engender, and the need for external control to prevent serious harm to others, makes the therapist a tacit participant.

Threats both to harm oneself or others are highly emotionally charged. Therefore, they may interfere with the objectivity of the supervisee, supervisor, and others involved. It is critical for the supervisor to acknowledge with the supervisee the anxiety and fear aroused by such behaviors. Only such honest reflection of the supervisor's feelings permits the supervisee to begin to express openly and thus to understand and cope with her or his own feelings. Sharing the feelings helps reduce the anxiety and makes it possible to consider therapeutic alternatives with the client.

Development as a Supervisor

A final phase of the supervisory process is to help the supervisee learn to be a supervisor. An important tool in learning to be an effective supervisor is to be able to have the experience of supervising others while being supervised oneself in that process.

The experience of being a supervisee does not automatically prepare one to function as a supervisor. Therefore, as the supervisee gains increasing skill and competence, additional learning can be achieved by continuing supervision of the nurse while he or she begins to supervise others. This provides opportunity for the supervisee to deal with the role of benign authority—to recognize the skills and insights he or she has developed and to use them in the service of helping others learn. This experience is particularly helpful in providing the supervisee with a view of supervision from a different perspective, that of the teacher rather than the learner. Such an experience inevitably further sensitizes the nurse not only to *his* or *her* feelings, but also to those of the other person.

The end goal of supervision is to help the supervisee achieve a level of understanding and clinical competence as close as possible to that of the supervisor. One of the rewards for supervisors is their own increased self-awareness, continued development, and refinement of clinical skills. Such growth is fostered by being in the position of helping others to work through clinical problems and understand their own feelings. Working through issues in this way continually reminds supervisors of issues they have themselves dealt with previously or may need to consider currently.

SUMMARY

Supervision has been discussed in terms of developmental learning toward the goal of enhanced clinical competency. The supervisor and the supervisee each bring responsibilities to the relationship. The supervisor is obligated to provide a nonthreatening, accepting relationship in which it is both expected and possible to examine in detail every clinical aspect affecting relationships with both clients and colleagues, including the therapist's feelings and responses.

The supervisee is obligated to make an honest effort to bring all details of clinical work to the discussion. Additionally, the trainee is expected to be open to learning new problem-solving methods using the following techniques: (1) careful observation, (2) precise reporting of data, (3) mutual hypothesis generation about causality and interventions, (4) agreement on the interventions used to test the hypothesis, (5) evaluation of the results, and (6) regeneration of new hypotheses, testing, and evaluation.

As a result of this process recurring over time, the supervisee is more likely to accept the safety and usefulness of self-disclosure to achieve learning. There comes a point of mutual recognition and satisfaction in the process about the growth of the supervisee and of new learning for the supervisor. Generally at this point the goals of increased awareness of self and others and enhanced clinical competency have been achieved to the satisfaction of both. They can then agree that learning more about psychotherapy with children, adolescents, and families would be enhanced by work with a different supervisor—one with different talents and who uses other approaches. In this way, the supervisee has a number of opportunities to learn different approaches to psychotherapy and how to deal with increasingly complex client issues. These abilities require refined self-scrutiny. At some point, the supervisee has become effective as a therapist with a variety of client combinations and no longer needs ongoing supervision. At such times it is appropriate to seek consultation with peers or colleagues at moments of crisis or therapeutic impasse.

For some, the question may still remain: Is supervision really necessary for psychiatric mental health clinical nursing practice? Whether one is working as a counselor, a therapist, or in a more traditional inpatient unit, one has the responsibility of seeking to learn and to grow in professional competence. One needs to search continually for greater understanding of one's own feelings, as well as those of others, and to use that understanding responsively. This is a responsibility not only to oneself but equally to one's clients.

Either supervision or consultation is necessary for the practicing psychiatric nurse. Although it is imperative for the beginning practitioner, it is equally valuable for the experienced nurse. Personal limitations create a need for assistance in remaining objective throughout the therapeutic process and the "normal" stresses it presents. Obviously, supervision is only as helpful as the skill of the supervisor, the openness of the supervisee, and the motivation of both to grow and learn.

REFERENCES

Doehrman, M. Parrallel process in supervision and psychotherapy. *Baltimore Menninger Clinic,* 1976, *40,* 9.

Gaoni, B., & Newmann, M. Supervision from the point of view of the supervisee. *American Journal of Psychotherapy,* 1974, *23,* 108–114.

Haller, L. Clinical psychiatric supervision. In C. R. Kneisl & H. S. Wilson (Eds.), *Current perspectives in psychiatric Nursing* (Vol. 1). St. Louis: C. V. Mosby, 1976.

Hora, T. Contribution to the phenomenology of the supervisory process. *American Journal of Psychotherapy,* 1957, *11,* 769–773.

Lewin, K. *Resolving social conflicts: Selected papers on group dynamics.* New York: Harper & Row, 1948.

Muslin, H. L., Burstein, A. G., Gedo, J. E., & Sado, L. Research on the supervisory process I. Supervisor's appraisal of the interview data. *Archives of General Psychiatry,* 1967, *16,* 427–431.

Sullivan, H. S. Basic concepts in the psychiatric interview. In H. S. Sullivan, *The psychiatric interview.* New York: W. W. Norton, 1954.

Szurek, S. A. Emotional factors in the use of authority. In E. L. Ginsburg (Ed.), *Public health is people.* New York: Commonwealth Fund, 1950.

BIBLIOGRAPHY

Aiken, L., & Aiken, J. A systematic approach to the evaluation of interpersonal relationships. *American Journal of Nursing,* 1973, *73,* 863.

Altucher, N. Constructive use of the supervisory relationship. *Journal of Counseling Psychology,* 1967, *14*(*2*), 165–170.

Arlow, J. A. The supervisory situation. *American Psychoanalytic Journal,* 1963, *11,* 576–594.

Berlin, I. N. Some implications of ego psychology for the supervisory process. *American Journal of Psychotherapy,* 1960, *14,* 536–544.

Bier, E. G. On supervision in psychotherapy. *Psychotherapy: Theory, Research and Practice,* 1964, *1,* 91–95.

Cherniss, C., & Egnatios, E. Clinical supervision in community mental health. *Social Work,* 1978, *23,* 219–223.

Chickering, A. W. *Education and identity.* San Francisco: Jossey Bass, 1969.

Ekstein, R., & Wallerstein, R. S. *The teaching and learning of psychotherapy* (2nd ed.). New York: International University Press, 1972.

Feather, R., & Bissel, B. Clinical supervision vs. psychotherapy: The psychiatric mental health supervisory process. *Perspectives in Psychiatric Care,* 1979, *17*(*6*), 266–272.

Gregg, D., Bregg, E., & Spring, F. Individual supervision: A method of teaching psychiatric concepts in nursing education. *Perspectives in Psychiatric Care,* 1976, *14*(*3*), 115–129.

Hogan, R. A. Issues and approaches in supervision. *Psychotherapy: Theory, Research and Practice,* 1964, *1,* 139–141.

Johnson, M. Self-disclosure: A variable in the nurse-client relationship. *Journal of Psychiatric Nursing,* 1980, *18*(*1*), 17.

Littrell, J. M., Lee-Borden, N., & Lorenz, J. Developmental framework for counseling supervision. *Counselor Education and Supervision,* 1979, *18,* 129–136.

Loganbill, C., Hardy, E., & Delworth, V. Supervision: A conceptual model. *The Counseling Psychologist,* 1981, *10*(*1*), 3–42.

Meerlo, J. Some psychological problems in supervision of therapists. *American Journal of Psychotherapy,* 1952, *6,* 467–483.

Morrison, E. Aspects of supervision in psychiatric nursing. In C. R. Kneisl & H. S. Wilson (Eds.), *Current perspectives in psychiatric nursing* (Vol. 1). St. Louis: C. V. Mosby, 1976.

Muecke, M. Video-tape recordings: A tool for psychiatric clinical supervision. *Perspectives in Psychiatric Care,* 1970, *8,* 200–208.

Mueller, W., & Kell, B. *Coping with conflict: Supervising counselors and psychotherapists.* New York: Appleton-Century-Crofts, 1972.

Nehren, J. G., & Larson, M. L. Supervised supervision. *Perspectives in Psychiatric Care,* 1968, *6,* 25–27.

Ornstein, P. S., Cicchetti, D. V., Levine, J., & Fierman, L. B. Some parameters of verbal behavior that reliably differentiate novice from experienced psychotherapists. *Journal of Abnormal Psychology,* 1968, *73,* 240–244.

Peitchinis, J. Therapeutic effectiveness of counseling by nursing personnel. *Nursing Research,* 1972, *21*(*2*), 138.

Searles, H. T. The informational value of the supervisor's emotional experience. *Collected papers on schizophrenia and related subjects.* New York: International Universities Press, 1975.

Sergiovanni, T. J., & Starratt, R. J. *Supervision: Human perspectives* (2nd ed.). New York: McGraw-Hill, 1979.

Termini, M., & Hauser, M. The process of the supervisory relationship. *Perspectives in Psychiatric Care,* 1973, *11*(*3*), 121–125.

Truax, C. B., Carkuff, R. R., & Doudo, J. Toward an integration of didactic and experiential approaches to training in counseling and psychotherapy. *Journal of Counseling Psychology,* 1964, *11,* 240–247.

Wolberg, L. R. Supervision of the psychotherapeutic process. *American Journal of Psychotherapy,* 1951, *5,* 141–171.

UNIT IV CONCLUDING ISSUES

PART SIX IMPLICATIONS FOR THE FUTURE

The contributors to this book exemplify the diversity, versatility, scholarship, and clinical acumen of nurses engaged in psychiatric mental health nursing. They have presented their individual viewpoints from their perspectives as theorists, researchers, and/or clinicians on the integration of knowledge from these three areas in ways uniquely meaningful to their particular nursing focus. Their writings carry implications for the future of psychiatric mental health nursing in two broad areas: those which affect specific aspects of the field and those in which future developments will affect the entire specialty. Possible implications derived from each of these perspectives for the future of advanced psychiatric mental health nursing are briefly considered.

CHAPTER

24 PSYCHIATRIC MENTAL HEALTH NURSING PERSPECTIVES

Deane L. Critchley
Judith T. Maurin

NURSING'S KNOWLEDGE BASE

Chapter 3 identifies those structures and functions within the central nervous system that are thought to be involved in the symptomatic behaviors of the mentally ill and perhaps in the etiologies of some mental illnesses. It proposes possibilities in which knowledge of those same structures and processes might be applied, by the clinician, to specific neurophysiological states thus bringing about relief for the client from symptomatic behaviors.

The rapid increase in knowledge about the biochemical interactions and processes at various sites within the brain will inevitably continue. Major new discoveries are on the horizon. As a result, knowledge regarding the neurochemical contribution to mental illness will become more specific and precise. When this occurs, research into the use of psychotropic medications to alter brain chemistry will undoubtedly result in increased therapeutic effectiveness with diminished untoward reactions. Increased knowledge may also permit sites within the brain to be stimulated so that individuals will produce their own endogenous chemicals as "medications." Production of one's own neurochemical substances would reduce the possibility of adverse effects while increasing the likelihood of drug compatibility for the individual. Chapter 3 predicts that, with further neurobiological discoveries, psychotherapeutic techniques will be refined until they are specific to the disease process for which they are used.

However, as Chapter 15 points out, no matter how the efficacy and specificity of psychotropic medications increase, there will always be those clients for whom their use is contraindicated. It is clear from current experience and research in the use of psychotropic medications that interpersonal interventions that alter behavior will still be required in addition to medication in order to achieve changes in behavior.

In the more autonomous therapist role described in the treatment chapters, a thorough understanding of the biochemical action and therapeutic use of psychotropic medications is required of the clinical specialist. Only when knowledge from neurophysiology and biochemical functioning is used together with psychosocial theories when making client assessments and planning treatment will clinical specialists be using the holistic framework that is the hallmark of nursing.

Psychiatric mental health clinical nurse specialists would quite likely have unchallenged access to work with clients refractory to the use of medication if they chose to do so. These clients are usually considered "too difficult," "too frustrating," or "unrewarding" by many of our mental health colleagues. As a result, clinical specialists would have a relatively free hand in planning, carrying out, and evaluating interpersonal, behavioral, and educational nursing interventions for clients not amenable to medication. Clinical specialists will have to assertively seize such opportunities when they arise. If they hang back because they believe these clients to be "uninteresting" or to carry "low status," the opportunity may be taken by other disciplines. This could be a tragedy for the clients and for the nursing profession. Most other disciplines do not have nursing's biopsychosocial base, so that once again care for the client will be fragmented and the nursing profession will have lost yet another chance to establish itself as particularly expert in a specific clinical area.

The implications of Chapter 3 go beyond psychopharmacology, however. The dynamic interaction between our social psychological experience and neurophysiology implies a circular feedback process. Our neurophysiology can affect our perceptions and thus social experience; our perception of social experiences can, in turn, affect our neurophysiological status. Potential intervention strategies for behavioral difficulties may be physical, social, or both. What are the neurophysical consequences of our social interventions? What are the perceptual and social consequences of physical interventions? The dynamics of the circular feedback process need description and further study.

A major barrier to utilizing the knowledge accumulating in the neurosciences and social sciences is the lack of communication between and among experts in these respective fields. These experts lack a shared understanding of one another's language. We challenge psychiatric mental health nurse specialists to begin interdisciplinary and internursing specialty dialogue with the goal of identifying biopsychosocial research questions. The task will be difficult, but the possibilities are exciting.

Chapter 2 discusses the need for psychiatric nursing to respond to the challenge and develop a body of nursing knowledge for clinical specialist practice. The issue is not whether that body of knowledge is "unique" but that it has nursing goals and concerns as its focus. Knowledge derived from other fields must be adapted so that its focus, too, will be nursing's focus, which encourages the most effective patient care.

There are currently several nursing conceptual models being used, modified, and evaluated for their helpfulness to clinical practice. Chapter 2 shows us how Orem's self-care deficit model might be helpful to psychiatric mental health nursing. However, it is pointed out that the model is too abstract to be helpful in providing specific explanations for the deficits identified. The model was not helpful in identifying interventions specific to the individual situation. Psychiatric mental health nurses would need to use other, more specific theories, such as crisis intervention, in combination with Orem's model, to make it more pragmatically and prognostically useful. Other perhaps more specifically clinically based theories could be combined with Orem's model and their combined use evaluated.

Others maintain that to facilitate communication with other disciplines psychiatric mental health nursing should use an already widely used interdisciplinary framework, the DSM-III. This belief, in fact, is the position taken by the Division on Psychiatric and Mental Health Nursing Practice of the American Nurses' Association. Williams and Wilson (1982) have proposed expanding Axes IV and V of the DSM-III, whereas Loomis and Wood (1983) see the diagnostic categories included in DSM-III as compatible with categories of actual or potential health problems that are or can be defined through the nursing diagnostic categories being developed by the North American Nursing Diagnosis Association.

The decision regarding whether to seek a unique nursing perspective or to use an interdisciplinary framework will not be easily determined. It is important that there is acceptance of the need for a theoretical framework. It is the fruitful combination of diagnostic methods that will provide us with a more comprehensive and meaningful diagnostic process in the future. The case study approach discussed in Chapter 4 could be particularly helpful in determining the strengths and limitations of the unique nursing perspective versus the interdisciplinary model. The case study method could be invaluable in helping nurses determine which framework provided the most accurate explanation of behavior and provide guidance for intervention while most fruitfully maintaining nursing's holistic perspective of the client. There is certainly a need to evaluate intervention modalities in terms of their short- and long-term effectiveness.

We are optimistic about the promise for continued theory development in psychiatric mental health nursing. There is a growing cohort of doctorally prepared nurses and an increasing number are being prepared in nursing. This fact, coupled with the growing sophistication with which nurse scholars are approaching theory development, bodes well for the future.

As this information becomes available, it requires constant circulation and reevaluation throughout the clinical arena. Chapter 5 discusses the point that dissemination and use of research findings clinically cannot be accomplished simply through publication in professional journals. It is a slow and complex process taking place over months and years via the classical process of assimilation and accommodation by the field. The whole research process including application of the findings is based on the assumption that those involved have the capacity to critically evaluate a theory or data and devise methods of testing them. Thus, in addition to scientific thinking, our colleagues must also trust their educated intuition in the evaluation process.

Clinical specialists can play a vital link in this communication chain. They have the theoretical orientation and research background to define clinical issues requiring systematic study and to test new practices. They have the ability to evaluate research in terms of its practical implications for usefulness in clinical practice or within an organizational structure. Clinical specialists also have the ability to translate research findings into activities that can be taught to others.

As a group, we would do well to rediscover and emulate the work of Hildegard Peplau. During the 1960s, she led countless workshops in state mental hospitals across the country teaching the dynamics and therapeutic uses of the nurse-patient relationship. Unfortunately, since that time, psychiatric mental health nurses have largely ignored the fact that for the most part the greatest number of contributors to the care of the mentally ill have been nurses, aides, and technicians largely unprepared for the work they are doing.

As a professional group, psychiatric mental health nurses have done little to try to increase the knowledge base or to enhance the quality of care this group provides. Rather, we seem to have focused on "doing our own thing," keeping ourselves apart from them.

We will need to close this gap and work more closely with our nursing colleagues in state institutions if we wish to truly have an impact on nursing care of the mentally ill. A group of nurses working together to improve the quality of care in such an institution has a far greater potential for such impact and affects the lives of a greater number of patients than the same number of nurses working independently and seeing a small number of private clients.

Clinical specialists need to take a more active role as knowledgeable consumers of research, as validators of the efficacy of the findings, and as participants and leaders in research activities. Equally important, clinical specialists need to become far more comfortable in discussing the theoretical links between their clinical activities and theoretical foci in formal and informal networks within and outside of nursing. They need to be prepared to be more openly critical and to use their clinical experience to both challenge and encourage research.

Psychiatric mental health nurses have always relied heavily on developmental theory as a basis for understanding and working with their clients throughout the life cycle. As more research data are available in the areas of developmental diagnosis and developmental deficits, application of these findings and their implications for treatment of clients of all ages becomes critical. Using this information, interventions will be increasingly more precise. The efforts will be to advance the client's developmental capacity and adaptive functioning. Treating individuals with early deficits who operate at concrete operational levels requires different approaches than those used with individuals who have achieved the stage of formal operational thought despite their developmental problems. Similar issues apply for elderly clients. Their current social and cognitive functioning needs to be assessed in order to determine appropriate interventions. Similar use of developmental diagnosis of ego function and other interpersonal developmental data can be applied to forming a more precise treatment plan for clients of any age.

The ongoing research on all developmental stages from infancy throughout the life span is making possible early intervention and prevention programs designed specifically to strengthen coping skills for individuals and families. This book does not deal with intervention with infants and the clinical specialist's already important role in early intervention and prevention in this area. There is every indication that this field will become even more important over time and offer opportunities for major involvement in such areas as parent education, infant screening, early intervention programs, and health education programs for children of all ages along with parents and educators.

Though taken for granted in our evaluation of clients, developmental data is becoming better integrated in these processes. New findings from physiological, cognitive, and psychosocial areas make it possible to assess developmental deficits and plan for treatment more precisely. The ability to integrate the information derived from these new developments will also enable the clinical specialist as therapist to plan more comprehensive client care and evaluate more specifically all factors involved in client behavior.

CLINICAL PRACTICE ISSUES

Chapter 16 identifies the knowledge required to work in an increasingly multicultural society. This information is complex but essential for anyone working with people. With individual clients and families, such information is required to help the therapist understand a client's cultural beliefs, which govern behavior. Only by understanding the cultural influences on the client's behavior will the therapist be able to alter the therapist role as necessary to meet these cultural expectations in a helpful manner.

Continuing research from different cultures negates old stereotypes and points to methods of using the inherent strengths and adaptive capacities of the culture as part of the healing process. No therapist can afford to neglect the new information about each culture. Nor can therapists ignore what we are learning about the effects of the dominant culture on the mental health of minorities.

There are several client populations discussed in this volume who can be described as minorities because of their characteristics of powerlessness, lack of unity, and autonomy. These groups include children, the elderly, the chronically mentally ill, and women.

Several authors discuss the problems involved for nurses in terms of the characteristics listed above as nursing is primarily a women's profession. Stereotyping and prejudice toward women both as clients and as mental health providers is an important issue for psychiatric mental health nurses to consider.

One of the problems within the profession has been the lack of support nurses give other nurses and the lack of unity in the field. This can be an equally serious problem for nurses who work with women as clients. As Chapter 18 discusses, women who work with women often have negative feelings toward them, holding the same stereotypes and prejudices towards them as are prevalent in society. Clinical specialists need to examine closely their attitudes toward women in general and especially their attitudes toward women as peers, superiors, and clients.

Women as members of a low-status, relatively powerless group are subjected to a multitude of stressors, many of them resulting from the economic, racial, and sexual discrimination that they experience on a daily basis. The higher incidence of supposed psychiatric disorders in women may well in part be a result of these constant stressors. Clinical specialists are a natural group among the mental health professions to seek to identify scientifically the stressors women experience in our society and their emotional and behavioral manifestations. Many clinical specialists are knowledgeable, clinically skilled women who have experienced many of these same stressors. They are in the unique position of being able to offer women clients both empathetic understanding as another woman and the therapeutic skills of a competent mental health professional. Their biophysical background gives psychiatric mental health nurses the ability to assess the stress-related effects in physical dysfunctions. Clinical specialists could become leaders in the assessment and treatment of stress-associated illnesses in women and in the area of women's health care. Despite the gains women have made in our society, stress-related health problems are far more likely to increase than to decrease. There are reasons for this phenomenon. First, though gains have been made, we all know that there is still much to accomplish to achieve parity for women in our society. Second, as women engage in greater risk-taking in their personal lives, professionally and politically they will experience other stressors and become subject to the stress-related illnesses that men in such situations have long experienced. It seems, then, that research into and a clinical focus on the field of stress-related illness in women could be professionally and personally satisfying for the clinical specialist.

Clients experiencing chronic mental illness are subjected to multiple stressors; those related directly to their illness such as symptomatic behaviors and lack of self-esteem and those related to their life circumstances, which are usually associated either directly or indirectly with their illness. Related stressors could include poor financial circumstances, limited social support systems, or often the inability to hold a job. Chapter 19 has identified several reasons why those who are chronically ill are perceived as less satisfying and less prestigious as clients. It makes the point that, if the therapist focuses not on curing clients but on helping them to improve the quality of their life experience, this group becomes less frustrating and more rewarding as clients.

Working with the chronically mentally ill is another area that holds opportunity for the psychiatric mental health clinical nurse specialist. Most of these clients require maintenance on medication. However, it is well known that without supportive treatment most will stop their medication when they feel they "don't need it," leading to symptom exacerbation and often hospitalization.

As Chapter 19 describes, clinical specialists can play a major therapeutic role with these clients by assisting them with the major stress-provoking areas in their lives, assisting them to accept their illness and concurrently establish and work towards adaptive, health-promoting goals. As therapists, clinical specialists need to accept and therapeutically use the client's perhaps prolonged dependence on the relationship. The therapist needs to be prepared to step out of the traditional therapist role and offer these clients supportive problem-solving and directive intervention. These clients often need strong advocates and direct assistance and support in dealing with agencies, organizations, and bureaucratic "red tape." Providing this kind of active assistance in solving the problems encountered in day-to-day living is well within the competence of the clinical specialist and can make the difference between living in the community or institutionalization for many of these clients.

Again, because of the "low status" in which these clients are regarded, it is likely that most disciplines would welcome the entry of the clinical specialist into the therapist role with these clients. Care of the chronically ill, whether mentally or physically, is also an area needing investigation. An interesting area of study would be to compare the effectiveness of providing information, teaching specific skills, problem solving, and goal setting in the vein described in Chapter 19 with the more traditional supportive treatment in terms of adaptive functioning of the client. Other possible areas for investigation are pointed out in this chapter. This information would make an invaluable contribution to the treatment of this troubled group of clients. Work with the chronically mentally ill and their families is a field that holds both opportunity and challenge for the clinical specialist.

Another area of potential expansion for psychiatric mental health nurses is in liaison and consultation. Chapter 17 has outlined the characteristics of each and their usefulness in a general hospital setting. However, liaison-consultation would be invaluable in other settings as well: home health care and visiting nurse agencies, hospice, extended care, residential care, and nursing homes, to name only a few possibilities. Clinical specialists with their background in health and medication assessment as well as their ability to assess and treat clients' families within the home can provide comprehensive services in a cost-effective manner compared to other disciplines. Clinical specialists need to actively develop ideas for pilot projects in these areas and "sell" their potential to health care providers for funding in order to demonstrate and document their services and their cost effectiveness.

The previous sections have identified possible future directions for specific aspects of psychiatric mental health nursing. Next, we will briefly discuss those issues in which progress, or lack thereof, has implications for the entire field.

THE VIABILITY OF PSYCHIATRIC MENTAL HEALTH NURSING—ITS FUTURE

Authors in this book as well as others have raised the issue of the viability of psychiatric mental health nursing. They cite the decreasing numbers of students in graduate programs in the field, the economic cutbacks in mental health care that have decreased the numbers and kinds of positions available, and the overall inability, despite some gains, for clinical specialists to receive direct third-party reimbursement. The concerns expressed are valid. Though it may seem impossible to some to think of nursing without a specialty in psychiatric mental health, others are concerned that nursing itself, at least as we know it today and would like to see it develop, will disappear.

What can be done to ensure nursing's viability and that of our specialty? First, clinical specialists need to become more involved in their specialty and their professional organization at the state and national level. Chapter 22 points out that, of approximately 6,000 master's-prepared psychiatric mental health nurses, roughly one-tenth of them belong to the Council of Specialists and fewer than 25% of all nurses belong to their national professional organization. Six thousand nurses may not seem a sizeable number compared to the total number of nurses. However, if all 6,000 of those nurses were actively involved in their profession, working together on issues and problems, it could make a profound difference. Necessary tasks include defining the clinical specialist role, providing supportive data on the efficacy and cost effectiveness of treatment of the mentally ill, and outlining early and maintenance strategies of intervention as well as prevention and education functions that clinical specialists are prepared to carry out.

Nurses need to have a more powerful voice in proposed legislative and professional efforts to modify health care funding and organization and distribution of health care. They need to be active rather than token members of decision-making bodies who deal with health care and reimbursement issues. Reports of actual treatment outcome studies in terms of interventions used, cost of care, and its effectiveness in preventing expensive hospitalization speak far more powerfully than simple rhetoric. Systematic data rather than anecdotal material is necessary about whether such care is possible, its quality, and its substitutability for more expensive treatment provided by other disciplines. Nurses have been effective in influencing legislative action when the effort is united even when carried out by a relatively small number. It was this kind of action by psychiatric mental health nurses in California in 1983 that resulted in passage of a law authorizing direct third-party reimbursement to master's-prepared psychiatric mental health nurses.

Another area of concern is the relatively small number of certified specialists in the area. Chapter 22 notes that little more than 800 of the total 6,000 nurses are certified at the specialist level. Again, this limited number is not impressive in establishing our credibility as professionals who choose to use the credentialing process as a means of expressing our interest in accountability and as an expression of our competence.

There is no absolute requirement for certification, yet there are certainly pragmatic reasons for it. It provides a way of attesting to those nurses who can be designated as therapists. As such, certification paves the way for third-party reimbursement in that it is an assurance to the public, to health care providers, and to other professions that clinical specialists are as prepared as members of other disciplines who receive direct reimbursement for comparable mental health services.

It is true that because of efforts at cost containment in health care and decreases in fund allocations the outlook for direct reimbursement to qualified nurses is not optimistic. Yet, if nurses do not take the steps outlined above reimbursement is even less likely to occur. Beyond the reasons already given, it would seem that clinicians within the field would want to have formal certification to demonstrate their professed concern for recognized competence and accountability and to protect their role and title.

To achieve those objectives outlined above as well as others that are sure to arise in the complex, ever-changing health care arena will take not only the involvement of those presently in the field but also assurance that others will continue to enter it. Steps need to be taken to counter the decreasing enrollment in graduate programs in psychiatric mental health nursing. Others have suggested that graduate psychiatric mental health nursing faculty must become more visible in teaching undergraduate nursing students. Clinical specialists in practice settings must also recognize their responsibility for contributing to the education of the profession's recruits. If psychiatric mental health nursing specialists were visable to undergraduate students of nursing, these same students would be more aware of the challenges and professional rewards to be found in psychiatric mental health nursing. Because of the currently limited appropriate nurse role models in clinical psychiatric nursing practice, these steps could be important in stimulating interest in working and pursuing graduate education in the field.

If clinical specialists did become more active and visible in clinical practice and organizational activities as previously described, this too would serve as a magnet to others, to both students and other nurses who wish to become a part of a productive, autonomous aspect of the profession that provides recognition and the possibility of satisfactory financial remuneration. We believe recruitment will not be a problem if those in the field effectively demonstrate the clinical opportunities and financial rewards of the specialty. Ultimately, the issue is whether psychiatric mental health nursing will remain a viable contributor to mental health care delivery. In order for this to happen, psychiatric mental health nursing needs to demonstrate its contribution and impact on mental health services in the ways described above. Additionally, the demonstration needs to come not from a few but from the entire population of clinical specialists. The diverse areas and means by which this demonstration can occur have only been touched on in this book. However, it is hoped that the contributors have stimulated those in the field to intensify their clinical and professional learning and participation, to increase their involvement in clinical research and theory development, and to speak out on issues critical to improving the quality and availability of mental health care.

The editors hope that each reader will be enriched by new learning. We also hope the readers will recognize that together with knowledge there is a responsibility to use that knowledge effectively. Effective use of one's talents and learning can only occur when clinical specialists assert their competence by convincing legislators that clinical specialist practice is important to making mental health care both affordable and highly effective. This is particularly true for underserved populations, be they ethnic minorities, women, children, the aged, or the chronically physically and mentally ill. Psychiatric mental health nursing is about to emerge into a new era of independent, effective patient care.

REFERENCES

Loomis, M. E., & Wood, D. J. Cure: The potential outcome of nursing care. *Image: The Journal of Nursing Scholarship,* 1983, *15,* 4–7.

Williams, J. B. W., & Wilson, H. S. A psychiatric nursing perspective on DSM III. *Journal of Psychosocial Nursing and Mental Health Services,* 1982, *20,* 14–20.

APPENDIX STANDARDS OF PSYCHIATRIC AND MENTAL HEALTH NURSING PRACTICE

INTRODUCTION

The purpose of *Standards of Psychiatric and Mental Health Nursing Practice* is to fulfill the profession's obligation to provide a means of improving the quality of care. The standards reflect the current state of knowledge in the field and are therefore provisional, dynamic, and subject to testing and subsequent change. Since standards represent agreed-upon levels of practice, they have been developed to characterize, to measure, and to provide guidance in achieving excellence in care.*

The standards presented here are a revision of the standards enunciated by the Division on Psychiatric and Mental Health Nursing Practice in 1973. They apply to any setting in which psychiatric and mental health nursing is practiced, and to both generalists and specialists in psychiatric and mental health nursing. Standards V-F (psychotherapy) and X (community health systems) apply specifically to the specialist. The standards are written within the framework of the nursing process, which includes data collection, diagnosis, planning, treatment, and evaluation.

The treatment or intervention phase of the nursing process is elaborated upon in order to highlight the specific interventions or nursing care activities commonly carried out by psychiatric and mental health nurses: therapeutic interventions, health teaching, activities of daily living, somatic therapies, therapeutic environment, and psychotherapy. In addition to the standards concerned with the nursing process are standards that address professional performance, such as use of theory, peer review, continuing education, interdisciplinary team collaboration, community health systems, and research. Accountability of the provider to the client, client rights, and client advocacy are implicit throughout the standards.

Standards of Psychiatric and Mental Health Nursing Practice should be used in conjunction with the following ANA publications: (1) *Standards of Nursing Practice,* (2) *Statement on Psychiatric and Mental Health Nursing Practice,* (3) *Nursing: A Social Policy Statement,* and (4) *Code for Nurses with Interpretive Statements.*

PROFESSIONAL PRACTICE STANDARDS

Standard I. Theory

The nurse applies appropriate theory that is scientifically sound as a basis for decisions regarding nursing practice.

This appendix is from the American Nurses' Association, *Standards of psychiatric and mental health nursing,* Kansas City, MO: American Nurses' Association, 1982, used with permission.

* American Nurses' Association. *A Plan for Implementation of the Standards of Nursing Practice.* Kansas City, MO: The American Nurses' Association, 1975, p. 4.

Rationale
Psychiatric and mental health nursing is characterized by the application of relevant theories to explain phenomena of concern to nurses, and to provide a basis for intervention and subsequent evaluation of that intervention. A primary source of knowledge for practice rests on the scholarly conceptualizations of psychiatric and mental health nursing practice and on research findings generated from intradisciplinary and cross-disciplinary studies of human behavior. The nurse's use of selected theories provides comprehensive, balanced perceptions of clients' characteristics, diagnoses, or presenting conditions.

Standard II. Data Collection

The nurse continuously collects data that are comprehensive, accurate, and systematic.

Rationale
Effective interviewing, behavioral observation, and physical and mental health assessment enable the nurse to reach sound conclusions and plan appropriate interventions with the client.

Standard III. Diagnosis

The nurse utilizes nursing diagnoses and/or standard classification of mental disorders to express conclusions supported by recorded assessment data and current scientific premises.

Rationale
Nursing's logical basis for providing care rests on the recognition and identification of those actual or potential health problems that are within the scope of nursing practice.

Standard IV. Planning

The nurse develops a nursing care plan with specific goals and interventions delineating nursing actions unique to each client's needs.

Rationale
The nursing care plan is used to guide therapeutic intervention and effectively achieve the desired outcomes.

Standard V. Intervention

The nurse intervenes as guided by the nursing care plan to implement nursing actions that promote, maintain, or restore physical and mental health, prevent illness, and effect rehabilitation.

Rationale
Mental health is one aspect of general health and well-being. Nursing actions reflect an appreciation for the hierarchy of human needs and include interventions for all aspects of physical and mental health and illness.

Standard V-A. Intervention: Psychotherapeutic Interventions

The nurse uses psychotherapeutic interventions to assist clients in regaining or improving their previous coping abilities and to prevent further disability.

Rationale

Individuals with and without mental health problems often respond to health problems in a dysfunctional manner. During counseling, interviewing, crisis or emergency intervention, or daily interaction, nurses diagnose dysfunctional behaviors, engage clients in noting such behaviors, and assist the client in modifying or eliminating those behaviors.

Standard V-B. Intervention: Health Teaching

The nurse assists clients, families, and groups to achieve satisfying and productive patterns of living through health teaching.

Rationale

Health teaching is an essential part of the nurse's role with those who have mental health problems. Every interaction can be utilized as a teaching-learning situation. Formal and informal teaching methods can be used in working with individuals, families, groups, and the community. Emphasis is on understanding principles of mental health as well as on developing ways of coping with mental health problems. Client adherence to treatment regimens increases when health teaching is an integral part of the client's care.

Standard V-C. Intervention: Activities of Daily Living

The nurse uses the activities of daily living in a goal-directed way to foster adequate self-care and physical and mental well-being of clients.

Rationale

A major portion of one's daily life is spent in some form of activity related to health and well-being. An individual's developmental and intellectual levels, emotional state, and physical limitations may be reflected in these activities. Nurses are the primary professional health care providers who interact with clients on a day-to-day basis regarding the tasks of daily living. Therefore, the nurse has a unique opportunity to assess and intervene in these processes in order to encourage constructive changes in the client's behavior so that each child, adolescent, and adult can realize his potential for growth and health or maintain that level previously achieved.

Standard V-D. Intervention: Somatic Therapies

The nurse uses knowledge of somatic therapies and applies related clinical skills in working with clients.

Rationale

Various treatment modalities may be needed by clients during the course of illness. Pertinent clinical observations and judgments are made concerning the effect of drugs and other somatic treatments used in the therapeutic program.

Standard V-E. Intervention: Therapeutic Environment

The nurse provides, structures, and maintains a therapeutic environment in collaboration with the client and other health care providers.

Rationale

The nurse works with clients in a variety of environmental settings such as inpatient, residential, day care, and home. The environment contributes in positive and negative ways to the state of health or illness of the client. When it serves the interest of the client as an inherent part of the overall nursing care plan, the setting is structured and/or altered.

Standard V-F. Intervention: Psychotherapy

The nurse utilizes advanced clinical expertise in individual, group, and family psychotherapy, child psychotherapy, and other treatment modalities to function as a psychotherapist, and recognizes professional accountability for nursing practice.

Rationale

Acceptance of the role of psychotherapist entails primary responsibility for the treatment of clients and entrance into a contractual agreement. This contract includes a commitment to see a client through the problem presented or to assist the client in finding other appropriate assistance. It also includes an explicit definition of the relationship, the respective role of each person in the relationship, and what can be realistically expected of each person.

Standard VI. Evaluation

The nurse evaluates client responses to nursing actions in order to revise the data base, nursing diagnoses, and nursing care plan.

Rationale

Nursing care is a dynamic process that implies alterations in data, diagnoses, or plans previously made.

PROFESSIONAL PERFORMANCE STANDARDS

Standard VII. Peer Review

The nurse participates in peer review and other means of evaluation to assure quality of nursing care provided for clients.

Rationale

Evaluation of the quality of nursing care through examination of the clinical practice of nurses is one way to fulfill the profession's obligation to ensure that consumers are provided excellence in care. Peer review and other quality assurance procedures are utilized in this endeavor.

Standard VIII. Continuing Education

The nurse assumes responsibility for continuing education and professional development and contributes to the professional growth of others.

Rationale
The scientific, cultural, social, and political changes characterizing our contemporary society require the nurse to be committed to the ongoing pursuit of knowledge that will enhance professional growth.

Standard IX. Interdisciplinary Collaboration

The nurse collaborates with other health care providers in assessing, planning, implementing, and evaluating programs and other mental health activities.

Rationale
Psychiatric nursing practice requires planning and sharing with others to deliver maximum mental health services to the client and the community. Through the collaborative process, different abilities of health care providers are utilized to communicate, plan, solve problems, and evaluate services delivered.

Standard X. Utilization of Community Health Systems

The nurse participates with other members of the community in assessing, planning, implementing, and evaluating mental health services and community systems that include the promotion of the broad continuum of primary, secondary, and tertiary prevention of mental illness.

Rationale
The high incidence of mental illness in our contemporary society requires increased effort to devise more effective treatment and prevention programs. Nurses must participate in programs that strengthen the existing health potential of all members of society. Such concepts as primary prevention and continuity of care are essential in planning to meet the mental health needs of the community. The nurse uses organizational, advisory, advocacy, and consultative skills to facilitate the development and implementation of mental health services.

Standard XI. Research

The nurse contributes to nursing and the mental health field through innovations in theory and practice and participation in research.

Rationale
Each professional has responsibility for the continuing development and refinement of knowledge in the mental health field through research and experimentation with new and creative approaches to practice.

INDEX